Place-of-Service Codes for Professional Claims

Listed below are place-of-service codes and descriptions. These codes should be used on professional claims to specify the entity where service(s) were rendered. Check with individual payers (eg, Medicare, Medica[...] .... for reimbursement policies regarding these codes. If you would like to comment on a code(s) [...] your request to posinfo@cms.hhs.gov.

Place of Service Code(s)	Place of Service Name	Place of Service Description
01	Pharmacy	A facility or location where drugs and other medically related items and services are sold, dispensed, or otherwise provided directly to patients. (effective 10/1/05)
02	Unassigned	N/A
03	School	A facility whose primary purpose is education.
04	Homeless shelter	A facility or location whose primary purpose is to provide temporary housing to homeless individuals (eg, emergency shelters, individual, or family shelters).
05	Indian Health Service freestanding facility	A facility or location, owned and operated by the Indian Health Service, that provides diagnostic, therapeutic (surgical and nonsurgical), and rehabilitation services to American Indians and Alaska Natives who do not require hospitalization.
06	Indian Health Service provider-based facility	A facility or location, owned and operated by the Indian Health Service, that provides diagnostic, therapeutic (surgical and nonsurgical), and rehabilitation services rendered by, or under the supervision of, physicians to American Indians and Alaska Natives admitted as inpatients or outpatients.
07	Tribal 638 freestanding facility	A facility or location, owned and operated by a federally recognized American Indian or Alaska Native tribe or tribal organization under a 638 agreement, that provides diagnostic, therapeutic (surgical and nonsurgical), and rehabilitation services to tribal members who do not require hospitalization.
08	Tribal 638 provider-based facility	A facility or location, owned and operated by a federally recognized American Indian or Alaska Native tribe or tribal organization under a 638 agreement, that provides diagnostic, therapeutic (surgical and nonsurgical), and rehabilitation services to tribal members admitted as inpatients or outpatients.
09	Prison-correctional facility	A prison, jail, reformatory, work farm, detention center, or any other similar facility maintained by federal, state, or local authorities for the purpose of confinement or rehabilitation of adult or juvenile criminal offenders. (effective 7/1/06)
10	Unassigned	N/A
11	Office	Location, other than a hospital, skilled nursing facility, military treatment facility, community health center, state or local public health clinic, or intermediate care facility, where the health professional routinely provides health examinations, diagnosis, and treatment of illness or injury on an ambulatory basis.
12	Home	Location, other than a hospital or other facility, where the patient receives care in a private residence.
13	Assisted living facility	Congregate residential facility with self-contained living units providing assessment of each resident's needs and on-site support 24 hours a day, seven days a week, with the capacity to deliver or arrange for services including some health care and other services. (effective 10/1/03)
14	Group home	A residence, with shared living areas, where clients receive supervision and other services such as social and/or behavioral services, custodial service, and minimal services (eg, medication administration) (effective 4/1/04)
15	Mobile unit	A facility or unit that moves from place to place and is equipped to provide preventive, screening, diagnostic, and/or treatment services.
16-19	Unassigned	N/A
20	Urgent care facility	Location, distinct from a hospital emergency department, an office, or a clinic, whose purpose is to diagnose and treat illness or injury for unscheduled, ambulatory patients seeking immediate medical attention.
21	Inpatient hospital	A facility, other than psychiatric, that primarily provides diagnostic, therapeutic (both surgical and nonsurgical), and rehabilitation services by, or under, the supervision of physicians to patients admitted for a variety of medical conditions.
22	Outpatient hospital	A portion of a hospital that provides diagnostic, therapeutic (both surgical and nonsurgical), and rehabilitation services to sick or injured persons who do not require hospitalization or institutionalization.
23	Emergency room—hospital	A portion of a hospital where emergency diagnosis and treatment of illness or injury is provided.
24	Ambulatory surgical center	A freestanding facility, other than a physician's office, where surgical and diagnostic services are provided on an ambulatory basis.
25	Birthing center	A facility, other than a hospital's maternity facilities or a physician's office, that provides a setting for labor, delivery, and immediate postpartum care as well as immediate care of newborn infants.
26	Military treatment facility	A medical facility operated by one or more of the uniformed services. Military treatment facility also refers to certain former US Public Health Service facilities now designated as uniformed service treatment facilities.
27-30	Unassigned	N/A
31	Skilled nursing facility	A facility that primarily provides inpatient skilled nursing care and related services to patients who require medical, nursing, or rehabilitative services but does not provide the level of care or treatment available in a hospital.

32	Nursing facility	A facility that primarily provides to residents skilled nursing care and related services for the rehabilitation of injured, disabled, or sick persons, or, on a regular basis, health-related care services above the level of custodial care to other than mentally retarded individuals.
33	Custodial care facility	A facility that provides room, board, and other personal assistance services, generally on a long-term basis, and does not include a medical component.
34	Hospice	A facility, other than a patient's home, in which palliative and supportive care for terminally ill patients and their families are provided.
35-40	Unassigned	N/A
41	Ambulance—land	A land vehicle specifically designed, equipped, and staffed for lifesaving and transporting the sick or injured.
42	Ambulance—air or water	An air or water vehicle specifically designed, equipped, and staffed for lifesaving and transporting the sick or injured.
43-48	Unassigned	N/A
49	Independent clinic	A location, not part of a hospital and not described by any other place-of-service code, that is organized and operated to provide preventive, diagnostic, therapeutic, rehabilitative, or palliative services to outpatients only. (effective 10/1/03)
50	Federally qualified health center	A facility located in a medically underserved area that provides Medicare beneficiaries preventive primary medical care under the general direction of a physician.
51	Inpatient psychiatric facility	A facility that provides inpatient psychiatric services for the diagnosis and treatment of mental illness on a 24-hour basis, by or under the supervision of a physician.
52	Psychiatric facility— partial hospitalization	A facility for the diagnosis and treatment of mental illness that provides a planned therapeutic program for patients who do not require full-time hospitalization but who need broader programs than are possible from outpatient visits to a hospital-based or hospital-affiliated facility.
53	Community mental health center	A facility that provides the following services: outpatient services, including specialized outpatient services for children, the elderly, individuals who are chronically ill, and residents of the community mental health center's mental health services area who have been discharged from inpatient treatment at a mental health facility; 24-hour-a-day emergency care services; day treatment, other partial hospitalization services, or psychosocial rehabilitation services; screening for patients being considered for admission to state mental health facilities to determine the appropriateness of such admission; and consultation and education services.
54	Intermediate care facility/mentally retarded	A facility that primarily provides health-related care and services above the level of custodial care to mentally retarded individuals but does not provide the level of care or treatment available in a hospital or skilled nursing facility.
55	Residential substance abuse treatment facility	A facility that provides treatment for substance (alcohol and drug) abuse to live-in residents who do not require acute medical care. Services include individual and group therapy and counseling, family counseling, laboratory tests, drugs and supplies, psychological testing, and room and board.
56	Psychiatric residential treatment center	A facility or distinct part of a facility for psychiatric care that provides a total 24-hour therapeutically planned and professionally staffed group living and learning environment.
57	Nonresidential substance abuse treatment facility	A location that provides treatment for substance (alcohol and drug) abuse on an ambulatory basis. Services include individual and group therapy and counseling, family counseling, laboratory tests, drugs and supplies, and psychological testing. (effective 10/1/03)
58-59	Unassigned	N/A
60	Mass immunization center	A location where providers administer pneumococcal pneumonia and influenza virus vaccinations and submit these services as electronic media claims or paper claims or by using the roster billing method. This generally takes place in a mass immunization setting, such as a public health center, pharmacy, or mall but may include a physician office setting.
61	Comprehensive inpatient rehabilitation facility	A facility that provides comprehensive rehabilitation services under the supervision of a physician to inpatients with physical disabilities. Services include physical therapy, occupational therapy, speech pathology, social or psychological services, and orthotics and prosthetics services.
62	Comprehensive outpatient rehabilitation facility	A facility that provides comprehensive rehabilitation services under the supervision of a physician to outpatients with physical disabilities. Services include physical therapy, occupational therapy, and speech pathology services.
63-64	Unassigned	N/A
65	End-stage renal disease treatment facility	A facility, other than a hospital, that provides dialysis treatment, maintenance, and/or training to patients or caregivers on an ambulatory or home-care basis.
66-70	Unassigned	N/A
71	Public health clinic	A facility maintained by either state or local health departments that provides ambulatory primary medical care under the general direction of a physician. (effective 10/1/03)
72	Rural health clinic	A certified facility located in a rural, medically underserved area that provides ambulatory primary medical care under the general direction of a physician.
73-80	Unassigned	N/A
81	Independent laboratory	A laboratory certified to perform diagnostic and/or clinical tests independent of an institution or a physician's office.
82-98	Unassigned	N/A
99	Other place of service	Other place of service not identified above.

Stay on top of critical CPT code changes

As the AMA's official communication tool for circulating accurate information and guidance on CPT codes and issues, this insightful monthly newsletter should be part of every compliance program. Each issue features articles used for answering day-to-day coding questions, appealing insurance denials and validating coding to auditors.

Enhance your coding proficiency—Case studies and clinical examples offer insight into confusing coding situations

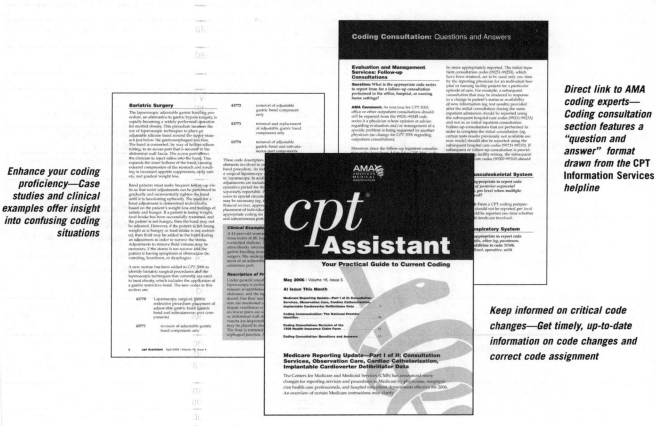

Direct link to AMA coding experts—Coding consultation section features a "question and answer" format drawn from the CPT Information Services helpline

Keep informed on critical code changes—Get timely, up-to-date information on code changes and correct code assignment

E-mail *amy.burgess@ama-assn.org* to request a free sample issue, and an issue will be e-mailed to you promptly.

AMERICAN
MEDICAL
ASSOCIATION

Understand the changes to *CPT® 2007* in detail and code CPT® accurately

An indispensable guide for CPT® Professional users.
CPT® Changes:An Insider's View provides the official AMA interpretations and explanations for each CPT code and guideline change in the *CPT 2007* codebook. Every new, revised, or deleted code, text and guideline change is listed along with a detailed rationale for the change.

***Organized by CPT®
code section and code
number, just like the
CPT® Professional book.***

***Detailed rationales
provide an explanation
as to why the code
change(s) occurred.***

***"At-a-glance" tabular
review of 2007 code, text
and guideline changes.***

***Useful clinical examples
and procedural descriptions
are presented to help you
understand the practical
application for that code.***

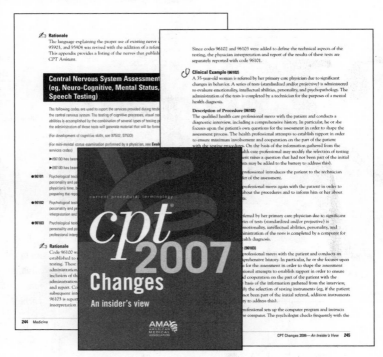

Order the 2007 edition today! Call (800) 621-8335.

Order #: OP512907CCW   Price: $64.95   AMA member price: $45.95

AMA
AMERICAN
MEDICAL
ASSOCIATION

current procedural terminology

cpt® 2007

Standard Edition

Michael Beebe
Joyce A. Dalton
Martha Espronceda, AAS
Desiree D. Evans, AAS
Rejina L. Glenn
Gloria Green, BA
DeHandro Hayden, BS

Anita Majerowicz, MS, RHIA
Janette Meggs, RHIA
Marie L. Mindeman, BA, RHIT
Karen E. O'Hara, BS, CCS-P
Mary R. O'Heron, RHIA, CCS-P
Danielle Pavloski, BS, RHIT, CCS-P
Desiree Rozell, MPA

Lianne Stancik, RHIT
Peggy Thompson, MS, RHIA, CCS
Susan Tracy, BA, RHIT
Jennifer Trajkovski, BS, RHIT
Ada Walker, CCA

AMA
AMERICAN
MEDICAL
ASSOCIATION

Standard ISBN: 1-57947-790-9
Standard ISBN: 978-1-57947-790-5
ISSN: 0276-8283

Foreword

Current Procedural Terminology (CPT®), Fourth Edition, is a listing of descriptive terms and identifying codes for reporting medical services and procedures performed by physicians. The purpose of the terminology is to provide a uniform language that will accurately describe medical, surgical, and diagnostic services, and will thereby provide an effective means for reliable nationwide communication among physicians, patients, and third parties. *CPT 2007* is the most recent revision of a work that first appeared in 1966.

CPT descriptive terms and identifying codes currently serve a wide variety of important functions in the field of medical nomenclature. The CPT codebook is useful for administrative management purposes such as claims processing and for the development of guidelines for medical care review. The uniform language is also applicable to medical education and outcomes, health services and quality research by providing a useful basis for local, regional, and national utilization comparisons. The CPT codebook is the most widely accepted nomenclature for the reporting of physician procedures and services under government and private health insurance programs. In 2000, the CPT code set was designated by the Department of Health and Human Services as the national coding standard for physician and other health care professional services and procedures under the Health Insurance Portability and Accountability Act (HIPAA). This means that for all financial and administrative health care transactions sent electronically, the CPT code set will need to be used.

The changes that appear in this revision have been prepared by the CPT Editorial Panel with the assistance of physicians representing all specialties of medicine, and with important contributions from many third-party payers and governmental agencies.

The American Medical Association trusts that this revision will continue the usefulness of its predecessors in identifying, describing, and coding medical, surgical, and diagnostic services.

Michael D. Maves, MD, MBA
Executive Vice President, CEO

Acknowledgments

Publication of the annual CPT codebook represents many challenges and opportunities. From reconciling the many differences of opinion about the best way to describe a procedure, to the last details on placement of a semicolon, many individuals and organizations devote their energies and expertise to the preparation of this revision.

The editorial staff wishes to express sincere thanks to the many national medical specialty societies, health insurance organizations and agencies, and individual physicians and other health professionals who have made contributions.

Thanks are due to Robert A. Musacchio, PhD, Sr VP, American Medical Association; Claudia Bonnell, Blue Cross and Blue Shield Association; Nelly Leon-Chisen, American Hospital Association; Tom Wilder, America's Health Insurance Plans; and Sue Bowman, RHIA, American Health Information Management Association, for their invaluable assistance in enhancing the CPT code set.

For their assistance in development of the CPT Category II codes:

Ronald A. Gabel, MD,
Darryl T Gray, MD, ScD
Trent T. Haywood, MD, JD
Peter A. Hollmann, MD
Susan M. Nedza, MD
Gregory Pawlson, MD, MPH
Sylvia Publ, RHIA, MBA
Phil Renner, MBA
Sam J. W. Romeo, MD, MBA
Paul M. Schyve, MD
Sharon Sprenger, RHIA, PHQ, MPA
Sally Turbyville, MA

We recognize the following people for efforts in working with the Physician Consortium for Performance Improvement and other quality measurement organizations:

Karen S. Kmetick, PhD
Heidi Bossley, MSN, MBA
Kendra Hanley, MS, CHE

Dedication

We dedicate *CPT 2007* to Karen Borman, MD. Her years of leadership as a Panel member and Vice-Chair of the CPT Editorial Panel were dedicated to setting high standards and improving the CPT code set. Her selfless and remarkable endeavors on behalf of the CPT process were critical to the movement of the CPT code set into the new millennium.

Dr Borman served as a CPT Advisor from 1995 to 2000, on the CPT Editorial Panel from 1997 to 2005, and as Vice-Chair from 2000 to 2005. She will have more time now to mentor her residents while continuing to pursue her interests in health policy.

AMA CPT Editorial Panel

Chair
Tracy R. Gordy, MD*
Vice-Chair
Karen R. Borman, MD*
William T. Thorwarth, Jr, MD* (10/05)
James S. Adamson, Jr, MD*
Joel F. Bradley, Jr, MD
Patrick J. Cafferty, MPAS, PA-C
Simon Philip Cohn, MD
Helene M. Fearon, PT*
Samuel Hassenbusch III, MD, PhD
M. Bradford Henley, MD, MBA† (10/05)
Lee Harold Hilborne, MD, MPH
Peter A. Hollmann, MD
Glenn D. Littenberg, MD
Andrea H. McGuire, MD
Bernard M. Rosof, MD, MACP† (4/06)
Kenneth B. Simon, MD, MBA
Stanley W. Stead, MD, MBA*
J. Martin Tucker, MD
Richard W. Waguespack, MD

Secretary
Michael Beebe
*Member of the CPT Executive Committee
†New Panel Member October 2005, April and June 2006
‡New Advisors

AMA CPT Advisory Committee

American Academy of Allergy, Asthma and Immunology
Donald W. Aaronson, MD
American Academy of Child & Adolescent Psychiatry
David I. Berland, MD
American Academy of Dermatology Association
Dirk M. Elston, MD
American Academy of Facial Plastic and Reconstructive Surgery
Mark V. Connelly, MD
American Academy of Family Physicians
David A. Ellington, MD
American Academy of Neurology
Marc Nuwer, MD, PhD
American Academy of Ophthalmology
Michael X. Repka, MD
American Academy of Orthopaedic Surgeons
M. Bradford Henley, MD
American Academy of Otolaryngic Allergy
Harold R. Wright, Jr, MD
American Academy of Otolaryngology-Head and Neck Surgery
Joseph E. Leonard, MD‡
American Academy of Pain Medicine
Eduardo M. Fraifeld, MD
American Academy of Pediatrics
Richard A. Molteni, MD
American Academy of Physical Medicine and Rehabilitation
Francis P. Lagattuta, MD
American Academy of Sleep Medicine
Samuel A. Fleishman, MD
American Association for Thoracic Surgery
James M. Levett, MD
Kirk R. Kanter, MD‡
American Association of Clinical Endocrinologists
Satti Sethu-Kumar Reddy, MD
Eric A. Orzek, MD, FACE, CDE‡
American Association of Electrodiagnostic Medicine
Kyle W. Ruffling, MD

American Association of Gynecologic Laparoscopists
Jodi Kaigh, MD
American Association of Neurological Surgeons
Jeffrey Cozzens, MD
American Association of Public Health Physicians
Arvind K. Goyal, MD, MPH
American Clinical Neurophysiology Society
Marc Nuwer, MD, PhD
American College of Allergy, Asthma and Immunology
Gary N. Gross, MD
American College of Cardiology
Diane E. Wallis, MD, FACC
American College of Chest Physicians
Steve G. Peters, MD
American College of Emergency Physicians
Peter L. Sawchuk, MD
Kenneth L. DeHart, MD, FACEP‡
American College of Gastroenterology
Robert B. Cameron, MD
American College of Medical Genetics
David B. Flannery, MD
American College of Medical Quality
Joel Grossman, MD
American College of Nuclear Physicians
Gary L. Dillehay, MD
American College of Obstetricians and Gynecologists
J. Craig Strafford, MD
Jordan G. Pritzker, MD, MBA, FACOG‡
American College of Occupational and Environmental Medicine
Elizabeth Genovese, MD, MBA
American College of Physicians
H. Christopher Alexander III, MD, MACR, FACP
American College of Preventive Medicine
Fred T. Nobrega, MD
American College of Radiation Oncology
Thomas J. Weatherall, Jr, MD
American College of Radiology
Richard Duszak, Jr, MD
American College of Rheumatology
Robert J. Lloyd, MD
American College of Surgeons
Albert E. Bothe, Jr, MD, FACS
American Dental Association
Charles A. Crago, MD, DMD
American Gastroenterological Association
Joel V. Brill, MD
American Geriatric Society
Robert A. Zorowitz, MD, MBA
American Institute of Ultrasound in Medicine
Harvey L. Nisenbaum, MD
American Medical Directors Association
Dennis L. Stone, MD, MBA
American Medical Group Association
Susan K. Turney, MD
David E. Hooper, MD‡
American Orthopaedic Association
Blair C. Filler, MD
American Orthopaedic Foot and Ankle Society
Walter J. Pedowitz, MD
American Osteopathic Association
Boyd R. Buser, DO
American Pediatric Surgical Association
John P. Crow, MD
American Psychiatric Association
Chester W. Schmidt, Jr, MD

American Roentgen Ray Society
Geraldine B. McGinty, MD, MBA
American Society for Aesthetic Plastic Surgery, Inc.
Paul R. Weiss, MD
American Society for Clinical Pathology
Mark S. Synovec, MD
American Society for Dermatologic Surgery
Pamela K. Phillips, MD
American Society for Gastrointestinal Endoscopy
Robert B. Cameron, MD‡
American Society for Reproductive Medicine
John T. Queenan, Jr, MD
American Society for Surgery of the Hand
Daniel J. Nagle, MD
American Society for Therapeutic Radiology and Oncology
Michael L. Steinberg, MD
American Society of Abdominal Surgeons
Louis F. Alfano, Jr, MD
American Society of Anesthesiologists
H. J. Przybylo, Jr, MD
American Society of Bariatric Physicians
Mary C. Vernon, MD
American Society of Cataract and Refractive Surgery
Stephen S. Lane, MD
American Society of Clinical Oncology
William C. Penley, MD
American Society of Colon and Rectal Surgeons
David A. Margolin, MD
Guy R. Orangio, MD, FACS, FASCRS‡
American Society of Cytopathology
Patricia A. Gregg, MD
American Society of General Surgeons
Charles Drueck III, MD, FACS
American Society of Hematology
Samuel M. Silver, MD, PhD
American Society of Neuroimaging
Mircea A. Morariu, Jr, MD
American Society of Neuroradiology
Robert A. Murray, MD
American Society of Ophthalmic Plastic and Reconstructive Surgery
L. Neal Freeman, MD, MBA, CCS-P, FACS
American Society of Plastic Surgeons
Raymond V. Janevicius, MD
American Thoracic Society
Stephen P. Hoffmann, MD
American Urological Association
Jeffrey A. Dann, MD
Association of University Radiologists
Bob W. Gayler, MD
College of American Pathologists
Stephen N. Bauer, MD
James P. Almas, MD, FCAP‡
Congress of Neurological Surgeons
R. Patrick Jacob, MD
Contact Lens Association of Ophthalmologists
Charles B. Slonim, MD, FACS
Infectious Disease Society of America
Lawrence P. Martinelli, MD
International Spinal Injection Society
Claire Tibiletti, MD
National Association of Medical Examiners
Paul A. Raslavicus, MD
North American Spine Society
William Mitchell, MD
Radiological Society of North America
Richard E. Fulton, MD

Renal Physicians Association
Richard J. Hamburger, MD
Society for Investigative Dermatology
Stephen P. Stone, MD
Society for Vascular Surgery
Anton N. Sidawy, MD
Society of American Gastrointestinal Endoscopic Surgeons
Paresh C. Shah, MD
Society of Critical Care Medicine
George A. Sample, MD
Society of Interventional Radiology
Katharine L. Krol, MD
Society of Nuclear Medicine
Kenneth A. McKusick, MD
Society of Radiologists in Ultrasound
Robert L. Bree, MD
Society of Thoracic Surgeons
Keith S. Naunheim, MD
Cameron D. Wright, MD‡
The Academy of Pharamaceutical Physicians and Investigators
Grant Bagley, MD
The Endocrine Society
Richard A. Guthrie, MD‡
The Triological Society
James H. Kelly, MD
United States and Canadian Academy of Pathology
David S. Wilkinson, MD, PhD

AMA Health Care Professionals Advisory Committee (HCPAC)

Tracy R. Gordy, MD, Co-Chair
AMA CPT Editorial Panel
Helene Fearon, PT, Co-Chair
AMA CPT Editorial Panel
American Academy of Physician Assistants
Terry E. Carlisle, PA-C, MPAS‡
American Association of Naturopathatic Physicians
Wendell B. Milliman, ND
American Association for Respiratory Care
Susan Rinaldo-Gallo, Med, RRT
American Chiropractic Association
Craig S. Little, DC
American Dietetic Association
Keith Thomas-Ayoob, EdD, RD, FADA, CSP
American Massage Therapy Association
Whitney W. Lowe
American Nurses Association
David Keepnews, PhD, JD, RN
American Occupational Therapy Association
Leslie F. Davison, MS, Ed, OTR/L
American Optometric Association
Douglas C. Morrow, OD
American Physical Therapy Association
Paul A. Rockar, Jr, PT, MS
American Podiatric Medical Association
Michael J. King, DPM
American Psychological Association
Antonio E. Puente, PhD
American Speech-Language Hearing Association
R. Wayne Holland, EdD
National Association of Social Workers
Nelda Spyres, ACSW, LCSW
National Society of Genetic Counselors
Debra L. Doyle, MS, CGC
Pharmacist Services Technical Advisory Coalition
Daniel E. Buffington, PharmD, MBA

Contents

Contents

Introduction

Current Procedural Terminology (*CPT®*), Fourth Edition, is a set of codes, descriptions, and guidelines intended to describe procedures and services performed by physicians and other health care providers. Each procedure or service is identified with a five-digit code. The use of CPT codes simplifies the reporting of services.

Inclusion of a descriptor and its associated five-digit code number in the CPT codebook is based on whether the procedure is consistent with contemporary medical practice and is performed by many practitioners in clinical practice in multiple locations. Inclusion in the CPT codebook does not represent endorsement by the American Medical Association (AMA) of any particular diagnostic or therapeutic procedure. Inclusion or exclusion of a procedure does not imply any health insurance coverage or reimbursement policy.

The CPT code set is published annually in the late summer or early fall as both electronic data files and books. The release of CPT data files on the Internet typically precedes the book by several weeks. In any case, January 1 is the effective date for use of the update of the CPT code set. The interval between the release of the update and the effective date is considered the implementation period and is intended to allow physicians and other providers, payers, and vendors to incorporate CPT changes into their systems. The exception to this schedule of release and effective dates are CPT Category III and vaccine product codes, which are released twice a year on January 1 or July 1 with effective dates for use six months later. The CPT Category II codes are released three times yearly with effective dates for use three months later.

The main body of the Category I material is listed in six sections. Each section is divided into subsections with anatomic, procedural, condition, or descriptor subheadings. The procedures and services with their identifying codes are presented in numeric order with one exception—the entire **Evaluation and Management** section (99201-99499) appears at the beginning of the listed procedures. These items are used by most physicians in reporting a significant portion of their services.

Section Numbers and Their Sequences

Category I

Evaluation and Management 99201-99499
Anesthesiology 00100-01999, 99100-99140
Surgery 10021-69990
Radiology (Including Nuclear Medicine and Diagnostic
    Ultrasound) 70010-79999
Pathology and Laboratory 80048-89356
Medicine
    (except Anesthesiology) . . 90281-99199, 99500-99602

Category II 0001F-6005F
Category III 0016T-0170T

The first and last code numbers and the subsection name of the items appear at the top margin of most pages (eg, "11010-11306 Surgery/Integumentary System"). The continuous pagination of the CPT codebook is found on the lower margin of each page along with explanation of any code symbols that are found on that page.

Instructions for Use of the CPT Codebook

Select the name of the procedure or service that accurately identifies the service performed. Do not select a CPT code that merely approximates the service provided. If no such procedure or service exists, then report the service using the appropriate unlisted procedure or service code. In surgery, it may be an operation; in medicine, a diagnostic or therapeutic procedure; in radiology, a radiograph. Other additional procedures performed or pertinent special services are also listed. When necessary, any modifying or extenuating circumstances are added. Any service or procedure should be adequately documented in the medical record.

It is important to recognize that the listing of a service or procedure and its code number in a specific section of this book does not restrict its use to a specific specialty group. Any procedure or service in any section of this book may be used to designate the services rendered by any qualified physician or other qualified health care professional.

Instructions, typically included as parenthetical notes, with selected codes indicate that a code should not be reported with another code or codes. These instructions are intended to prevent errors of significant probability and are not all inclusive. For example, the code with such instructions may be a component of another code and therefore it would be incorrect to report both codes even when the component service is performed. These instructions are not intended as a listing of all possible code combinations that should not be reported, nor to indicate all possible code combinations that are appropriately reported. When reporting codes for services provided, it is important to ensure the accuracy and quality of coding through verification of the intent of the code by use of the related guidelines, parenthetical instructions, and coding resources, including *CPT Assistant* and other publications resulting from collaborative efforts of the American Medical Association with the medical specialty societies (eg, *Clinical Examples in Radiology*).

Format of the Terminology

The CPT code set has been developed as stand-alone descriptions of medical procedures. However, some of the procedures in the CPT codebook are not printed in their entirety but refer back to a common portion of the procedure listed in a preceding entry. This is evident when an entry is followed by one or more indentations. This is done in an effort to conserve space.

Example

25100 Arthrotomy, wrist joint; with biopsy

25105   with synovectomy

Note that the common part of code 25100 (the part before the semicolon) should be considered part of code 25105. Therefore, the full procedure represented by code 25105 should read:

25105 Arthrotomy, wrist joint; with synovectomy

Requests to Update the CPT Nomenclature

The effectiveness of the CPT nomenclature depends on constant updating to reflect changes in medical practice. This can only be accomplished through the interest and timely suggestions of practicing physicians, medical specialty societies, state medical associations, and other organizations and agencies. Accordingly, the AMA welcomes correspondence, inquiries, and suggestions concerning old and new procedures, as well as other matters such as codes and indices.

To submit a suggestion to add, delete, or revise procedures contained in the CPT codebook, please contact:
CPT Editorial Research & Development
American Medical Association
515 North State Street
Chicago, Illinois 60610

Coding change request forms are available at the AMA's CPT Web site: www.ama-assn.org/ama/pub/category/3866.html.

All proposed changes of the CPT codebook will be considered by the CPT Editorial Panel with consultation of appropriate medical specialty societies.

Guidelines

Specific guidelines are presented at the beginning of each of the six sections. These guidelines define items that are necessary to appropriately interpret and report the procedures and services contained in that section. For example, in the **Medicine** section, specific instructions are provided for handling unlisted services or procedures, special reports, and supplies and materials provided. Guidelines also provide explanations regarding terms that apply only to a particular section. For instance, **Radiology Guidelines** provide a definition of the unique term, "radiological supervision and interpretation." While in **Anesthesia**, a discussion of reporting time is included.

Add-on Codes

Some of the listed procedures are commonly carried out in addition to the primary procedure performed. These additional or supplemental procedures are designated as add-on codes with the "✚" symbol and they are listed in **Appendix D** of the CPT codebook. Add-on codes in *CPT 2007* can be readily identified by specific descriptor nomenclature that includes phrases such as "each additional" or "(List separately in addition to primary procedure)."

The add-on code concept in *CPT 2007* applies only to add-on procedures or services performed by the same physician. Add-on codes describe additional intra-service work associated with the primary procedure, eg, additional digit(s), lesion(s), neurorrhaphy(s), vertebral segment(s), tendon(s), joint(s).

Add-on codes are always performed in addition to the primary service or procedure and must never be reported as a stand-alone code. All add-on codes found in the CPT codebook are exempt from the multiple procedure concept (see the modifier 51 definition in **Appendix A**).

Modifiers

A modifier provides the means by which the reporting physician can indicate that a service or procedure that has been performed has been altered by some specific circumstance but not changed in its definition or code. The judicious application of modifiers obviates the necessity for separate procedure listings that may describe the modifying circumstance. Modifiers may be used to indicate to the recipient of a report that:

- A service or procedure had both a professional and technical component.

- A service or procedure was performed by more than one physician and/or in more than one location.

- A service or procedure was increased or reduced.

- Only part of a service was performed.

- An adjunctive service was performed.

- A bilateral procedure was performed.

- A service or procedure was provided more than once.

- Unusual events occurred.

Example

A physician providing diagnostic or therapeutic radiology services, ultrasound, or nuclear medicine services in a hospital would add modifier 26 to report the professional component.

73090 with modifier 26 = Professional component only for an X ray of the forearm

Example

Two surgeons may be required to manage a specific surgical problem. When two surgeons work together as primary surgeons performing distinct part(s) of a procedure, each surgeon should report his/her distinct operative work by adding modifier 62 to the procedure code and any associated code(s) for that procedure as long as both surgeons continue to work together as primary surgeons. Each surgeon should report the co-surgery once using the same procedure code. Modifier 62 would be applicable. For instance, a neurological surgeon and an otolaryngologist are working as co-surgeons in performing transphenoidal excision of a pituitary neoplasm.

The first surgeon would report:

61548 with modifier 62 = Hypophysectomy or excision of pituitary tumor, transnasal or transseptal approach, nonstereotactic + two surgeons modifier

AND the second surgeon would report:

61548 with modifier 62 = Hypophysectomy or excision of pituitary tumor, transnasal or transseptal approach, nonstereotactic + two surgeons modifier

If additional procedure(s) (including add-on procedure[s]) are performed during the same surgical session, separate code(s) may also be reported with modifier 62 added. It should be noted that if a co-surgeon acts as an assistant in the performance of additional procedure(s) during the same surgical session, those services may be reported using separate procedure code(s) with modifier 80 or modifier 82 added, as appropriate. A complete listing of modifiers is found in **Appendix A**.

Unlisted Procedure or Service

It is recognized that there may be services or procedures performed by physicians that are not found in the CPT codebook. Therefore, a number of specific code numbers have been designated for reporting unlisted procedures. When an unlisted procedure number is used, the service or procedure should be described. Each of these unlisted procedural code numbers (with the appropriate accompanying topical entry) relates to a specific section of the book and is presented in the guidelines of that section.

Special Report

A service that is rarely provided, unusual, variable, or new may require a special report in determining medical appropriateness of the service. Pertinent information should include an adequate definition or description of the nature, extent, and need for the procedure and the time, effort, and equipment necessary to provide the service. Additional items may include complexity of symptoms, final diagnosis, pertinent physical findings, diagnostic and therapeutic procedures, concurrent problems, and follow-up care.

Code Symbols

A summary listing of additions, deletions, and revisions applicable to the CPT codebook is found in **Appendix B**. New procedure numbers added to the CPT codebook are identified throughout the text with the symbol ● placed before the code number. In instances where a code revision has resulted in a substantially altered procedure

descriptor, the symbol ▲ is placed before the code number. The symbols ► ◄ are used to indicate new and revised text other than the procedure descriptors. These symbols indicate CPT Editorial Panel actions. The AMA reserves the right to correct typographical error and make stylistic improvements. CPT add-on codes are annotated by the symbol + and are listed in **Appendix D**. The symbol ⊘ is used to identify codes that are exempt from the use of modifier 51 but have not been designated as CPT add-on procedures or services. A list of codes exempt from modifier 51 usage is included in **Appendix E**. The symbol ⊙ is used to identify codes that include moderate sedation (see **Appendix G**). The symbol ⚯ is used to identify codes for vaccines that are pending FDA approval (see **Appendix K**).

Alphabetical Reference Index

This codebook features an expanded alphabetical index that includes listings by procedure and anatomic site. Procedures and services commonly known by their eponyms or other designations are also included.

CPT 2007 in Electronic Formats

CPT 2007 procedure codes and descriptions are available on CD-ROM as data files and electronic software. Data files are available in ASCII and EBCDIC formats and can be imported into any billing and claims reporting software that accepts a text (TXT) file format. *CPT 2007 Electronic Professional* software, now with *Netter's Atlas of Human Anatomy for CPT Coding*, provides access to the entire *CPT 2007 Professional Edition* codebook on your desktop. Easy-to-use and fully searchable, this invaluable software contains all of the favorite *CPT Professional* features plus quick linking access between CPT codes, guidelines, modifiers, appendixes, index, and more. For more information call 800 621-8335 or visit www.amabookstore.com.

Additional CPT Resources

The AMA publishes additional CPT coding books and software to ensure your practice has current, complete, and compliant coding resources.

CPT® Assistant Newsletter

As the AMA's official communication tool for circulating accurate information and guidance on CPT codes and issues, this insightful monthly newsletter should be part of every compliance program. Each issue features articles used for answering day-to-day coding questions, appealing insurance denials, and validating coding to auditors. *CPT® Assistant* keeps you informed on critical code changes, enhances your coding proficiency through case studies and clinical examples, and provides a coding consultation section featuring questions and answers drawn from the *CPT® Information Services*.

E-mail amy.burgess@ama-assn.org to request a free sample issue.

Subscriptions to *CPT® Assistant* can be purchased by calling the AMA's Unified Services Center at 800 621-8335. Individual back issues are available for purchase and immediate download at www.amabookstore.com.

CPT® Assistant Archives 1990–2006 (Available February 2007)

Enjoy convenient access to 17 years of *CPT® Assistant* newsletter articles on your computer desktop. Search past issues of the AMA's authoritative coding newsletter by keyword, phrase, CPT code number, newsletter issue, article index, or codebook table of contents. The new edition of this product offers simple search capabilities, menu screens, a cumulative index of article titles, and a complete historical CPT code list from 1990-2006 that references when a code was added, deleted, and/or revised. Call 800 621-8335 or visit www.amabookstore.com for more information.

Clinical Examples in Radiology Newsletter

Understand the correct application of radiology CPT codes with this authoritative guide from the AMA and the American College of Radiology (ACR). A quarterly newsletter, it provides expert advice and guidance of especially high value to the day-to-day needs of radiology coding professionals. Each issue features clinical examples, radiology coding FAQs, a documentation challenge, and a radiology test case. Special report bulletins are also mailed throughout the year covering important news and issues related to radiology coding. Email amy.burgess@ama-assn.org to request a free sample issue.

CPT® Changes 2007: An Insider's View

An indispensable guide for CPT codebook users. This book provides the official AMA interpretations and rationales for every new, revised, and deleted CPT code and guideline change. This valuable resource provides useful clinical examples and procedural descriptions to help explain the practical application for each new CPT code, and an "at-a-glance" tabular review of 2007 changes helps you easily determine the level to which your particular field has been affected by the changes. Call 800 621-8335 or visit www.amabookstore.com for more information.

CPT® Changes Archives 2000–2007

Access current and historical CPT code and guideline changes on your computer desktop. An invaluable electronic library, use it to search the AMA's best-selling *CPT® Changes: An Insider's View* by keyword, phrase, CPT code number, edition, and CPT codebook table of contents. This product offers simple, intuitive search capabilities and a complete historical CPT code list from 1990-2007 that references when a code was added, deleted, and/or revised. Call 800 621-8335 or visit www.amabookstore.com for more information.

More AMA Coding Resources

Check out these additional AMA coding resources at www.amabookstore.com:

- New—*CPT® Reference of Clinical Examples: Official Coding Scenarios for Correct Coding*
- New—*Netter's Atlas of Anatomy for CPT® and ICD-9-CM Coding: Musculoskeletal*
- *CPT® for Outpatient Services*
- *Practical E/M: Documentation and Coding Solutions for Quality Patient Care*
- *Coding with Modifiers: A Guide to Correct CPT® and HCPCS Level II Modifier Usage*
- *Principles of CPT® Coding*
- *Netter's Atlas of Human Anatomy for CPT® Coding*
- *CPT® Coding Workbook: Coding Challenges and Exercises for Instructors and Students*
- *CPT® Specialty Resources*
- *CodeManager®* software

Additional References

For best coding results, you will need to use other reference materials in addition to your coding books. These references include a medical dictionary and one or more anatomy books that can be purchased from the American Medical Association by calling 800 621-8335.

Medical Dictionaries

Merriam-Webster's Medical Desk Dictionary. Springfield, Mass: Merriam Webster. OP941493

Stedman's Medical Dictionary, 27th ed. Baltimore, Md: Williams & Wilkins; 2000. OP982900

Anatomy References

Kirschner, CG. *Netter's Atlas of Anatomy for CPT® and ICD-9-CM Coding Series: Musculoskeletal.* Chicago, Ill: American Medical Association; *Coming Soon.* OP492206

Kirschner, CG. *Netter's Atlas of Human Anatomy for CPT® Coding.* Chicago, Ill: American Medical Association; 2005. OP490605

Netter, FH. *Atlas of Human Anatomy.* 3rd ed. East Hanover, NJ: Novartis; 2003. OP936798

Evaluation and Management (E/M) Services Guidelines

In addition to the information presented in the Introduction, several other items unique to this section are defined or identified here.

Classification of Evaluation and Management (E/M) Services

The E/M section is divided into broad categories such as office visits, hospital visits, and consultations. Most of the categories are further divided into two or more subcategories of E/M services. For example, there are two subcategories of office visits (new patient and established patient) and there are two subcategories of hospital visits (initial and subsequent). The subcategories of E/M services are further classified into levels of E/M services that are identified by specific codes. This classification is important because the nature of physician work varies by type of service, place of service, and the patient's status.

The basic format of the levels of E/M services is the same for most categories. First, a unique code number is listed. Second, the place and/or type of service is specified, eg, office consultation. Third, the content of the service is defined, eg, comprehensive history and comprehensive examination. (See "Levels of E/M Services," page 3, for details on the content of E/M services.) Fourth, the nature of the presenting problem(s) usually associated with a given level is described. Fifth, the time typically required to provide the service is specified. (A detailed discussion of time is provided on page 4.)

Definitions of Commonly Used Terms

Certain key words and phrases are used throughout the E/M section. The following definitions are intended to reduce the potential for differing interpretations and to increase the consistency of reporting by physicians in differing specialties.

New and Established Patient

Solely for the purposes of distinguishing between new and established patients, **professional services** are those face-to-face services rendered by a physician and reported by a specific CPT code(s). A new patient is one who has not received any professional services from the physician

or another physician of the same specialty who belongs to the same group practice, within the past three years.

An established patient is one who has received professional services from the physician or another physician of the same specialty who belongs to the same group practice, within the past three years.

In the instance where a physician is on call for or covering for another physician, the patient's encounter will be classified as it would have been by the physician who is not available.

No distinction is made between new and established patients in the emergency department. E/M services in the emergency department category may be reported for any new or established patient who presents for treatment in the emergency department.

▶The decision tree on page 2 is provided to aid in determining whether to report the E/M service provided as a new or an established patient encounter.◀

Chief Complaint
A chief complaint is a concise statement describing the symptom, problem, condition, diagnosis, or other factor that is the reason for the encounter, usually stated in the patient's words.

Concurrent Care
Concurrent care is the provision of similar services, eg, hospital visits, to the same patient by more than one physician on the same day. When concurrent care is provided, no special reporting is required. Modifier 75 has been deleted.

Counseling
Counseling is a discussion with a patient and/or family concerning one or more of the following areas:

- Diagnostic results, impressions, and/or recommended diagnostic studies
- Prognosis
- Risks and benefits of management (treatment) options
- Instructions for management (treatment) and/or follow-up
- Importance of compliance with chosen management (treatment) options
- Risk factor reduction
- Patient and family education

(For psychotherapy, see 90804-90857)

Evaluation and Management Guidelines

Decision Tree for New vs Established Patients

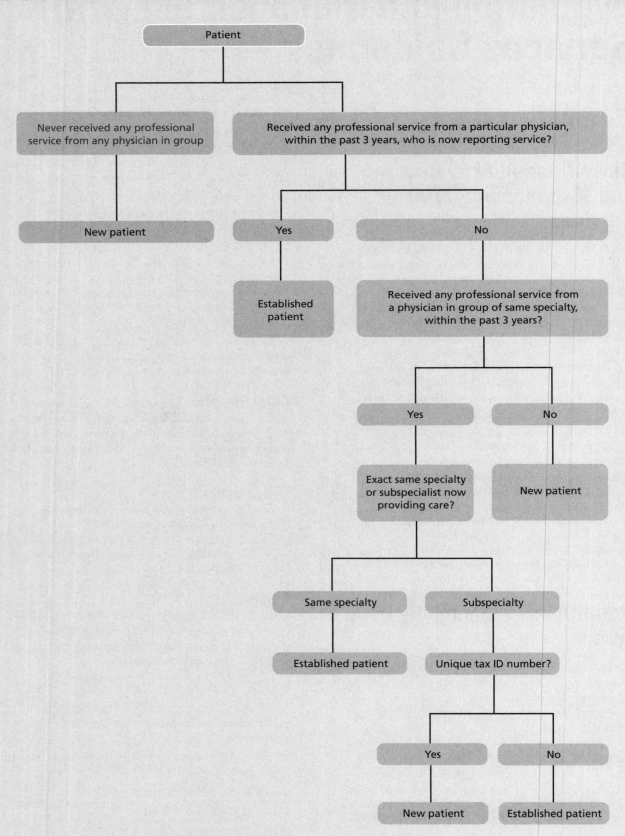

☉=Moderate sedation   ✚=Add-on code   ✗=FDA approval pending

Family History

A review of medical events in the patient's family that includes significant information about:

- The health status or cause of death of parents, siblings, and children

- Specific diseases related to problems identified in the Chief Complaint or History of the Present Illness, and/or System Review

- Diseases of family members that may be hereditary or place the patient at risk

History of Present Illness

A chronological description of the development of the patient's present illness from the first sign and/or symptom to the present. This includes a description of location, quality, severity, timing, context, modifying factors, and associated signs and symptoms significantly related to the presenting problem(s).

Levels of E/M Services

Within each category or subcategory of E/M service, there are three to five levels of E/M services available for reporting purposes. Levels of E/M services are **not** interchangeable among the different categories or subcategories of service. For example, the first level of E/M services in the subcategory of office visit, new patient, does not have the same definition as the first level of E/M services in the subcategory of office visit, established patient.

The levels of E/M services include examinations, evaluations, treatments, conferences with or concerning patients, preventive pediatric and adult health supervision, and similar medical services, such as the determination of the need and/or location for appropriate care. Medical screening includes the history, examination, and medical decision-making required to determine the need and/or location for appropriate care and treatment of the patient (eg, office and other outpatient setting, emergency department, nursing facility). The levels of E/M services encompass the wide variations in skill, effort, time, responsibility, and medical knowledge required for the prevention or diagnosis and treatment of illness or injury and the promotion of optimal health. Each level of E/M services may be used by all physicians.

The descriptors for the levels of E/M services recognize seven components, six of which are used in defining the levels of E/M services. These components are:

- History
- Examination
- Medical decision making
- Counseling
- Coordination of care
- Nature of presenting problem
- Time

The first three of these components (history, examination, and medical decision making) are considered the **key** components in selecting a level of E/M services. (See "Determine the Extent of History Obtained," page 6.)

The next three components (counseling, coordination of care, and the nature of the presenting problem) are considered **contributory** factors in the majority of encounters. Although the first two of these contributory factors are important E/M services, it is not required that these services be provided at every patient encounter.

Coordination of care with other providers or agencies without a patient encounter on that day is reported using the case management codes.

The final component, time, is discussed in detail (see page 4).

Any specifically identifiable procedure (ie, identified with a specific CPT code) performed on or subsequent to the date of initial or subsequent E/M services should be reported separately.

The actual performance and/or interpretation of diagnostic tests/studies ordered during a patient encounter are not included in the levels of E/M services. Physician performance of diagnostic tests/studies for which specific CPT codes are available may be reported separately, in addition to the appropriate E/M code. The physician's interpretation of the results of diagnostic tests/studies (ie, professional component) with preparation of a separate distinctly identifiable signed written report may also be reported separately, using the appropriate CPT code with modifier 26 appended.

The physician may need to indicate that on the day a procedure or service identified by a CPT code was performed, the patient's condition required a significant separately identifiable E/M service above and beyond other services provided or beyond the usual preservice and postservice care associated with the procedure that was performed. The E/M service may be caused or prompted by the symptoms or condition for which the procedure and/or service was provided. This circumstance may be reported by adding modifier 25 to the appropriate level of E/M service. As such, different diagnoses are not required for reporting of the procedure and the E/M services on the same date.

Nature of Presenting Problem

A presenting problem is a disease, condition, illness, injury, symptom, sign, finding, complaint, or other reason for encounter, with or without a diagnosis being established at the time of the encounter. The E/M codes recognize five types of presenting problems that are defined as follows:

Minimal: A problem that may not require the presence of the physician, but service is provided under the physician's supervision.

Self-limited or minor: A problem that runs a definite and prescribed course, is transient in nature, and is not likely to permanently alter health status OR has a good prognosis with management/compliance.

Low severity: A problem where the risk of morbidity without treatment is low; there is little to no risk of mortality without treatment; full recovery without functional impairment is expected.

Moderate severity: A problem where the risk of morbidity without treatment is moderate; there is moderate risk of mortality without treatment; uncertain prognosis OR increased probability of prolonged functional impairment.

High severity: A problem where the risk of morbidity without treatment is high to extreme; there is a moderate to high risk of mortality without treatment OR high probability of severe, prolonged functional impairment.

Past History

A review of the patient's past experiences with illnesses, injuries, and treatments that includes significant information about:

- Prior major illnesses and injuries
- Prior operations
- Prior hospitalizations
- Current medications
- Allergies (eg, drug, food)
- Age appropriate immunization status
- Age appropriate feeding/dietary status

Social History

An age appropriate review of past and current activities that includes significant information about:

- Marital status and/or living arrangements
- Current employment
- Occupational history
- Use of drugs, alcohol, and tobacco
- Level of education
- Sexual history
- Other relevant social factors

System Review (Review of Systems)

An inventory of body systems obtained through a series of questions seeking to identify signs and/or symptoms that the patient may be experiencing or has experienced. For the purposes of the CPT codebook the following elements of a system review have been identified:

- Constitutional symptoms (fever, weight loss, etc)
- Eyes
- Ears, nose, mouth, throat
- Cardiovascular

- Respiratory
- Gastrointestinal
- Genitourinary
- Musculoskeletal
- Integumentary (skin and/or breast)
- Neurological
- Psychiatric
- Endocrine
- Hematologic/lymphatic
- Allergic/immunologic

The review of systems helps define the problem, clarify the differential diagnosis, identify needed testing, or serves as baseline data on other systems that might be affected by any possible management options.

Time

The inclusion of time in the definitions of levels of E/M services has been implicit in prior editions of the CPT codebook. The inclusion of time as an explicit factor beginning in *CPT 1992* is done to assist physicians in selecting the most appropriate level of E/M services. It should be recognized that the specific times expressed in the visit code descriptors are averages and, therefore, represent a range of times that may be higher or lower depending on actual clinical circumstances.

Time is **not** a descriptive component for the emergency department levels of E/M services because emergency department services are typically provided on a variable intensity basis, often involving multiple encounters with several patients over an extended period of time. Therefore, it is often difficult for physicians to provide accurate estimates of the time spent face-to-face with the patient.

Studies to establish levels of E/M services employed surveys of practicing physicians to obtain data on the amount of time and work associated with typical E/M services. Since "work" is not easily quantifiable, the codes must rely on other objective, verifiable measures that correlate with physicians' estimates of their "work." It has been demonstrated that physicians' estimations of **intraservice** time (as explained on the next page), both within and across specialties, is a variable that is predictive of the "work" of E/M services. This same research has shown there is a strong relationship between intraservice time and total time for E/M services. Intraservice time, rather than total time, was chosen for inclusion with the codes because of its relative ease of measurement and because of its direct correlation with measurements of the total amount of time and work associated with typical E/M services.

Intraservice times are defined as **face-to-face** time for office and other outpatient visits and as **unit/floor** time for hospital and other inpatient visits. This distinction is necessary because most of the work of typical office visits takes place during the face-to-face time with the patient, while most of the work of typical hospital visits takes place during the time spent on the patient's floor or unit.

Face-to-face time (office and other outpatient visits and office consultations): For coding purposes, face-to-face time for these services is defined as only that time that the physician spends face-to-face with the patient and/or family. This includes the time in which the physician performs such tasks as obtaining a history, performing an examination, and counseling the patient.

Physicians also spend time doing work before or after the face-to-face time with the patient, performing such tasks as reviewing records and tests, arranging for further services, and communicating further with other professionals and the patient through written reports and telephone contact.

This **non-face-to-face** time for office services—also called pre- and postencounter time—is not included in the time component described in the E/M codes. However, the pre- and post-face-to-face work associated with an encounter was included in calculating the total work of typical services in physician surveys.

Thus, the face-to-face time associated with the services described by any E/M code is a valid proxy for the total work done before, during, and after the visit.

Unit/floor time (hospital observation services, inpatient hospital care, initial and follow-up hospital consultations, nursing facility): For reporting purposes, intraservice time for these services is defined as unit/floor time, which includes the time that the physician is present on the patient's hospital unit and at the bedside rendering services for that patient. This includes the time in which the physician establishes and/or reviews the patient's chart, examines the patient, writes notes, and communicates with other professionals and the patient's family.

In the hospital, pre- and post-time includes time spent off the patient's floor performing such tasks as reviewing pathology and radiology findings in another part of the hospital.

This pre- and postvisit time is not included in the time component described in these codes. However, the pre- and postwork performed during the time spent off the floor or unit was included in calculating the total work of typical services in physician surveys.

Thus, the unit/floor time associated with the services described by any code is a valid proxy for the total work done before, during, and after the visit.

Unlisted Service

An E/M service may be provided that is not listed in this section of the CPT codebook. When reporting such a service, the appropriate "Unlisted" code may be used to indicate the service, identifying it by "Special Report," as discussed in the following paragraph. The "Unlisted Services" and accompanying codes for the E/M section are as follows:

99429   **Unlisted preventive** medicine service

99499   **Unlisted evaluation and management** service

►Results/Testing/Reports◄

►Results are the technical component of a service. Testing leads to results; results lead to interpretation. Reports are the work product of the interpretation of numerous test results.◄

Special Report

An unlisted service or one that is unusual, variable, or new may require a special report demonstrating the medical appropriateness of the service. Pertinent information should include an adequate definition or description of the nature, extent, and need for the procedure and the time, effort, and equipment necessary to provide the service. Additional items that may be included are complexity of symptoms, final diagnosis, pertinent physical findings, diagnostic and therapeutic procedures, concurrent problems, and follow-up care.

Clinical Examples

Clinical examples of the codes for E/M services are provided to assist physicians in understanding the meaning of the descriptors and selecting the correct code. The clinical examples are listed in Appendix C. Each example was developed by physicians in the specialties shown.

The same problem, when seen by physicians in different specialties, may involve different amounts of work. Therefore, the appropriate level of encounter should be reported using the descriptors rather than the examples.

The examples have been tested for validity and approved by the CPT Editorial Panel. Physicians were given the examples and asked to assign a code or assess the amount of time and work involved. Only examples that were rated consistently have been included in Appendix C.

Table 1
Categories and Subcategories of Service

Category/Subcategory	Code Numbers	Category/Subcategory	Code Numbers
Office or Other Outpatient Services		Domiciliary, Rest Home or	
New Patient	99201-99205	Custodial Care Services	
Established Patient	99211-99215	New Patient	99324-99328
Hospital Observation Services		Established Patient	99334-99337
Hospital Observation Discharge Services	99217	Domiciliary, Rest Home (eg, Assisted	
Initial Hospital Observation Services	99218-99220	Living Facility), or Home Care Plan	
Hospital Observation or Inpatient Care		Oversight Services	99339-99340
Services (Including Admission and		Home Services	
Discharge Services)	99234-99236	New Patient	99341-99345
Hospital Inpatient Services		Established Patient	99347-99350
Initial Hospital Care	99221-99223	Prolonged Services	
Subsequent Hospital Care	99231-99233	With Direct Patient Contact	99354-99357
Hospital Discharge Services	99238-99239	Without Direct Patient Contact	99358-99359
Consultations		Standby Services	99360
Office Consultations	99241-99245	Case Management Services	
Initial Inpatient Consultations	99251-99255	Team Conferences	99361-99362
Emergency Department Services	99281-99288	Telephone Calls	99371-99373
Pediatric Patient Transport	99289-99290	Care Plan Oversight Services	99374-99380
Critical Care Services		Preventive Medicine Services	
Adult (over 24 months of age)	99291-99292	New Patient	99381-99387
Pediatric	99293-99294	Established Patient	99391-99397
Neonatal	99295-99296	Individual Counseling	99401-99404
Continuing Intensive Care Services	99298-99300	Group Counseling	99411-99412
Nursing Facility Services		Other	99420-99429
Initial Nursing Facility Care	99304-99306	Newborn Care	99431-99440
Subsequent Nursing Facility Care	99307-99310	Special E/M Services	99450-99456
Nursing Facility Discharge Services	99315-99316	Other E/M Services	99499
Other Nursing Facility Services	99318		

Instructions for Selecting a Level of E/M Service

Identify the Category and Subcategory of Service

The categories and subcategories of codes available for reporting E/M services are shown in Table 1.

Review the Reporting Instructions for the Selected Category or Subcategory

Most of the categories and many of the subcategories of service have special guidelines or instructions unique to that category or subcategory. Where these are indicated, eg, "Inpatient Hospital Care," special instructions will be presented preceding the levels of E/M services.

Review the Level of E/M Service Descriptors and Examples in the Selected Category or Subcategory

The descriptors for the levels of E/M services recognize seven components, six of which are used in defining the levels of E/M services. These components are:

- History
- Examination
- Medical decision making
- Counseling
- Coordination of care
- Nature of presenting problem
- Time

The first three of these components (ie, history, examination, and medical decision making) should be considered the **key** components in selecting the level of E/M services. An exception to this rule is in the case of visits that consist predominantly of counseling or coordination of care (see numbered paragraph 3, page 8).

The nature of the presenting problem and time are provided in some levels to assist the physician in determining the appropriate level of E/M service.

Determine the Extent of History Obtained

The extent of the history is dependent upon clinical judgment and on the nature of the presenting problems(s). The levels of E/M services recognize four types of history that are defined as follows:

Problem focused: Chief complaint; brief history of present illness or problem.

Expanded problem focused: Chief complaint; brief history of present illness; problem pertinent system review.

Detailed: Chief complaint; extended history of present illness; problem pertinent system review extended to include a review of a limited number of additional systems; **pertinent** past, family, and/or social history **directly related to the patient's problems.**

Comprehensive: Chief complaint; extended history of present illness; review of systems that is directly related to the problem(s) identified in the history of the present illness plus a review of all additional body systems; **complete** past, family, and social history.

The comprehensive history obtained as part of the preventive medicine E/M service is not problem-oriented and does not involve a chief complaint or present illness. It does, however, include a comprehensive system review and comprehensive or interval past, family, and social history as well as a comprehensive assessment/history of pertinent risk factors.

Determine the Extent of Examination Performed

The extent of the examination performed is dependent on clinical judgment and on the nature of the presenting problem(s). The levels of E/M services recognize four types of examination that are defined as follows:

Problem focused: A limited examination of the affected body area or organ system.

Expanded problem focused: A limited examination of the affected body area or organ system and other symptomatic or related organ system(s).

Detailed: An extended examination of the affected body area(s) and other symptomatic or related organ system(s).

Comprehensive: A general multisystem examination or a complete examination of a single organ system. **Note:** The comprehensive examination performed as part of the preventive medicine E/M service is multisystem, but its extent is based on age and risk factors identified.

For the purposes of these CPT definitions, the following body areas are recognized:

- Head, including the face
- Neck
- Chest, including breasts and axilla
- Abdomen
- Genitalia, groin, buttocks
- Back
- Each extremity

For the purposes of these CPT definitions, the following organ systems are recognized:

- Eyes
- Ears, nose, mouth, and throat
- Cardiovascular
- Respiratory
- Gastrointestinal
- Genitourinary
- Musculoskeletal
- Skin
- Neurologic
- Psychiatric
- Hematologic/lymphatic/immunologic

Determine the Complexity of Medical Decision Making

Medical decision making refers to the complexity of establishing a diagnosis and/or selecting a management option as measured by:

- The number of possible diagnoses and/or the number of management options that must be considered

- The amount and/or complexity of medical records, diagnostic tests, and/or other information that must be obtained, reviewed, and analyzed

- The risk of significant complications, morbidity, and/or mortality, as well as comorbidities, associated with the patient's presenting problems(s), the diagnostic procedure(s), and/or the possible management options

Four types of medical decision making are recognized: straightforward, low complexity, moderate complexity, and high complexity. To qualify for a given type of decision making, two of the three elements in Table 2 must be met or exceeded.

Comorbidities/underlying diseases, in and of themselves, are not considered in selecting a level of E/M services *unless* their presence significantly increases the complexity of the medical decision making.

Select the Appropriate Level of E/M Services Based on the Following

1. For the following categories/subcategories, **all of the key components,** ie, history, examination, and medical decision making, must meet or exceed the stated requirements to qualify for a particular level of E/M service: office, new patient; hospital observation services; initial hospital care; office consultations; initial inpatient consultations; emergency department services; initial nursing facility care; domiciliary care, new patient; and home, new patient.

Evaluation and Management Guidelines *(side margin)*

Table 2
Complexity of Medical Decision Making

Number of Diagnoses or Management Options	Amount and/or Complexity of Data to be Reviewed	Risk of Complications and/or Morbidity or Mortality	Type of Decision Making
minimal	minimal or none	minimal	**straightforward**
limited	limited	low	**low complexity**
multiple	moderate	moderate	**moderate complexity**
extensive	extensive	high	**high complexity**

2. For the following categories/subcategories, **two of the three key components** (ie, history, examination, and medical decision making) must meet or exceed the stated requirements to qualify for a particular level of E/M services: office, established patient; subsequent hospital care; subsequent nursing facility care; domiciliary care, established patient; and home, established patient.

3. When counseling and/or coordination of care dominates (more than 50%) the physician/patient and/or family encounter (face-to-face time in the office or other outpatient setting or floor/unit time in the hospital or nursing facility), then **time** may be considered the key or controlling factor to qualify for a particular level of E/M services. This includes time spent with parties who have assumed responsibility for the care of the patient or decision making whether or not they are family members (eg, foster parents, person acting in locum parentis, legal guardian). The extent of counseling and/or coordination of care must be documented in the medical record.

Evaluation and Management

Office or Other Outpatient Services

The following codes are used to report evaluation and management services provided in the physician's office or in an outpatient or other ambulatory facility. A patient is considered an outpatient until inpatient admission to a health care facility occurs.

To report services provided to a patient who is admitted to a hospital or nursing facility in the course of an encounter in the office or other ambulatory facility, see the notes for initial hospital inpatient care (page 11) or initial nursing facility care (page 21).

For services provided by physicians in the emergency department, see 99281-99285.

For observation care, see 99217-99220.

For observation or inpatient care services (including admission and discharge services), see 99234-99236.

New Patient

99201   **Office or other outpatient visit** for the evaluation and management of a new patient, which requires these three key components:

- **A problem focused history;**
- **A problem focused examination;**
- **Straightforward medical decision making.**

Counseling and/or coordination of care with other providers or agencies are provided consistent with the nature of the problem(s) and the patient's and/or family's needs.

Usually, the presenting problem(s) are self limited or minor. Physicians typically spend 10 minutes face-to-face with the patient and/or family.

99202   **Office or other outpatient visit** for the evaluation and management of a new patient, which requires these three key components:

- **An expanded problem focused history;**
- **An expanded problem focused examination;**
- **Straightforward medical decision making.**

Counseling and/or coordination of care with other providers or agencies are provided consistent with the nature of the problem(s) and the patient's and/or family's needs.

Usually, the presenting problem(s) are of low to moderate severity. Physicians typically spend 20 minutes face-to-face with the patient and/or family.

99203   **Office or other outpatient visit** for the evaluation and management of a new patient, which requires these three key components:

- **A detailed history;**
- **A detailed examination;**
- **Medical decision making of low complexity.**

Counseling and/or coordination of care with other providers or agencies are provided consistent with the nature of the problem(s) and the patient's and/or family's needs.

Usually, the presenting problem(s) are of moderate severity. Physicians typically spend 30 minutes face-to-face with the patient and/or family.

99204   **Office or other outpatient visit** for the evaluation and management of a new patient, which requires these three key components:

- **A comprehensive history;**
- **A comprehensive examination;**
- **Medical decision making of moderate complexity.**

Counseling and/or coordination of care with other providers or agencies are provided consistent with the nature of the problem(s) and the patient's and/or family's needs.

Usually, the presenting problem(s) are of moderate to high severity. Physicians typically spend 45 minutes face-to-face with the patient and/or family.

99205   **Office or other outpatient visit** for the evaluation and management of a new patient, which requires these three key components:

- **A comprehensive history;**
- **A comprehensive examination;**
- **Medical decision making of high complexity.**

Counseling and/or coordination of care with other providers or agencies are provided consistent with the nature of the problem(s) and the patient's and/or family's needs.

Usually, the presenting problem(s) are of moderate to high severity. Physicians typically spend 60 minutes face-to-face with the patient and/or family.

Established Patient

99211   **Office or other outpatient visit** for the evaluation and management of an established patient, that may not require the presence of a physician. Usually, the presenting problem(s) are minimal. Typically, 5 minutes are spent performing or supervising these services.

99212   **Office or other outpatient visit** for the evaluation and management of an established patient, which requires at least two of these three key components:

- **A problem focused history;**

- **A problem focused examination;**

- **Straightforward medical decision making.**

Counseling and/or coordination of care with other providers or agencies are provided consistent with the nature of the problem(s) and the patient's and/or family's needs.

Usually, the presenting problem(s) are self limited or minor. Physicians typically spend 10 minutes face-to-face with the patient and/or family.

99213   **Office or other outpatient visit** for the evaluation and management of an established patient, which requires at least two of these three key components:

- **An expanded problem focused history;**

- **An expanded problem focused examination;**

- **Medical decision making of low complexity.**

Counseling and coordination of care with other providers or agencies are provided consistent with the nature of the problem(s) and the patient's and/or family's needs.

Usually, the presenting problem(s) are of low to moderate severity. Physicians typically spend 15 minutes face-to-face with the patient and/or family.

99214   **Office or other outpatient visit** for the evaluation and management of an established patient, which requires at least two of these three key components:

- **A detailed history;**

- **A detailed examination;**

- **Medical decision making of moderate complexity.**

Counseling and/or coordination of care with other providers or agencies are provided consistent with the nature of the problem(s) and the patient's and/or family's needs.

Usually, the presenting problem(s) are of moderate to high severity. Physicians typically spend 25 minutes face-to-face with the patient and/or family.

99215   **Office or other outpatient visit** for the evaluation and management of an established patient, which requires at least two of these three key components:

- **A comprehensive history;**

- **A comprehensive examination;**

- **Medical decision making of high complexity.**

Counseling and/or coordination of care with other providers or agencies are provided consistent with the nature of the problem(s) and the patient's and/or family's needs.

Usually, the presenting problem(s) are of moderate to high severity. Physicians typically spend 40 minutes face-to-face with the patient and/or family.

Hospital Observation Services

The following codes are used to report evaluation and management services provided to patients designated/admitted as "observation status" in a hospital. It is not necessary that the patient be located in an observation area designated by the hospital.

If such an area does exist in a hospital (as a separate unit in the hospital, in the emergency department, etc), these codes are to be utilized if the patient is placed in such an area.

For definitions of key components and commonly used terms, please see **Evaluation and Management Services Guidelines.**

Typical times have not yet been established for this category of services.

Observation Care Discharge Services

Observation care discharge of a patient from "observation status" includes final examination of the patient, discussion of the hospital stay, instructions for continuing care, and preparation of discharge records. For observation or inpatient hospital care including the admission and discharge of the patient on the same date, see codes 99234-99236 as appropriate.

99217   **Observation care discharge** day management (This code is to be utilized by the physician to report all services provided to a patient on discharge from "observation status" if the discharge is on other than the initial date of "observation status." To report services to a patient designated as "observation status" or "inpatient status" and discharged on the same date, use the codes for Observation or Inpatient Care Services [including Admission and Discharge Services, 99234-99236 as appropriate.])

Initial Observation Care

New or Established Patient

The following codes are used to report the encounter(s) by the supervising physician with the patient when designated as "observation status." This refers to the initiation of observation status, supervision of the care plan for observation and performance of periodic reassessments. For observation encounters by other physicians, see Office or Other Outpatient Consultation codes (99241-99245).

To report services provided to a patient who is admitted to the hospital after receiving hospital observation care services on the same date, see the notes for initial hospital inpatient care (page 12). For a patient admitted to the hospital on a date subsequent to the date of observation status, the hospital admission would be reported with the appropriate Initial Hospital Care code (99221-99223). For a patient admitted and discharged from observation or inpatient status on the same date, the services should be reported with codes 99234-99236 as appropriate. Do not report observation discharge (99217) in conjunction with a hospital admission.

When "observation status" is initiated in the course of an encounter in another site of service (eg, hospital emergency department, physician's office, nursing facility) all evaluation and management services provided by the supervising physician in conjunction with initiating "observation status" are considered part of the initial observation care when performed on the same date. The observation care level of service reported by the supervising physician should include the services related to initiating "observation status" provided in the other sites of service as well as in the observation setting.

Evaluation and management services on the same date provided in sites that are related to initiating "observation status" should NOT be reported separately.

These codes may not be utilized for post-operative recovery if the procedure is considered part of the surgical "package." These codes apply to all evaluation and management services that are provided on the same date of initiating "observation status."

99218   **Initial observation care,** per day, for the evaluation and management of a patient which requires these three key components:

- **A detailed or comprehensive history;**

- **A detailed or comprehensive examination; and**

- **Medical decision making that is straightforward or of low complexity.**

Counseling and/or coordination of care with other providers or agencies are provided consistent with the nature of the problem(s) and the patient's and/or family's needs.

Usually, the problem(s) requiring admission to "observation status" are of low severity.

99219   **Initial observation care,** per day, for the evaluation and management of a patient, which requires these three key components:

- **A comprehensive history;**

- **A comprehensive examination; and**

- **Medical decision making of moderate complexity.**

Counseling and/or coordination of care with other providers or agencies are provided consistent with the nature of the problem(s) and the patient's and/or family's needs.

Usually, the problem(s) requiring admission to "observation status" are of moderate severity.

99220   **Initial observation care,** per day, for the evaluation and management of a patient, which requires these three key components:

- **A comprehensive history;**

- **A comprehensive examination; and**

- **Medical decision making of high complexity.**

Counseling and/or coordination of care with other providers or agencies are provided consistent with the nature of the problem(s) and the patient's and/or family's needs.

Usually, the problem(s) requiring admission to "observation status" are of high severity.

Hospital Inpatient Services

The following codes are used to report evaluation and management services provided to hospital inpatients. Hospital inpatient services include those services provided to patients in a "partial hospital" setting. These codes are to be used to report these partial hospitalization services. See also psychiatry notes in the full text of CPT codebook.

For definitions of key components and commonly used terms, please see **Evaluation and Management Services Guidelines.** For Hospital Observation Services, see 99218-99220. For a patient admitted and discharged from observation or inpatient status on the same date, the services should be reported with codes 99234-99236 as appropriate.

Evaluation and Management

Initial Hospital Care

New or Established Patient

The following codes are used to report the first hospital inpatient encounter with the patient by the admitting physician.

For initial inpatient encounters by physicians other than the admitting physician, see initial inpatient consultation codes (99251-99255) or subsequent hospital care codes (99231-99233) as appropriate.

When the patient is admitted to the hospital as an inpatient in the course of an encounter in another site of service (eg, hospital emergency department, observation status in a hospital, physician's office, nursing facility) all evaluation and management services provided by that physician in conjunction with that admission are considered part of the initial hospital care when performed on the same date as the admission. The inpatient care level of service reported by the admitting physician should include the services related to the admission he/she provided in the other sites of service as well as in the inpatient setting.

Evaluation and management services on the same date provided in sites that are related to the admission "observation status" should NOT be reported separately. For a patient admitted and discharged from observation or inpatient status on the same date, the services should be reported with codes 99234-99236 as appropriate.

99221   **Initial hospital care,** per day, for the evaluation and management of a patient, which requires these three key components:

- **A detailed or comprehensive history;**
- **A detailed or comprehensive examination; and**
- **Medical decision making that is straightforward or of low complexity.**

Counseling and/or coordination of care with other providers or agencies are provided consistent with the nature of the problem(s) and the patient's and/or family's needs.

Usually, the problem(s) requiring admission are of low severity. Physicians typically spend 30 minutes at the bedside and on the patient's hospital floor or unit.

99222   **Initial hospital care,** per day, for the evaluation and management of a patient, which requires these three key components:

- **A comprehensive history;**
- **A comprehensive examination; and**
- **Medical decision making of moderate complexity.**

Counseling and/or coordination of care with other providers or agencies are provided consistent with the nature of the problem(s) and the patient's and/or family's needs.

Usually, the problem(s) requiring admission are of moderate severity. Physicians typically spend 50 minutes at the bedside and on the patient's hospital floor or unit.

99223   **Initial hospital care,** per day, for the evaluation and management of a patient, which requires these three key components:

- **A comprehensive history;**
- **A comprehensive examination; and**
- **Medical decision making of high complexity.**

Counseling and/or coordination of care with other providers or agencies are provided consistent with the nature of the problem(s) and the patient's and/or family's needs.

Usually, the problem(s) requiring admission are of high severity. Physicians typically spend 70 minutes at the bedside and on the patient's hospital floor or unit.

Subsequent Hospital Care

All levels of subsequent hospital care include reviewing the medical record and reviewing the results of diagnostic studies and changes in the patient's status (ie, changes in history, physical condition and response to management) since the last assessment by the physician.

99231   **Subsequent hospital care,** per day, for the evaluation and management of a patient, which requires at least two of these three key components:

- **A problem focused interval history;**
- **A problem focused examination;**
- **Medical decision making that is straightforward or of low complexity.**

Counseling and/or coordination of care with other providers or agencies are provided consistent with the nature of the problem(s) and the patient's and/or family's needs.

Usually, the patient is stable, recovering or improving. Physicians typically spend 15 minutes at the bedside and on the patient's hospital floor or unit.

99232   **Subsequent hospital care,** per day, for the evaluation and management of a patient, which requires at least two of these three key components:

- **An expanded problem focused interval history;**
- **An expanded problem focused examination;**
- **Medical decision making of moderate complexity.**

Counseling and/or coordination of care with other providers or agencies are provided consistent with the nature of the problem(s) and the patient's and/or family's needs.

Usually, the patient is responding inadequately to therapy or has developed a minor complication. Physicians typically spend 25 minutes at the bedside and on the patient's hospital floor or unit.

99233   **Subsequent hospital care,** per day, for the evaluation and management of a patient, which requires at least two of these three key components:

- **A detailed interval history;**

- **A detailed examination;**

- **Medical decision making of high complexity.**

Counseling and/or coordination of care with other providers or agencies are provided consistent with the nature of the problem(s) and the patient's and/or family's needs.

Usually, the patient is unstable or has developed a significant complication or a significant new problem. Physicians typically spend 35 minutes at the bedside and on the patient's hospital floor or unit.

Observation or Inpatient Care Services (Including Admission and Discharge Services)

The following codes are used to report observation or inpatient hospital care services provided to patients admitted and discharged on the same date of service. When a patient is admitted to the hospital from observation status on the same date, the physician should report only the initial hospital care code. The initial hospital care code reported by the admitting physician should include the services related to the observation status services he/she provided on the same date of inpatient admission.

When "observation status" is initiated in the course of an encounter in another site of service (eg, hospital emergency department, physician's office, nursing facility) all evaluation and management services provided by the supervising physician in conjunction with initiating "observation status" are considered part of the initial observation care when performed on the same date. The observation care level of service should include the services related to initiating "observation status" provided in the other sites of service as well as in the observation setting when provided by the same physician.

For patients admitted to observation or inpatient care and discharged on a different date, see codes 99218-99220 and 99217, or 99221-99223 and 99238, 99239.

99234   **Observation or inpatient hospital care,** for the evaluation and management of a patient including admission and discharge on the same date which requires these three key components:

- **A detailed or comprehensive history;**

- **A detailed or comprehensive examination; and**

- **Medical decision making that is straightforward or of low complexity.**

Counseling and/or coordination of care with other providers or agencies are provided consistent with the nature of the problem(s) and the patient's and/or family's needs.

Usually the presenting problem(s) requiring admission are of low severity.

99235   **Observation or inpatient hospital care,** for the evaluation and management of a patient including admission and discharge on the same date which requires these three key components:

- **A comprehensive history;**

- **A comprehensive examination; and**

- **Medical decision making of moderate complexity.**

Counseling and/or coordination of care with other providers or agencies are provided consistent with the nature of the problem(s) and the patient's and/or family's needs.

Usually the presenting problem(s) requiring admission are of moderate severity.

99236   **Observation or inpatient hospital care,** for the evaluation and management of a patient including admission and discharge on the same date which requires these three key components:

- **A comprehensive history;**

- **A comprehensive examination; and**

- **Medical decision making of high complexity.**

Counseling and/or coordination of care with other providers or agencies are provided consistent with the nature of the problem(s) and the patient's and/or family's needs.

Usually the presenting problem(s) requiring admission are of high severity.

Evaluation and Management

Hospital Discharge Services

The hospital discharge day management codes are to be used to report the total duration of time spent by a physician for final hospital discharge of a patient. The codes include, as appropriate, final examination of the patient, discussion of the hospital stay, even if the time spent by the physician on that date is not continuous, instructions for continuing care to all relevant caregivers, and preparation of discharge records, prescriptions and referral forms. For a patient admitted and discharged from observation or inpatient status on the same date, the services should be reported with codes 99234-99236 as appropriate.

99238   **Hospital discharge day management;** 30 minutes or less

99239   more than 30 minutes

(These codes are to be utilized by the physician to report all services provided to a patient on the date of discharge, if other than the initial date of inpatient status. To report services to a patient who is admitted as an inpatient, and discharged on the same date, see codes 99234-99236 for observation or inpatient hospital care including the admission and discharge of the patient on the same date. To report concurrent care services provided by a physician(s) other than the attending physician, use subsequent hospital care codes (99231-99233) on the day of discharge.)

(For Observation Care Discharge, use 99217)

(For observation or inpatient hospital care including the admission and discharge of the patient on the same date, see 99234-99236)

(For Nursing Facility Care Discharge, see 99315, 99316)

(For discharge services provided to newborns admitted and discharged on the same date, use 99435)

Consultations

A consultation is a type of service provided by a physician whose opinion or advice regarding evaluation and/or management of a specific problem is requested by another physician or other appropriate source.

A physician consultant may initiate diagnostic and/or therapeutic services at the same or subsequent visit.

The written or verbal request for a consult may be made by a physician or other appropriate source and documented in the patient's medical record. The consultant's opinion and any services that were ordered or performed must also be documented in the patient's medical record and communicated by written report to the requesting physician or other appropriate source.

▶A "consultation" initiated by a patient and/or family, and not requested by a physician or other appropriate source (eg, physician assistant, nurse practitioner, doctor of chiropractic, physical therapist, occupational therapist, speech-language pathologist, psychologist, social worker, lawyer, or insurance company), is not reported using the consultation codes but may be reported using the office visit, home service, or domiciliary/rest home care codes.◀

If a consultation is mandated, eg, by a third-party payer, modifier 32 should also be reported.

Any specifically identifiable procedure (ie, identified with a specific CPT code) performed on or subsequent to the date of the initial consultation should be reported separately.

▶If subsequent to the completion of a consultation the consultant assumes responsibility for management of a portion or all of the patient's condition(s), the appropriate **Evaluation and Management** services code for the site of service should be reported. In the hospital or nursing facility setting, the consulting physician should use the appropriate inpatient consultation code for the initial encounter and then subsequent hospital or nursing facility care codes. In the office setting, the physician should use the appropriate office or other outpatient consultation codes and then the established patient office or other outpatient services codes.◀

For definitions of key components and commonly used terms, please see **Evaluation and Management Services Guidelines.**

Office or Other Outpatient Consultations

New or Established Patient

▶The following codes are used to report consultations provided in the physician's office or in an outpatient or other ambulatory facility, including hospital observation services, home services, domiciliary, rest home, or emergency department (see the preceding consultation definition above). Follow-up visits in the consultant's office or other outpatient facility that are initiated by the physician consultant or patient are reported using the appropriate codes for established patients, office visits (99211-99215), domiciliary, rest home (99334-99337), or home (99347-99350). If an additional request for an opinion or advice regarding the same or a new problem is received from another physician or other appropriate source and documented in the medical record, the office consultation codes may be used again.◀

99241   **Office consultation** for a new or established patient, which requires these three key components:

- **A problem focused history;**

- **A problem focused examination; and**

- **Straightforward medical decision making.**

Counseling and/or coordination of care with other providers or agencies are provided consistent with the nature of the problem(s) and the patient's and/or family's needs.

Usually, the presenting problem(s) are self limited or minor. Physicians typically spend 15 minutes face-to-face with the patient and/or family.

99242   **Office consultation** for a new or established patient, which requires these three key components:

- **An expanded problem focused history;**

- **An expanded problem focused examination; and**

- **Straightforward medical decision making.**

Counseling and/or coordination of care with other providers or agencies are provided consistent with the nature of the problem(s) and the patient's and/or family's needs.

Usually, the presenting problem(s) are of low severity. Physicians typically spend 30 minutes face-to-face with the patient and/or family.

99243   **Office consultation** for a new or established patient, which requires these three key components:

- **A detailed history;**

- **A detailed examination; and**

- **Medical decision making of low complexity.**

Counseling and/or coordination of care with other providers or agencies are provided consistent with the nature of the problem(s) and the patient's and/or family's needs.

Usually, the presenting problem(s) are of moderate severity. Physicians typically spend 40 minutes face-to-face with the patient and/or family.

99244   **Office consultation** for a new or established patient, which requires these three key components:

- **A comprehensive history;**

- **A comprehensive examination; and**

- **Medical decision making of moderate complexity.**

Counseling and/or coordination of care with other providers or agencies are provided consistent with the nature of the problem(s) and the patient's and/or family's needs.

Usually, the presenting problem(s) are of moderate to high severity. Physicians typically spend 60 minutes face-to-face with the patient and/or family.

99245   **Office consultation** for a new or established patient, which requires these three key components:

- **A comprehensive history;**

- **A comprehensive examination; and**

- **Medical decision making of high complexity.**

Counseling and/or coordination of care with other providers or agencies are provided consistent with the nature of the problem(s) and the patient's and/or family's needs.

Usually, the presenting problem(s) are of moderate to high severity. Physicians typically spend 80 minutes face-to-face with the patient and/or family.

►Inpatient Consultations◄

New or Established Patient

►The following codes are used to report physician consultations provided to hospital inpatients, residents of nursing facilities, or patients in a partial hospital setting. Only one consultation should be reported by a consultant per admission. Subsequent services during the same admission are reported using Subsequent Hospital Care codes (99231-99233) or Subsequent Nursing Facility Care codes (99307-99310), including services to complete the initial consultation, monitor progress, revise recommendations, or address a new problem.◄

▲ **99251**   **Inpatient consultation** for a new or established patient, which requires these three key components:

- **A problem focused history;**

- **A problem focused examination; and**

- **Straightforward medical decision making.**

Counseling and/or coordination of care with other providers or agencies are provided consistent with the nature of the problem(s) and the patient's and/or family's needs.

Usually, the presenting problem(s) are self limited or minor. Physicians typically spend 20 minutes at the bedside and on the patient's hospital floor or unit.

▲ **99252**   **Inpatient consultation** for a new or established patient, which requires these three key components:

- **An expanded problem focused history;**

- **An expanded problem focused examination; and**

- **Straightforward medical decision making.**

Counseling and/or coordination of care with other providers or agencies are provided consistent with the nature of the problem(s) and the patient's and/or family's needs.

Usually, the presenting problem(s) are of low severity. Physicians typically spend 40 minutes at the bedside and on the patient's hospital floor or unit.

Evaluation and Management

▲ 99253   **Inpatient consultation** for a new or established patient, which requires these three key components:

- **A detailed history;**
- **A detailed examination; and**
- **Medical decision making of low complexity.**

Counseling and/or coordination of care with other providers or agencies are provided consistent with the nature of the problem(s) and the patient's and/or family's needs.

Usually, the presenting problem(s) are of moderate severity. Physicians typically spend 55 minutes at the bedside and on the patient's hospital floor or unit.

▲ 99254   **Inpatient consultation** for a new or established patient, which requires these three key components:

- **A comprehensive history;**
- **A comprehensive examination; and**
- **Medical decision making of moderate complexity.**

Counseling and/or coordination of care with other providers or agencies are provided consistent with the nature of the problem(s) and the patient's and/or family's needs.

Usually, the presenting problem(s) are of moderate to high severity. Physicians typically spend 80 minutes at the bedside and on the patient's hospital floor or unit.

▲ 99255   **Inpatient consultation** for a new or established patient, which requires these three key components:

- **A comprehensive history;**
- **A comprehensive examination; and**
- **Medical decision making of high complexity.**

Counseling and/or coordination of care with other providers or agencies are provided consistent with the nature of the problem(s) and the patient's and/or family's needs.

Usually, the presenting problem(s) are of moderate to high severity. Physicians typically spend 110 minutes at the bedside and on the patient's hospital floor or unit.

Emergency Department Services

New or Established Patient

The following codes are used to report evaluation and management services provided in the emergency department. No distinction is made between new and established patients in the emergency department.

An emergency department is defined as an organized hospital-based facility for the provision of unscheduled episodic services to patients who present for immediate medical attention. The facility must be available 24 hours a day.

For critical care services provided in the emergency department, see Critical Care notes and 99291, 99292.

For evaluation and management services provided to a patient in an observation area of a hospital, see 99217-99220.

For observation or inpatient care services (including admission and discharge services), see 99234-99236.

99281   **Emergency department visit** for the evaluation and management of a patient, which requires these three key components:

- **A problem focused history;**
- **A problem focused examination; and**
- **Straightforward medical decision making.**

Counseling and/or coordination of care with other providers or agencies are provided consistent with the nature of the problem(s) and the patient's and/or family's needs.

Usually, the presenting problem(s) are self limited or minor.

99282   **Emergency department visit** for the evaluation and management of a patient, which requires these three key components:

- **An expanded problem focused history;**
- **An expanded problem focused examination; and**
- **Medical decision making of low complexity.**

Counseling and/or coordination of care with other providers or agencies are provided consistent with the nature of the problem(s) and the patient's and/or family's needs.

Usually, the presenting problem(s) are of low to moderate severity.

99283   **Emergency department visit** for the evaluation and management of a patient, which requires these three key components:

- **An expanded problem focused history;**
- **An expanded problem focused examination; and**
- **Medical decision making of moderate complexity.**

Counseling and/or coordination of care with other providers or agencies are provided consistent with the nature of the problem(s) and the patient's and/or family's needs.

Usually, the presenting problem(s) are of moderate severity.

99284   **Emergency department visit** for the evaluation and management of a patient, which requires these three key components:

- **A detailed history;**

- **A detailed examination; and**

- **Medical decision making of moderate complexity.**

Counseling and/or coordination of care with other providers or agencies are provided consistent with the nature of the problem(s) and the patient's and/or family's needs.

Usually, the presenting problem(s) are of high severity, and require urgent evaluation by the physician but do not pose an immediate significant threat to life or physiologic function.

99285   **Emergency department visit** for the evaluation and management of a patient, which requires these three key components within the constraints imposed by the urgency of the patient's clinical condition and/or mental status:

- **A comprehensive history;**

- **A comprehensive examination; and**

- **Medical decision making of high complexity.**

Counseling and/or coordination of care with other providers or agencies are provided consistent with the nature of the problem(s) and the patient's and/or family's needs.

Usually, the presenting problem(s) are of high severity and pose an immediate significant threat to life or physiologic function.

Other Emergency Services

In physician directed emergency care, advanced life support, the physician is located in a hospital emergency or critical care department, and is in two-way voice communication with ambulance or rescue personnel outside the hospital. The physician directs the performance of necessary medical procedures, including but not limited to: telemetry of cardiac rhythm; cardiac and/or pulmonary resuscitation; endotracheal or esophageal obturator airway intubation; administration of intravenous fluids and/or administration of intramuscular, intratracheal or subcutaneous drugs; and/or electrical conversion of arrhythmia.

99288   **Physician direction of** emergency medical systems (EMS) emergency care, advanced life support

Pediatric Critical Care Patient Transport

The following codes 99289 and 99290 are used to report the physical attendance and direct face-to-face care by a physician during the interfacility transport of a critically ill or critically injured pediatric patient. For the purpose of reporting codes 99289 and 99290, face-to-face care begins when the physician assumes primary responsibility of the pediatric patient at the referring hospital/facility, and ends when the receiving hospital/facility accepts responsibility for the pediatric patient's care. Only the time the physician spends in direct face-to-face contact with the patient during the transport should be reported. Pediatric patient transport services involving less than 30 minutes of face-to-face physician care should not be reported using codes 99289, 99290. Procedure(s) or service(s) performed by other members of the transporting team may not be reported by the supervising physician.

►The following services are included when performed during the pediatric patient transport by the physician providing critical care and may not be reported separately: routine monitoring evaluations (eg, heart rate, respiratory rate, blood pressure, and pulse oximetry), the interpretation of cardiac output measurements (93561, 93562), chest x-rays (71010, 71015, 71020), pulse oximetry (94760, 94761, 94762), blood gases and information data stored in computers (eg, ECGs, blood pressures, hematologic data) (99090), gastric intubation (43752, 91105), temporary transcutaneous pacing (92953), ventilatory management (94002-94004, 94660, 94662) and vascular access procedures (36000, 36400, 36405, 36406, 36410, 36415, 36540, 36600). Any services performed which are not listed above should be reported separately.◄

Critical care is the direct delivery by a physician(s) of medical care for a critically ill or critically injured patient. A critical illness or injury acutely impairs one or more vital organ systems such that there is a high probability of imminent or life threatening deterioration in the patient's condition. Critical care involves high complexity decision making to assess, manipulate, and support vital system function(s) to treat single or multiple vital organ system failure and/or to prevent further life threatening deterioration of the patient's condition. Examples of vital organ system failure include, but are not limited to: central nervous system failure, circulatory failure, shock, renal, hepatic, metabolic, and/or respiratory failure.

Providing medical care to a critically ill, injured, or post-operative patient qualifies as a critical care service only if both the illness or injury and the treatment being provided meet the above requirements.

Evaluation and Management

The direction of emergency care to transporting staff by a physician located in a hospital or other facility by two-way communication is not considered direct face-to-face care and should not be reported with codes 99289, 99290. Physician directed emergency care through outside voice communication to transporting staff personnel is reported with code 99288.

The emergency department services codes (99281-99285), initial hospital care codes (99221-99223), hourly critical care codes (99291, 99292), or initial date neonatal intensive care code (99295) are only reported after the patient has been admitted to the emergency department, the inpatient floor or the critical care unit of the receiving facility.

Code 99289 is used to report the first 30-74 minutes of direct face-to-face time with the transport pediatric patient and should be reported only once on a given date. Code 99290 is used to report each additional 30 minutes provided on a given date. Face-to-face services less than 30 minutes should not be reported with these codes.

99289   Critical care services delivered by a physician, face-to-face, during an interfacility transport of critically ill or critically injured pediatric patient, 24 months of age or less; first 30-74 minutes of hands on care during transport

+ 99290   each additional 30 minutes (List separately in addition to code for primary service)

(Use 99290 in conjunction with 99289)

(Critical care of less than 30 minutes total duration should be reported with the appropriate E/M code)

Critical Care Services

Critical care is the direct delivery by a physician(s) of medical care for a critically ill or critically injured patient. A critical illness or injury acutely impairs one or more vital organ systems such that there is a high probability of imminent or life threatening deterioration in the patient's condition. Critical care involves high complexity decision making to assess, manipulate, and support vital system function(s) to treat single or multiple vital organ system failure and/or to prevent further life threatening deterioration of the patient's condition. Examples of vital organ system failure include, but are not limited to: central nervous system failure, circulatory failure, shock, renal, hepatic, metabolic, and/or respiratory failure. Although critical care typically requires interpretation of multiple physiologic parameters and/or application of advanced technology(s), critical care may be provided in life threatening situations when these elements are not present. Critical care may be provided on multiple days, even if no changes are made in the treatment rendered to the patient, provided that the patient's condition continues to require the level of physician attention described above.

Providing medical care to a critically ill, injured, or post-operative patient qualifies as a critical care service only if both the illness or injury and the treatment being provided meet the above requirements. Critical care is usually, but not always, given in a critical care area, such as the coronary care unit, intensive care unit, pediatric intensive care unit, respiratory care unit, or the emergency care facility.

Inpatient critical care services provided to infants 29 days through 24 months of age are reported with pediatric critical care codes 99293 and 99294. The pediatric critical care codes are reported as long as the infant/young child qualifies for critical care services during the hospital stay through 24 months of age. Inpatient critical care services provided to neonates (28 days of age or less) are reported with the neonatal critical care codes 99295 and 99296. The neonatal critical care codes are reported as long as the neonate qualifies for critical care services during the hospital stay through the 28th postnatal day. The reporting of the pediatric and neonatal critical care services is not based on time or the type of unit (eg, pediatric or neonatal critical care unit) and it is not dependent upon the type of provider delivering the care. To report critical care services provided in the outpatient setting (eg, emergency department or office), for neonates and pediatric patients up through 24 months of age, see the hourly Critical Care codes 99291, 99292. If the same physician provides critical care services for a neonatal or pediatric patient in both the outpatient and inpatient settings on the same day, report only the appropriate Neonatal or Pediatric Critical Care code (99293-99296) for all critical care services provided on that day. For additional instructions on reporting these services, see the Neonatal and Pediatric Critical Care section and codes 99293-99296.

Services for a patient who is not critically ill but happens to be in a critical care unit are reported using other appropriate E/M codes.

Critical care and other E/M services may be provided to the same patient on the same date by the same physician.

▶The following services are included in reporting critical care when performed during the critical period by the physician(s) providing critical care: the interpretation of cardiac output measurements (93561, 93562), chest x-rays (71010, 71015, 71020), pulse oximetry (94760, 94761, 94762), blood gases, and information data stored in computers (eg, ECGs, blood pressures, hematologic data (99090)); gastric intubation (43752, 91105); temporary transcutaneous pacing (92953); ventilatory management (94002-94004, 94660, 94662); and vascular access procedures (36000, 36410, 36415, 36540, 36600). Any services performed which are not listed above should be reported separately.◀

Codes 99291, 99292 should be reported for the physician's attendance during the transport of critically ill or critically injured patients over 24 months of age to or from a facility or hospital. For physician transport services of critically ill or critically injured pediatric patients 24 months of age or less see 99289, 99290.

The critical care codes 99291 and 99292 are used to report the total duration of time spent by a physician providing critical care services to a critically ill or critically injured patient, even if the time spent by the physician on that date is not continuous. For any given period of time spent providing critical care services, the physician must devote his or her full attention to the patient and, therefore, cannot provide services to any other patient during the same period of time.

Time spent with the individual patient should be recorded in the patient's record. The time that can be reported as critical care is the time spent engaged in work directly related to the individual patient's care whether that time was spent at the immediate bedside or elsewhere on the floor or unit. For example, time spent on the unit or at the nursing station on the floor reviewing test results or imaging studies, discussing the critically ill patient's care with other medical staff or documenting critical care services in the medical record would be reported as critical care, even though it does not occur at the bedside. Also, when the patient is unable or clinically incompetent to participate in discussions, time spent on the floor or unit with family members or surrogate decision makers obtaining a medical history, reviewing the patient's condition or prognosis, or discussing treatment or limitation(s) of treatment may be reported as critical care, provided that the conversation bears directly on the management of the patient.

Time spent in activities that occur outside of the unit or off the floor (eg, telephone calls, whether taken at home, in the office, or elsewhere in the hospital) may not be reported as critical care since the physician is not immediately available to the patient. Time spent in activities that do not directly contribute to the treatment of the patient may not be reported as critical care, even if they are performed in the critical care unit (eg, participation in administrative meetings or telephone calls to discuss other patients). Time spent performing separately reportable procedures or services should not be included in the time reported as critical care time.

Code 99291 is used to report the first 30-74 minutes of critical care on a given date. It should be used only once per date even if the time spent by the physician is not continuous on that date. Critical care of less than 30 minutes total duration on a given date should be reported with the appropriate E/M code.

Code 99292 is used to report additional block(s) of time, of up to 30 minutes each beyond the first 74 minutes. (See table below.)

The following examples illustrate the correct reporting of critical care services:

Total Duration of Critical Care	Codes
less than 30 minutes (less than 30 minutes)	appropriate E/M codes
30-74 minutes (30 minutes - 1 hr. 14 min.)	99291 X 1
75-104 minutes (1 hr. 15 min. - 1 hr. 44 min.)	99291 X 1 AND 99292 X 1
105-134 minutes (1 hr. 45 min. - 2 hr. 14 min.)	99291 X 1 AND 99292 X 2
135 - 164 minutes (2 hr. 15 min. - 2 hr. 44 min.)	99291 X 1 AND 99292 X 3
165 - 194 minutes (2 hr. 45 min. - 3 hr. 14 min.)	99291 X 1 AND 99292 X 4
194 minutes or longer (3 hr. 14 min. - etc.)	99291 and 99292 as appropriate (see illustrated reporting examples above)

99291   **Critical care, evaluation and management** of the critically ill or critically injured patient; first 30-74 minutes

+ **99292**   each additional 30 minutes (List separately in addition to code for primary service)

(Use 99292 in conjunction with 99291)

Inpatient Neonatal and Pediatric Critical Care Services

The following codes (99293-99296) are used to report services provided by a physician directing the inpatient care of a critically ill neonate/infant. The same definitions for critical care services apply for the adult, child, and neonate.

The initial day neonatal critical care code (99295) can be used in addition to codes 99360, 99436 or 99440 as appropriate, when the physician is present for the delivery (99360 or 99436) and newborn resuscitation (99440) is required. Other procedures performed as a necessary part of the resuscitation (eg, endotracheal intubation (31500)) are also reported separately when performed as part of the pre-admission delivery room care. In order to report these procedures separately, they must be performed as a necessary component of the resuscitation and not simply as a convenience before admission to the neonatal intensive care unit.

Evaluation and Management

Codes 99295, 99296 are used to report services provided by a physician directing the inpatient care of a critically ill neonate through the first 28 days of life. They represent care starting with the date of admission (99295) and subsequent day(s) (99296) and may be reported only once per day, per patient.

Codes 99293, 99294 are used to report services provided by a physician directing the inpatient care of a critically ill infant or young child from 29 days of postnatal age through 24 months of age. They represent care starting with the date of admission (99293) and subsequent day(s) (99294) and may be reported by a single physician only once per day, per patient in a given setting. The critically ill or critically injured child older than 24 months of age would be reported with hourly critical care service codes (99291, 99292).

When a neonate or infant is not critically ill, but requires intensive observation, frequent interventions and other intensive care services, the Continuing Intensive Care Services codes (99298, 99299, 99300) should be used to report services for those neonates/infants with present body weight of 5000 grams or less. When the present body weight of those neonates/infants exceeds 5000 grams, the Subsequent Hospital Care Services codes (99231-99233) should be used.

To report critical care services provided in the outpatient setting (eg, emergency department or office) for neonates and pediatric patients up through 24 months of age, see the hourly Critical Care codes 99291, 99292. If the same physician provides critical care services for a neonatal or pediatric patient in both the outpatient and inpatient settings on the same day, report only the appropriate Neonatal or Pediatric Critical Care code (99293-99296) for all critical care services provided on that day.

Care rendered under 99293-99296 includes management, monitoring, and treatment of the patient including respiratory, pharmacologic control of the circulatory system, enteral and parenteral nutrition, metabolic and hematologic maintenance, parent/family counseling, case management services, and personal direct supervision of the health care team in the performance of cognitive and procedural activities.

▶The pediatric and neonatal critical care codes include those procedures listed above for the hourly critical care codes (99291, 99292). In addition, the following procedures are also included in the bundled (global) pediatric and neonatal critical care service codes (99293-99296): umbilical venous (36510) and umbilical arterial catheters (36660), other arterial catheters (36140, 36620), central (36555) or peripheral vessel catheterization (36000), vascular access procedures (36400, 36405, 36406), vascular punctures (36420, 36600), oral or nasogastric tube placement (43752), endotracheal intubation (31500), lumbar puncture (62270), suprapubic bladder aspiration (51000), bladder catheterization (51701, 51702), ventilatory management

(94002-94004), continuous positive airway pressure (CPAP) (94660), surfactant administration (94610), intravascular fluid administration (90760-90761), transfusion of blood components (36430, 36440), invasive or non-invasive electronic monitoring of vital signs, bedside pulmonary function testing (94375), and/or monitoring or interpretation of blood gases or oxygen saturation (94760-94762). Any services performed which are not listed above should be reported separately.◄

For additional instructions, see descriptions listed for 99293-99296

Inpatient Pediatric Critical Care

99293 **Initial inpatient pediatric critical care,** per day, for the evaluation and management of a critically ill infant or young child, 29 days through 24 months of age

99294 **Subsequent inpatient pediatric critical care,** per day, for the evaluation and management of a critically ill infant or young child, 29 days through 24 months of age

Inpatient Neonatal Critical Care

99295 **Initial inpatient neonatal critical care,** per day, for the evaluation and management of a critically ill neonate, 28 days of age or less

This code is reserved for the date of admission for neonates who are critically ill. Critically ill neonates require cardiac and/or respiratory support (including ventilator or nasal CPAP when indicated), continuous or frequent vital sign monitoring, laboratory and blood gas interpretations, follow-up physician reevaluations, and constant observation by the health care team under direct physician supervision. Immediate preoperative evaluation and stabilization of neonates with life threatening surgical or cardiac conditions are included under this code. Neonates with life threatening surgical or cardiac conditions are included under this code.

Care for neonates who require an intensive care setting but who are not critically ill is reported using the initial hospital care codes (99221-99223).

99296 **Subsequent inpatient neonatal critical care,** per day, for the evaluation and management of a critically ill neonate, 28 days of age or less

A critically ill neonate will require cardiac and/or respiratory support (including ventilator or nasal CPAP when indicated), continuous or frequent vital sign monitoring, laboratory and blood gas interpretations, follow-up physician re-evaluations throughout a 24-hour period, and constant observation by the health care team under direct physician supervision.

(Subsequent care for neonates who require an intensive setting but who are not critically ill is reported using either the intensive low birth weight services codes (99298, 99299) or the subsequent hospital care codes (99231-99233))

Continuing Intensive Care Services

Codes 99298, 99299, 99300 are used to report services subsequent to the day of admission provided by a physician directing the continuing intensive care of the low birth weight (LBW, 1500-2500 grams present body weight) infant, very low birth weight (VLBW, less than 1500 grams present body weight) infant, or normal weight (2501-5000 grams present body weight) newborn who do not meet the definition of critically ill but continue to require intensive observation, frequent interventions, and other intensive services. Codes 99298, 99299, 99300 represent subsequent day(s) of care and may be reported only once per calendar day, per patient and are global codes with the same services bundled as outlined under codes 99293-99296.

For additional instructions, see descriptions listed for 99298, 99299, 99300.

99298   **Subsequent intensive care,** per day, for the evaluation and management of the recovering very low birth weight infant (present body weight less than 1500 g)

Infants with present body weight less than 1500 grams who are not critically ill but continue to require intensive cardiac and respiratory monitoring, continuous and/or frequent vital sign monitoring, heat maintenance, enteral and/or parenteral nutritional adjustments, laboratory and oxygen monitoring and constant observation by the health care team under direct physician supervision.

99299   **Subsequent intensive care,** per day, for the evaluation and management of the recovering low birth weight infant (present body weight of 1500-2500 g)

Infants with present body weight of 1500-2500 grams who are not critically ill but continue to require intensive cardiac and respiratory monitoring, continuous and/or frequent vital sign monitoring, heat maintenance, enteral and/or parenteral nutritional adjustments, laboratory and oxygen monitoring, and constant observation by the health care team under direct physician supervision.

99300   Subsequent intensive care, per day, for the evaluation and management of the recovering infant (present body weight of 2501-5000 g)

Infants with present body weight of 2501-5000 grams who are not critically ill but continue to require intensive cardiac and respiratory monitoring, continuous and/or frequent vital sign monitoring, heat maintenance, enteral and/or parenteral nutritional adjustments, laboratory and oxygen monitoring, and constant observation by the health care team under direct physician supervision.

Nursing Facility Services

The following codes are used to report evaluation and management services to patients in Nursing Facilities (formerly called Skilled Nursing Facilities (SNFs), Intermediate Care Facilities (ICFs), or Long-Term Care Facilities (LTCFs)).

These codes should also be used to report evaluation and management services provided to a patient in a psychiatric residential treatment center (a facility or a distinct part of a facility for psychiatric care, which provides a 24-hour therapeutically planned and professionally staffed group living and learning environment). If procedures such as medical psychotherapy are provided in addition to evaluation and management services, these should be reported in addition to the evaluation and management services provided.

Nursing facilities that provide convalescent, rehabilitative, or long term care are required to conduct comprehensive, accurate, standardized, and reproducible assessments of each resident's functional capacity using a Resident Assessment Instrument (RAI). All RAIs include the Minimum Data Set (MDS), Resident Assessment Protocols (RAPs) and utilization guidelines. The MDS is the primary screening and assessment tool; the RAPs trigger the identification of potential problems and provide guidelines for follow-up assessments.

Physicians have a central role in assuring that all residents receive thorough assessments and that medical plans of care are instituted or revised to enhance or maintain the residents' physical and psychosocial functioning. This role includes providing input in the development of the MDS and a multi-disciplinary plan of care, as required by regulations pertaining to the care of nursing facility residents.

Two major subcategories of nursing facility services are recognized: Initial Nursing Facility Care and Subsequent Nursing Facility Care. Both subcategories apply to new or established patients.

For definitions of key components and commonly used terms, please see **Evaluation and Management Services Guidelines.**

(For care plan oversight services provided to nursing facility residents, see 99379-99380)

Initial Nursing Facility Care

New or Established Patient

When the patient is admitted to the nursing facility in the course of an encounter in another site of service (eg, hospital emergency department, physician's office), all evaluation and management services provided by that physician in conjunction with that admission are considered part of the initial nursing facility care when performed on the same date as the admission or readmission. The nursing facility care level of service reported by the admitting physician should include the services related to the admission he/she provided in the other sites of service as well as in the nursing facility setting.

Hospital discharge or observation discharge services performed on the same date of nursing facility admission or readmission may be reported separately. For a patient discharged from inpatient status on the same date of nursing facility admission or readmission, the hospital discharge services should be reported with codes 99238, 99239 as appropriate. For a patient discharged from observation status on the same date of nursing facility admission or readmission, the observation care discharge services should be reported with code 99217. For a patient admitted and discharged from observation or inpatient status on the same date, see codes 99234-99236.

(For nursing facility care discharge, see 99315, 99316)

Typical unit times have not been established for 99304-99306.

(99301-99303 have been deleted)

99304   Initial nursing facility care, per day, for the evaluation and management of a patient which requires these three key components:

- **A detailed or comprehensive history;**
- **A detailed or comprehensive examination; and**
- **Medical decision making that is straightforward or of low complexity.**

Counseling and/or coordination of care with other providers or agencies are provided consistent with the nature of the problem(s) and the patient's and/or family's needs.

Usually, the problem(s) requiring admission are of low severity.

99305   Initial nursing facility care, per day, for the evaluation and management of a patient which requires these three key components:

- **A comprehensive history;**
- **A comprehensive examination; and**
- **Medical decision making of moderate complexity.**

Counseling and/or coordination of care with other providers or agencies are provided consistent with the nature of the problem(s) and the patient's and/or family's needs.

Usually, the problem(s) requiring admission are of moderate severity.

99306   Initial nursing facility care, per day, for the evaluation and management of a patient, which requires these three key components:

- **A comprehensive history;**
- **A comprehensive examination; and**
- **Medical decision making of high complexity.**

Counseling and/or coordination of care with other providers or agencies are provided consistent with the nature of the problem(s) and the patient's and/or family's needs.

Usually, the problem(s) requiring admission are of high severity.

Subsequent Nursing Facility Care

All levels of subsequent nursing facility care include reviewing the medical record and reviewing the results of diagnostic studies and changes in the patient's status (ie, changes in history, physical condition, and response to management) since the last assessment by the physician.

99307   Subsequent nursing facility care, per day, for the evaluation and management of a patient, which requires at least two of these three key components:

- **A problem focused interval history;**
- **A problem focused examination;**
- **Straightforward medical decision making.**

Counseling and/or coordination of care with other providers or agencies are provided consistent with the nature of the problem(s) and the patient's and/or family's needs.

Usually, the patient is stable, recovering, or improving.

99308   Subsequent nursing facility care, per day, for the evaluation and management of a patient, which requires at least two of these three key components:

- **An expanded problem focused interval history;**
- **An expanded problem focused examination;**
- **Medical decision making of low complexity.**

Counseling and/or coordination of care with other providers or agencies are provided consistent with the nature of the problem(s) and the patient's and/or family's needs.

Usually, the patient is responding inadequately to therapy or has developed a minor complication.

99309   Subsequent nursing facility care, per day, for the evaluation and management of a patient, which requires at least two of these three key components:

- **A detailed interval history;**
- **A detailed examination;**
- **Medical decision making of moderate complexity.**

Counseling and/or coordination of care with other providers or agencies are provided consistent with the nature of the problem(s) and the patient's and/or family's needs.

Usually, the patient has developed a significant complication or a significant new problem.

99310   Subsequent nursing facility care, per day, for the evaluation and management of a patient, which requires at least two of these three key components:

- **A comprehensive interval history;**

- **A comprehensive examination;**

- **Medical decision making of high complexity.**

Counseling and/or coordination of care with other providers or agencies are provided consistent with the nature of the problem(s) and the patient's and/or family's needs.

The patient may be unstable or may have developed a significant new problem requiring immediate physician attention.

(99311-99313 have been deleted)

Nursing Facility Discharge Services

The nursing facility discharge day management codes are to be used to report the total duration of time spent by a physician for the final nursing facility discharge of a patient. The codes include, as appropriate, final examination of the patient, discussion of the nursing facility stay, even if the time spent by the physician on that date is not continuous. Instructions are given for continuing care to all relevant caregivers, and preparation of discharge records, prescriptions and referral forms.

99315   Nursing facility discharge day management; 30 minutes or less

99316   more than 30 minutes

Other Nursing Facility Services

99318   Evaluation and management of a patient involving an annual nursing facility assessment, which requires these three key components:

- **A detailed interval history;**

- **A comprehensive examination; and**

- **Medical decision making that is of low to moderate complexity.**

Counseling and/or coordination of care with other providers or agencies are provided consistent with the nature of the problem(s) and the patient's and/or family's needs.

Usually, the patient is stable, recovering, or improving.

(Do not report 99318 on the same date of service as nursing facility services codes 99304-99316)

Domiciliary, Rest Home (eg, Boarding Home), or Custodial Care Services

The following codes are used to report evaluation and management services in a facility which provides room, board and other personal assistance services, generally on a long-term basis. They also are used to report evaluation and management services in an assisted living facility.

The facility's services do not include a medical component.

For definitions of key components and commonly used terms, please see **Evaluation and Management Services Guidelines.**

(For care plan oversight services provided to a patient in a domiciliary facility under the care of a home health agency, see 99374-99375)

(For care plan oversight services provided to a patient in a domiciliary facility under the individual supervision of a physician, see 99339, 99340)

New Patient

(99321-99323 have been deleted)

99324   Domiciliary or rest home visit for the evaluation and management of a new patient, which requires these three key components:

- **A problem focused history;**

- **A problem focused examination; and**

- **Straightforward medical decision making.**

Counseling and/or coordination of care with other providers or agencies are provided consistent with the nature of the problem(s) and the patient's and/or family's needs.

Usually, the presenting problem(s) are of low severity. Physicians typically spend 20 minutes with the patient and/or family or caregiver.

99325   Domiciliary or rest home visit for the evaluation and management of a new patient, which requires these three key components:

- **An expanded problem focused history;**

- **An expanded problem focused examination; and**

- **Medical decision making of low complexity.**

Counseling and/or coordination of care with other providers or agencies are provided consistent with the nature of the problem(s) and the patient's and/or family's needs.

Usually, the presenting problem(s) are of moderate severity. Physicians typically spend 30 minutes with the patient and/or family or caregiver.

Evaluation and Management

Evaluation and Management

99326 Domiciliary or rest home visit for the evaluation and management of a new patient, which requires these three key components:

- **A detailed history;**

- **A detailed examination; and**

- **Medical decision making of moderate complexity.**

Counseling and/or coordination of care with other providers or agencies are provided consistent with the nature of the problem(s) and the patient's and/or family's needs.

Usually, the presenting problem(s) are of moderate to high severity. Physicians typically spend 45 minutes with the patient and/or family or caregiver.

99327 Domiciliary or rest home visit for the evaluation and management of a new patient, which requires these three key components:

- **A comprehensive history;**

- **A comprehensive examination; and**

- **Medical decision making of moderate complexity.**

Counseling and/or coordination of care with other providers or agencies are provided consistent with the nature of the problem(s) and the patient's and/or family's needs.

Usually, the presenting problem(s) are of high severity. Physicians typically spend 60 minutes with the patient and/or family or caregiver.

99328 Domiciliary or rest home visit for the evaluation and management of a new patient, which requires these three key components:

- **A comprehensive history;**

- **A comprehensive examination; and**

- **Medical decision making of high complexity.**

Counseling and/or coordination of care with other providers or agencies are provided consistent with the nature of the problem(s) and the patient's and/or family's needs.

Usually, the patient is unstable or has developed a significant new problem requiring immediate physician attention. Physicians typically spend 75 minutes with the patient and/or family or caregiver.

Established Patient

(99331-99333 have been deleted)

99334 Domiciliary or rest home visit for the evaluation and management of an established patient, which requires at least two of these three key components:

- **A problem focused interval history;**

- **A problem focused examination;**

- **Straightforward medical decision making.**

Counseling and/or coordination of care with other providers or agencies are provided consistent with the nature of the problem(s) and the patient's and/or family's needs.

Usually, the presenting problem(s) are self-limited or minor. Physicians typically spend 15 minutes with the patient and/or family or caregiver.

99335 Domiciliary or rest home visit for the evaluation and management of an established patient, which requires at least two of these three key components:

- **An expanded problem focused interval history;**

- **An expanded problem focused examination;**

- **Medical decision making of low complexity.**

Counseling and/or coordination of care with other providers or agencies are provided consistent with the nature of the problem(s) and the patient's and/or family's needs.

Usually, the presenting problem(s) are of low to moderate severity. Physicians typically spend 25 minutes with the patient and/or family or caregiver.

99336 Domiciliary or rest home visit for the evaluation and management of an established patient, which requires at least two of these three key components:

- **A detailed interval history;**

- **A detailed examination;**

- **Medical decision making of moderate complexity.**

Counseling and/or coordination of care with other providers or agencies are provided consistent with the nature of the problem(s) and the patient's and/or family's needs.

Usually, the presenting problem(s) are of moderate to high severity. Physicians typically spend 40 minutes with the patient and/or family or caregiver.

99337 Domiciliary or rest home visit for the evaluation and management of an established patient, which requires at least two of these three key components:

- **A comprehensive interval history;**

- **A comprehensive examination;**

- **Medical decision making of moderate to high complexity.**

Counseling and/or coordination of care with other providers or agencies are provided consistent with the nature of the problem(s) and the patient's and/or family's needs.

Usually, the presenting problem(s) are of moderate to high severity. The patient may be unstable or may have developed a significant new problem requiring immediate physician attention. Physicians typically spend 60 minutes with the patient and/or family or caregiver.

Domiciliary, Rest Home (eg, Assisted Living Facility), or Home Care Plan Oversight Services

(For instructions on the use of 99339, 99340, see introductory notes for 99374-99380)

(For care plan oversight services for patients under the care of a home health agency, hospice, or nursing facility, see 99374-99380)

99339   Individual physician supervision of a patient (patient not present) in home, domiciliary or rest home (eg, assisted living facility) requiring complex and multidisciplinary care modalities involving regular physician development and/or revision of care plans, review of subsequent reports of patient status, review of related laboratory and other studies, communication (including telephone calls) for purposes of assessment or care decisions with health care professional(s), family member(s), surrogate decision maker(s) (eg, legal guardian) and/or key caregiver(s) involved in patient's care, integration of new information into the medical treatment plan and/or adjustment of medical therapy, within a calendar month; 15-29 minutes

99340   30 minutes or more

(Do not report 99339, 99340 for patients under the care of a home health agency, enrolled in a hospice program, or for nursing facility residents)

Home Services

The following codes are used to report evaluation and management services provided in a private residence.

For definitions of key components and commonly used terms, please see **Evaluation and Management Services Guidelines.**

(For care plan oversight services provided to a patient in the home under the care of a home health agency, see 99374-99375)

(For care plan oversight services provided to a patient in the home under the individual supervision of a physician, see 99339, 99340)

New Patient

99341   **Home visit** for the evaluation and management of a new patient, which requires these three key components:

- **A problem focused history;**
- **A problem focused examination; and**
- **Straightforward medical decision making.**

Counseling and/or coordination of care with other providers or agencies are provided consistent with the nature of the problem(s) and the patient's and/or family's needs.

Usually, the presenting problem(s) are of low severity. Physicians typically spend 20 minutes face-to-face with the patient and/or family.

99342   **Home visit** for the evaluation and management of a new patient, which requires these three key components:

- **An expanded problem focused history;**
- **An expanded problem focused examination; and**
- **Medical decision making of low complexity.**

Counseling and/or coordination of care with other providers or agencies are provided consistent with the nature of the problem(s) and the patient's and/or family's needs.

Usually, the presenting problem(s) are of moderate severity. Physicians typically spend 30 minutes face-to-face with the patient and/or family.

99343   **Home visit** for the evaluation and management of a new patient, which requires these three key components:

- **A detailed history;**
- **A detailed examination; and**
- **Medical decision making of moderate complexity.**

Counseling and/or coordination of care with other providers or agencies are provided consistent with the nature of the problem(s) and the patient's and/or family's needs.

Usually, the presenting problem(s) are of moderate to high severity. Physicians typically spend 45 minutes face-to-face with the patient and/or family.

99344   **Home visit** for the evaluation and management of a new patient, which requires these three components:

- **A comprehensive history;**
- **A comprehensive examination; and**
- **Medical decision making of moderate complexity.**

Counseling and/or coordination of care with other providers or agencies are provided consistent with the nature of the problem(s) and the patient's and/or family's needs.

Usually, the presenting problem(s) are of high severity. Physicians typically spend 60 minutes face-to-face with the patient and/or family.

99345 **Home visit** for the evaluation and management of a new patient, which requires these three key components:

- **A comprehensive history;**
- **A comprehensive examination; and**
- **Medical decision making of high complexity.**

Counseling and/or coordination of care with other providers or agencies are provided consistent with the nature of the problem(s) and the patient's and/or family's needs.

Usually, the patient is unstable or has developed a significant new problem requiring immediate physician attention. Physicians typically spend 75 minutes face-to-face with the patient and/or family.

Established Patient

99347 **Home visit** for the evaluation and management of an established patient, which requires at least two of these three key components:

- **A problem focused interval history;**
- **A problem focused examination;**
- **Straightforward medical decision making.**

Counseling and/or coordination of care with other providers or agencies are provided consistent with the nature of the problem(s) and the patient's and/or family's needs.

Usually, the presenting problem(s) are self limited or minor. Physicians typically spend 15 minutes face-to-face with the patient and/or family.

99348 **Home visit** for the evaluation and management of an established patient, which requires at least two of these three key components:

- **An expanded problem focused interval history;**
- **An expanded problem focused examination;**
- **Medical decision making of low complexity.**

Counseling and/or coordination of care with other providers or agencies are provided consistent with the nature of the problem(s) and the patient's and/or family's needs.

Usually, the presenting problem(s) are of low to moderate severity. Physicians typically spend 25 minutes face-to-face with the patient and/or family.

99349 **Home visit** for the evaluation and management of an established patient, which requires at least two of these three key components:

- **A detailed interval history;**
- **A detailed examination;**
- **Medical decision making of moderate complexity.**

Counseling and/or coordination of care with other providers or agencies are provided consistent with the nature of the problem(s) and the patient's and/or family's needs.

Usually, the presenting problem(s) are moderate to high severity. Physicians typically spend 40 minutes face-to-face with the patient and/or family.

99350 **Home visit** for the evaluation and management of an established patient, which requires at least two of these three key components:

- **A comprehensive interval history;**
- **A comprehensive examination;**
- **Medical decision making of moderate to high complexity.**

Counseling and/or coordination of care with other providers or agencies are provided consistent with the nature of the problem(s) and the patient's and/or family's needs.

Usually, the presenting problem(s) are of moderate to high severity. The patient may be unstable or may have developed a significant new problem requiring immediate physician attention. Physicians typically spend 60 minutes face-to-face with the patient and/or family.

Prolonged Services

Prolonged Physician Service With Direct (Face-To-Face) Patient Contact

Codes 99354-99357 are used when a physician provides prolonged service involving direct (face-to-face) patient contact that is beyond the usual service in either the inpatient or outpatient setting. This service is reported in addition to other physician services, including evaluation and management services at any level. Appropriate codes should be selected for supplies provided or procedures performed in the care of the patient during this period.

Codes 99354-99357 are used to report the total duration of face-to-face time spent by a physician on a given date providing prolonged service, even if the time spent by the physician on that date is not continuous.

Code 99354 or 99356 is used to report the first hour of prolonged service on a given date, depending on the place of service.

Either code also may be used to report a total duration of prolonged service of 30-60 minutes on a given date. Either code should be used only once per date, even if the time spent by the physician is not continuous on that date. Prolonged service of less than 30 minutes total duration on a given date is not separately reported because the work involved is included in the total work of the evaluation and management codes.

Code 99355 or 99357 is used to report each additional 30 minutes beyond the first hour, depending on the place of service. Either code may also be used to report the final 15-30 minutes of prolonged service on a given date. Prolonged service of less than 15 minutes beyond the first hour or less than 15 minutes beyond the final 30 minutes is not reported separately.

The following examples illustrate the correct reporting of prolonged physician service with direct patient contact in the office setting:

Total Duration of Prolonged Services	Code(s)
less than 30 minutes (less than 30 minutes)	Not reported separately
30-74 minutes (30 minutes - 1 hr. 14 min.)	99354 X 1
75-104 minutes (1 hr. 15 min. - 1 hr. 44 min.)	99354 X 1 AND 99355 X 1
105-134 minutes (1 hr. 45 min. - 2 hr. 14 min.)	99354 X 1 AND 99355 X 2
135-164 minutes (2 hr. 15 min. - 2 hr. 44 min.)	99354 X 1 AND 99355 X 3
165-194 minutes (2 hr. 45 min. - 3 hr. 14 min.)	99354 X 1 AND 99355 X 4

+ **99354**   Prolonged physician service in the office or other outpatient setting requiring direct (face-to-face) patient contact beyond the usual service (eg, prolonged care and treatment of an acute asthmatic patient in an outpatient setting); first hour (List separately in addition to code for office or other outpatient **Evaluation and Management** service)

      (Use 99354 in conjunction with 99201-99215, 99241-99245, 99304-99350)

+ **99355**   each additional 30 minutes (List separately in addition to code for prolonged physician service)

      (Use 99355 in conjunction with 99354)

+ **99356**   Prolonged physician service in the inpatient setting, requiring direct (face-to-face) patient contact beyond the usual service (eg, maternal fetal monitoring for high risk delivery or other physiological monitoring, prolonged care of an acutely ill inpatient); first hour (List separately in addition to code for inpatient Evaluation and Management service)

      (Use 99356 in conjunction with 99221-99233, 99251-99255)

+ **99357**   each additional 30 minutes (List separately in addition to code for prolonged physician service)

      (Use 99357 in conjunction with 99356)

Prolonged Physician Service Without Direct (Face-To-Face) Patient Contact

Codes 99358 and 99359 are used when a physician provides prolonged service not involving direct (face-to-face) care that is beyond the usual service in either the inpatient or outpatient setting.

This service is to be reported in addition to other physician service, including evaluation and management services at any level.

Codes 99358 and 99359 are used to report the total duration of non-face-to-face time spent by a physician on a given date providing prolonged service, even if the time spent by the physician on that date is not continuous. Code 99358 is used to report the first hour of prolonged service on a given date regardless of the place of service.

It may also be used to report a total duration of prolonged service of 30-60 minutes on a given date. It should be used only once per date even if the time spent by the physician is not continuous on that date.

Prolonged service of less than 30 minutes total duration on a given date is not separately reported.

Code 99359 is used to report each additional 30 minutes beyond the first hour regardless of the place of service. It may also be used to report the final 15-30 minutes of prolonged service on a given date.

Prolonged service of less than 15 minutes beyond the first hour or less than 15 minutes beyond the final 30 minutes is not reported separately.

+ **99358**   **Prolonged evaluation and management service** before and/or after direct (face-to-face) patient care (eg, review of extensive records and tests, communication with other professionals and/or the patient/family); first hour (List separately in addition to code(s) for other physician service(s) and/or inpatient or outpatient Evaluation and Management service)

+ **99359**   each additional 30 minutes (List separately in addition to code for prolonged physician service)

      (Use 99359 in conjunction with 99358)

      (To report telephone calls, see 99371-99373)

Evaluation and Management

Evaluation and Management

Physician Standby Services

Code 99360 is used to report physician standby service that is requested by another physician and that involves prolonged physician attendance without direct (face-to-face) patient contact. The physician may not be providing care or services to other patients during this period. This code is not used to report time spent proctoring another physician. It is also not used if the period of standby ends with the performance of a procedure subject to a "surgical" package by the physician who was on standby.

Code 99360 is used to report the total duration of time spent by a physician on a given date on standby. Standby service of less than 30 minutes total duration on a given date is not reported separately.

Second and subsequent periods of standby beyond the first 30 minutes may be reported only if a full 30 minutes of standby was provided for each unit of service reported.

99360   **Physician standby service,** requiring prolonged physician attendance, each 30 minutes (eg, operative standby, standby for frozen section, for cesarean/high risk delivery, for monitoring EEG)

        (For hospital mandated on call services, see 99026, 99027)

        (99360 may be reported in addition to 99431, 99440 as appropriate)

        (Do not report 99360 in conjunction with 99436)

Case Management Services

Physician case management is a process in which a physician is responsible for direct care of a patient, and for coordinating and controlling access to or initiating and/or supervising other health care services needed by the patient.

Team Conferences

99361   **Medical conference** by a physician with interdisciplinary team of health professionals or representatives of community agencies to coordinate activities of patient care (patient not present); approximately 30 minutes

99362   approximately 60 minutes

►Anticoagulant Management◄

►Anticoagulant services are intended to describe the outpatient management of warfarin therapy, including ordering, review, and interpretation of International Normalized Ratio (INR) testing, communication with patient, and dosage adjustments as appropriate.

When reporting these services, the work of anticoagulant management may not be used as a basis for reporting an Evaluation and Management service or Care Plan Oversight time during the reporting period. Do not report these services with 99371-99373, 0074T when telephone or on-line services address anticoagulation with warfarin management. If a significant, separately identifiable E/M service is performed, report the appropriate E/M service code using modifier 25.

These services are outpatient services only. When anticoagulation therapy is initiated or continued in the inpatient or observation setting, a new period begins after discharge and is reported with 99364. Do not report 99363-99364 with 99217-99239, 99291-99300, 99304-99318 or other code(s) for physician review, interpretation, and patient management of home INR testing for a patient with mechanical heart valve(s).

Any period less than 60 continuous outpatient days is not reported. If less than the specified minimum number of services per period are performed, do not report the anticoagulant management services (99363-99364).◄

● **99363**   Anticoagulant management for an outpatient taking warfarin, physician review and interpretation of International Normalized Ratio (INR) testing, patient instructions, dosage adjustment (as needed), and ordering of additional tests; initial 90 days of therapy (must include a minimum of 8 INR measurements)

● **99364**   each subsequent 90 days of therapy (must include a minimum of 3 INR measurements)

Telephone Calls

99371   **Telephone call** by a physician to patient or for consultation or medical management or for coordinating medical management with other health care professionals (eg, nurses, therapists, social workers, nutritionists, physicians, pharmacists); simple or brief (eg, to report on tests and/or laboratory results, to clarify or alter previous instructions, to integrate new information from other health professionals into the medical treatment plan, or to adjust therapy)

99372   intermediate (eg, to provide advice to an established patient on a new problem, to initiate therapy that can be handled by telephone, to discuss test results in detail, to coordinate medical management of a new problem in an established patient, to discuss and evaluate new information and details, or to initiate new plan of care)

99373   complex or lengthy (eg, lengthy counseling session with anxious or distraught patient, detailed or prolonged discussion with family members regarding seriously ill patient, lengthy communication necessary to coordinate complex services of several different health professionals working on different aspects of the total patient care plan)

Care Plan Oversight Services

Care Plan Oversight Services are reported separately from codes for office/outpatient, hospital, home, nursing facility or domiciliary services. The complexity and approximate physician time of the care plan oversight services provided within a 30-day period determine code selection. Only one physician may report services for a given period of time, to reflect that physician's sole or predominant supervisory role with a particular patient. These codes should not be reported for supervision of patients in nursing facilities or under the care of home health agencies unless they require recurrent supervision of therapy.

The work involved in providing very low intensity or infrequent supervision services is included in the pre- and post-encounter work for home, office/outpatient and nursing facility or domiciliary visit codes.

> (For care plan oversight services of patients in the home, domiciliary, or rest home (eg, assisted living facility) under the individual supervision of a physician, see 99339, 99340)

99374   **Physician supervision** of a patient under care of home health agency (patient not present) in home, domiciliary or equivalent environment (eg, Alzheimer's facility) requiring complex and multidisciplinary care modalities involving regular physician development and/or revision of care plans, review of subsequent reports of patient status, review of related laboratory and other studies, communication (including telephone calls) for purposes of assessment or care decisions with health care professional(s), family member(s), surrogate decision maker(s) (eg, legal guardian) and/or key caregiver(s) involved in patient's care, integration of new information into the medical treatment plan and/or adjustment of medical therapy, within a calendar month; 15-29 minutes

99375   30 minutes or more

99377   **Physician supervision** of a hospice patient (patient not present) requiring complex and multidisciplinary care modalities involving regular physician development and/or revision of care plans, review of subsequent reports of patient status, review of related laboratory and other studies, communication (including telephone calls) for purposes of assessment or care decisions with health care professional(s), family member(s), surrogate decision maker(s) (eg, legal guardian) and/or key caregiver(s) involved in patient's care, integration of new information into the medical treatment plan and/or adjustment of medical therapy, within a calendar month; 15-29 minutes

99378   30 minutes or more

99379   **Physician supervision** of a nursing facility patient (patient not present) requiring complex and multidisciplinary care modalities involving regular physician development and/or revision of care plans, review of subsequent reports of patient status, review of related laboratory and other studies, communication (including telephone calls) for purposes of assessment or care decisions with health care professional(s), family member(s), surrogate decision maker(s) (eg, legal guardian) and/or key caregiver(s) involved in patient's care, integration of new information into the medical treatment plan and/or adjustment of medical therapy, within a calendar month; 15-29 minutes

99380   30 minutes or more

Preventive Medicine Services

The following codes are used to report the preventive medicine evaluation and management of infants, children, adolescents and adults.

The extent and focus of the services will largely depend on the age of the patient.

If an abnormality/ies is encountered or a preexisting problem is addressed in the process of performing this preventive medicine evaluation and management service, and if the problem/abnormality is significant enough to require additional work to perform the key components of a problem-oriented E/M service, then the appropriate Office/Outpatient code 99201-99215 should also be reported. Modifier 25 should be added to the Office/Outpatient code to indicate that a significant, separately identifiable Evaluation and Management service was provided by the same physician on the same day as the preventive medicine service. The appropriate preventive medicine service is additionally reported.

An insignificant or trivial problem/abnormality that is encountered in the process of performing the preventive medicine evaluation and management service and which does not require additional work and the performance of the key components of a problem-oriented E/M service should not be reported.

The "comprehensive" nature of the Preventive Medicine Services codes 99381-99397 reflects an age and gender appropriate history/exam and is NOT synonymous with the "comprehensive" examination required in Evaluation and Management codes 99201-99350.

Codes 99381-99397 include counseling/anticipatory guidance/risk factor reduction interventions which are provided at the time of the initial or periodic comprehensive preventive medicine examination. (Refer to codes 99401-99412 for reporting those counseling/anticipatory guidance/risk factor reduction interventions that are provided at an encounter separate from the preventive medicine examination.)

Immunizations and ancillary studies involving laboratory, radiology, other procedures, or screening tests identified with a specific CPT code are reported separately. For immunizations, see 90465-90474 and 90476-90749.

New Patient

99381   **Initial comprehensive preventive medicine** evaluation and management of an individual including an age and gender appropriate history, examination, counseling/anticipatory guidance/risk factor reduction interventions, and the ordering of appropriate immunization(s), laboratory/diagnostic procedures, new patient; infant (age younger than 1 year)

99382   early childhood (age 1 through 4 years)

99383   late childhood (age 5 through 11 years)

99384   adolescent (age 12 through 17 years)

99385   18-39 years

99386   40-64 years

99387   65 years and older

Established Patient

99391   **Periodic comprehensive preventive medicine** reevaluation and management of an individual including an age and gender appropriate history, examination, counseling/anticipatory guidance/risk factor reduction interventions, and the ordering of appropriate immunization(s), laboratory/diagnostic procedures, established patient; infant (age younger than 1 year)

99392   early childhood (age 1 through 4 years)

99393   late childhood (age 5 through 11 years)

99394   adolescent (age 12 through 17 years)

99395   18-39 years

99396   40-64 years

99397   65 years and older

Counseling and/or Risk Factor Reduction Intervention

New or Established Patient

These codes are used to report services provided to individuals at a separate encounter for the purpose of promoting health and preventing illness or injury.

Preventive medicine counseling and risk factor reduction interventions provided as a separate encounter will vary with age and should address such issues as family problems, diet and exercise, substance abuse, sexual practices, injury prevention, dental health, and diagnostic and laboratory test results available at the time of the encounter.

These codes are not to be used to report counseling and risk factor reduction interventions provided to patients with symptoms or established illness. For counseling individual patients with symptoms or established illness, use the appropriate office, hospital or consultation or other evaluation and management codes. For counseling groups of patients with symptoms or established illness, use 99078.

Preventive Medicine, Individual Counseling

99401   **Preventive medicine counseling** and/or risk factor reduction intervention(s) provided to an individual (separate procedure); approximately 15 minutes

99402   approximately 30 minutes

99403   approximately 45 minutes

99404   approximately 60 minutes

Preventive Medicine, Group Counseling

99411   **Preventive medicine counseling** and/or risk factor reduction intervention(s) provided to individuals in a group setting (separate procedure); approximately 30 minutes

99412   approximately 60 minutes

Other Preventive Medicine Services

99420   **Administration and interpretation** of health risk assessment instrument (eg, health hazard appraisal)

99429   **Unlisted preventive** medicine service

Newborn Care

The following codes are used to report the services provided to newborns in several different settings.

For newborn hospital discharge services provided on a date subsequent to the admission date of the newborn, use 99238.

For discharge services provided to newborns admitted and discharged on the same date, use 99435.

99431   **History and examination** of the normal newborn infant, initiation of diagnostic and treatment programs and preparation of hospital records. (This code should also be used for birthing room deliveries.)

99432   **Normal newborn care** in other than hospital or birthing room setting, including physical examination of baby and conference(s) with parent(s)

99433   **Subsequent hospital care,** for the evaluation and management of a normal newborn, per day

99435   **History and examination** of the normal newborn infant, including the preparation of medical records. (This code should only be used for newborns assessed and discharged from the hospital or birthing room on the same date.)

99436   **Attendance** at delivery (when requested by delivering physician) and initial stabilization of newborn

(99436 may be reported in addition to 99431)

(Do not report 99436 in conjunction with 99440)

99440   **Newborn resuscitation**: provision of positive pressure ventilation and/or chest compressions in the presence of acute inadequate ventilation and/or cardiac output

Special Evaluation and Management Services

The following codes are used to report evaluations performed to establish baseline information prior to life or disability insurance certificates being issued. This service is performed in the office or other setting, and applies to both new and established patients. When using these codes, no active management of the problem(s) is undertaken during the encounter.

If other evaluation and management services and/or procedures are performed on the same date, the appropriate E/M or procedure code(s) should be reported in addition to these codes.

Basic Life and/or Disability Evaluation Services

99450   **Basic life** and/or disability examination that includes:

- **Measurement of height, weight and blood pressure;**

- **Completion of a medical history following a life insurance pro forma;**

- **Collection of blood sample and/or urinalysis complying with "chain of custody" protocols; and**

- **Completion of necessary documentation/certificates.**

Work Related or Medical Disability Evaluation Services

99455   **Work related** or medical disability examination by the treating physician that includes:

- **Completion of a medical history commensurate with the patient's condition;**

- **Performance of an examination commensurate with the patient's condition;**

- **Formulation of a diagnosis, assessment of capabilities and stability, and calculation of impairment;**

- **Development of future medical treatment plan; and**

- **Completion of necessary documentation/certificates and report.**

99456   **Work related** or medical disability examination by other than the treating physician that includes:

- **Completion of a medical history commensurate with the patient's condition;**

- **Performance of an examination commensurate with the patient's condition;**

- **Formulation of a diagnosis, assessment of capabilities and stability, and calculation of impairment;**

- **Development of future medical treatment plan; and**

- **Completion of necessary documentation/certificates and report.**

(Do not report 99455, 99456 in conjunction with 99080 for the completion of Workman's Compensation forms)

Other Evaluation and Management Services

99499   **Unlisted evaluation and management** service

Notes

Anesthesia Guidelines

Services involving administration of anesthesia are reported by the use of the anesthesia five-digit procedure code (00100-01999) plus modifier codes (defined under "Anesthesia Modifiers" later in these Guidelines).

The reporting of anesthesia services is appropriate by or under the responsible supervision of a physician. These services may include but are not limited to general, regional, supplementation of local anesthesia, or other supportive services in order to afford the patient the anesthesia care deemed optimal by the anesthesiologist during any procedure. These services include the usual preoperative and postoperative visits, the anesthesia care during the procedure, the administration of fluids and/or blood and the usual monitoring services (eg, ECG, temperature, blood pressure, oximetry, capnography, and mass spectrometry). Unusual forms of monitoring (eg, intra-arterial, central venous, and Swan-Ganz) are not included.

Items used by all physicians in reporting their services are presented in the **Introduction.** Some of the commonalities are repeated in this section for the convenience of those physicians referring to this section on **Anesthesia.** Other definitions and items unique to anesthesia are also listed.

To report moderate (conscious) sedation provided by a physician also performing the service for which conscious sedation is being provided, see codes 99143-99145.

For the procedures listed in Appendix G, when a second physician other than the health care professional performing the diagnostic or therapeutic services provides moderate (conscious) sedation in the facility setting (eg, hospital, outpatient hospital/ambulatory surgery center, skilled nursing facility), the second physician reports the associated moderate sedation procedure/service 99148-99150; when these services are performed by the second physician in the nonfacility setting (eg, physician office, freestanding imaging center), codes 99148-99150 would not be reported. Moderate sedation does not include minimal sedation (anxiolysis), deep sedation, or monitored anesthesia care (00100-01999).

To report regional or general anesthesia provided by a physician also performing the services for which the anesthesia is being provided, see modifier 47 in Appendix A.

Time Reporting

Time for anesthesia procedures may be reported as is customary in the local area. Anesthesia time begins when the anesthesiologist begins to prepare the patient for the induction of anesthesia in the operating room or in an equivalent area and ends when the anesthesiologist is no longer in personal attendance, that is, when the patient may be safely placed under postoperative supervision.

Physician's Services

Physician's services rendered in the office, home, or hospital; consultation; and other medical services are listed in the section titled **Evaluation and Management Services** (99201-99499 series) found on page 1. "Special Services and Reporting" (99000-99091 series) are listed in the **Medicine** section.

Materials Supplied by Physician

Supplies and materials provided by the physician (eg, sterile trays, drugs) over and above those usually included with the office visit or other services rendered may be listed separately. Drugs, tray supplies, and materials provided should be listed and identified with 99070 or the appropriate supply code.

Separate or Multiple Procedures

When multiple surgical procedures are performed during a single anesthetic administration, the anesthesia code representing the most complex procedure is reported. The time reported is the combined total for all procedures.

▶Results/Testing/Reports◀

▶Results are the technical component of a service. Testing leads to results; results lead to interpretation. Reports are the work product of the interpretation of numerous test results.◀

Special Report

A service that is rarely provided, unusual, variable, or new may require a special report in determining medical appropriateness of the service. Pertinent information should include an adequate definition or description of the nature, extent, and need for the procedure and the time, effort, and equipment necessary to provide the service. Additional items may include:

- Complexity of symptoms
- Final diagnosis
- Pertinent physical findings
- Diagnostic and therapeutic procedures
- Concurrent problems
- Follow-up care

Anesthesia Modifiers

All anesthesia services are reported by use of the anesthesia five-digit procedure code (00100-01999) plus the addition of a physical status modifier. The use of other optional modifiers may be appropriate.

Physical Status Modifiers

Physical Status modifiers are represented by the initial letter 'P' followed by a single digit from 1 to 6 as defined in the following list.

P1: A normal healthy patient

P2: A patient with mild systemic disease

P3: A patient with severe systemic disease

P4: A patient with severe systemic disease that is a constant threat to life

P5: A moribund patient who is not expected to survive without the operation

P6: A declared brain-dead patient whose organs are being removed for donor purposes

These six levels are consistent with the American Society of Anesthesiologists (ASA) ranking of patient physical status. Physical status is included in the CPT codebook to distinguish among various levels of complexity of the anesthesia service provided.

Example: 00100-P1

Qualifying Circumstances

More than one qualifying circumstance may be selected.

Many anesthesia services are provided under particularly difficult circumstances, depending on factors such as extraordinary condition of patient, notable operative conditions, and/or unusual risk factors. This section includes a list of important qualifying circumstances that significantly affect the character of the anesthesia service provided. These procedures would not be reported alone but would be reported as additional procedure numbers qualifying an anesthesia procedure or service.

+ 99100 Anesthesia for patient of extreme age, younger than 1 year and older than 70 (List separately in addition to code for primary anesthesia procedure)

(For procedure performed on infants younger than 1 year of age at time of surgery, see 00326, 00561, 00834, 00836)

+ 99116 Anesthesia complicated by utilization of total body hypothermia (List separately in addition to code for primary anesthesia procedure)

+ 99135 Anesthesia complicated by utilization of controlled hypotension (List separately in addition to code for primary anesthesia procedure)

+ 99140 Anesthesia complicated by emergency conditions (specify) (List separately in addition to code for primary anesthesia procedure)

(An emergency is defined as existing when delay in treatment of the patient would lead to a significant increase in the threat to life or body part.)

Anesthesia

Head

00100 Anesthesia for procedures on salivary glands, including biopsy

00102 Anesthesia for procedures involving plastic repair of cleft lip

00103 Anesthesia for reconstructive procedures of eyelid (eg, blepharoplasty, ptosis surgery)

00104 Anesthesia for electroconvulsive therapy

00120 Anesthesia for procedures on external, middle, and inner ear including biopsy; not otherwise specified

00124   otoscopy

00126   tympanotomy

00140 Anesthesia for procedures on eye; not otherwise specified

00142   lens surgery

00144   corneal transplant

00145   vitreoretinal surgery

00147   iridectomy

00148   ophthalmoscopy

00160 Anesthesia for procedures on nose and accessory sinuses; not otherwise specified

00162   radical surgery

00164   biopsy, soft tissue

00170 Anesthesia for intraoral procedures, including biopsy; not otherwise specified

00172   repair of cleft palate

00174   excision of retropharyngeal tumor

00176   radical surgery

00190 Anesthesia for procedures on facial bones or skull; not otherwise specified

00192   radical surgery (including prognathism)

00210 Anesthesia for intracranial procedures; not otherwise specified

00212   subdural taps

00214   burr holes, including ventriculography

00215   cranioplasty or elevation of depressed skull fracture, extradural (simple or compound)

00216   vascular procedures

00218   procedures in sitting position

00220   cerebrospinal fluid shunting procedures

00222   electrocoagulation of intracranial nerve

Neck

00300 Anesthesia for all procedures on the integumentary system, muscles and nerves of head, neck, and posterior trunk, not otherwise specified

00320 Anesthesia for all procedures on esophagus, thyroid, larynx, trachea and lymphatic system of neck; not otherwise specified, age 1 year or older

00322   needle biopsy of thyroid

(For procedures on cervical spine and cord, see 00600, 00604, 00670)

00326 Anesthesia for all procedures on the larynx and trachea in children younger than 1 year of age

(Do not report 00326 in conjunction with 99100)

00350 Anesthesia for procedures on major vessels of neck; not otherwise specified

00352   simple ligation

(For arteriography, use 01916)

Thorax (Chest Wall and Shoulder Girdle)

00400 Anesthesia for procedures on the integumentary system on the extremities, anterior trunk and perineum; not otherwise specified

00402   reconstructive procedures on breast (eg, reduction or augmentation mammoplasty, muscle flaps)

00404   radical or modified radical procedures on breast

00406   radical or modified radical procedures on breast with internal mammary node dissection

00410   electrical conversion of arrhythmias

00450 Anesthesia for procedures on clavicle and scapula; not otherwise specified

00452   radical surgery

00454   biopsy of clavicle

00470 Anesthesia for partial rib resection; not otherwise specified

00472   thoracoplasty (any type)

00474   radical procedures (eg, pectus excavatum)

Anesthesia

Intrathoracic

00500	Anesthesia for all procedures on esophagus
00520	Anesthesia for closed chest procedures; (including bronchoscopy) not otherwise specified
00522	needle biopsy of pleura
00524	pneumocentesis
00528	mediastinoscopy and diagnostic thoracoscopy not utilizing one lung ventilation
	(For tracheobronchial reconstruction, use 00539)
00529	mediastinoscopy and diagnostic thoracoscopy utilizing one lung ventilation
00530	Anesthesia for permanent transvenous pacemaker insertion
00532	Anesthesia for access to central venous circulation
00534	Anesthesia for transvenous insertion or replacement of pacing cardioverter-defibrillator
	(For transthoracic approach, use 00560)
00537	Anesthesia for cardiac electrophysiologic procedures including radiofrequency ablation
00539	Anesthesia for tracheobronchial reconstruction
00540	Anesthesia for thoracotomy procedures involving lungs, pleura, diaphragm, and mediastinum (including surgical thoracoscopy); not otherwise specified
00541	utilizing one lung ventilation
	►(For thoracic spine and cord anesthesia procedures via an anterior transthoracic approach, see 00625-00626)◄
00542	decortication
00546	pulmonary resection with thoracoplasty
00548	intrathoracic procedures on the trachea and bronchi
00550	Anesthesia for sternal debridement
00560	Anesthesia for procedures on heart, pericardial sac, and great vessels of chest; without pump oxygenator
00561	with pump oxygenator, younger than one year of age
	(Do not report 00561 in conjunction with 99100, 99116, and 99135)
00562	with pump oxygenator
00563	with pump oxygenator with hypothermic circulatory arrest
00566	Anesthesia for direct coronary artery bypass grafting without pump oxygenator
00580	Anesthesia for heart transplant or heart/lung transplant

Spine and Spinal Cord

00600	Anesthesia for procedures on cervical spine and cord; not otherwise specified
	(For myelography and discography, see radiological procedures 01905)
00604	procedures with patient in the sitting position
00620	Anesthesia for procedures on thoracic spine and cord; not otherwise specified
00622	thoracolumbar sympathectomy
● **00625**	Anesthesia for procedures on the thoracic spine and cord, via an anterior transthoracic approach; not utilizing one lung ventilation
● **00626**	utilizing one lung ventilation
	►(For anesthesia for thoracotomy procedures other than spinal, see 00540-00541)◄
00630	Anesthesia for procedures in lumbar region; not otherwise specified
00632	lumbar sympathectomy
00634	chemonucleolysis
00635	diagnostic or therapeutic lumbar puncture
00640	Anesthesia for manipulation of the spine or for closed procedures on the cervical, thoracic or lumbar spine
00670	Anesthesia for extensive spine and spinal cord procedures (eg, spinal instrumentation or vascular procedures)

Upper Abdomen

00700	Anesthesia for procedures on upper anterior abdominal wall; not otherwise specified
00702	percutaneous liver biopsy
00730	Anesthesia for procedures on upper posterior abdominal wall
00740	Anesthesia for upper gastrointestinal endoscopic procedures, endoscope introduced proximal to duodenum
00750	Anesthesia for hernia repairs in upper abdomen; not otherwise specified
00752	lumbar and ventral (incisional) hernias and/or wound dehiscence
00754	omphalocele
00756	transabdominal repair of diaphragmatic hernia
00770	Anesthesia for all procedures on major abdominal blood vessels
00790	Anesthesia for intraperitoneal procedures in upper abdomen including laparoscopy; not otherwise specified
00792	partial hepatectomy or management of liver hemorrhage (excluding liver biopsy)

00794   pancreatectomy, partial or total (eg, Whipple procedure)

00796   liver transplant (recipient)

(For harvesting of liver, use 01990)

00797   gastric restrictive procedure for morbid obesity

Lower Abdomen

00800   Anesthesia for procedures on lower anterior abdominal wall; not otherwise specified

00802   panniculectomy

00810   Anesthesia for lower intestinal endoscopic procedures, endoscope introduced distal to duodenum

00820   Anesthesia for procedures on lower posterior abdominal wall

00830   Anesthesia for hernia repairs in lower abdomen; not otherwise specified

00832   ventral and incisional hernias

(For hernia repairs in the infant 1 year of age or younger, see 00834, 00836)

00834   Anesthesia for hernia repairs in the lower abdomen not otherwise specified, younger than 1 year of age

(Do not report 00834 in conjunction with 99100)

00836   Anesthesia for hernia repairs in the lower abdomen not otherwise specified, infants younger than 37 weeks gestational age at birth and younger than 50 weeks gestational age at time of surgery

(Do not report 00836 in conjunction with 99100)

00840   Anesthesia for intraperitoneal procedures in lower abdomen including laparoscopy; not otherwise specified

00842   amniocentesis

00844   abdominoperineal resection

00846   radical hysterectomy

00848   pelvic exenteration

00851   tubal ligation/transection

00860   Anesthesia for extraperitoneal procedures in lower abdomen, including urinary tract; not otherwise specified

00862   renal procedures, including upper one-third of ureter, or donor nephrectomy

00864   total cystectomy

00865   radical prostatectomy (suprapubic, retropubic)

00866   adrenalectomy

00868   renal transplant (recipient)

(For donor nephrectomy, use 00862)

(For harvesting kidney from brain-dead patient, use 01990)

00870   cystolithotomy

00872   Anesthesia for lithotripsy, extracorporeal shock wave; with water bath

00873   without water bath

00880   Anesthesia for procedures on major lower abdominal vessels; not otherwise specified

00882   inferior vena cava ligation

Perineum

(For perineal procedures on integumentary system, muscles and nerves, see 00300, 00400)

00902   Anesthesia for; anorectal procedure

00904   radical perineal procedure

00906   vulvectomy

00908   perineal prostatectomy

00910   Anesthesia for transurethral procedures (including urethrocystoscopy); not otherwise specified

00912   transurethral resection of bladder tumor(s)

00914   transurethral resection of prostate

00916   post-transurethral resection bleeding

00918   with fragmentation, manipulation and/or removal of ureteral calculus

00920   Anesthesia for procedures on male genitalia (including open urethral procedures); not otherwise specified

00921   vasectomy, unilateral or bilateral

00922   seminal vesicles

00924   undescended testis, unilateral or bilateral

00926   radical orchiectomy, inguinal

00928   radical orchiectomy, abdominal

00930   orchiopexy, unilateral or bilateral

00932   complete amputation of penis

00934   radical amputation of penis with bilateral inguinal lymphadenectomy

00936   radical amputation of penis with bilateral inguinal and iliac lymphadenectomy

00938   insertion of penile prosthesis (perineal approach)

00940   Anesthesia for vaginal procedures (including biopsy of labia, vagina, cervix or endometrium); not otherwise specified

00942   colpotomy, vaginectomy, colporrhaphy, and open urethral procedures

00944   vaginal hysterectomy

00948   cervical cerclage

00950   culdoscopy

00952   hysteroscopy and/or hysterosalpingography

Anesthesia

Pelvis (Except Hip)

01112	Anesthesia for bone marrow aspiration and/or biopsy, anterior or posterior iliac crest
01120	Anesthesia for procedures on bony pelvis
01130	Anesthesia for body cast application or revision
01140	Anesthesia for interpelviabdominal (hindquarter) amputation
01150	Anesthesia for radical procedures for tumor of pelvis, except hindquarter amputation
01160	Anesthesia for closed procedures involving symphysis pubis or sacroiliac joint
01170	Anesthesia for open procedures involving symphysis pubis or sacroiliac joint
01173	Anesthesia for open repair of fracture disruption of pelvis or column fracture involving acetabulum
01180	Anesthesia for obturator neurectomy; extrapelvic
01190	intrapelvic

Upper Leg (Except Knee)

01200	Anesthesia for all closed procedures involving hip joint
01202	Anesthesia for arthroscopic procedures of hip joint
01210	Anesthesia for open procedures involving hip joint; not otherwise specified
01212	hip disarticulation
01214	total hip arthroplasty
01215	revision of total hip arthroplasty
01220	Anesthesia for all closed procedures involving upper two-thirds of femur
01230	Anesthesia for open procedures involving upper two-thirds of femur; not otherwise specified
01232	amputation
01234	radical resection
01250	Anesthesia for all procedures on nerves, muscles, tendons, fascia, and bursae of upper leg
01260	Anesthesia for all procedures involving veins of upper leg, including exploration
01270	Anesthesia for procedures involving arteries of upper leg, including bypass graft; not otherwise specified
01272	femoral artery ligation
01274	femoral artery embolectomy

Knee and Popliteal Area

01320	Anesthesia for all procedures on nerves, muscles, tendons, fascia, and bursae of knee and/or popliteal area
01340	Anesthesia for all closed procedures on lower one-third of femur
01360	Anesthesia for all open procedures on lower one-third of femur
01380	Anesthesia for all closed procedures on knee joint
01382	Anesthesia for diagnostic arthroscopic procedures of knee joint
01390	Anesthesia for all closed procedures on upper ends of tibia, fibula, and/or patella
01392	Anesthesia for all open procedures on upper ends of tibia, fibula, and/or patella
01400	Anesthesia for open or surgical arthroscopic procedures on knee joint; not otherwise specified
01402	total knee arthroplasty
01404	disarticulation at knee
01420	Anesthesia for all cast applications, removal, or repair involving knee joint
01430	Anesthesia for procedures on veins of knee and popliteal area; not otherwise specified
01432	arteriovenous fistula
01440	Anesthesia for procedures on arteries of knee and popliteal area; not otherwise specified
01442	popliteal thromboendarterectomy, with or without patch graft
01444	popliteal excision and graft or repair for occlusion or aneurysm

Lower Leg (Below Knee, Includes Ankle and Foot)

01462	Anesthesia for all closed procedures on lower leg, ankle, and foot
01464	Anesthesia for arthroscopic procedures of ankle and/or foot
01470	Anesthesia for procedures on nerves, muscles, tendons, and fascia of lower leg, ankle, and foot; not otherwise specified
01472	repair of ruptured Achilles tendon, with or without graft
01474	gastrocnemius recession (eg, Strayer procedure)
01480	Anesthesia for open procedures on bones of lower leg, ankle, and foot; not otherwise specified
01482	radical resection (including below knee amputation)

01484	osteotomy or osteoplasty of tibia and/or fibula
01486	total ankle replacement
01490	Anesthesia for lower leg cast application, removal, or repair
01500	Anesthesia for procedures on arteries of lower leg, including bypass graft; not otherwise specified
01502	embolectomy, direct or with catheter
01520	Anesthesia for procedures on veins of lower leg; not otherwise specified
01522	venous thrombectomy, direct or with catheter

Shoulder and Axilla

Includes humeral head and neck, sternoclavicular joint, acromioclavicular joint, and shoulder joint.

01610	Anesthesia for all procedures on nerves, muscles, tendons, fascia, and bursae of shoulder and axilla
01620	Anesthesia for all closed procedures on humeral head and neck, sternoclavicular joint, acromioclavicular joint, and shoulder joint
01622	Anesthesia for diagnostic arthroscopic procedures of shoulder joint
01630	Anesthesia for open or surgical arthroscopic procedures on humeral head and neck, sternoclavicular joint, acromioclavicular joint, and shoulder joint; not otherwise specified
01632	radical resection
01634	shoulder disarticulation
01636	interthoracoscapular (forequarter) amputation
01638	total shoulder replacement
01650	Anesthesia for procedures on arteries of shoulder and axilla; not otherwise specified
01652	axillary-brachial aneurysm
01654	bypass graft
01656	axillary-femoral bypass graft
01670	Anesthesia for all procedures on veins of shoulder and axilla
01680	Anesthesia for shoulder cast application, removal or repair; not otherwise specified
01682	shoulder spica

Upper Arm and Elbow

01710	Anesthesia for procedures on nerves, muscles, tendons, fascia, and bursae of upper arm and elbow; not otherwise specified
01712	tenotomy, elbow to shoulder, open
01714	tenoplasty, elbow to shoulder
01716	tenodesis, rupture of long tendon of biceps
01730	Anesthesia for all closed procedures on humerus and elbow
01732	Anesthesia for diagnostic arthroscopic procedures of elbow joint
01740	Anesthesia for open or surgical arthroscopic procedures of the elbow; not otherwise specified
01742	osteotomy of humerus
01744	repair of nonunion or malunion of humerus
01756	radical procedures
01758	excision of cyst or tumor of humerus
01760	total elbow replacement
01770	Anesthesia for procedures on arteries of upper arm and elbow; not otherwise specified
01772	embolectomy
01780	Anesthesia for procedures on veins of upper arm and elbow; not otherwise specified
01782	phleborrhaphy

Forearm, Wrist, and Hand

01810	Anesthesia for all procedures on nerves, muscles, tendons, fascia, and bursae of forearm, wrist, and hand
01820	Anesthesia for all closed procedures on radius, ulna, wrist, or hand bones
01829	Anesthesia for diagnostic arthroscopic procedures on the wrist
01830	Anesthesia for open or surgical arthroscopic/endoscopic procedures on distal radius, distal ulna, wrist, or hand joints; not otherwise specified
01832	total wrist replacement
01840	Anesthesia for procedures on arteries of forearm, wrist, and hand; not otherwise specified
01842	embolectomy
01844	Anesthesia for vascular shunt, or shunt revision, any type (eg, dialysis)
01850	Anesthesia for procedures on veins of forearm, wrist, and hand; not otherwise specified
01852	phleborrhaphy
01860	Anesthesia for forearm, wrist, or hand cast application, removal, or repair

Anesthesia

Radiological Procedures

01905   Anesthesia for myelography, discography, vertebroplasty

01916   Anesthesia for diagnostic arteriography/venography

(Do not report 01916 in conjunction with therapeutic codes 01924-01926, 01930-01933)

01920   Anesthesia for cardiac catheterization including coronary angiography and ventriculography (not to include Swan-Ganz catheter)

01922   Anesthesia for non-invasive imaging or radiation therapy

01924   Anesthesia for therapeutic interventional radiologic procedures involving the arterial system; not otherwise specified

01925   carotid or coronary

01926   intracranial, intracardiac, or aortic

01930   Anesthesia for therapeutic interventional radiologic procedures involving the venous/lymphatic system (not to include access to the central circulation); not otherwise specified

01931   intrahepatic or portal circulation (eg, transcutaneous porto-caval shunt (TIPS))

01932   intrathoracic or jugular

01933   intracranial

Burn Excisions or Debridement

01951   Anesthesia for second and third degree burn excision or debridement with or without skin grafting, any site, for total body surface area (TBSA) treated during anesthesia and surgery; less than four percent total body surface area

01952   between four and nine percent of total body surface area

+ 01953   each additional nine percent total body surface area or part thereof (List separately in addition to code for primary procedure)

(Use 01953 in conjunction with 01952)

Obstetric

01958   Anesthesia for external cephalic version procedure

01960   Anesthesia for vaginal delivery only

01961   Anesthesia for cesarean delivery only

01962   Anesthesia for urgent hysterectomy following delivery

01963   Anesthesia for cesarean hysterectomy without any labor analgesia/anesthesia care

(01964 has been deleted. To report, see 01965, 01966)

01965   Anesthesia for incomplete or missed abortion procedures

01966   Anesthesia for induced abortion procedures

01967   Neuraxial labor analgesia/anesthesia for planned vaginal delivery (this includes any repeat subarachnoid needle placement and drug injection and/or any necessary replacement of an epidural catheter during labor)

+ 01968   Anesthesia for cesarean delivery following neuraxial labor analgesia/anesthesia (List separately in addition to code for primary procedure performed)

(Use 01968 in conjunction with 01967)

+ 01969   Anesthesia for cesarean hysterectomy following neuraxial labor analgesia/anesthesia (List separately in addition to code for primary procedure performed)

(Use 01969 in conjunction with 01967)

Other Procedures

01990   Physiological support for harvesting of organ(s) from brain-dead patient

01991   Anesthesia for diagnostic or therapeutic nerve blocks and injections (when block or injection is performed by a different provider); other than the prone position

01992   prone position

(Do not report 01991 or 01992 in conjunction with 99143-99150)

▶(When regional intravenous administration of local anesthetic agent or other medication in the upper or lower extremity is used as the anesthetic for a surgical procedure, report the appropriate anesthesia code. To report a Bier block for pain management, use 64999. For intra-arterial or intravenous injections, see 90773, 90774)◀

▶(For intra-arterial or intravenous therapy for pain management, see 90773, 90774)◀

▶(01995 has been deleted)◀

01996   Daily hospital management of epidural or subarachnoid continuous drug administration

(Report code 01996 for daily hospital management of continuous epidural or subarachnoid drug administration performed after insertion of an epidural or subarachnoid catheter)

01999   Unlisted anesthesia procedure(s)

Surgery Guidelines

Items used by all physicians in reporting their services are presented in the **Introduction.** Some of the commonalities are repeated here for the convenience of those physicians referring to this section on **Surgery.** Other definitions and items unique to Surgery are also listed.

Physicians' Services

Physicians' services rendered in the office, home, or hospital, consultations, and other medical services are listed in the section entitled **Evaluation and Management Services** (99201-99499) found in the front of the book, beginning on page 9. "Special Services and Reports" (99000 series) is presented in the **Medicine** section.

CPT Surgical Package Definition

The services provided by the physician to any patient by their very nature are variable. The CPT codes that represent a readily identifiable surgical procedure thereby include, on a procedure-by-procedure basis, a variety of services. In defining the specific services "included" in a given CPT surgical code, the following services are always included in addition to the operation per se:

- Local infiltration, metacarpal/metatarsal/digital block or topical anesthesia
- Subsequent to the decision for surgery, one related E/M encounter on the date immediately prior to or on the date of procedure (including history and physical)
- Immediate postoperative care, including dictating operative notes, talking with the family and other physicians
- Writing orders
- Evaluating the patient in the postanesthesia recovery area
- Typical postoperative follow-up care

Follow-Up Care for Diagnostic Procedures

Follow-up care for diagnostic procedures (eg, endoscopy, arthroscopy, injection procedures for radiography) includes only that care related to recovery from the diagnostic procedure itself. Care of the condition for which the diagnostic procedure was performed or of other concomitant conditions is not included and may be listed separately.

Follow-Up Care for Therapeutic Surgical Procedures

Follow-up care for therapeutic surgical procedures includes only that care which is usually a part of the surgical service. Complications, exacerbations, recurrence, or the presence of other diseases or injuries requiring additional services should be separately reported.

Materials Supplied by Physician

Supplies and materials provided by the physician (eg, sterile trays/drugs), over and above those usually included with the procedure(s) rendered are reported separately. List drugs, trays, supplies, and materials provided. Identify as 99070 or specific supply code.

Reporting More Than One Procedure/Service

When a physician performs more than one procedure/service on the same date, same session or during a post-operative period (subject to the "surgical package" concept), several CPT modifiers may apply (see Appendix A for definition).

27 Multiple Outpatient Hospital E/M Encounters on the Same Date

For hospital outpatient reporting purposes, utilization of hospital resources related to separate and distinct E/M encounters performed in multiple outpatient hospital settings on the same date may be reported by adding modifier 27 to each appropriate level outpatient and/or emergency department E/M code(s). This modifier provides a means of reporting circumstances involving evaluation and management services provided by physician(s) in more than one (multiple) outpatient hospital setting(s) (eg, hospital emergency department, clinic). **Note:** This modifier is not to be used for physician reporting of multiple E/M services performed by the same physician on the same date. For physician reporting of all outpatient evaluation and management services provided by the same physician on the same date and performed in multiple outpatient setting(s) (eg, hospital emergency department, clinic), see **Evaluation and Management, Emergency Department,** or **Preventive Medicine Services** codes.

51 Multiple Procedures

When multiple procedures/services (other than evaluation and management) are performed at the same session, report the most significant procedure first, with all other procedures listed with modifier 51 appended. For a list of procedures exempt from the use of modifier 51, see Appendices D and E.

58 Staged or Related Procedure or Service by the Same Physician During the Postoperative Period

When a procedure(s) is prospectively planned as a staged procedure, or when the secondary and subsequent procedure(s) is more extensive, or to indicate therapy following a diagnostic surgical procedure, use modifier 58 with the staged procedure(s).

59 Distinct Procedural Service

For procedure(s)/service(s) not ordinarily performed or encountered on the same day by the same physician, but appropriate under certain circumstances (eg, different site or organ system, separate excision or lesion), use modifier 59.

76 Repeat Procedure by Same Physician

When a procedure or service is repeated by the same physician subsequent to the original service, use modifier 76.

77 Repeat Procedure by Another Physician

When a procedure is repeated by another physician subsequent to the original service, use modifier 77.

78 Return to the Operating Room for a Related Procedure During the Postoperative Period

When a procedure, related to the initial procedure, requires a return to the operating room during the postoperative period of that initial procedure, use modifier 78.

79 Unrelated Procedure or Service by the Same Physician During the Postoperative Period

When a procedure, unrelated to the initial procedure, is performed by the same physician during the post-operative period of the initial procedure, use modifier 79.

91 Repeat Clinical Diagnostic Laboratory Test

In the course of treatment of the patient, it may be necessary to repeat the same laboratory test on the same day to obtain subsequent (multiple) test results. Under these circumstances, the laboratory test performed can be identified by its usual procedure number and the addition of modifier 91. **Note:** This modifier may not be used when tests are rerun to confirm initial results; due to testing problems with specimens or equipment; or for any other reason when a normal, one-time, reportable result is all that is required. This modifier may not be used when other code(s) describe a series of test results (eg, glucose tolerance tests, evocative/suppression testing). This modifier may only be used for laboratory test(s) performed more than once on the same day on the same patient.

Separate Procedure

Some of the procedures or services listed in the CPT codebook that are commonly carried out as an integral component of a total service or procedure have been identified by the inclusion of the term "separate procedure." The codes designated as "separate procedure" should not be reported in addition to the code for the total procedure or service of which it is considered an integral component.

However, when a procedure or service that is designated as a "separate procedure" is carried out independently or considered to be unrelated or distinct from other procedures/services provided at that time, it may be reported by itself, or in addition to other procedures/services by appending modifier 59 to the specific "separate procedure" code to indicate that the procedure is not considered to be a component of another procedure, but is a distinct, independent procedure. This may represent a different session or patient encounter, different procedure or surgery, different site or organ system, separate incision/excision, separate lesion, or separate injury (or area of injury in extensive injuries).

Subsection Information

Several of the subheadings or subsections have special needs or instructions unique to that section. Where these are indicated (eg, "Maternity Care and Delivery"), special **"Notes"** will be presented preceding those procedural terminology listings, referring to that subsection specifically. If there is an "Unlisted Procedure" code number (see below) for the individual subsection, it will also be shown. Those subsections within the **Surgery** section that have **"Notes"** are as follows:

Biopsy 11100-11101

Removal of Skin Tags. 11200-11201

Shaving of Lesions. 11300-11313

Excision—Benign Lesions 11400-11471

Excision—Malignant Lesions 11600-11646

Repair (Closure) 12001-13160

Adjacent Tissue Transfer or
Rearrangement 14000-14350

▶Skin Replacement Surgery and
Skin Substitutes. . . . . 15002-15431◀

  Allograft and Tissue Cultured Allogeneic Skin
  Substitutes 15300-15366

  Xenograft. 15400-15431

Flaps (Skin and/or Deep Tissue) 15570-15999

Burns, Local Treatment 16000-16036

Destruction 17000-17286

▶Mohs Micrographic Surgery . . . . . . 17311-17315◀

Breast—Excision 19100-19272

Musculoskeletal 20000-29999

Wound Exploration—Trauma 20100-20103

Grafts (or Implants). 20900-20999

Introduction or Removal 21076-21116

Spine: (Vertebral Column). 22100-22855

Spine: Excision 22100-22116

Spine: Osteotomy 22210-22226

Spine: Fracture/Dislocation 22305-22328

Spine: Arthrodesis 22548-22812

Spine: Exploration 22830

Spinal Instrumentation 22840-22855

Casting and Strapping. 29000-29750

Musculoskeletal:
Endoscopy/Arthroscopy 29800-29999

Respiratory: Endoscopy 31231-31294, 31505-
             31579, 31615-31656, 32601-32665

Cardiovascular System. 33010-37799

Pacing Cardioverter-Pacemaker
or Defibrillator 33202-33249

▶Electrophysiologic Procedures . . . . 33250-33266◀

Venous—CABG. 33510-33516

Arteries and Veins 34001-35907

Endovascular Repair of Abdominal
Aortic Aneurysm 34800-34826

Endovascular Repair of
Illiac Aneurysm 34900

Transluminal Angioplasty 35450-35476

Transluminal Atherectomy 35480-35495

Bypass Graft 35500-35572

Composite Grafts. 35681-35683

Adjuvant Techniques 35685-35686

Vascular Injection Procedures:
Intravenous 36000-36015

Central Venous Access Procedures . . . 36555-36597

Transcatheter Procedures:
Intravenous 37195-37216

Intravascular Ultrasound. 37250-37251

Bone Marrow or Stem Cell
Services/Procedures 38204-38242

Hemic and Lymphatic Systems:
Laparoscopy 38570-38589

Digestive:
Endoscopy/Laparoscopy. 43200-43272,
        43280-43289, 43651-43659, 43770-43774,
        44180-44238, 44360-44397, 44970-44979,
        45300-45387, 45395-45397, 45400-45402,
        46600-46615, 47370-47379, 47550-47556,
        47560-47562, 49320-49329, 49650-49659

Pancreas Transplantation. 48550-48556

Herniotomy. 49491-49611

Renal Transplantation 50300-50380

Urodynamics 51725-51798

Endoscopy/Laparoscopy

  Urinary. 50541-50545, 50945-50980,
                          51990-52648

  Male Genital   54690-54699, 55550-55559, 55866

  Female Genital 58545-58579, 58660-58679

  Endocrine 60650-60659

Maternity Care and Delivery 59000-59899

Nervous System:
Surgery of Skull Base. 61580-61619

Neurostimulators (Intracranial) 61850-61888,
                           62160-62319

Neurostimulators (Spinal) 63650-63688

Neurostimulators (Peripheral Nerve) . 64553-64595

Secondary Implants(s) 65125-65175

Removal Cataract 66830-66999

Prophylaxis 67141-67145

Excision 67800-67820

Reconstruction 67930-67999

Operating Microscope 69990

Unlisted Service or Procedure

A service or procedure may be provided that is not listed in this edition of the CPT codebook. When reporting such a service, the appropriate "Unlisted Procedure" code may be used to indicate the service, identifying it by "Special Report" as discussed in the section below. The "Unlisted Procedures" and accompanying codes for **Surgery** are as follows:

15999 Unlisted procedure, excision pressure ulcer

17999 Unlisted procedure, skin, mucous membrane and subcutaneous tissue

19499 Unlisted procedure, breast

20999 Unlisted procedure, musculoskeletal system, general

21089 Unlisted maxillofacial prosthetic procedure

21299 Unlisted craniofacial and maxillofacial procedure

21499 Unlisted musculoskeletal procedure, head

21899 Unlisted procedure, neck or thorax

22899 Unlisted procedure, spine

22999 Unlisted procedure, abdomen, musculoskeletal system

23929 Unlisted procedure, shoulder

24999 Unlisted procedure, humerus or elbow

25999 Unlisted procedure, forearm or wrist

26989 Unlisted procedure, hands or fingers

27299 Unlisted procedure, pelvis or hip joint

27599 Unlisted procedure, femur or knee

27899 Unlisted procedure, leg or ankle

28899 Unlisted procedure, foot or toes

29799 Unlisted procedure, casting or strapping

29999 Unlisted procedure, arthroscopy

30999 Unlisted procedure, nose

31299 Unlisted procedure, accessory sinuses

31599 Unlisted procedure, larynx

31899 Unlisted procedure, trachea, bronchi

32999 Unlisted procedure, lungs and pleura

33999 Unlisted procedure, cardiac surgery

36299 Unlisted procedure, vascular injection

37501 Unlisted vascular endoscopy procedure

37799 Unlisted procedure, vascular surgery

38129 Unlisted laparoscopy procedure, spleen

38589 Unlisted laparoscopy procedure, lymphatic system

38999 Unlisted procedure, hemic or lymphatic system

39499 Unlisted procedure, mediastinum

39599 Unlisted procedure, diaphragm

40799 Unlisted procedure, lips

40899 Unlisted procedure, vestibule of mouth

41599 Unlisted procedure, tongue, floor of mouth

41899 Unlisted procedure, dentoalveolar structures

42299 Unlisted procedure, palate, uvula

42699 Unlisted procedure, salivary glands or ducts

42999 Unlisted procedure, pharynx, adenoids, or tonsils

43289 Unlisted laparoscopy procedure, esophagus

43499 Unlisted procedure, esophagus

43659 Unlisted laparoscopy procedure, stomach

43999 Unlisted procedure, stomach

44238 Unlisted laparoscopy procedure, intestine (except rectum)

44799 Unlisted procedure, intestine

44899 Unlisted procedure, Meckel's diverticulum and the mesentery

44979 Unlisted laparoscopy procedure, appendix

45499 Unlisted laparoscopy procedure, rectum

45999 Unlisted procedure, rectum

46999 Unlisted procedure, anus

47379 Unlisted laparoscopic procedure, liver

47399 Unlisted procedure, liver

47579 Unlisted laparoscopy procedure, biliary tract

47999 Unlisted procedure, biliary tract

48999 Unlisted procedure, pancreas

49329 Unlisted laparoscopy procedure, abdomen, peritoneum and omentum

49659 Unlisted laparoscopy procedure, hernioplasty, herniorrhaphy, herniotomy

49999 Unlisted procedure, abdomen, peritoneum and omentum

50549 Unlisted laparoscopy procedure, renal

50949 Unlisted laparoscopy procedure, ureter

51999 Unlisted laparoscopy procedure, bladder

53899 Unlisted procedure, urinary system

54699 Unlisted laparoscopy procedure, testis

55559	Unlisted laparoscopy procedure, spermatic cord
55899	Unlisted procedure, male genital system
58578	Unlisted laparoscopy procedure, uterus
58579	Unlisted hysteroscopy procedure, uterus
58679	Unlisted laparoscopy procedure, oviduct, ovary
58999	Unlisted procedure, female genital system (nonobstetrical)
59897	Unlisted fetal invasive procedure, including ultrasound guidance
59898	Unlisted laparoscopy procedure, maternity care and delivery
59899	Unlisted procedure, maternity care and delivery
60659	Unlisted laparoscopy procedure, endocrine system
60699	Unlisted procedure, endocrine system
64999	Unlisted procedure, nervous system
66999	Unlisted procedure, anterior segment of eye
67299	Unlisted procedure, posterior segment
67399	Unlisted procedure, ocular muscle
67599	Unlisted procedure, orbit
67999	Unlisted procedure, eyelids
68399	Unlisted procedure, conjunctiva
68899	Unlisted procedure, lacrimal system
69399	Unlisted procedure, external ear
69799	Unlisted procedure, middle ear
69949	Unlisted procedure, inner ear
69979	Unlisted procedure, temporal bone, middle fossa approach

- Complexity of symptoms
- Final diagnosis
- Pertinent physical findings (such as size, locations, and number of lesion(s), if appropriate)
- Diagnostic and therapeutic procedures (including major and supplementary surgical procedures, if appropriate)
- Concurrent problems
- Follow-up care

Surgical Destruction

Surgical destruction is a part of a surgical procedure and different methods of destruction are not ordinarily listed separately unless the technique substantially alters the standard management of a problem or condition. Exceptions under special circumstances are provided for by separate code numbers.

►Results/Testing/Reports◄

►Results are the technical component of a service. Testing leads to results; results lead to interpretation. Reports are the work product of the interpretation of numerous test results.◄

Special Report

A service that is rarely provided, unusual, variable, or new may require a special report in determining medical appropriateness of the service. Pertinent information should include an adequate definition or description of the nature, extent, and need for the procedure, and the time, effort, and equipment necessary to provide the service. Additional items which may be included are:

Notes

⊙ =Moderate sedation   ✚ =Add-on code   ✔ =FDA approval pending

Surgery

General

10021 Fine needle aspiration; without imaging guidance

10022   with imaging guidance

▶(For radiological supervision and interpretation, see 76942, 77002, 77012, 77021)◀

(For percutaneous needle biopsy other than fine needle aspiration, see 20206 for muscle, 32400 for pleura, 32405 for lung or mediastinum, 42400 for salivary gland, 47000, 47001 for liver, 48102 for pancreas, 49180 for abdominal or retroperitoneal mass, 60100 for thyroid, 62269 for spinal cord)

(For evaluation of fine needle aspirate, see 88172, 88173)

Integumentary System

Skin, Subcutaneous and Accessory Structures

Incision and Drainage

(For excision, see 11400, et seq)

10040 Acne surgery (eg, marsupialization, opening or removal of multiple milia, comedones, cysts, pustules)

10060 Incision and drainage of abscess (eg, carbuncle, suppurative hidradenitis, cutaneous or subcutaneous abscess, cyst, furuncle, or paronychia); simple or single

10061   complicated or multiple

10080 Incision and drainage of pilonidal cyst; simple

10081   complicated

(For excision of pilonidal cyst, see 11770-11772)

10120 Incision and removal of foreign body, subcutaneous tissues; simple

10121   complicated

(To report wound exploration due to penetrating trauma without laparotomy or thoracotomy, see 20100-20103, as appropriate)

(To report debridement associated with open fracture(s) and/or dislocation(s), use 11010-11012, as appropriate)

10140 Incision and drainage of hematoma, seroma or fluid collection

▶(If imaging guidance is performed, see 76942, 77012, 77021)◀

10160 Puncture aspiration of abscess, hematoma, bulla, or cyst

▶(If imaging guidance is performed, see 76942, 77012, 77021)◀

10180 Incision and drainage, complex, postoperative wound infection

(For secondary closure of surgical wound, see 12020, 12021, 13160)

Excision—Debridement

(For dermabrasions, see 15780-15783)

(For nail debridement, see 11720-11721)

(For burn(s), see 16000-16035)

11000 Debridement of extensive eczematous or infected skin; up to 10% of body surface

(For abdominal wall or genitalia debridement for necrotizing soft tissue infection, see 11004-11006)

+ 11001   each additional 10% of the body surface (List separately in addition to code for primary procedure)

(Use 11001 in conjunction with 11000)

11004 Debridement of skin, subcutaneous tissue, muscle and fascia for necrotizing soft tissue infection; external genitalia and perineum

11005   abdominal wall, with or without fascial closure

11006   external genitalia, perineum and abdominal wall, with or without fascial closure

+ 11008 Removal of prosthetic material or mesh, abdominal wall for necrotizing soft tissue infection (List separately in addition to code for primary procedure)

(Use 11008 in conjunction with 11004-11006)

(Do not report 11008 in conjunction with 11000-11001, 11010-11044)

(Report skin grafts or flaps separately when performed for closure at the same session as 11004-11008)

(When insertion of mesh is used for closure, use 49568)

(If orchiectomy is performed, use 54520)

(If testicular transplantation is performed, use 54680)

11010 Debridement including removal of foreign material associated with open fracture(s) and/or dislocation(s); skin and subcutaneous tissues

11011   skin, subcutaneous tissue, muscle fascia, and muscle

11012   skin, subcutaneous tissue, muscle fascia, muscle, and bone

11040 Debridement; skin, partial thickness

11041   skin, full thickness

Surgery: Integumentary System

Surgery: Integumentary System

11042   skin, and subcutaneous tissue

11043   skin, subcutaneous tissue, and muscle

11044   skin, subcutaneous tissue, muscle, and bone

     (Do not report 11040-11044 in conjunction with 97597-97602)

Paring or Cutting

     (To report destruction, see 17000-17004)

11055   Paring or cutting of benign hyperkeratotic lesion (eg, corn or callus); single lesion

11056   two to four lesions

11057   more than four lesions

Biopsy

During certain surgical procedures in the integumentary system, such as excision, destruction, or shave removals, the removed tissue is often submitted for pathologic examination. The obtaining of tissue for pathology during the course of these procedures is a routine component of such procedures. This obtaining of tissue is not considered a separate biopsy procedure and is not separately reported. The use of a biopsy procedure code (eg, 11100, 11101) indicates that the procedure to obtain tissue for pathologic examination was performed independently, or was unrelated or distinct from other procedures/services provided at that time. Such biopsies are not considered components of other procedures when performed on different lesions or different sites on the same date, and are to be reported separately.

     (For biopsy of conjunctiva, use 68100; eyelid, use 67810)

11100   Biopsy of skin, subcutaneous tissue and/or mucous membrane (including simple closure), unless otherwise listed; single lesion

+ 11101   each separate/additional lesion (List separately in addition to code for primary procedure)

     (Use 11101 in conjunction with 11100)

Removal of Skin Tags

Removal by scissoring or any sharp method, ligature strangulation, electrosurgical destruction or combination of treatment modalities including chemical or electrocauterization of wound, with or without local anesthesia.

11200   Removal of skin tags, multiple fibrocutaneous tags, any area; up to and including 15 lesions

+ 11201   each additional ten lesions (List separately in addition to code for primary procedure)

     (Use 11201 in conjunction with 11200)

Shaving of Epidermal or Dermal Lesions

Shaving is the sharp removal by transverse incision or horizontal slicing to remove epidermal and dermal lesions without a full-thickness dermal excision. This includes local anesthesia, chemical or electrocauterization of the wound. The wound does not require suture closure.

11300   Shaving of epidermal or dermal lesion, single lesion, trunk, arms or legs; lesion diameter 0.5 cm or less

11301   lesion diameter 0.6 to 1.0 cm

11302   lesion diameter 1.1 to 2.0 cm

11303   lesion diameter over 2.0 cm

11305   Shaving of epidermal or dermal lesion, single lesion, scalp, neck, hands, feet, genitalia; lesion diameter 0.5 cm or less

11306   lesion diameter 0.6 to 1.0 cm

11307   lesion diameter 1.1 to 2.0 cm

11308   lesion diameter over 2.0 cm

11310   Shaving of epidermal or dermal lesion, single lesion, face, ears, eyelids, nose, lips, mucous membrane; lesion diameter 0.5 cm or less

11311   lesion diameter 0.6 to 1.0 cm

11312   lesion diameter 1.1 to 2.0 cm

11313   lesion diameter over 2.0 cm

Excision—Benign Lesions

Excision (including simple closure) of benign lesions of skin (eg, neoplasm, cicatricial, fibrous, inflammatory, congenital, cystic lesions), includes local anesthesia. See appropriate size and area below. For shave removal, see 11300 et seq., and for electrosurgical and other methods see 17000 et seq.

Excision is defined as full-thickness (through the dermis) removal of a lesion, including margins, and includes simple (non-layered) closure when performed. Report separately each benign lesion excised. Code selection is determined by measuring the greatest clinical diameter of the apparent lesion plus that margin required for complete excision (lesion diameter plus the most narrow margins required equals the excised diameter). The margins refer to the most narrow margin required to adequately excise the lesion, based on the physician's judgment. The measurement of lesion plus margin is made prior to excision. The excised diameter is the same whether the surgical defect is repaired in a linear fashion, or reconstructed (eg, with a skin graft).

The closure of defects created by incision, excision, or trauma may require intermediate or complex closure. Repair by intermediate or complex closure should be reported separately. For excision of benign lesions requiring more than simple closure, ie, requiring intermediate or complex closure, report 11400-11446 in addition to appropriate intermediate (12031-12057) or complex closure (13100-13153) codes. For reconstructive closure, see 14000-14300, 15002-15261, 15570-15770. See page 51 for definition of intermediate or complex closure.

11400	Excision, benign lesion including margins, except skin tag (unless listed elsewhere), trunk, arms or legs; excised diameter 0.5 cm or less
11401	excised diameter 0.6 to 1.0 cm
11402	excised diameter 1.1 to 2.0 cm
11403	excised diameter 2.1 to 3.0 cm
11404	excised diameter 3.1 to 4.0 cm
11406	excised diameter over 4.0 cm

(For unusual or complicated excision, add modifier 22)

11420	Excision, benign lesion including margins, except skin tag (unless listed elsewhere), scalp, neck, hands, feet, genitalia; excised diameter 0.5 cm or less
11421	excised diameter 0.6 to 1.0 cm
11422	excised diameter 1.1 to 2.0 cm
11423	excised diameter 2.1 to 3.0 cm
11424	excised diameter 3.1 to 4.0 cm
11426	excised diameter over 4.0 cm

(For unusual or complicated excision, add modifier 22)

11440	Excision, other benign lesion including margins, except skin tag (unless listed elsewhere), face, ears, eyelids, nose, lips, mucous membrane; excised diameter 0.5 cm or less
11441	excised diameter 0.6 to 1.0 cm
11442	excised diameter 1.1 to 2.0 cm
11443	excised diameter 2.1 to 3.0 cm
11444	excised diameter 3.1 to 4.0 cm
11446	excised diameter over 4.0 cm

(For unusual or complicated excision, add modifier 22)

(For eyelids involving more than skin, see also 67800 et seq)

11450	Excision of skin and subcutaneous tissue for hidradenitis, axillary; with simple or intermediate repair
11451	with complex repair
11462	Excision of skin and subcutaneous tissue for hidradenitis, inguinal; with simple or intermediate repair
11463	with complex repair
11470	Excision of skin and subcutaneous tissue for hidradenitis, perianal, perineal, or umbilical; with simple or intermediate repair
11471	with complex repair

(When skin graft or flap is used for closure, use appropriate procedure code in addition)

(For bilateral procedure, add modifier 50)

Excision—Malignant Lesions

Excision (including simple closure) of malignant lesions of skin (eg, basal cell carcinoma, squamous cell carcinoma, melanoma) includes local anesthesia. (See appropriate size and body area below.) For destruction of malignant lesions of skin, see destruction codes 17260-17286.

Excision is defined as full-thickness (through the dermis) removal of a lesion including margins, and includes simple (non-layered) closure when performed. Report separately each malignant lesion excised. Code selection is determined by measuring the greatest clinical diameter of the apparent lesion plus that margin required for complete excision (lesion diameter plus the most narrow margins required equals the excised diameter). The margins refer to the most narrow margin required to adequately excise the lesion, based on the physician's judgment. The measurement of lesion plus margin is made prior to excision. The excised diameter is the same whether the surgical defect is repaired in a linear fashion, or reconstructed (eg, with a skin graft).

The closure of defects created by incision, excision, or trauma may require intermediate or complex closure. Repair by intermediate or complex closure should be reported separately. For excision of malignant lesions requiring more than simple closure, ie, requiring intermediate or complex closure, report 11600-11646 in addition to appropriate intermediate (12031-12057) or complex closure (13100-13153) codes. For reconstructive closure, see 14000-14300, 15002-15261, 15570-15770. See page 51 for definition of intermediate or complex closure.

When frozen section pathology shows the margins of excision were not adequate, an additional excision may be necessary for complete tumor removal. Use only one code to report the additional excision and re-excision(s) based on the final widest excised diameter required for complete tumor removal at the same operative session. To report a re-excision procedure performed to widen margins at a subsequent operative session, see codes 11600-11646, as appropriate. Append modifier 58 if the re-excision procedure is performed during the postoperative period of the primary excision procedure.

11600	Excision, malignant lesion including margins, trunk, arms, or legs; excised diameter 0.5 cm or less
11601	excised diameter 0.6 to 1.0 cm
11602	excised diameter 1.1 to 2.0 cm
11603	excised diameter 2.1 to 3.0 cm
11604	excised diameter 3.1 to 4.0 cm
11606	excised diameter over 4.0 cm

11620 Excision, malignant lesion including margins, scalp, neck, hands, feet, genitalia; excised diameter 0.5 cm or less

11621 excised diameter 0.6 to 1.0 cm

11622 excised diameter 1.1 to 2.0 cm

11623 excised diameter 2.1 to 3.0 cm

11624 excised diameter 3.1 to 4.0 cm

11626 excised diameter over 4.0 cm

11640 Excision, malignant lesion including margins, face, ears, eyelids, nose, lips; excised diameter 0.5 cm or less

11641 excised diameter 0.6 to 1.0 cm

11642 excised diameter 1.1 to 2.0 cm

11643 excised diameter 2.1 to 3.0 cm

11644 excised diameter 3.1 to 4.0 cm

11646 excised diameter over 4.0 cm

(For eyelids involving more than skin, see also 67800 et seq)

Nails

(For drainage of paronychia or onychia, see 10060, 10061)

11719 Trimming of nondystrophic nails, any number

11720 Debridement of nail(s) by any method(s); one to five

11721 six or more

11730 Avulsion of nail plate, partial or complete, simple; single

✚ 11732 each additional nail plate (List separately in addition to code for primary procedure)

(Use 11732 in conjunction with 11730)

11740 Evacuation of subungual hematoma

11750 Excision of nail and nail matrix, partial or complete, (eg, ingrown or deformed nail) for permanent removal;

11752 with amputation of tuft of distal phalanx

(For skin graft, if used, use 15050)

11755 Biopsy of nail unit (eg, plate, bed, matrix, hyponychium, proximal and lateral nail folds) (separate procedure)

11760 Repair of nail bed

11762 Reconstruction of nail bed with graft

11765 Wedge excision of skin of nail fold (eg, for ingrown toenail)

Pilonidal Cyst

11770 Excision of pilonidal cyst or sinus; simple

11771 extensive

11772 complicated

(For incision of pilonidal cyst, see 10080, 10081)

Introduction

11900 Injection, intralesional; up to and including seven lesions

11901 more than seven lesions

(11900, 11901 are not to be used for preoperative local anesthetic injection)

(For veins, see 36470, 36471)

(For intralesional chemotherapy administration, see 96405, 96406)

11920 Tattooing, intradermal introduction of insoluble opaque pigments to correct color defects of skin, including micropigmentation; 6.0 sq cm or less

11921 6.1 to 20.0 sq cm

✚ 11922 each additional 20.0 sq cm (List separately in addition to code for primary procedure)

(Use 11922 in conjunction with 11921)

11950 Subcutaneous injection of filling material (eg, collagen); 1 cc or less

11951 1.1 to 5.0 cc

11952 5.1 to 10.0 cc

11954 over 10.0 cc

11960 Insertion of tissue expander(s) for other than breast, including subsequent expansion

(For breast reconstruction with tissue expander(s), use 19357)

11970 Replacement of tissue expander with permanent prosthesis

11971 Removal of tissue expander(s) without insertion of prosthesis

11975 Insertion, implantable contraceptive capsules

11976 Removal, implantable contraceptive capsules

11977 Removal with reinsertion, implantable contraceptive capsules

11980 Subcutaneous hormone pellet implantation (implantation of estradiol and/or testosterone pellets beneath the skin)

11981 Insertion, non-biodegradable drug delivery implant

11982 Removal, non-biodegradable drug delivery implant

11983 Removal with reinsertion, non-biodegradable drug delivery implant

Repair (Closure)

Use the codes in this section to designate wound closure utilizing sutures, staples, or tissue adhesives (eg, 2-cyanoacrylate), either singly or in combination with each other, or in combination with adhesive strips. Wound closure utilizing adhesive strips as the sole repair material should be coded using the appropriate E/M code.

Definitions

The repair of wounds may be classified as Simple, Intermediate, or Complex.

Simple repair is used when the wound is superficial; eg, involving primarily epidermis or dermis, or subcutaneous tissues without significant involvement of deeper structures, and requires simple one layer closure. This includes local anesthesia and chemical or electrocauterization of wounds not closed.

Intermediate repair includes the repair of wounds that, in addition to the above, require layered closure of one or more of the deeper layers of subcutaneous tissue and superficial (non-muscle) fascia, in addition to the skin (epidermal and dermal) closure. Single-layer closure of heavily contaminated wounds that have required extensive cleaning or removal of particulate matter also constitutes intermediate repair.

Complex repair includes the repair of wounds requiring more than layered closure, viz., scar revision, debridement (eg, traumatic lacerations or avulsions), extensive undermining, stents or retention sutures. Necessary preparation includes creation of a defect for repairs (eg, excision of a scar requiring a complex repair) or the debridement of complicated lacerations or avulsions. Complex repair does not include excision of benign (11400-11446) or malignant (11600-11646) lesions.

Instructions for listing services at time of wound repair:

1. The repaired wound(s) should be measured and recorded in centimeters, whether curved, angular, or stellate.

2. When multiple wounds are repaired, add together the lengths of those in the same classification (see above) and from all anatomic sites that are grouped together into the same code descriptor. For example, add together the lengths of intermediate repairs to the trunk and extremities. Do not add lengths of repairs from different groupings of anatomic sites (eg, face and extremities). Also, do not add together lengths of different classifications (eg, intermediate and complex repairs).

When more than one classification of wounds is repaired, list the more complicated as the primary procedure and the less complicated as the secondary procedure, using modifier 51.

3. Decontamination and/or debridement: Debridement is considered a separate procedure only when gross contamination requires prolonged cleansing, when appreciable amounts of devitalized or contaminated tissue are removed, or when debridement is carried out separately without immediate primary closure. (For extensive debridement of soft tissue and/or bone, see 11040-11044.)

(For extensive debridement of soft tissue and/or bone, not associated with open fracture(s) and/or dislocation(s) resulting from penetrating and/or blunt trauma, see 11040-11044.)

(For extensive debridement of subcutaneous tissue, muscle fascia, muscle, and/or bone associated with open fracture(s) and/or dislocation(s), see 11010-11012.)

4. Involvement of nerves, blood vessels and tendons: Report under appropriate system (Nervous, Cardiovascular, Musculoskeletal) for repair of these structures. The repair of these associated wounds is included in the primary procedure unless it qualifies as a complex wound, in which case modifier 51 applies.

Simple ligation of vessels in an open wound is considered as part of any wound closure.

Simple "exploration" of nerves, blood vessels or tendons exposed in an open wound is also considered part of the essential treatment of the wound and is not a separate procedure unless appreciable dissection is required. If the wound requires enlargement, extension of dissection (to determine penetration), debridement, removal of foreign body(s), ligation or coagulation of minor subcutaneous and/or muscular blood vessel(s) of the subcutaneous tissue, muscle fascia, and/or muscle, not requiring thoracotomy or laparotomy, use codes 20100-20103, as appropriate.

Repair—Simple

Sum of lengths of repairs for each group of anatomic sites.

12001	Simple repair of superficial wounds of scalp, neck, axillae, external genitalia, trunk and/or extremities (including hands and feet); 2.5 cm or less
12002	2.6 cm to 7.5 cm
12004	7.6 cm to 12.5 cm
12005	12.6 cm to 20.0 cm
12006	20.1 cm to 30.0 cm
12007	over 30.0 cm
12011	Simple repair of superficial wounds of face, ears, eyelids, nose, lips and/or mucous membranes; 2.5 cm or less
12013	2.6 cm to 5.0 cm
12014	5.1 cm to 7.5 cm
12015	7.6 cm to 12.5 cm
12016	12.6 cm to 20.0 cm
12017	20.1 cm to 30.0 cm
12018	over 30.0 cm

Surgery: Integumentary System

12020   Treatment of superficial wound dehiscence; simple closure

12021   with packing

(For extensive or complicated secondary wound closure, use 13160)

Repair—Intermediate

Sum of lengths of repairs for each group of anatomic sites.

12031   Layer closure of wounds of scalp, axillae, trunk and/or extremities (excluding hands and feet); 2.5 cm or less

12032   2.6 cm to 7.5 cm

12034   7.6 cm to 12.5 cm

12035   12.6 cm to 20.0 cm

12036   20.1 cm to 30.0 cm

12037   over 30.0 cm

12041   Layer closure of wounds of neck, hands, feet and/or external genitalia; 2.5 cm or less

12042   2.6 cm to 7.5 cm

12044   7.6 cm to 12.5 cm

12045   12.6 cm to 20.0 cm

12046   20.1 cm to 30.0 cm

12047   over 30.0 cm

12051   Layer closure of wounds of face, ears, eyelids, nose, lips and/or mucous membranes; 2.5 cm or less

12052   2.6 cm to 5.0 cm

12053   5.1 cm to 7.5 cm

12054   7.6 cm to 12.5 cm

12055   12.6 cm to 20.0 cm

12056   20.1 cm to 30.0 cm

12057   over 30.0 cm

Repair—Complex

Reconstructive procedures, complicated wound closure.

Sum of lengths of repairs for each group of anatomic sites.

(For full thickness repair of lip or eyelid, see respective anatomical subsections)

13100   Repair, complex, trunk; 1.1 cm to 2.5 cm

(For 1.0 cm or less, see simple or intermediate repairs)

13101   2.6 cm to 7.5 cm

+ 13102   each additional 5 cm or less (List separately in addition to code for primary procedure)

(Use 13102 in conjunction with 13101)

13120   Repair, complex, scalp, arms, and/or legs; 1.1 cm to 2.5 cm

(For 1.0 cm or less, see simple or intermediate repairs)

13121   2.6 cm to 7.5 cm

+ 13122   each additional 5 cm or less (List separately in addition to code for primary procedure)

(Use 13122 in conjunction with 13121)

13131   Repair, complex, forehead, cheeks, chin, mouth, neck, axillae, genitalia, hands and/or feet; 1.1 cm to 2.5 cm

(For 1.0 cm or less, see simple or intermediate repairs)

13132   2.6 cm to 7.5 cm

+ 13133   each additional 5 cm or less (List separately in addition to code for primary procedure)

(Use 13133 in conjunction with 13132)

13150   Repair, complex, eyelids, nose, ears and/or lips; 1.0 cm or less

(See also 40650-40654, 67961-67975)

13151   1.1 cm to 2.5 cm

13152   2.6 cm to 7.5 cm

+ 13153   each additional 5 cm or less (List separately in addition to code for primary procedure)

(Use 13153 in conjunction with 13152)

13160   Secondary closure of surgical wound or dehiscence, extensive or complicated

(For packing or simple secondary wound closure, see 12020, 12021)

Adjacent Tissue Transfer or Rearrangement

For full thickness repair of lip or eyelid, see respective anatomical subsections.

Excision (including lesion) and/or repair by adjacent tissue transfer or rearrangement (eg, Z-plasty, W-plasty, V-Y plasty, rotation flap, advancement flap, double pedicle flap). When applied in repairing lacerations, the procedures listed must be developed by the surgeon to accomplish the repair. They do not apply when direct closure or rearrangement of traumatic wounds incidentally result in these configurations.

Skin graft necessary to close secondary defect is considered an additional procedure. For purposes of code selection, the term "defect" includes the primary and secondary defects. The primary defect resulting from the excision and the secondary defect resulting from flap design to perform the reconstruction are measured together to determine the code.

14000   Adjacent tissue transfer or rearrangement, trunk; defect 10 sq cm or less

14001   defect 10.1 sq cm to 30.0 sq cm

14020   Adjacent tissue transfer or rearrangement, scalp, arms and/or legs; defect 10 sq cm or less

14021   defect 10.1 sq cm to 30.0 sq cm

14040   Adjacent tissue transfer or rearrangement, forehead, cheeks, chin, mouth, neck, axillae, genitalia, hands and/or feet; defect 10 sq cm or less

14041   defect 10.1 sq cm to 30.0 sq cm

14060   Adjacent tissue transfer or rearrangement, eyelids, nose, ears and/or lips; defect 10 sq cm or less

14061   defect 10.1 sq cm to 30.0 sq cm

       (For eyelid, full thickness, see 67961 et seq)

14300   Adjacent tissue transfer or rearrangement, more than 30 sq cm, unusual or complicated, any area

14350   Filleted finger or toe flap, including preparation of recipient site

Skin Replacement Surgery and Skin Substitutes

Identify by size and location of the defect (recipient area) and the type of graft or skin substitute; includes simple debridement of granulation tissue or recent avulsion.

When a primary procedure such as orbitectomy, radical mastectomy, or deep tumor removal requires skin graft for definitive closure, see appropriate anatomical subsection for primary procedure and this section for skin graft or skin substitute.

►Use 15002-15005 for initial wound recipient site preparation.◄

Use 15100-15261 for autologous skin grafts. For autologous tissue-cultured epidermal grafts, use 15150-15157. For harvesting of autologous keratinocytes and dermal tissue for tissue-cultured skin grafts, use 15040. Procedures are coded by recipient site. Use 15170-15176 for acellular dermal replacement. Use modifier 58 for staged application procedure(s).

Repair of donor site requiring skin graft or local flaps is to be added as an additional procedure.

►Codes 15002-15005 describe burn and wound preparation or incisional or excisional release of scar contracture resulting in an open wound requiring a skin graft. Codes 15100-15431 describe the application of skin replacements and skin substitutes. The following definition should be applied to those codes that reference "100 sq cm or 1% of body area of infants and children" when determining the involvement of body size: The measurement of 100 sq cm is applicable to adults and children age 10 and older; percentages of body surface area apply to infants and children younger than the age of 10.

These codes are not intended to be reported for simple graft application alone or application stabilized with dressings (eg, by simple gauze wrap). The skin substitute/graft is anchored using the surgeon's choice of fixation. When services are performed in the office, the supply of the skin substitute/graft should be reported separately. Routine dressing supplies are not reported separately.◄

(For microvascular flaps, see 15756-15758)

Surgical Preparation

►(15000, 15001 have been deleted. To report, see 15002-15005)◄

● **15002**   Surgical preparation or creation of recipient site by excision of open wounds, burn eschar, or scar (including subcutaneous tissues), or incisional release of scar contracture, trunk, arms, legs; first 100 sq cm or 1% of body area of infants and children

+● **15003**   each additional 100 sq cm or each additional 1% of body area of infants and children (List separately in addition to code for primary procedure)

       ►(Use 15003 in conjunction with 15002)◄

● **15004**   Surgical preparation or creation of recipient site by excision of open wounds, burn eschar, or scar (including subcutaneous tissues), or incisional release of scar contracture, face, scalp, eyelids, mouth, neck, ears, orbits, genitalia, hands, feet and/or multiple digits; first 100 sq cm or 1% of body area of infants and children

+● **15005**   each additional 100 sq cm or each additional 1% of body area of infants and children (List separately in addition to code for primary procedure)

       ►(Use 15005 in conjunction with 15004)◄

       ►(Report 15002-15005 in conjunction with code for appropriate skin grafts or replacements [15050-15261, 15330-15336]. List the graft or replacement separately by its procedure number when the graft, immediate or delayed, is applied)◄

       ►(For excision of benign lesions, see 11400-11471)◄

       ►(For excision of malignant lesions, see 11600-11646)◄

       ►(For excision to prepare or create recipient site with dressings or materials not listed in 15040-15431, use 15002-15005 only)◄

       ►(For excision with immediate skin grafting, use 15002-15005 in conjunction with 15050-15261)◄

       ►(For excision with immediate allograft skin placement, use 15002-15005 in conjunction with 15300-15336 and 15360-15366)◄

       ►(For excision with immediate xenogeneic dermis placement, use 15002-15005 in conjunction with 15400-15421)◄

Surgery: Integumentary System

Surgery: Integumentary System

Grafts

Autograft/Tissue Cultured Autograft

15040 Harvest of skin for tissue cultured skin autograft, 100 sq cm or less

15050 Pinch graft, single or multiple, to cover small ulcer, tip of digit, or other minimal open area (except on face), up to defect size 2 cm diameter

15100 Split-thickness autograft, trunk, arms, legs; first 100 sq cm or less, or 1% of body area of infants and children (except 15050)

+ 15101 each additional 100 sq cm, or each additional 1% of body area of infants and children, or part thereof (List separately in addition to code for primary procedure)

(Use 15101 in conjunction with 15100)

15110 Epidermal autograft, trunk, arms, legs; first 100 sq cm or less, or 1% of body area of infants and children

+ 15111 each additional 100 sq cm, or each additional 1% of body area of infants and children, or part thereof (List separately in addition to code for primary procedure)

(Use 15111 in conjunction with 15110)

15115 Epidermal autograft, face, scalp, eyelids, mouth, neck, ears, orbits, genitalia, hands, feet, and/or multiple digits; first 100 sq cm or less, or 1% of body area of infants and children

+ 15116 each additional 100 sq cm, or each additional 1% of body area of infants and children, or part thereof (List separately in addition to code for primary procedure)

(Use 15116 in conjunction with 15115)

15120 Split-thickness autograft, face, scalp, eyelids, mouth, neck, ears, orbits, genitalia, hands, feet, and/or multiple digits; first 100 sq cm or less, or 1% of body area of infants and children (except 15050)

+ 15121 each additional 100 sq cm, or each additional 1% of body area of infants and children, or part thereof (List separately in addition to code for primary procedure)

(Use 15121 in conjunction with 15120)

(For eyelids, see also 67961 et seq)

15130 Dermal autograft, trunk, arms, legs; first 100 sq cm or less, or 1% of body area of infants and children

+ 15131 each additional 100 sq cm, or each additional 1% of body area of infants and children, or part thereof (List separately in addition to code for primary procedure)

(Use 15131 in conjunction with 15130)

15135 Dermal autograft, face, scalp, eyelids, mouth, neck, ears, orbits, genitalia, hands, feet, and/or multiple digits; first 100 sq cm or less, or 1% of body area of infants and children

+ 15136 each additional 100 sq cm, or each additional 1% of body area of infants and children, or part thereof (List separately in addition to code for primary procedure)

(Use 15136 in conjunction with 15135)

15150 Tissue cultured epidermal autograft, trunk, arms, legs; first 25 sq cm or less

+ 15151 additional 1 sq cm to 75 sq cm (List separately in addition to code for primary procedure)

(Do not report 15151 more than once per session)

(Use 15151 in conjunction with 15150)

+ 15152 each additional 100 sq cm, or each additional 1% of body area of infants and children, or part thereof (List separately in addition to code for primary procedure)

(Use 15152 in conjunction with 15151)

15155 Tissue cultured epidermal autograft, face, scalp, eyelids, mouth, neck, ears, orbits, genitalia, hands, feet, and/or multiple digits; first 25 sq cm or less

+ 15156 additional 1 sq cm to 75 sq cm (List separately in addition to code for primary procedure)

(Do not report 15156 more than once per session)

(Use 15156 in conjunction with 15155)

+ 15157 each additional 100 sq cm, or each additional 1% of body area of infants and children, or part thereof (List separately in addition to code for primary procedure)

(Use 15157 in conjunction with 15156)

Acellular Dermal Replacement

15170 Acellular dermal replacement, trunk, arms, legs; first 100 sq cm or less, or 1% of body area of infants and children

+ 15171 each additional 100 sq cm, or each additional 1% of body area of infants and children, or part thereof (List separately in addition to code for primary procedure)

(Use 15171 in conjunction with 15170)

15175 Acellular dermal replacement, face, scalp, eyelids, mouth, neck, ears, orbits, genitalia, hands, feet, and/or multiple digits; first 100 sq cm or less, or 1% of body area of infants and children

+ 15176 each additional 100 sq cm, or each additional 1% of body area of infants and children, or part thereof (List separately in addition to code for primary procedure)

(Use 15176 in conjunction with 15175)

15200   Full thickness graft, free, including direct closure of donor site, trunk; 20 sq cm or less

+ 15201   each additional 20 sq cm (List separately in addition to code for primary procedure)

        (Use 15201 in conjunction with 15200)

15220   Full thickness graft, free, including direct closure of donor site, scalp, arms, and/or legs; 20 sq cm or less

+ 15221   each additional 20 sq cm (List separately in addition to code for primary procedure)

        (Use 15221 in conjunction with 15220)

15240   Full thickness graft, free, including direct closure of donor site, forehead, cheeks, chin, mouth, neck, axillae, genitalia, hands, and/or feet; 20 sq cm or less

        (For finger tip graft, use 15050)

        (For repair of syndactyly, fingers, see 26560-26562)

+ 15241   each additional 20 sq cm (List separately in addition to code for primary procedure)

        (Use 15241 in conjunction with 15240)

15260   Full thickness graft, free, including direct closure of donor site, nose, ears, eyelids, and/or lips; 20 sq cm or less

+ 15261   each additional 20 sq cm (List separately in addition to code for primary procedure)

        (Use 15261 in conjunction with 15260)

        (For eyelids, see also 67961 et seq)

        (Repair of donor site requiring skin graft or local flaps, to be added as additional separate procedure)

Allograft/Tissue Cultured Allogeneic Skin Substitute

Application of a non-autologous human skin graft (ie, homograft) from a donor to a part of the recipient's body to resurface an area damaged by burns, traumatic injury, soft tissue infection and/or tissue necrosis or surgery.

15300   Allograft skin for temporary wound closure, trunk, arms, legs; first 100 sq cm or less, or 1% of body area of infants and children

+ 15301   each additional 100 sq cm, or each additional 1% of body area of infants and children, or part thereof (List separately in addition to code for primary procedure)

        (Use 15301 in conjunction with 15300)

15320   Allograft skin for temporary wound closure, face, scalp, eyelids, mouth, neck, ears, orbits, genitalia, hands, feet, and/or multiple digits; first 100 sq cm or less, or 1% of body area of infants and children

+ 15321   each additional 100 sq cm, or each additional 1% of body area of infants and children, or part thereof (List separately in addition to code for primary procedure)

        (Use 15321 in conjunction with 15320)

15330   Acellular dermal allograft, trunk, arms, legs; first 100 sq cm or less, or 1% of body area of infants and children

+ 15331   each additional 100 sq cm, or each additional 1% of body area of infants and children, or part thereof (List separately in addition to code for primary procedure)

        (Use 15331 in conjunction with 15330)

15335   Acellular dermal allograft, face, scalp, eyelids, mouth, neck, ears, orbits, genitalia, hands, feet, and/or multiple digits; first 100 sq cm or less, or 1% of body area of infants and children

+ 15336   each additional 100 sq cm, or each additional 1% of body area of infants and children, or part thereof (List separately in addition to code for primary procedure)

        (Use 15336 in conjunction with 15335)

15340   Tissue cultured allogeneic skin substitute; first 25 sq cm or less

+ 15341   each additional 25 sq cm

        (Use 15341 in conjunction with 15340)

        ►(Do not report 15340, 15341 in conjunction with 11040-11042, 15002-15005)◄

        (15342 has been deleted. To report, see 15170, 15175, 15340, 15360, 15365)

        (15343 has been deleted. To report, see 15171, 15176, 15341, 15361, 15366)

        (15350 has been deleted. To report, see 15300, 15320, 15330, 15335)

        (15351 has been deleted. To report, see 15301, 15321, 15331, 15336)

15360   Tissue cultured allogeneic dermal substitute, trunk, arms, legs; first 100 sq cm or less, or 1% of body area of infants and children

+ 15361   each additional 100 sq cm, or each additional 1% of body area of infants and children, or part thereof (List separately in addition to code for primary procedure)

        (Use 15361 in conjunction with 15360)

15365   Tissue cultured allogeneic dermal substitute, face, scalp, eyelids, mouth, neck, ears, orbits, genitalia, hands, feet, and/or multiple digits; first 100 sq cm or less, or 1% of body area of infants and children

+ 15366   each additional 100 sq cm, or each additional 1% of body area of infants and children, or part thereof (List separately in addition to code for primary procedure)

        (Use 15366 in conjunction with 15365)

Surgery: Integumentary System

Surgery: Integumentary System

Xenograft

Application of a non-human skin graft or biologic wound dressing (eg, porcine tissue or pigskin) to a part of the recipient's body following debridement of the burn wound or area of traumatic injury, soft tissue infection and/or tissue necrosis, or surgery.

15400 Xenograft, skin (dermal), for temporary wound closure, trunk, arms, legs; first 100 sq cm or less, or 1% of body area of infants and children

+ 15401 each additional 100 sq cm, or each additional 1% of body area of infants and children, or part thereof (List separately in addition to code for primary procedure)

(Use 15401 in conjunction with 15400)

15420 Xenograft skin (dermal), for temporary wound closure, face, scalp, eyelids, mouth, neck, ears, orbits, genitalia, hands, feet, and/or multiple digits; first 100 sq cm or less, or 1% of body area of infants and children

+ 15421 each additional 100 sq cm, or each additional 1% of body area of infants and children, or part thereof (List separately in addition to code for primary procedure)

(Use 15421 in conjunction with 15420)

15430 Acellular xenograft implant; first 100 sq cm or less, or 1% of body area of infants and children

+ 15431 each additional 100 sq cm, or each additional 1% of body area of infants and children, or part thereof (List separately in addition to code for primary procedure)

(Use 15431 in conjunction with 15430)

►(Do not report 15430, 15431 in conjunction with 11040-11042, 15002-15005, 0170T)◄

Flaps (Skin and/or Deep Tissues)

Regions listed refer to recipient area (not donor site) when flap is being attached in transfer or to final site.

Regions listed refer to donor site when tube is formed for later or when "delay" of flap is prior to transfer.

Procedures 15570-15738 do not include extensive immobilization (eg, large plaster casts and other immobilizing devices are considered additional separate procedures).

Repair of donor site requiring skin graft or local flaps is considered an additional separate procedure.

(For microvascular flaps, see 15756-15758)

►(For flaps without inclusion of a vascular pedicle, see 15570-15576)◄

►(For adjacent tissue transfer flaps, see 14000-14300)◄

15570 Formation of direct or tubed pedicle, with or without transfer; trunk

15572 scalp, arms, or legs

15574 forehead, cheeks, chin, mouth, neck, axillae, genitalia, hands or feet

15576 eyelids, nose, ears, lips, or intraoral

15600 Delay of flap or sectioning of flap (division and inset); at trunk

15610 at scalp, arms, or legs

15620 at forehead, cheeks, chin, neck, axillae, genitalia, hands, or feet

15630 at eyelids, nose, ears, or lips

15650 Transfer, intermediate, of any pedicle flap (eg, abdomen to wrist, Walking tube), any location

(For eyelids, nose, ears, or lips, see also anatomical area)

(For revision, defatting or rearranging of transferred pedicle flap or skin graft, see 13100-14300)

(Procedures 15732-15738 are described by donor site of the muscle, myocutaneous, or fasciocutaneous flap)

● **15731** Forehead flap with preservation of vascular pedicle (eg, axial pattern flap, paramedian forehead flap)

►(For muscle, myocutaneous, or fasciocutaneous flap of the head or neck, use 15732)◄

15732 Muscle, myocutaneous, or fasciocutaneous flap; head and neck (eg, temporalis, masseter muscle, sternocleidomastoid, levator scapulae)

►(For forehead flap with preservation of vascular pedicle, use 15731)◄

15734 trunk

15736 upper extremity

15738 lower extremity

Other Flaps and Grafts

Repair of donor site requiring skin graft or local flaps should be reported as an additional procedure.

15740 Flap; island pedicle

15750 neurovascular pedicle

15756 Free muscle or myocutaneous flap with microvascular anastomosis

(Do not report code 69990 in addition to code 15756)

15757 Free skin flap with microvascular anastomosis

(Do not report code 69990 in addition to code 15757)

15758 Free fascial flap with microvascular anastomosis

(Do not report code 69990 in addition to code 15758)

15760 Graft; composite (eg, full thickness of external ear or nasal ala), including primary closure, donor area

15770 derma-fat-fascia

15775   Punch graft for hair transplant; 1 to 15 punch grafts

15776   more than 15 punch grafts

        (For strip transplant, use 15220)

Other Procedures

15780   Dermabrasion; total face (eg, for acne scarring, fine wrinkling, rhytids, general keratosis)

15781   segmental, face

15782   regional, other than face

15783   superficial, any site, (eg, tattoo removal)

15786   Abrasion; single lesion (eg, keratosis, scar)

+ **15787**   each additional four lesions or less (List separately in addition to code for primary procedure)

        (Use 15787 in conjunction with 15786)

15788   Chemical peel, facial; epidermal

15789   dermal

15792   Chemical peel, nonfacial; epidermal

15793   dermal

        (15810, 15811 have been deleted)

15819   Cervicoplasty

15820   Blepharoplasty, lower eyelid;

15821   with extensive herniated fat pad

15822   Blepharoplasty, upper eyelid;

15823   with excessive skin weighting down lid

        (For bilateral blepharoplasty, add modifier 50)

15824   Rhytidectomy; forehead

        (For repair of brow ptosis, use 67900)

15825   neck with platysmal tightening (platysmal flap, P-flap)

15826   glabellar frown lines

15828   cheek, chin, and neck

15829   superficial musculoaponeurotic system (SMAS) flap

        (For bilateral rhytidectomy, add modifier 50)

● **15830**   Excision, excessive skin and subcutaneous tissue (includes lipectomy); abdomen, infraumbilical panniculectomy

        ▶(Do not report 15830 in conjunction with 12031, 12032, 12034, 12035, 12036, 12037, 13100, 13101, 13102, 14000-14001, 14300)◀

        ▶(15831 has been deleted. To report abdominoplasty with panniculectomy, use 15830 in conjunction with 15847. To report other abdominoplasty, use 17999)◀

15832   thigh

15833   leg

15834   hip

15835   buttock

15836   arm

15837   forearm or hand

15838   submental fat pad

15839   other area

        (For bilateral procedure, add modifier 50)

15840   Graft for facial nerve paralysis; free fascia graft (including obtaining fascia)

        (For bilateral procedure, add modifier 50)

15841   free muscle graft (including obtaining graft)

15842   free muscle flap by microsurgical technique

        (Do not report code 69990 in addition to code 15842)

15845   regional muscle transfer

        (For intravenous fluorescein examination of blood flow in graft or flap, use 15860)

        (For nerve transfers, decompression, or repair, see 64831-64876, 64905, 64907, 69720, 69725, 69740, 69745, 69955)

+● **15847**   Excision, excessive skin and subcutaneous tissue (includes lipectomy), abdomen (eg, abdominoplasty) (includes umbilical transposition and fascial plication) (List separately in addition to code for primary procedure)

        ▶(Use 15847 in conjunction with 15830)◀

        ▶(For abdominal wall hernia repair, see 49491-49587)◀

        ▶(To report other abdominoplasty, use 17999)◀

15850   Removal of sutures under anesthesia (other than local), same surgeon

15851   Removal of sutures under anesthesia (other than local), other surgeon

15852   Dressing change (for other than burns) under anesthesia (other than local)

15860   Intravenous injection of agent (eg, fluorescein) to test vascular flow in flap or graft

15876   Suction assisted lipectomy; head and neck

15877   trunk

15878   upper extremity

15879   lower extremity

Pressure Ulcers (Decubitus Ulcers)

15920   Excision, coccygeal pressure ulcer, with coccygectomy; with primary suture

15922   with flap closure

15931   Excision, sacral pressure ulcer, with primary suture;

15933   with ostectomy

Surgery: Integumentary System

15934 Excision, sacral pressure ulcer, with skin flap closure;

15935 with ostectomy

15936 Excision, sacral pressure ulcer, in preparation for muscle or myocutaneous flap or skin graft closure;

15937 with ostectomy

(For repair of defect using muscle or myocutaneous flap, use code(s) 15734 and/or 15738 in addition to 15936, 15937. For repair of defect using split skin graft, use codes 15100 and/or 15101 in addition to 15936, 15937)

15940 Excision, ischial pressure ulcer, with primary suture;

15941 with ostectomy (ischiectomy)

15944 Excision, ischial pressure ulcer, with skin flap closure;

15945 with ostectomy

15946 Excision, ischial pressure ulcer, with ostectomy, in preparation for muscle or myocutaneous flap or skin graft closure

(For repair of defect using muscle or myocutaneous flap, use code(s) 15734 and/or 15738 in addition to 15946. For repair of defect using split skin graft, use codes 15100 and/or 15101 in addition to 15946)

15950 Excision, trochanteric pressure ulcer, with primary suture;

15951 with ostectomy

15952 Excision, trochanteric pressure ulcer, with skin flap closure;

15953 with ostectomy

15956 Excision, trochanteric pressure ulcer, in preparation for muscle or myocutaneous flap or skin graft closure;

15958 with ostectomy

(For repair of defect using muscle or myocutaneous flap, use code(s) 15734 and/or 15738 in addition to 15956, 15958. For repair of defect using split skin graft, use codes 15100 and/or 15101 in addition to 15956, 15958)

15999 Unlisted procedure, excision pressure ulcer

▶(For free skin graft to close ulcer or donor site, see 15002 et seq)◀

Burns, Local Treatment

Procedures 16000-16036 refer to local treatment of burned surface only. Codes 16020-16030 include the application of materials (eg, dressings) not described in 15100-15431.

List percentage of body surface involved and depth of burn.

For necessary related medical services (eg, hospital visits, detention) in management of burned patients, see appropriate services in **Evaluation and Management** and **Medicine** sections.

For the application of skin grafts or skin substitutes, see 15100-15650.

16000 Initial treatment, first degree burn, when no more than local treatment is required

(16010, 16015 have been deleted. To report, see 16020-16030)

16020 Dressings and/or debridement of partial-thickness burns, initial or subsequent; small (less than 5% total body surface area)

16025 medium (eg, whole face or whole extremity, or 5% to 10% total body surface area)

16030 large (eg, more than one extremity, or greater than 10% total body surface area)

16035 Escharotomy; initial incision

+ 16036 each additional incision (List separately in addition to code for primary procedure)

(Use 16036 in conjunction with 16035)

(For debridement, curettement of burn wound, see 16020-16030)

Destruction

Destruction means the ablation of benign, premalignant or malignant tissues by any method, with or without curettement, including local anesthesia, and not usually requiring closure.

Any method includes electrosurgery, cryosurgery, laser and chemical treatment. Lesions include condylomata, papillomata, molluscum contagiosum, herpetic lesions, warts (ie, common, plantar, flat), milia, or other benign, premalignant (eg, actinic keratoses), or malignant lesions.

(For destruction of lesion(s) in specific anatomic sites, see 40820, 46900-46917, 46924, 54050-54057, 54065, 56501, 56515, 57061, 57065, 67850, 68135)

(For paring or cutting of benign hyperkeratotic lesions (eg, corns or calluses), see 11055-11057)

(For sharp removal or electrosurgical destruction of skin tags and fibrocutaneous tags, see 11200, 11201)

(For cryotherapy of acne, use 17340)

(For initiation or follow-up care of topical chemotherapy (eg, 5-FU or similar agents), see appropriate office visits)

(For shaving of epidermal or dermal lesions, see 11300-11313)

Destruction, Benign or Premalignant Lesions

▲ **17000** Destruction (eg, laser surgery, electrosurgery, cryosurgery, chemosurgery, surgical curettement), premalignant lesions (eg, actinic keratoses); first lesion

+ 17003 second through 14 lesions, each (List separately in addition to code for first lesion)

(Use 17003 in conjunction with 17000)

▶(For destruction of common or plantar warts, see 17110, 17111)◀

⊘▲ **17004**   Destruction (eg, laser surgery, electrosurgery, cryosurgery, chemosurgery, surgical curettement), premalignant lesions (eg, actinic keratoses), 15 or more lesions

(Do not report 17004 in conjunction with 17000-17003)

17106   Destruction of cutaneous vascular proliferative lesions (eg, laser technique); less than 10 sq cm

17107   10.0 to 50.0 sq cm

17108   over 50.0 sq cm

▲ **17110**   Destruction (eg, laser surgery, electrosurgery, cryosurgery, chemosurgery, surgical curettement), of benign lesions other than skin tags or cutaneous vascular lesions; up to 14 lesions

17111   15 or more lesions

17250   Chemical cauterization of granulation tissue (proud flesh, sinus or fistula)

(17250 is not to be used with removal or excision codes for the same lesion)

Destruction, Malignant Lesions, Any Method

17260   Destruction, malignant lesion (eg, laser surgery, electrosurgery, cryosurgery, chemosurgery, surgical curettement), trunk, arms or legs; lesion diameter 0.5 cm or less

17261   lesion diameter 0.6 to 1.0 cm

17262   lesion diameter 1.1 to 2.0 cm

17263   lesion diameter 2.1 to 3.0 cm

17264   lesion diameter 3.1 to 4.0 cm

17266   lesion diameter over 4.0 cm

17270   Destruction, malignant lesion (eg, laser surgery, electrosurgery, cryosurgery, chemosurgery, surgical curettement), scalp, neck, hands, feet, genitalia; lesion diameter 0.5 cm or less

17271   lesion diameter 0.6 to 1.0 cm

17272   lesion diameter 1.1 to 2.0 cm

17273   lesion diameter 2.1 to 3.0 cm

17274   lesion diameter 3.1 to 4.0 cm

17276   lesion diameter over 4.0 cm

17280   Destruction, malignant lesion (eg, laser surgery, electrosurgery, cryosurgery, chemosurgery, surgical curettement), face, ears, eyelids, nose, lips, mucous membrane; lesion diameter 0.5 cm or less

17281   lesion diameter 0.6 to 1.0 cm

17282   lesion diameter 1.1 to 2.0 cm

17283   lesion diameter 2.1 to 3.0 cm

17284   lesion diameter 3.1 to 4.0 cm

17286   lesion diameter over 4.0 cm

Mohs Micrographic Surgery

▶Mohs micrographic surgery is a technique for the removal of complex or ill-defined skin cancer with histologic examination of 100% of the surgical margins. It requires a single physician to act in two integrated but separate and distinct capacities: surgeon and pathologist. If either of these responsibilities is delegated to another physician who reports the services separately, these codes should not be reported. The Mohs surgeon removes the tumor tissue and maps and divides the tumor specimen into pieces, and each piece is embedded into an individual tissue block for histopathologic examination. Thus a tissue block in Mohs surgery is defined as an individual tissue piece embedded in a mounting medium for sectioning.◀

If repair is performed, use separate repair, flap, or graft codes. If a biopsy of a suspected skin cancer is performed on the same day as Mohs surgery because there was no prior pathology confirmation of a diagnosis, then report diagnostic skin biopsy (11100, 11101) and frozen section pathology (88331) with modifier 59 to distinguish from the subsequent definitive surgical procedure of Mohs surgery.

▶(17304-17310 have been deleted. To report, see 17311-17315)◀

(If additional special pathology procedures, stains or immunostains are required, use 88311-88314, 88342)

▶(Do not report 88314 in conjunction with 17311-17315 for routine frozen section stain (eg, hematoxylin and eosin, toluidine blue) performed during Mohs surgery. When a nonroutine histochemical stain on frozen tissue is utilized, report 88314 with modifier 59)◀

▶(Do not report 88302-88309 on the same specimen as part of the Mohs surgery)◀

● **17311**   Mohs micrographic technique, including removal of all gross tumor, surgical excision of tissue specimens, mapping, color coding of specimens, microscopic examination of specimens by the surgeon, and histopathologic preparation including routine stain(s) (eg, hematoxylin and eosin, toluidine blue), head, neck, hands, feet, genitalia, or any location with surgery directly involving muscle, cartilage, bone, tendon, major nerves, or vessels; first stage, up to 5 tissue blocks

+● **17312**   each additional stage after the first stage, up to 5 tissue blocks (List separately in addition to code for primary procedure)

▶(Use 17312 in conjunction with 17311)◀

Surgery: Integumentary System

● **17313** Mohs micrographic technique, including removal of all gross tumor, surgical excision of tissue specimens, mapping, color coding of specimens, microscopic examination of specimens by the surgeon, and histopathologic preparation including routine stain(s) (eg, hematoxylin and eosin, toluidine blue), of the trunk, arms, or legs; first stage, up to 5 tissue blocks

+● **17314** each additional stage after the first stage, up to 5 tissue blocks (List separately in addition to code for primary procedure)

►(Use 17314 in conjunction with 17313)◄

+● **17315** Mohs micrographic technique, including removal of all gross tumor, surgical excision of tissue specimens, mapping, color coding of specimens, microscopic examination of specimens by the surgeon, and histopathologic preparation including routine stain(s) (eg, hematoxylin and eosin, toluidine blue), each additional block after the first 5 tissue blocks, any stage (List separately in addition to code for primary procedure)

►(Use 17315 in conjunction with 17311-17314)◄

Other Procedures

17340 Cryotherapy (CO_2 slush, liquid N_2) for acne

17360 Chemical exfoliation for acne (eg, acne paste, acid)

17380 Electrolysis epilation, each 30 minutes

(For actinotherapy, use 96900)

17999 Unlisted procedure, skin, mucous membrane and subcutaneous tissue

Breast

Incision

19000 Puncture aspiration of cyst of breast;

+ **19001** each additional cyst (List separately in addition to code for primary procedure)

(Use 19001 in conjunction with 19000)

►(If imaging guidance is performed, see 76942, 77021, 77031, 77032)◄

19020 Mastotomy with exploration or drainage of abscess, deep

19030 Injection procedure only for mammary ductogram or galactogram

►(For radiological supervision and interpretation, see 77053, 77054)◄

(For catheter lavage of mammary ducts for collection of cytology specimens, use Category III codes 0046T, 0047T)

Excision

(To report bilateral procedures, report modifier 50 with the procedure code)

Excisional breast surgery includes certain biopsy procedures, the removal of cysts or other benign or malignant tumors or lesions, and the surgical treatment of breast and chest wall malignancies. Biopsy procedures may be percutaneous or open, and they involve the removal of differing amounts of tissue for diagnosis.

Breast biopsies are reported using codes 19100-19103. The open excision of breast lesions (eg, lesions of the breast ducts, cysts, benign or malignant tumors), without specific attention to adequate surgical margins, with or without the preoperative placement of radiological markers, is reported using codes 19110-19126. Partial mastectomy procedures (eg, lumpectomy, tylectomy, quadrantectomy, or segmentectomy) describe open excisions of breast tissue with specific attention to adequate surgical margins.

Partial mastectomy procedures are reported using codes 19301 or 19302 as appropriate. Documentation for partial mastectomy procedures includes attention to the removal of adequate surgical margins surrounding the breast mass or lesion.

Total mastectomy procedures include simple mastectomy, complete mastectomy, subcutaneous mastectomy, modified radical mastectomy, radical mastectomy, and more extended procedures (eg, Urban type operation). Total mastectomy procedures are reported using codes 19303-19307 as appropriate.

Excisions or resections of chest wall tumors including ribs, with or without reconstruction, with or without mediastinal lymphadenectomy, are reported using codes 19260, 19271, or 19272. Codes 19260-19272 are not restricted to breast tumors and are used to report resections of chest wall tumors originating from any chest wall component. (For excision of lung or pleura, see 32310 et seq.)

19100 Biopsy of breast; percutaneous, needle core, not using imaging guidance (separate procedure)

(For fine needle aspiration, use 10021)

(For image guided breast biopsy, see 19102, 19103, 10022)

19101 open, incisional

19102 percutaneous, needle core, using imaging guidance

(For placement of percutaneous localization clip, use 19295)

19103 percutaneous, automated vacuum assisted or rotating biopsy device, using imaging guidance

►(For imaging guidance performed in conjunction with 19102, 19103, see 76942, 77012, 77021, 77031, 77032)◄

(For placement of percutaneous localization clip, use 19295)

● **19105**   Ablation, cryosurgical, of fibroadenoma, including ultrasound guidance, each fibroadenoma

►(Do not report 19105 in conjunction with 76940, 76942)◄

►(For adjacent lesions treated with one cryoprobe insertion, report once)◄

19110   Nipple exploration, with or without excision of a solitary lactiferous duct or a papilloma lactiferous duct

19112   Excision of lactiferous duct fistula

▲ **19120**   Excision of cyst, fibroadenoma, or other benign or malignant tumor, aberrant breast tissue, duct lesion, nipple or areolar lesion (except 19300), open, male or female, one or more lesions

19125   Excision of breast lesion identified by preoperative placement of radiological marker, open; single lesion

+ **19126**   each additional lesion separately identified by a preoperative radiological marker (List separately in addition to code for primary procedure)

(Use 19126 in conjunction with 19125)

►(19140-19240 have been deleted. To report, see 19300-19307)◄

19260   Excision of chest wall tumor including ribs

19271   Excision of chest wall tumor involving ribs, with plastic reconstruction; without mediastinal lymphadenectomy

19272   with mediastinal lymphadenectomy

(Do not report 19260, 19271, 19272 in conjunction with 32002, 32020, 32100, 32503, 32504)

Introduction

19290   Preoperative placement of needle localization wire, breast;

+ **19291**   each additional lesion (List separately in addition to code for primary procedure)

(Use 19291 in conjunction with 19290)

►(For radiological supervision and interpretation, see 76942, 77031, 77032)◄

+ **19295**   Image guided placement, metallic localization clip, percutaneous, during breast biopsy (List separately in addition to code for primary procedure)

(Use 19295 in conjunction with 19102, 19103)

19296   Placement of radiotherapy afterloading balloon catheter into the breast for interstitial radioelement application following partial mastectomy, includes imaging guidance; on date separate from partial mastectomy

+ **19297**   concurrent with partial mastectomy (List separately in addition to code for primary procedure)

(Use 19297 in conjunction with 19301 or 19302)

⊙ **19298**   Placement of radiotherapy afterloading brachytherapy catheters (multiple tube and button type) into the breast for interstitial radioelement application following (at the time of or subsequent to) partial mastectomy, includes imaging guidance

►Mastectomy Procedures◄

● **19300**   Mastectomy for gynecomastia

● **19301**   Mastectomy, partial (eg, lumpectomy, tylectomy, quadrantectomy, segmentectomy);

● **19302**   with axillary lymphadenectomy

►(For placement of radiotherapy afterloading balloon/brachytherapy catheters, see 19296-19298)◄

● **19303**   Mastectomy, simple, complete

►(For immediate or delayed insertion of implant, see 19340, 19342)◄

►(For gynecomastia, use 19300)◄

● **19304**   Mastectomy, subcutaneous

►(For immediate or delayed insertion of implant, see 19340, 19342)◄

● **19305**   Mastectomy, radical, including pectoral muscles, axillary lymph nodes

►(For immediate or delayed insertion of implant, see 19340, 19342)◄

● **19306**   Mastectomy, radical, including pectoral muscles, axillary and internal mammary lymph nodes (Urban type operation)

►(For immediate or delayed insertion of implant, see 19340, 19342)◄

● **19307**   Mastectomy, modified radical, including axillary lymph nodes, with or without pectoralis minor muscle, but excluding pectoralis major muscle

►(For immediate or delayed insertion of implant, see 19340, 19342)◄

Repair and/or Reconstruction

(To report bilateral procedures, report modifier 50 with the procedure code)

19316   Mastopexy

19318   Reduction mammaplasty

19324   Mammaplasty, augmentation; without prosthetic implant

19325   with prosthetic implant

(For flap or graft, use also appropriate number)

Surgery: Integumentary System

19328	Removal of intact mammary implant
19330	Removal of mammary implant material
19340	Immediate insertion of breast prosthesis following mastopexy, mastectomy or in reconstruction
19342	Delayed insertion of breast prosthesis following mastopexy, mastectomy or in reconstruction

(For supply of implant, use 99070)

(For preparation of custom breast implant, use 19396)

19350	Nipple/areola reconstruction
19355	Correction of inverted nipples
19357	Breast reconstruction, immediate or delayed, with tissue expander, including subsequent expansion
▲ **19361**	Breast reconstruction with latissimus dorsi flap, without prosthetic implant

►(For insertion of prosthesis, use also 19340)◄

19364	Breast reconstruction with free flap

(Do not report code 69990 in addition to code 19364)

(19364 includes harvesting of the flap, microvascular transfer, closure of the donor site, and inset shaping the flap into a breast)

19366	Breast reconstruction with other technique

(For operating microscope, use 69990)

(For insertion of prosthesis, use also 19340 or 19342)

19367	Breast reconstruction with transverse rectus abdominis myocutaneous flap (TRAM), single pedicle, including closure of donor site;
19368	with microvascular anastomosis (supercharging)

(Do not report code 69990 in addition to code 19368)

19369	Breast reconstruction with transverse rectus abdominis myocutaneous flap (TRAM), double pedicle, including closure of donor site
19370	Open periprosthetic capsulotomy, breast
19371	Periprosthetic capsulectomy, breast
19380	Revision of reconstructed breast
19396	Preparation of moulage for custom breast implant

Other Procedures

(For microwave thermotherapy of the breast, use Category III code 0061T)

19499	Unlisted procedure, breast

⊙=Moderate sedation ✚=Add-on code ✗=FDA approval pending

Surgery: Integumentary System

Musculoskeletal System

Cast and strapping procedures appear at the end of this section.

The services listed below include the application and removal of the first cast or traction device only. Subsequent replacement of cast and/or traction device may require an additional listing.

Definitions

The terms "closed treatment," "open treatment," and "percutaneous skeletal fixation" have been carefully chosen to accurately reflect current orthopaedic procedural treatments.

Closed treatment specifically means that the fracture site is not surgically opened (exposed to the external environment and directly visualized). This terminology is used to describe procedures that treat fractures by three methods: 1) without manipulation; 2) with manipulation; or 3) with or without traction.

Open treatment is used when the fractured bone is either: 1) surgically opened (exposed to the external environment) and the fracture (bone ends) visualized and internal fixation may be used; or 2) the fractured bone is opened remote from the fracture site in order to insert an intramedullary nail across the fracture site (the fracture site is not opened and visualized).

Percutaneous skeletal fixation describes fracture treatment which is neither open nor closed. In this procedure, the fracture fragments are not visualized, but fixation (eg, pins) is placed across the fracture site, usually under X-ray imaging.

The type of fracture (eg, open, compound, closed) does not have any coding correlation with the type of treatment (eg, closed, open, or percutaneous) provided.

The codes for treatment of fractures and joint injuries (dislocations) are categorized by the type of manipulation (reduction) and stabilization (fixation or immobilization). These codes can apply to either open (compound) or closed fractures or joint injuries.

Skeletal traction is the application of a force (distracting or traction force) to a limb segment through a wire, pin, screw, or clamp that is attached (eg, penetrates) to bone.

Skin traction is the application of a force (longitudinal) to a limb using felt or strapping applied directly to skin only.

External fixation is the usage of skeletal pins plus an attaching mechanism/device used for temporary or definitive treatment of acute or chronic bony deformity.

Codes for obtaining autogenous bone grafts, cartilage, tendon, fascia lata grafts or other tissues through separate incisions are to be used only when the graft is not already listed as part of the basic procedure.

Re-reduction of a fracture and/or dislocation performed by the primary physician may be identified by the addition of the modifier 76 to the usual procedure number to indicate "Repeat Procedure by Same Physician." (See guidelines.)

Codes for external fixation are to be used only when external fixation is not already listed as part of the basic procedure.

All codes for suction irrigation have been deleted. To report, list only the primary surgical procedure performed (eg, sequestrectomy, deep incision).

Manipulation is used throughout the musculoskeletal fracture and dislocation subsections to specifically mean the attempted reduction or restoration of a fracture or joint dislocation to its normal anatomic alignment by the application of manually applied forces.

(For computer-assisted musculoskeletal surgical navigational orthopedic procedures, report 0054T-0056T)

General

Incision

20000	Incision of soft tissue abscess (eg, secondary to osteomyelitis); superficial
20005	deep or complicated

Wound Exploration—Trauma (eg, Penetrating Gunshot, Stab Wound)

20100-20103 relate to wound(s) resulting from penetrating trauma. These codes describe surgical exploration and enlargement of the wound, extension of dissection (to determine penetration), debridement, removal of foreign body(s), ligation or coagulation of minor subcutaneous and/or muscular blood vessel(s), of the subcutaneous tissue, muscle fascia, and/or muscle, not requiring thoracotomy or laparotomy. If a repair is done to major structure(s) or major blood vessel(s) requiring thoracotomy or laparotomy, then those specific code(s) would supersede the use of codes 20100-20103. To report Simple, Intermediate, or Complex repair of wound(s) that do not require enlargement of the wound, extension of dissection, etc., as stated above, use specific Repair code(s) in the **Integumentary System** section.

20100	Exploration of penetrating wound (separate procedure); neck
20101	chest
20102	abdomen/flank/back
20103	extremity

Excision

20150 Excision of epiphyseal bar, with or without autogenous soft tissue graft obtained through same fascial incision

(For aspiration of bone marrow, use 38220)

20200 Biopsy, muscle; superficial

20205 deep

20206 Biopsy, muscle, percutaneous needle

►(If imaging guidance is performed, see 76942, 77012, 77021)◄

(For fine needle aspiration, use 10021 or 10022)

(For evaulation of fine needle aspirate, see 88172-88173)

(For excision of muscle tumor, deep, see specific anatomic section)

20220 Biopsy, bone, trocar, or needle; superficial (eg, ilium, sternum, spinous process, ribs)

20225 deep (eg, vertebral body, femur)

(For bone marrow biopsy, use 38221)

►(For radiologic supervision and interpretation, see 77002, 77012, 77021)◄

20240 Biopsy, bone, open; superficial (eg, ilium, sternum, spinous process, ribs, trochanter of femur)

20245 deep (eg, humerus, ischium, femur)

20250 Biopsy, vertebral body, open; thoracic

20251 lumbar or cervical

(For sequestrectomy, osteomyelitis or drainage of bone abscess, see anatomical area)

Introduction or Removal

(For injection procedure for arthrography, see anatomical area)

20500 Injection of sinus tract; therapeutic (separate procedure)

20501 diagnostic (sinogram)

(For radiological supervision and interpretation, use 76080)

20520 Removal of foreign body in muscle or tendon sheath; simple

20525 deep or complicated

20526 Injection, therapeutic (eg, local anesthetic, corticosteroid), carpal tunnel

20550 Injection(s); single tendon sheath, or ligament, aponeurosis (eg, plantar "fascia")

20551 single tendon origin/insertion

20552 Injection(s); single or multiple trigger point(s), one or two muscle(s)

20553 single or multiple trigger point(s), three or more muscle(s)

►(If imaging guidance is performed, see 76942, 77002, 77021)◄

20600 Arthrocentesis, aspiration and/or injection; small joint or bursa (eg, fingers, toes)

20605 intermediate joint or bursa (eg, temporomandibular, acromioclavicular, wrist, elbow or ankle, olecranon bursa)

20610 major joint or bursa (eg, shoulder, hip, knee joint, subacromial bursa)

►(If imaging guidance is performed, see 76942, 77002, 77012, 77021)◄

20612 Aspiration and/or injection of ganglion cyst(s) any location

(To report multiple ganglion cyst aspirations/injections, use 20612 and append modifier 59)

20615 Aspiration and injection for treatment of bone cyst

20650 Insertion of wire or pin with application of skeletal traction, including removal (separate procedure)

⊘ **20660** Application of cranial tongs, caliper, or stereotactic frame, including removal (separate procedure)

20661 Application of halo, including removal; cranial

20662 pelvic

20663 femoral

20664 Application of halo, including removal, cranial, 6 or more pins placed, for thin skull osteology (eg, pediatric patients, hydrocephalus, osteogenesis imperfecta), requiring general anesthesia

20665 Removal of tongs or halo applied by another physician

20670 Removal of implant; superficial, (eg, buried wire, pin or rod) (separate procedure)

20680 deep (eg, buried wire, pin, screw, metal band, nail, rod or plate)

⊘ **20690** Application of a uniplane (pins or wires in one plane), unilateral, external fixation system

⊘ **20692** Application of a multiplane (pins or wires in more than one plane), unilateral, external fixation system (eg, Ilizarov, Monticelli type)

20693 Adjustment or revision of external fixation system requiring anesthesia (eg, new pin(s) or wire(s) and/or new ring(s) or bar(s))

20694 Removal, under anesthesia, of external fixation system

Replantation

20802   Replantation, arm (includes surgical neck of humerus through elbow joint), complete amputation

(To report replantation of incomplete arm amputation, see specific code(s) for repair of bone(s), ligament(s), tendon(s), nerve(s), or blood vessel(s) with modifier 52)

20805   Replantation, forearm (includes radius and ulna to radial carpal joint), complete amputation

(To report replantation of incomplete forearm amputation, see specific code(s) for repair of bone(s), ligament(s), tendon(s), nerve(s), or blood vessel(s) with modifier 52)

20808   Replantation, hand (includes hand through metacarpophalangeal joints), complete amputation

(To report replantation of incomplete hand amputation, see specific code(s) for repair of bone(s), ligament(s), tendon(s), nerve(s), or blood vessel(s) with modifier 52)

20816   Replantation, digit, excluding thumb (includes metacarpophalangeal joint to insertion of flexor sublimis tendon), complete amputation

(To report replantation of incomplete digit amputation, excluding thumb, see specific code(s) for repair of bone(s), ligament(s), tendon(s), nerve(s), or blood vessel(s) with modifier 52)

20822   Replantation, digit, excluding thumb (includes distal tip to sublimis tendon insertion), complete amputation

(To report replantation of incomplete digit amputation, excluding thumb, see specific code(s) for repair of bone(s), ligament(s), tendon(s), nerve(s), or blood vessel(s) with modifier 52)

20824   Replantation, thumb (includes carpometacarpal joint to MP joint), complete amputation

(To report replantation of incomplete thumb amputation, see specific code(s) for repair of bone(s), ligament(s), tendon(s), nerve(s), or blood vessel(s) with modifier 52)

20827   Replantation, thumb (includes distal tip to MP joint), complete amputation

(To report replantation of incomplete thumb amputation, see specific code(s) for repair of bone(s), ligament(s), tendon(s), nerve(s), or blood vessel(s) with modifier 52)

(To report replantation of complete leg amputation, see specific code(s) for repair of bone(s), ligament(s), tendon(s), nerve(s), or blood vessel(s) with modifier 52)

(To report replantation of incomplete leg amputation, see specific code(s) for repair of bone(s), ligament(s), tendon(s), nerve(s), or blood vessel(s) with modifier 52)

20838   Replantation, foot, complete amputation

(To report replantation of incomplete foot amputation, see specific code(s) for repair of bone(s), ligament(s), tendon(s), nerve(s), or blood vessel(s) with modifier 52)

Grafts (or Implants)

Codes for obtaining autogenous bone, cartilage, tendon, fascia lata grafts, or other tissues through separate skin/fascial incisions should be reported separately unless the code descriptor references the harvesting of the graft or implant (eg, includes obtaining graft).

Do not append modifier 62 to bone graft codes 20900-20938.

(For spinal surgery bone graft(s) see codes 20930-20938)

⊘ **20900**   Bone graft, any donor area; minor or small (eg, dowel or button)

⊘ **20902**   major or large

⊘ **20910**   Cartilage graft; costochondral

⊘ **20912**   nasal septum

(For ear cartilage, use 21235)

⊘ **20920**   Fascia lata graft; by stripper

⊘ **20922**   by incision and area exposure, complex or sheet

⊘ **20924**   Tendon graft, from a distance (eg, palmaris, toe extensor, plantaris)

⊘ **20926**   Tissue grafts, other (eg, paratenon, fat, dermis)

(Codes 20930-20938 are reported in addition to codes for the definitive procedure(s) without modifier 51)

⊘ **20930**   Allograft for spine surgery only; morselized

⊘ **20931**   structural

⊘ **20936**   Autograft for spine surgery only (includes harvesting the graft); local (eg, ribs, spinous process, or laminar fragments) obtained from same incision

⊘ **20937**   morselized (through separate skin or fascial incision)

⊘ **20938**   structural, bicortical or tricortical (through separate skin or fascial incision)

(For needle aspiration of bone marrow for the purpose of bone grafting, use 38220)

Other Procedures

20950   Monitoring of interstitial fluid pressure (includes insertion of device, eg, wick catheter technique, needle manometer technique) in detection of muscle compartment syndrome

20955   Bone graft with microvascular anastomosis; fibula

20956   iliac crest

20957   metatarsal

20962   other than fibula, iliac crest, or metatarsal

(Do not report code 69990 in addition to codes 20955-20962)

Surgery: Musculoskeletal System

20969 Free osteocutaneous flap with microvascular anastomosis; other than iliac crest, metatarsal, or great toe

20970 iliac crest

20972 metatarsal

20973 great toe with web space

(Do not report code 69990 in addition to codes 20969-20973)

(For great toe, wrap-around procedure, use 26551)

⊘ **20974** Electrical stimulation to aid bone healing; noninvasive (nonoperative)

⊘ **20975** invasive (operative)

20979 Low intensity ultrasound stimulation to aid bone healing, noninvasive (nonoperative)

⊙ **20982** Ablation, bone tumor(s) (eg, osteoid osteoma, metastasis) radiofrequency, percutaneous, including computed tomographic guidance

▶(Do not report 20982 in conjunction with 77013)◀

20999 Unlisted procedure, musculoskeletal system, general

Head

Skull, facial bones, and temporomandibular joint.

Incision

(For drainage of superficial abscess and hematoma, use 20000)

(For removal of embedded foreign body from dentoalveolar structure, see 41805, 41806)

21010 Arthrotomy, temporomandibular joint

(To report bilateral procedures, report 21010 with modifier 50)

Excision

21015 Radical resection of tumor (eg, malignant neoplasm), soft tissue of face or scalp

(To report excision of skull tumor for osteomyelitis, use 61501)

21025 Excision of bone (eg, for osteomyelitis or bone abscess); mandible

21026 facial bone(s)

21029 Removal by contouring of benign tumor of facial bone (eg, fibrous dysplasia)

21030 Excision of benign tumor or cyst of maxilla or zygoma by enucleation and curettage

21031 Excision of torus mandibularis

21032 Excision of maxillary torus palatinus

21034 Excision of malignant tumor of maxilla or zygoma

21040 Excision of benign tumor or cyst of mandible, by enucleation and/or curettage

(For enucleation and/or curettage of benign cysts or tumors of mandible not requiring osteotomy, use 21040)

(For excision of benign tumor or cyst of mandible requiring osteotomy, see 21046-21047)

21044 Excision of malignant tumor of mandible;

21045 radical resection

(For bone graft, use 21215)

21046 Excision of benign tumor or cyst of mandible; requiring intra-oral osteotomy (eg, locally aggressive or destructive lesion(s))

21047 requiring extra-oral osteotomy and partial mandibulectomy (eg, locally aggressive or destructive lesion(s))

21048 Excision of benign tumor or cyst of maxilla; requiring intra-oral osteotomy (eg, locally aggressive or destructive lesion(s))

21049 requiring extra-oral osteotomy and partial maxillectomy (eg, locally aggressive or destructive lesion(s))

21050 Condylectomy, temporomandibular joint (separate procedure)

(For bilateral procedures, report 21050 with modifier 50)

21060 Meniscectomy, partial or complete, temporomandibular joint (separate procedure)

(For bilateral procedures, report 21060 with modifier 50)

21070 Coronoidectomy (separate procedure)

(For bilateral procedures, report 21070 with modifier 50)

▶Head Prosthesis◀

(For application or removal of caliper or tongs, see 20660, 20665.) Codes 21076-21089 describe professional services for the rehabilitation of patients with oral, facial or other anatomical deficiencies by means of prostheses such as an artificial eye, ear, or nose or intraoral obturator to close a cleft. Codes 21076-21089 should only be used when the physician actually designs and prepares the prosthesis (ie, not prepared by an outside laboratory).

21076 Impression and custom preparation; surgical obturator prosthesis

21077 orbital prosthesis

21079 interim obturator prosthesis

21080 definitive obturator prosthesis

21081 mandibular resection prosthesis

21082 palatal augmentation prosthesis

21083 palatal lift prosthesis

21084	speech aid prosthesis
21085	oral surgical splint
21086	auricular prosthesis
21087	nasal prosthesis
21088	facial prosthesis

►Other Procedures◄

21089 Unlisted maxillofacial prosthetic procedure

►Introduction or Removal◄

21100 Application of halo type appliance for maxillofacial fixation, includes removal (separate procedure)

21110 Application of interdental fixation device for conditions other than fracture or dislocation, includes removal

(For removal of interdental fixation by another physician, see 20670-20680)

21116 Injection procedure for temporomandibular joint arthrography

►(For radiological supervision and interpretation, use 70332. Do not report 77002 in conjunction with 70332)◄

Repair, Revision, and/or Reconstruction

(For cranioplasty, see 21179, 21180 and 62116, 62120, 62140-62147)

21120 Genioplasty; augmentation (autograft, allograft, prosthetic material)

21121 sliding osteotomy, single piece

21122 sliding osteotomies, two or more osteotomies (eg, wedge excision or bone wedge reversal for asymmetrical chin)

21123 sliding, augmentation with interpositional bone grafts (includes obtaining autografts)

21125 Augmentation, mandibular body or angle; prosthetic material

21127 with bone graft, onlay or interpositional (includes obtaining autograft)

21137 Reduction forehead; contouring only

21138 contouring and application of prosthetic material or bone graft (includes obtaining autograft)

21139 contouring and setback of anterior frontal sinus wall

21141 Reconstruction midface, LeFort I; single piece, segment movement in any direction (eg, for Long Face Syndrome), without bone graft

21142 two pieces, segment movement in any direction, without bone graft

21143 three or more pieces, segment movement in any direction, without bone graft

21145 single piece, segment movement in any direction, requiring bone grafts (includes obtaining autografts)

21146 two pieces, segment movement in any direction, requiring bone grafts (includes obtaining autografts) (eg, ungrafted unilateral alveolar cleft)

21147 three or more pieces, segment movement in any direction, requiring bone grafts (includes obtaining autografts) (eg, ungrafted bilateral alveolar cleft or multiple osteotomies)

21150 Reconstruction midface, LeFort II; anterior intrusion (eg, Treacher-Collins Syndrome)

21151 any direction, requiring bone grafts (includes obtaining autografts)

21154 Reconstruction midface, LeFort III (extracranial), any type, requiring bone grafts (includes obtaining autografts); without LeFort I

21155 with LeFort I

21159 Reconstruction midface, LeFort III (extra and intracranial) with forehead advancement (eg, mono bloc), requiring bone grafts (includes obtaining autografts); without LeFort I

21160 with LeFort I

21172 Reconstruction superior-lateral orbital rim and lower forehead, advancement or alteration, with or without grafts (includes obtaining autografts)

(For frontal or parietal craniotomy performed for craniosynostosis, use 61556)

21175 Reconstruction, bifrontal, superior-lateral orbital rims and lower forehead, advancement or alteration (eg, plagiocephaly, trigonocephaly, brachycephaly), with or without grafts (includes obtaining autografts)

(For bifrontal craniotomy performed for craniosynostosis, use 61557)

21179 Reconstruction, entire or majority of forehead and/or supraorbital rims; with grafts (allograft or prosthetic material)

21180 with autograft (includes obtaining grafts)

(For extensive craniectomy for multiple suture craniosynostosis, use only 61558 or 61559)

21181 Reconstruction by contouring of benign tumor of cranial bones (eg, fibrous dysplasia), extracranial

21182 Reconstruction of orbital walls, rims, forehead, nasoethmoid complex following intra- and extracranial excision of benign tumor of cranial bone (eg, fibrous dysplasia), with multiple autografts (includes obtaining grafts); total area of bone grafting less than 40 sq cm

21183 total area of bone grafting greater than 40 sq cm but less than 80 sq cm

21184 total area of bone grafting greater than 80 sq cm

(For excision of benign tumor of cranial bones, see 61563, 61564)

21188   Reconstruction midface, osteotomies (other than LeFort type) and bone grafts (includes obtaining autografts)

21193   Reconstruction of mandibular rami, horizontal, vertical, C, or L osteotomy; without bone graft

21194   with bone graft (includes obtaining graft)

21195   Reconstruction of mandibular rami and/or body, sagittal split; without internal rigid fixation

21196   with internal rigid fixation

21198   Osteotomy, mandible, segmental;

21199   with genioglossus advancement

(To report total osteotomy of the maxilla, see 21141-21160)

21206   Osteotomy, maxilla, segmental (eg, Wassmund or Schuchard)

21208   Osteoplasty, facial bones; augmentation (autograft, allograft, or prosthetic implant)

21209   reduction

21210   Graft, bone; nasal, maxillary or malar areas (includes obtaining graft)

(For cleft palate repair, see 42200-42225)

21215   mandible (includes obtaining graft)

21230   Graft; rib cartilage, autogenous, to face, chin, nose or ear (includes obtaining graft)

21235   ear cartilage, autogenous, to nose or ear (includes obtaining graft)

(To report graft augmentation of facial bones, use 21208)

21240   Arthroplasty, temporomandibular joint, with or without autograft (includes obtaining graft)

21242   Arthroplasty, temporomandibular joint, with allograft

21243   Arthroplasty, temporomandibular joint, with prosthetic joint replacement

21244   Reconstruction of mandible, extraoral, with transosteal bone plate (eg, mandibular staple bone plate)

21245   Reconstruction of mandible or maxilla, subperiosteal implant; partial

21246   complete

21247   Reconstruction of mandibular condyle with bone and cartilage autografts (includes obtaining grafts) (eg, for hemifacial microsomia)

21248   Reconstruction of mandible or maxilla, endosteal implant (eg, blade, cylinder); partial

21249   complete

(To report midface reconstruction, see 21141-21160)

21255   Reconstruction of zygomatic arch and glenoid fossa with bone and cartilage (includes obtaining autografts)

21256   Reconstruction of orbit with osteotomies (extracranial) and with bone grafts (includes obtaining autografts) (eg, micro-ophthalmia)

21260   Periorbital osteotomies for orbital hypertelorism, with bone grafts; extracranial approach

21261   combined intra- and extracranial approach

21263   with forehead advancement

21267   Orbital repositioning, periorbital osteotomies, unilateral, with bone grafts; extracranial approach

21268   combined intra- and extracranial approach

21270   Malar augmentation, prosthetic material

(For malar augmentation with bone graft, use 21210)

21275   Secondary revision of orbitocraniofacial reconstruction

21280   Medial canthopexy (separate procedure)

(For medial canthoplasty, use 67950)

21282   Lateral canthopexy

21295   Reduction of masseter muscle and bone (eg, for treatment of benign masseteric hypertrophy); extraoral approach

21296   intraoral approach

Other Procedures

21299   Unlisted craniofacial and maxillofacial procedure

Fracture and/or Dislocation

▶(For operative repair of skull fracture, see 62000-62010)◀

▶(21300 has been deleted)◀

▶(To report closed treatment of skull fracture, use the appropriate Evaluation and Management code)◀

21310   Closed treatment of nasal bone fracture without manipulation

21315   Closed treatment of nasal bone fracture; without stabilization

21320   with stabilization

21325   Open treatment of nasal fracture; uncomplicated

21330   complicated, with internal and/or external skeletal fixation

21335   with concomitant open treatment of fractured septum

21336   Open treatment of nasal septal fracture, with or without stabilization

21337   Closed treatment of nasal septal fracture, with or without stabilization

21338   Open treatment of nasoethmoid fracture; without external fixation

21339   with external fixation

21340   Percutaneous treatment of nasoethmoid complex fracture, with splint, wire or headcap fixation, including repair of canthal ligaments and/or the nasolacrimal apparatus

21343   Open treatment of depressed frontal sinus fracture

21344   Open treatment of complicated (eg, comminuted or involving posterior wall) frontal sinus fracture, via coronal or multiple approaches

21345   Closed treatment of nasomaxillary complex fracture (LeFort II type), with interdental wire fixation or fixation of denture or splint

21346   Open treatment of nasomaxillary complex fracture (LeFort II type); with wiring and/or local fixation

21347   requiring multiple open approaches

21348   with bone grafting (includes obtaining graft)

21355   Percutaneous treatment of fracture of malar area, including zygomatic arch and malar tripod, with manipulation

21356   Open treatment of depressed zygomatic arch fracture (eg, Gillies approach)

21360   Open treatment of depressed malar fracture, including zygomatic arch and malar tripod

21365   Open treatment of complicated (eg, comminuted or involving cranial nerve foramina) fracture(s) of malar area, including zygomatic arch and malar tripod; with internal fixation and multiple surgical approaches

21366   with bone grafting (includes obtaining graft)

21385   Open treatment of orbital floor blowout fracture; transantral approach (Caldwell-Luc type operation)

21386   periorbital approach

21387   combined approach

21390   periorbital approach, with alloplastic or other implant

21395   periorbital approach with bone graft (includes obtaining graft)

21400   Closed treatment of fracture of orbit, except blowout; without manipulation

21401   with manipulation

21406   Open treatment of fracture of orbit, except blowout; without implant

21407   with implant

21408   with bone grafting (includes obtaining graft)

21421   Closed treatment of palatal or maxillary fracture (LeFort I type), with interdental wire fixation or fixation of denture or splint

21422   Open treatment of palatal or maxillary fracture (LeFort I type);

21423   complicated (comminuted or involving cranial nerve foramina), multiple approaches

21431   Closed treatment of craniofacial separation (LeFort III type) using interdental wire fixation of denture or splint

21432   Open treatment of craniofacial separation (LeFort III type); with wiring and/or internal fixation

21433   complicated (eg, comminuted or involving cranial nerve foramina), multiple surgical approaches

21435   complicated, utilizing internal and/or external fixation techniques (eg, head cap, halo device, and/or intermaxillary fixation)

(For removal of internal or external fixation device, use 20670)

21436   complicated, multiple surgical approaches, internal fixation, with bone grafting (includes obtaining graft)

21440   Closed treatment of mandibular or maxillary alveolar ridge fracture (separate procedure)

21445   Open treatment of mandibular or maxillary alveolar ridge fracture (separate procedure)

21450   Closed treatment of mandibular fracture; without manipulation

21451   with manipulation

21452   Percutaneous treatment of mandibular fracture, with external fixation

21453   Closed treatment of mandibular fracture with interdental fixation

21454   Open treatment of mandibular fracture with external fixation

21461   Open treatment of mandibular fracture; without interdental fixation

21462   with interdental fixation

21465   Open treatment of mandibular condylar fracture

21470   Open treatment of complicated mandibular fracture by multiple surgical approaches including internal fixation, interdental fixation, and/or wiring of dentures or splints

21480   Closed treatment of temporomandibular dislocation; initial or subsequent

21485   complicated (eg, recurrent requiring intermaxillary fixation or splinting), initial or subsequent

21490   Open treatment of temporomandibular dislocation

(For interdental wire fixation, use 21497)

(21493 and 21494 have been deleted. To report, use the applicable Evaluation and Management codes)

21495   Open treatment of hyoid fracture

(For laryngoplasty with open reduction of fracture, use 31584)

(To report treatment of closed fracture of larynx, use the applicable Evaluation and Management codes)

21497   Interdental wiring, for condition other than fracture

Surgery: Musculoskeletal System

Other Procedures

21499   Unlisted musculoskeletal procedure, head

(For unlisted craniofacial or maxillofacial procedure, use 21299)

Neck (Soft Tissues) and Thorax

(For cervical spine and back, see 21920 et seq)

(For injection of fracture site or trigger point, use 20550)

Incision

(For incision and drainage of abscess or hematoma, superficial, see 10060, 10140)

21501   Incision and drainage, deep abscess or hematoma, soft tissues of neck or thorax;

(For posterior spine subfascial incision and drainage, see 22010-22015)

21502   with partial rib ostectomy

21510   Incision, deep, with opening of bone cortex (eg, for osteomyelitis or bone abscess), thorax

Excision

(For bone biopsy, see 20220-20251)

21550   Biopsy, soft tissue of neck or thorax

(For needle biopsy of soft tissue, use 20206)

21555   Excision tumor, soft tissue of neck or thorax; subcutaneous

21556   deep, subfascial, intramuscular

21557   Radical resection of tumor (eg, malignant neoplasm), soft tissue of neck or thorax

21600   Excision of rib, partial

(For radical resection of chest wall and rib cage for tumor, use 19260)

(For radical debridement of chest wall and rib cage for injury, see 11040-11044)

21610   Costotransversectomy (separate procedure)

21615   Excision first and/or cervical rib;

21616   with sympathectomy

21620   Ostectomy of sternum, partial

21627   Sternal debridement

(For debridement and closure, use 21750)

21630   Radical resection of sternum;

21632   with mediastinal lymphadenectomy

Repair, Revision, and/or Reconstruction

(For superficial wound, see **Integumentary System** section under Repair—Simple)

21685   Hyoid myotomy and suspension

21700   Division of scalenus anticus; without resection of cervical rib

21705   with resection of cervical rib

21720   Division of sternocleidomastoid for torticollis, open operation; without cast application

(For transection of spinal accessory and cervical nerves, see 63191, 64722)

21725   with cast application

21740   Reconstructive repair of pectus excavatum or carinatum; open

21742   minimally invasive approach (Nuss procedure), without thoracoscopy

21743   minimally invasive approach (Nuss procedure), with thoracoscopy

21750   Closure of median sternotomy separation with or without debridement (separate procedure)

Fracture and/or Dislocation

21800   Closed treatment of rib fracture, uncomplicated, each

21805   Open treatment of rib fracture without fixation, each

21810   Treatment of rib fracture requiring external fixation (flail chest)

21820   Closed treatment of sternum fracture

21825   Open treatment of sternum fracture with or without skeletal fixation

(For sternoclavicular dislocation, see 23520-23532)

Other Procedures

21899   Unlisted procedure, neck or thorax

Back and Flank

Excision

21920   Biopsy, soft tissue of back or flank; superficial

21925   deep

(For needle biopsy of soft tissue, use 20206)

21930   Excision, tumor, soft tissue of back or flank

21935   Radical resection of tumor (eg, malignant neoplasm), soft tissue of back or flank

Surgery: Musculoskeletal System

Spine (Vertebral Column)

Cervical, thoracic, and lumbar spine.

Within the SPINE section, bone grafting procedures are reported separately and in addition to arthrodesis. For bone grafts in other Musculoskeletal sections, see specific code(s) descriptor(s) and/or accompanying guidelines.

To report bone grafts performed after arthrodesis, see codes 20930-20938. Bone graft codes are reported without modifier 51 (multiple procedure). Do not append modifier 62 to bone graft codes 20900-20938.

Example:

Posterior arthrodesis of L5-S1 for degenerative disc disease utilizing morselized autogenous iliac bone graft harvested through a separate fascial incision.

Report as 22612 and 20937.

Within the SPINE section, instrumentation is reported separately and in addition to arthrodesis. To report instrumentation procedures performed with definitive vertebral procedure(s), see codes 22840-22855. Instrumentation procedure codes 22840-22848 and 22851 are reported in addition to the definitive procedure(s) without modifier 51. Modifier 62 may not be appended to the definitive or add-on spinal instrumentation procedure code(s) 22840-22848 and 22850-22852.

Example:

Posterior arthrodesis of L4-S1, utilizing morselized autogenous iliac bone graft harvested through separate fascial incision, and pedicle screw fixation.

Report as 22612, 22614, 22842, and 20937.

Vertebral procedures are sometimes followed by arthrodesis and in addition may include bone grafts and instrumentation.

When arthrodesis is performed in addition to another procedure, the arthrodesis should be reported in addition to the original procedure with modifier 51 (multiple procedures). Examples are after osteotomy, fracture care, vertebral corpectomy and laminectomy. Since bone grafts and instrumentation are never performed without arthrodesis, modifier 51 (multiple procedures) is not used.

Arthrodesis, however, may be performed in the absence of other procedures and therefore when it is combined with another definitive procedure, modifier 51 (multiple procedure) is appropriate.

Example:

Treatment of a burst fracture of L2 by corpectomy followed by arthrodesis of L1-L3, utilizing anterior instrumentation L1-L3 and structural allograft.

Report as 63090, 22558-51, 22585, 22845, and 20931.

When two surgeons work together as primary surgeons performing distinct part(s) of a single reportable procedure, each surgeon should report his/her distinct operative work by appending modifier 62 to the single definitive procedure code. If additional procedure(s) (including add-on procedure(s)) are performed during the same surgical session, separate code(s) may be reported by each co-surgeon, with modifier 62 appended (see Appendix A).

Example:

A 42-year-old male with a history of posttraumatic degenerative disc disease at L3-4 and L4-5 (internal disc disruption) underwent surgical repair. Surgeon A performed an anterior exposure of the spine with mobilization of the great vessels. Surgeon B performed anterior (minimal) discectomy and fusion at L3-4 and L4-5 using anterior interbody technique.

Report surgeon A: 22558 append modifier 62, 22585 append modifier 62
Report surgeon B: 22558 append modifier 62, 22585 append modifier 62, 20931

> (Do not append modifier 62 to bone graft code 20931)
>
> (For injection procedure for myelography, use 62284)
>
> (For injection procedure for discography, see 62290, 62291)
>
> (For injection procedure, chemonucleolysis, single or multiple levels, use 62292)
>
> (For injection procedure for facet joints, see 64470-64476, 64622-64627)
>
> (For needle or trocar biopsy, see 20220-20225)

Incision

22010   Incision and drainage, open, of deep abscess (subfascial), posterior spine; cervical, thoracic, or cervicothoracic

22015   lumbar, sacral, or lumbosacral

> (Do not report 22015 in conjunction with 22010)
>
> (Do not report 22015 in conjunction with instrumentation removal, 10180, 22850, 22852)
>
> (For incision and drainage of abscess or hematoma, superficial, see 10060, 10140)

Surgery: Musculoskeletal System

Excision

For the following codes, when two surgeons work together as primary surgeons performing distinct part(s) of partial vertebral body excision, each surgeon should report his/her distinct operative work by appending modifier 62 to the procedure code. In this situation, modifier 62 may be appended to the procedure code(s) 22100-22102, 22110-22114 and, as appropriate, to the associated additional vertebral segment add-on code(s) 22103, 22116 as long as both surgeons continue to work together as primary surgeons.

(For bone biopsy, see 20220-20251)

(To report soft tissue biopsy of back or flank, see 21920-21925)

(For needle biopsy of soft tissue, use 20206)

(To report excision of soft tissue tumor of back or flank, use 21930)

22100	Partial excision of posterior vertebral component (eg, spinous process, lamina or facet) for intrinsic bony lesion, single vertebral segment; cervical
22101	thoracic
22102	lumbar
+ 22103	each additional segment (List separately in addition to code for primary procedure)

(Use 22103 in conjunction with 22100, 22101, 22102)

22110	Partial excision of vertebral body, for intrinsic bony lesion, without decompression of spinal cord or nerve root(s), single vertebral segment; cervical
22112	thoracic
22114	lumbar
+ 22116	each additional vertebral segment (List separately in addition to code for primary procedure)

(Use 22116 in conjunction with 22110, 22112, 22114)

(For complete or near complete resection of vertebral body, see vertebral corpectomy, 63081-63091)

(For spinal reconstruction with bone graft (autograft, allograft) and/or methylmethacrylate of cervical vertebral body, use 63081 and 22554 and 20931 or 20938)

(For spinal reconstruction with bone graft (autograft, allograft) and/or methylmethacrylate of thoracic vertebral body, use 63085 or 63087 and 22556 and 20931 or 20938)

(For spinal reconstruction with bone graft (autograft, allograft) and/or methylmethacrylate of lumbar vertebral body, use 63087 or 63090 and 22558 and 20931 or 20938)

(For spinal reconstruction following vertebral body resection, use 63082 or 63086 or 63088 or 63091, and 22585)

(For harvest of bone autograft for vertebral reconstruction, see 20931 or 20938)

(For cervical spinal reconstruction with prosthetic replacement of resected vertebral bodies, see codes 63081 and 22554 and 20931 or 20938 and 22851)

(For thoracic spinal reconstruction with prosthetic replacement of resected vertebral bodies, see codes 63085 or 63087 and 22556 and 20931 or 20938 and 22851)

(For lumbar spinal reconstruction with prosthetic replacement of resected vertebral bodies, see codes 63087 or 63090 and 22558, and 20931 or 20938 and 22851)

(For osteotomy of spine, see 22210-22226)

Osteotomy

To report arthrodesis, see codes 22590-22632. (Report in addition to code(s) for the definitive procedure with modifier 51.)

To report instrumentation procedures, see codes 22840-22855. (Report in addition to code(s) for the definitive procedure(s) without modifier 51.) Do not append modifier 62 to spinal instrumentation codes 22840-22848 and 22850-22852.

To report bone graft procedures, see codes 20930-20938. (Report in addition to code(s) for the definitive procedure(s) without modifier 51.) Do not append modifier 62 to bone graft codes 20900-20938.

For the following codes, when two surgeons work together as primary surgeons performing distinct part(s) of an anterior spine osteotomy, each surgeon should report his/her distinct operative work by appending modifier 62 to the procedure code. In this situation, modifier 62 may be appended to the procedure code(s) 22210-22214, 22220-22224 and, as appropriate, to associated additional segment add-on code(s) 22216, 22226 as long as both surgeons continue to work together as primary surgeons.

22210	Osteotomy of spine, posterior or posterolateral approach, one vertebral segment; cervical
22212	thoracic
22214	lumbar
+ 22216	each additional vertebral segment (List separately in addition to primary procedure)

(Use 22216 in conjunction with 22210, 22212, 22214)

22220	Osteotomy of spine, including discectomy, anterior approach, single vertebral segment; cervical
22222	thoracic
22224	lumbar
+ 22226	each additional vertebral segment (List separately in addition to code for primary procedure)

(Use 22226 in conjunction with 22220, 22222, 22224)

(For vertebral corpectomy, see 63081-63091)

Fracture and/or Dislocation

To report arthrodesis, see codes 22590-22632. (Report in addition to code(s) for the definitive procedure with modifier 51.)

To report instrumentation procedures, see codes 22840-22855. (Report in addition to code(s) for the definitive procedure(s) without modifier 51.) Do not append modifier 62 to spinal instrumentation codes 22840-22848 and 22850-22852.

To report bone graft procedures, see codes 20930-20938. (Report in addition to code(s) for the definitive procedure(s) without modifier 51.) Do not append modifier 62 to bone graft codes 20900-20938.

For the following codes, when two surgeons work together as primary surgeons performing distinct part(s) of open fracture and/or dislocation procedure(s), each surgeon should report his/her distinct operative work by appending modifier 62 to the procedure code. In this situation, modifier 62 may be appended to the procedure code(s) 22318-22327 and, as appropriate, the associated additional fracture vertebrae or dislocated segment add-on code 22328 as long as both surgeons continue to work together as primary surgeons.

22305   Closed treatment of vertebral process fracture(s)

22310   Closed treatment of vertebral body fracture(s), without manipulation, requiring and including casting or bracing

22315   Closed treatment of vertebral fracture(s) and/or dislocation(s) requiring casting or bracing, with and including casting and/or bracing, with or without anesthesia, by manipulation or traction

     (For spinal subluxation, use 97140)

22318   Open treatment and/or reduction of odontoid fracture(s) and or dislocation(s) (including os odontoideum), anterior approach, including placement of internal fixation; without grafting

22319   with grafting

22325   Open treatment and/or reduction of vertebral fracture(s) and/or dislocation(s), posterior approach, one fractured vertebrae or dislocated segment; lumbar

22326   cervical

22327   thoracic

+ 22328   each additional fractured vertebrae or dislocated segment (List separately in addition to code for primary procedure)

     (Use 22328 in conjunction with 22325, 22326, 22327)

     (For treatment of vertebral fracture by the anterior approach, see corpectomy 63081-63091, and appropriate arthrodesis, bone graft and instrument codes)

     (For decompression of spine following fracture, see 63001-63091; for arthrodesis of spine following fracture, see 22548-22632)

Manipulation

     (For spinal manipulation without anesthesia, use 97140)

22505   Manipulation of spine requiring anesthesia, any region

Vertebral Body, Embolization or Injection

22520   Percutaneous vertebroplasty, one vertebral body, unilateral or bilateral injection; thoracic

22521   lumbar

+ 22522   each additional thoracic or lumbar vertebral body (List separately in addition to code for primary procedure)

     (Use 22522 in conjunction with 22520, 22521 as appropriate)

     ▶(For radiological supervision and interpretation, see 72291, 72292)◀

22523   Percutaneous vertebral augmentation, including cavity creation (fracture reduction and bone biopsy included when performed) using mechanical device, one vertebral body, unilateral or bilateral cannulation (eg, kyphoplasty); thoracic

22524   lumbar

+ 22525   each additional thoracic or lumbar vertebral body (List separately in addition to code for primary procedure)

     (Do not report 22525 in conjunction with 20225 when performed at the same level as 22523-22525)

     (Use 22525 in conjunction with 22523, 22524)

     ▶(For radiological supervision and interpretation, see 72291, 72292)◀

⊙● **22526**   Percutaneous intradiscal electrothermal annuloplasty, unilateral or bilateral including fluoroscopic guidance; single level

⊙+● **22527**   one or more additional levels (List separately in addition to code for primary procedure)

     ▶(Do not report codes 22526, 22527 in conjunction with 77002, 77003)◀

     ▶(For percutaneous intradiscal annuloplasty using method other than electrothermal, see 0062T, 0063T)◀

Arthrodesis

Arthrodesis may be performed in the absence of other procedures and therefore when it is combined with another definitive procedure (eg, osteotomy, fracture care, vertebral corpectomy or laminectomy), modifier 51 is appropriate. However, arthrodesis codes 22585, 22614, and 22632 are considered add-on procedure codes and should not be used with modifier 51.

To report instrumentation procedures, see 22840-22855. (Codes 22840-22848, 22851 are reported in conjunction with code(s) for the definitive procedure(s) without modifier 51. When instrumentation reinsertion or

---

Surgery: Musculoskeletal System

removal is reported in conjunction with other definitive procedures including arthrodesis, decompression, and exploration of fusion, append modifier 51 to 22849, 22850, 22852, and 22855.) To report exploration of fusion, use 22830. (When exploration is reported in conjunction with other definitive procedures, including arthrodesis and decompression, append modifier 51 to 22830.) Do not append modifier 62 to spinal instrumentation codes 22840-22848 and 22850-22852.

To report bone graft procedures, see codes 20930-20938. (Report in addition to code(s) for the definitive procedure(s) without modifier 51.) Do not append modifier 62 to bone graft codes 20900-20938.

Lateral Extracavitary Approach Technique

22532 Arthrodesis, lateral extracavitary technique, including minimal discectomy to prepare interspace (other than for decompression); thoracic

22533 lumbar

+ 22534 thoracic or lumbar, each additional vertebral segment (List separately in addition to code for primary procedure)

(Use 22534 in conjunction with 22532 and 22533)

Anterior or Anterolateral Approach Technique

Procedure codes 22554-22558 are for SINGLE interspace; for additional interspaces, use 22585. A vertebral interspace is the non-bony compartment between two adjacent vertebral bodies, which contains the intervertebral disc, and includes the nucleus pulposus, annulus fibrosus, and two cartilagenous endplates.

For the following codes, when two surgeons work together as primary surgeons performing distinct part(s) of an anterior interbody arthrodesis, each surgeon should report his/her distinct operative work by appending modifier 62 to the procedure code. In this situation, modifier 62 may be appended to the procedure code(s) 22548-22558 and, as appropriate, to the associated additional interspace add-on code 22585 as long as both surgeons continue to work together as primary surgeons.

22548 Arthrodesis, anterior transoral or extraoral technique, clivus-C1-C2 (atlas-axis), with or without excision of odontoid process

(For intervertebral disc excision by laminotomy or laminectomy, see 63020-63042)

22554 Arthrodesis, anterior interbody technique, including minimal discectomy to prepare interspace (other than for decompression); cervical below C2

22556 thoracic

22558 lumbar

+ 22585 each additional interspace (List separately in addition to code for primary procedure)

(Use 22585 in conjunction with 22554, 22556, 22558)

Posterior, Posterolateral or Lateral Transverse Process Technique

To report instrumentation procedures, see codes 22840-22855. (Report in addition to code(s) for the definitive procedure(s) without modifier 51.) Do not append modifier 62 to spinal instrumentation codes 22840-22848 and 22850-22852.

To report bone graft procedures, see codes 20930-20938. (Report in addition to code(s) for the definitive procedure(s) without modifier 51.) Do not append modifier 62 to bone graft codes 20900-20938.

A vertebral segment describes the basic constituent part into which the spine may be divided. It represents a single complete vertebral bone with its associated articular processes and laminae. A vertebral interspace is the non-bony compartment between two adjacent vertebral bodies which contains the intervertebral disc, and includes the nucleus pulposus, annulus fibrosus, and two cartilagenous endplates.

22590 Arthrodesis, posterior technique, craniocervical (occiput-C2)

22595 Arthrodesis, posterior technique, atlas-axis (C1-C2)

22600 Arthrodesis, posterior or posterolateral technique, single level; cervical below C2 segment

22610 thoracic (with or without lateral transverse technique)

22612 lumbar (with or without lateral transverse technique)

+ 22614 each additional vertebral segment (List separately in addition to code for primary procedure)

(Use 22614 in conjunction with 22600, 22610, 22612)

22630 Arthrodesis, posterior interbody technique, including laminectomy and/or discectomy to prepare interspace (other than for decompression), single interspace; lumbar

+ 22632 each additional interspace (List separately in addition to code for primary procedure)

(Use 22632 in conjunction with 22630)

Spine Deformity (eg, Scoliosis, Kyphosis)

To report instrumentation procedures, see codes 22840-22855. (Report in addition to code(s) for the definitive procedure(s) without modifier 51.) Do not append modifier 62 to spinal instrumentation codes 22840-22848 and 22850-22852.

To report bone graft procedures, see codes 20930-20938. (Report in addition to code(s) for the definitive procedure(s) without modifier 51.) Do not append modifier 62 to bone graft codes 20900-20938.

A vertebral segment describes the basic constituent part into which the spine may be divided. It represents a single complete vertebral bone with its associated articular processes and laminae.

For the following codes, when two surgeons work together as primary surgeons performing distinct part(s) of an arthrodesis for spinal deformity, each surgeon should report his/her distinct operative work by appending modifier 62 to the procedure code. In this situation, modifier 62 may be appended to procedure code(s) 22800-22819 as long as both surgeons continue to work together as primary surgeons.

22800   Arthrodesis, posterior, for spinal deformity, with or without cast; up to 6 vertebral segments

22802   7 to 12 vertebral segments

22804   13 or more vertebral segments

22808   Arthrodesis, anterior, for spinal deformity, with or without cast; 2 to 3 vertebral segments

22810   4 to 7 vertebral segments

22812   8 or more vertebral segments

22818   Kyphectomy, circumferential exposure of spine and resection of vertebral segment(s) (including body and posterior elements); single or 2 segments

22819   3 or more segments

         (To report arthrodesis, see 22800-22804 and add modifier 51)

Exploration

To report instrumentation procedures, see 22840-22855. (Codes 22840-22848, 22851 are reported in conjunction with code(s) for the definitive procedure(s) without modifier 51. When instrumentation reinsertion or removal is reported in conjunction with other definitive procedures including arthrodesis, decompression, and exploration of fusion, append modifier 51 to 22849, 22850, 22852 and 22855.) To report exploration of fusion, see 22830. (When exploration is reported in conjunction with other definitive procedures, including arthrodesis and decompression, append modifier 51 to 22830.)

         (To report bone graft procedures, see 20930-20938)

22830   Exploration of spinal fusion

Spinal Instrumentation

Segmental instrumentation is defined as fixation at each end of the construct and at least one additional interposed bony attachment.

Non-segmental instrumentation is defined as fixation at each end of the construct and may span several vertebral segments without attachment to the intervening segments.

Insertion of spinal instrumentation is reported separately and in addition to arthrodesis. Instrumentation procedure codes 22840-22848, 22851 are reported in addition to the definitive procedure(s) without modifier 51. Do not append modifier 62 to spinal instrumentation codes 22840-22848 and 22850-22852.

To report bone graft procedures, see codes 20930-20938. (Report in addition to code(s) for definitive procedure(s) without modifier 51.) Do not append modifier 62 to bone graft codes 20900-20938.

A vertebral segment describes the basic constituent part into which the spine may be divided. It represents a single complete vertebral bone with its associated articular processes and laminae. A vertebral interspace is the non-bony compartment between two adjacent vertebral bodies, which contains the intervertebral disc, and includes the nucleus pulposus, annulus fibrosus, and two cartilagenous endplates.

▶List 22840-22855 separately, in conjunction with code(s) for fracture, dislocation, arthrodesis or exploration of fusion of the spine 22325-22328, 22532-22534, 22548-22812, and 22830. Codes 22840-22848, 22851 are reported in conjunction with code(s) for the definitive procedure(s) without modifier 51. Codes 22849, 22850, 22852, and 22855 are subject to modifier 51 if reported with other definitive procedure(s), including arthrodesis, decompression, and exploration of fusion. Code 22849 should not be reported with 22850, 22852, and 22855 at the same spinal levels.◀

⊘ **22840**   Posterior non-segmental instrumentation (eg, Harrington rod technique, pedicle fixation across one interspace, atlantoaxial transarticular screw fixation, sublaminar wiring at C1, facet screw fixation)

⊘ **22841**   Internal spinal fixation by wiring of spinous processes

⊘ **22842**   Posterior segmental instrumentation (eg, pedicle fixation, dual rods with multiple hooks and sublaminar wires); 3 to 6 vertebral segments

⊘ **22843**   7 to 12 vertebral segments

⊘ **22844**   13 or more vertebral segments

⊘ **22845**   Anterior instrumentation; 2 to 3 vertebral segments

⊘ **22846**   4 to 7 vertebral segments

⊘ **22847**   8 or more vertebral segments

⊘ **22848**   Pelvic fixation (attachment of caudal end of instrumentation to pelvic bony structures) other than sacrum

22849   Reinsertion of spinal fixation device

22850   Removal of posterior nonsegmental instrumentation (eg, Harrington rod)

⊘ **22851**   Application of intervertebral biomechanical device(s) (eg, synthetic cage(s), threaded bone dowel(s), methylmethacrylate) to vertebral defect or interspace

22852   Removal of posterior segmental instrumentation

22855   Removal of anterior instrumentation

● **22857**   Total disc arthroplasty (artificial disc), anterior approach, including discectomy to prepare interspace (other than for decompression), lumbar, single interspace

▶(Do not report 22857 in conjunction with 22558, 22845, 22851, 49010 when performed at the same level)◀

▶(For additional interspace, use Category III code 0163T)◀

● **22862**   Revision including replacement of total disc arthroplasty (artificial disc) anterior approach, lumbar, single interspace

▶(Do not report 22862 in conjunction with 22558, 22845, 22851, 22865, 49010 when performed at the same level)◀

▶(For additional interspace, use Category III code 0165T)◀

● **22865**   Removal of total disc arthroplasty (artificial disc), anterior approach, lumbar, single interspace

▶(Do not report 22865 in conjunction with 49010)◀

▶(For additional interspace, see Category III code 0164T)◀

▶(22857-22865 include fluoroscopy when performed)◀

▶(For decompression, see 63001-63048)◀

Other Procedures

22899   Unlisted procedure, spine

Abdomen

Excision

22900   Excision, abdominal wall tumor, subfascial (eg, desmoid)

Other Procedures

22999   Unlisted procedure, abdomen, musculoskeletal system

Shoulder

Clavicle, scapula, humerus head and neck, sterno-clavicular joint, acromioclavicular joint and shoulder joint.

Incision

23000   Removal of subdeltoid calcareous deposits, open

(For arthroscopic removal of bursal deposits, use 29999)

23020   Capsular contracture release (eg, Sever type procedure)

(For incision and drainage procedures, superficial, see 10040-10160)

23030   Incision and drainage, shoulder area; deep abscess or hematoma

23031   infected bursa

23035   Incision, bone cortex (eg, osteomyelitis or bone abscess), shoulder area

23040   Arthrotomy, glenohumeral joint, including exploration, drainage, or removal of foreign body

23044   Arthrotomy, acromioclavicular, sternoclavicular joint, including exploration, drainage, or removal of foreign body

Excision

23065   Biopsy, soft tissue of shoulder area; superficial

23066   deep

(For needle biopsy of soft tissue, use 20206)

23075   Excision, soft tissue tumor, shoulder area; subcutaneous

23076   deep, subfascial, or intramuscular

23077   Radical resection of tumor (eg, malignant neoplasm), soft tissue of shoulder area

23100   Arthrotomy, glenohumeral joint, including biopsy

23101   Arthrotomy, acromioclavicular joint or sternoclavicular joint, including biopsy and/or excision of torn cartilage

23105   Arthrotomy; glenohumeral joint, with synovectomy, with or without biopsy

23106   sternoclavicular joint, with synovectomy, with or without biopsy

23107   Arthrotomy, glenohumeral joint, with joint exploration, with or without removal of loose or foreign body

23120   Claviculectomy; partial

(For arthroscopic procedure, use 29824)

23125   total

23130   Acromioplasty or acromionectomy, partial, with or without coracoacromial ligament release

23140   Excision or curettage of bone cyst or benign tumor of clavicle or scapula;

23145   with autograft (includes obtaining graft)

23146   with allograft

23150   Excision or curettage of bone cyst or benign tumor of proximal humerus;

23155   with autograft (includes obtaining graft)

23156   with allograft

23170   Sequestrectomy (eg, for osteomyelitis or bone abscess), clavicle

23172   Sequestrectomy (eg, for osteomyelitis or bone abscess), scapula

23174   Sequestrectomy (eg, for osteomyelitis or bone abscess), humeral head to surgical neck

23180   Partial excision (craterization, saucerization, or diaphysectomy) bone (eg, osteomyelitis), clavicle

23182   Partial excision (craterization, saucerization, or diaphysectomy) bone (eg, osteomyelitis), scapula

23184   Partial excision (craterization, saucerization, or diaphysectomy) bone (eg, osteomyelitis), proximal humerus

23190   Ostectomy of scapula, partial (eg, superior medial angle)

23195   Resection, humeral head

(For replacement with implant, use 23470)

23200   Radical resection for tumor; clavicle

23210   scapula

23220   Radical resection of bone tumor, proximal humerus;

23221   with autograft (includes obtaining graft)

23222   with prosthetic replacement

Introduction or Removal

(For arthrocentesis or needling of bursa, use 20610)

(For K-wire or pin insertion or removal, see 20650, 20670, 20680)

23330   Removal of foreign body, shoulder; subcutaneous

23331   deep (eg, Neer hemiarthroplasty removal)

23332   complicated (eg, total shoulder)

23350   Injection procedure for shoulder arthrography or enhanced CT/MRI shoulder arthrography

►(For radiographic arthrography, radiological supervision and interpretation, use 73040. Fluoroscopy [77002] is inclusive of radiographic arthrography)◄

►(When fluoroscopic guided injection is performed for enhanced CT arthrography, use 23350, 77002, and 73201 or 73202)◄

►(When fluoroscopic guided injection is performed for enhanced MR arthrography, use 23350, 77002, and 73222 or 73223)◄

►(For enhanced CT or enhanced MRI arthrography, use 77002 and either 73201, 73202, 73222, or 73223)◄

(To report biopsy of the shoulder and joint, see 29805-29826)

Repair, Revision, and/or Reconstruction

23395   Muscle transfer, any type, shoulder or upper arm; single

23397   multiple

23400   Scapulopexy (eg, Sprengels deformity or for paralysis)

23405   Tenotomy, shoulder area; single tendon

23406   multiple tendons through same incision

23410   Repair of ruptured musculotendinous cuff (eg, rotator cuff) open; acute

23412   chronic

(For arthroscopic procedure, use 29827)

23415   Coracoacromial ligament release, with or without acromioplasty

(For arthroscopic procedure, use 29826)

23420   Reconstruction of complete shoulder (rotator) cuff avulsion, chronic (includes acromioplasty)

23430   Tenodesis of long tendon of biceps

23440   Resection or transplantation of long tendon of biceps

23450   Capsulorrhaphy, anterior; Putti-Platt procedure or Magnuson type operation

(To report arthroscopic thermal capsulorrhaphy, use 29999)

23455   with labral repair (eg, Bankart procedure)

(For arthroscopic procedure, use 29806)

23460   Capsulorrhaphy, anterior, any type; with bone block

23462   with coracoid process transfer

(To report open thermal capsulorrhaphy, use 23929)

23465   Capsulorrhaphy, glenohumeral joint, posterior, with or without bone block

(For sternoclavicular and acromioclavicular reconstruction, see 23530, 23550)

23466   Capsulorrhaphy, glenohumeral joint, any type multi-directional instability

23470   Arthroplasty, glenohumeral joint; hemiarthroplasty

23472   total shoulder (glenoid and proximal humeral replacement (eg, total shoulder))

(For removal of total shoulder implants, see 23331, 23332)

(For osteotomy, proximal humerus, use 24400)

23480   Osteotomy, clavicle, with or without internal fixation;

23485   with bone graft for nonunion or malunion (includes obtaining graft and/or necessary fixation)

23490   Prophylactic treatment (nailing, pinning, plating or wiring) with or without methylmethacrylate; clavicle

23491   proximal humerus

Fracture and/or Dislocation

23500   Closed treatment of clavicular fracture; without manipulation

23505   with manipulation

23515   Open treatment of clavicular fracture, with or without internal or external fixation

23520   Closed treatment of sternoclavicular dislocation; without manipulation

23525   with manipulation

23530   Open treatment of sternoclavicular dislocation, acute or chronic;

23532   with fascial graft (includes obtaining graft)

23540   Closed treatment of acromioclavicular dislocation; without manipulation

23545   with manipulation

23550   Open treatment of acromioclavicular dislocation, acute or chronic;

23552   with fascial graft (includes obtaining graft)

23570   Closed treatment of scapular fracture; without manipulation

23575   with manipulation, with or without skeletal traction (with or without shoulder joint involvement)

23585   Open treatment of scapular fracture (body, glenoid or acromion) with or without internal fixation

23600   Closed treatment of proximal humeral (surgical or anatomical neck) fracture; without manipulation

23605   with manipulation, with or without skeletal traction

23615   Open treatment of proximal humeral (surgical or anatomical neck) fracture, with or without internal or external fixation, with or without repair of tuberosity(s);

23616   with proximal humeral prosthetic replacement

23620   Closed treatment of greater humeral tuberosity fracture; without manipulation

23625   with manipulation

23630   Open treatment of greater humeral tuberosity fracture, with or without internal or external fixation

23650   Closed treatment of shoulder dislocation, with manipulation; without anesthesia

23655   requiring anesthesia

23660   Open treatment of acute shoulder dislocation

(Repairs for recurrent dislocations, see 23450-23466)

23665   Closed treatment of shoulder dislocation, with fracture of greater humeral tuberosity, with manipulation

23670   Open treatment of shoulder dislocation, with fracture of greater humeral tuberosity, with or without internal or external fixation

23675   Closed treatment of shoulder dislocation, with surgical or anatomical neck fracture, with manipulation

23680   Open treatment of shoulder dislocation, with surgical or anatomical neck fracture, with or without internal or external fixation

Manipulation

23700   Manipulation under anesthesia, shoulder joint, including application of fixation apparatus (dislocation excluded)

Arthrodesis

23800   Arthrodesis, glenohumeral joint;

23802   with autogenous graft (includes obtaining graft)

Amputation

23900   Interthoracoscapular amputation (forequarter)

23920   Disarticulation of shoulder;

23921   secondary closure or scar revision

Other Procedures

23929   Unlisted procedure, shoulder

Humerus (Upper Arm) and Elbow

Elbow area includes head and neck of radius and olecranon process.

Incision

(For incision and drainage procedures, superficial, see 10040-10160)

23930   Incision and drainage, upper arm or elbow area; deep abscess or hematoma

23931   bursa

23935   Incision, deep, with opening of bone cortex (eg, for osteomyelitis or bone abscess), humerus or elbow

24000   Arthrotomy, elbow, including exploration, drainage, or removal of foreign body

24006   Arthrotomy of the elbow, with capsular excision for capsular release (separate procedure)

Excision

24065   Biopsy, soft tissue of upper arm or elbow area; superficial

24066   deep (subfascial or intramuscular)

(For needle biopsy of soft tissue, use 20206)

24075   Excision, tumor, soft tissue of upper arm or elbow area; subcutaneous

24076   deep (subfascial or intramuscular)

24077   Radical resection of tumor (eg, malignant neoplasm), soft tissue of upper arm or elbow area

24100 Arthrotomy, elbow; with synovial biopsy only

24101   with joint exploration, with or without biopsy, with or without removal of loose or foreign body

24102   with synovectomy

24105 Excision, olecranon bursa

24110 Excision or curettage of bone cyst or benign tumor, humerus;

24115   with autograft (includes obtaining graft)

24116   with allograft

24120 Excision or curettage of bone cyst or benign tumor of head or neck of radius or olecranon process;

24125   with autograft (includes obtaining graft)

24126   with allograft

24130 Excision, radial head

(For replacement with implant, use 24366)

24134 Sequestrectomy (eg, for osteomyelitis or bone abscess), shaft or distal humerus

24136 Sequestrectomy (eg, for osteomyelitis or bone abscess), radial head or neck

24138 Sequestrectomy (eg, for osteomyelitis or bone abscess), olecranon process

24140 Partial excision (craterization, saucerization, or diaphysectomy) bone (eg, osteomyelitis), humerus

24145 Partial excision (craterization, saucerization, or diaphysectomy) bone (eg, osteomyelitis), radial head or neck

24147 Partial excision (craterization, saucerization, or diaphysectomy) bone (eg, osteomyelitis), olecranon process

24149 Radical resection of capsule, soft tissue, and heterotopic bone, elbow, with contracture release (separate procedure)

(For capsular and soft tissue release only, use 24006)

24150 Radical resection for tumor, shaft or distal humerus;

24151   with autograft (includes obtaining graft)

24152 Radical resection for tumor, radial head or neck;

24153   with autograft (includes obtaining graft)

24155 Resection of elbow joint (arthrectomy)

Introduction or Removal

(For K-wire or pin insertion or removal, see 20650, 20670, 20680)

(For arthrocentesis or needling of bursa or joint, use 20605)

24160 Implant removal; elbow joint

24164   radial head

24200 Removal of foreign body, upper arm or elbow area; subcutaneous

24201   deep (subfascial or intramuscular)

24220 Injection procedure for elbow arthrography

▶(For radiological supervision and interpretation, use 73085. Do not report 77002 in conjunction with 73085)◀

(For injection for tennis elbow, use 20550)

Repair, Revision, and/or Reconstruction

24300 Manipulation, elbow, under anesthesia

(For application of external fixation, see 20690 or 20692)

24301 Muscle or tendon transfer, any type, upper arm or elbow, single (excluding 24320-24331)

24305 Tendon lengthening, upper arm or elbow, each tendon

24310 Tenotomy, open, elbow to shoulder, each tendon

24320 Tenoplasty, with muscle transfer, with or without free graft, elbow to shoulder, single (Seddon-Brookes type procedure)

24330 Flexor-plasty, elbow (eg, Steindler type advancement);

24331   with extensor advancement

24332 Tenolysis, triceps

24340 Tenodesis of biceps tendon at elbow (separate procedure)

24341 Repair, tendon or muscle, upper arm or elbow, each tendon or muscle, primary or secondary (excludes rotator cuff)

24342 Reinsertion of ruptured biceps or triceps tendon, distal, with or without tendon graft

24343 Repair lateral collateral ligament, elbow, with local tissue

24344 Reconstruction lateral collateral ligament, elbow, with tendon graft (includes harvesting of graft)

24345 Repair medial collateral ligament, elbow, with local tissue

24346 Reconstruction medial collateral ligament, elbow, with tendon graft (includes harvesting of graft)

24350 Fasciotomy, lateral or medial (eg, tennis elbow or epicondylitis);

24351   with extensor origin detachment

24352   with annular ligament resection

24354   with stripping

24356   with partial ostectomy

24360 Arthroplasty, elbow; with membrane (eg, fascial)

24361   with distal humeral prosthetic replacement

24362   with implant and fascia lata ligament reconstruction

24363   with distal humerus and proximal ulnar prosthetic replacement (eg, total elbow)

Surgery: Musculoskeletal System

24365   Arthroplasty, radial head;

24366   with implant

24400   Osteotomy, humerus, with or without internal fixation

24410   Multiple osteotomies with realignment on intramedullary rod, humeral shaft (Sofield type procedure)

24420   Osteoplasty, humerus (eg, shortening or lengthening) (excluding 64876)

24430   Repair of nonunion or malunion, humerus; without graft (eg, compression technique)

24435   with iliac or other autograft (includes obtaining graft)

(For proximal radius and/or ulna, see 25400-25420)

24470   Hemiepiphyseal arrest (eg, cubitus varus or valgus, distal humerus)

24495   Decompression fasciotomy, forearm, with brachial artery exploration

24498   Prophylactic treatment (nailing, pinning, plating or wiring), with or without methylmethacrylate, humeral shaft

Fracture and/or Dislocation

24500   Closed treatment of humeral shaft fracture; without manipulation

24505   with manipulation, with or without skeletal traction

24515   Open treatment of humeral shaft fracture with plate/screws, with or without cerclage

24516   Treatment of humeral shaft fracture, with insertion of intramedullary implant, with or without cerclage and/or locking screws

24530   Closed treatment of supracondylar or transcondylar humeral fracture, with or without intercondylar extension; without manipulation

24535   with manipulation, with or without skin or skeletal traction

24538   Percutaneous skeletal fixation of supracondylar or transcondylar humeral fracture, with or without intercondylar extension

24545   Open treatment of humeral supracondylar or transcondylar fracture, with or without internal or external fixation; without intercondylar extension

24546   with intercondylar extension

24560   Closed treatment of humeral epicondylar fracture, medial or lateral; without manipulation

24565   with manipulation

24566   Percutaneous skeletal fixation of humeral epicondylar fracture, medial or lateral, with manipulation

24575   Open treatment of humeral epicondylar fracture, medial or lateral, with or without internal or external fixation

24576   Closed treatment of humeral condylar fracture, medial or lateral; without manipulation

24577   with manipulation

24579   Open treatment of humeral condylar fracture, medial or lateral, with or without internal or external fixation

(To report closed treatment of fractures without manipulation, see 24530, 24560, 24576, 24650, 24670)

(To report closed treatment of fractures with manipulation, see 24535, 24565, 24577, 24675)

24582   Percutaneous skeletal fixation of humeral condylar fracture, medial or lateral, with manipulation

24586   Open treatment of periarticular fracture and/or dislocation of the elbow (fracture distal humerus and proximal ulna and/or proximal radius);

24587   with implant arthroplasty

(See also 24361)

24600   Treatment of closed elbow dislocation; without anesthesia

24605   requiring anesthesia

24615   Open treatment of acute or chronic elbow dislocation

24620   Closed treatment of Monteggia type of fracture dislocation at elbow (fracture proximal end of ulna with dislocation of radial head), with manipulation

24635   Open treatment of Monteggia type of fracture dislocation at elbow (fracture proximal end of ulna with dislocation of radial head), with or without internal or external fixation

24640   Closed treatment of radial head subluxation in child, nursemaid elbow, with manipulation

24650   Closed treatment of radial head or neck fracture; without manipulation

24655   with manipulation

24665   Open treatment of radial head or neck fracture, with or without internal fixation or radial head excision;

24666   with radial head prosthetic replacement

24670   Closed treatment of ulnar fracture, proximal end (olecranon process); without manipulation

24675   with manipulation

24685   Open treatment of ulnar fracture proximal end (olecranon process), with or without internal or external fixation

Arthrodesis

24800   Arthrodesis, elbow joint; local

24802   with autogenous graft (includes obtaining graft)

Surgery: Musculoskeletal System

Amputation

24900   Amputation, arm through humerus; with primary closure

24920   open, circular (guillotine)

24925   secondary closure or scar revision

24930   re-amputation

24931   with implant

24935   Stump elongation, upper extremity

24940   Cineplasty, upper extremity, complete procedure

Other Procedures

24999   Unlisted procedure, humerus or elbow

Forearm and Wrist

Radius, ulna, carpal bones, and joints.

Incision

25000   Incision, extensor tendon sheath, wrist (eg, deQuervains disease)

(For decompression median nerve or for carpal tunnel syndrome, use 64721)

25001   Incision, flexor tendon sheath, wrist (eg, flexor carpi radialis)

25020   Decompression fasciotomy, forearm and/or wrist, flexor OR extensor compartment; without debridement of nonviable muscle and/or nerve

25023   with debridement of nonviable muscle and/or nerve

(For decompression fasciotomy with brachial artery exploration, use 24495)

(For incision and drainage procedures, superficial, see 10060-10160)

(For debridement, see also 11000-11044)

25024   Decompression fasciotomy, forearm and/or wrist, flexor AND extensor compartment; without debridement of nonviable muscle and/or nerve

25025   with debridement of nonviable muscle and/or nerve

25028   Incision and drainage, forearm and/or wrist; deep abscess or hematoma

25031   bursa

25035   Incision, deep, bone cortex, forearm and/or wrist (eg, osteomyelitis or bone abscess)

25040   Arthrotomy, radiocarpal or midcarpal joint, with exploration, drainage, or removal of foreign body

Excision

25065   Biopsy, soft tissue of forearm and/or wrist; superficial

25066   deep (subfascial or intramuscular)

(For needle biopsy of soft tissue, use 20206)

25075   Excision, tumor, soft tissue of forearm and/or wrist area; subcutaneous

25076   deep (subfascial or intramuscular)

25077   Radical resection of tumor (eg, malignant neoplasm), soft tissue of forearm and/or wrist area

25085   Capsulotomy, wrist (eg, contracture)

25100   Arthrotomy, wrist joint; with biopsy

25101   with joint exploration, with or without biopsy, with or without removal of loose or foreign body

25105   with synovectomy

25107   Arthrotomy, distal radioulnar joint including repair of triangular cartilage, complex

● **25109**   Excision of tendon, forearm and/or wrist, flexor or extensor, each

25110   Excision, lesion of tendon sheath, forearm and/or wrist

25111   Excision of ganglion, wrist (dorsal or volar); primary

25112   recurrent

(For hand or finger, use 26160)

25115   Radical excision of bursa, synovia of wrist, or forearm tendon sheaths (eg, tenosynovitis, fungus, Tbc, or other granulomas, rheumatoid arthritis); flexors

25116   extensors, with or without transposition of dorsal retinaculum

(For finger synovectomies, use 26145)

25118   Synovectomy, extensor tendon sheath, wrist, single compartment;

25119   with resection of distal ulna

25120   Excision or curettage of bone cyst or benign tumor of radius or ulna (excluding head or neck of radius and olecranon process);

(For head or neck of radius or olecranon process, see 24120-24126)

25125   with autograft (includes obtaining graft)

25126   with allograft

25130   Excision or curettage of bone cyst or benign tumor of carpal bones;

25135   with autograft (includes obtaining graft)

25136   with allograft

25145   Sequestrectomy (eg, for osteomyelitis or bone abscess), forearm and/or wrist

Surgery: Musculoskeletal System

25150 Partial excision (craterization, saucerization, or diaphysectomy) of bone (eg, for osteomyelitis); ulna

25151 radius

(For head or neck of radius or olecranon process, see 24145, 24147)

25170 Radical resection for tumor, radius or ulna

25210 Carpectomy; one bone

(For carpectomy with implant, see 25441-25445)

25215 all bones of proximal row

25230 Radial styloidectomy (separate procedure)

25240 Excision distal ulna partial or complete (eg, Darrach type or matched resection)

(For implant replacement, distal ulna, use 25442)

(For obtaining fascia for interposition, see 20920, 20922)

Introduction or Removal

(For K-wire, pin or rod insertion or removal, see 20650, 20670, 20680)

25246 Injection procedure for wrist arthrography

▶(For radiological supervision and interpretation, use 73115. Do not report 77002 in conjunction with 73115)◀

(For foreign body removal, superficial use 20520)

25248 Exploration with removal of deep foreign body, forearm or wrist

25250 Removal of wrist prosthesis; (separate procedure)

25251 complicated, including total wrist

25259 Manipulation, wrist, under anesthesia

(For application of external fixation, see 20690 or 20692)

Repair, Revision, and/or Reconstruction

25260 Repair, tendon or muscle, flexor, forearm and/or wrist; primary, single, each tendon or muscle

25263 secondary, single, each tendon or muscle

25265 secondary, with free graft (includes obtaining graft), each tendon or muscle

25270 Repair, tendon or muscle, extensor, forearm and/or wrist; primary, single, each tendon or muscle

25272 secondary, single, each tendon or muscle

25274 secondary, with free graft (includes obtaining graft), each tendon or muscle

25275 Repair, tendon sheath, extensor, forearm and/or wrist, with free graft (includes obtaining graft) (eg, for extensor carpi ulnaris subluxation)

25280 Lengthening or shortening of flexor or extensor tendon, forearm and/or wrist, single, each tendon

25290 Tenotomy, open, flexor or extensor tendon, forearm and/or wrist, single, each tendon

25295 Tenolysis, flexor or extensor tendon, forearm and/or wrist, single, each tendon

25300 Tenodesis at wrist; flexors of fingers

25301 extensors of fingers

25310 Tendon transplantation or transfer, flexor or extensor, forearm and/or wrist, single; each tendon

25312 with tendon graft(s) (includes obtaining graft), each tendon

25315 Flexor origin slide (eg, for cerebral palsy, Volkmann contracture), forearm and/or wrist;

25316 with tendon(s) transfer

25320 Capsulorrhaphy or reconstruction, wrist, open (eg, capsulodesis, ligament repair, tendon transfer or graft) (includes synovectomy, capsulotomy and open reduction) for carpal instability

25332 Arthroplasty, wrist, with or without interposition, with or without external or internal fixation

(For obtaining fascia for interposition, see 20920, 20922)

(For prosthetic replacement arthroplasty, see 25441-25446)

25335 Centralization of wrist on ulna (eg, radial club hand)

25337 Reconstruction for stabilization of unstable distal ulna or distal radioulnar joint, secondary by soft tissue stabilization (eg, tendon transfer, tendon graft or weave, or tenodesis) with or without open reduction of distal radioulnar joint

(For harvesting of fascia lata graft, see 20920, 20922)

25350 Osteotomy, radius; distal third

25355 middle or proximal third

25360 Osteotomy; ulna

25365 radius AND ulna

25370 Multiple osteotomies, with realignment on intramedullary rod (Sofield type procedure); radius OR ulna

25375 radius AND ulna

25390 Osteoplasty, radius OR ulna; shortening

25391 lengthening with autograft

25392 Osteoplasty, radius AND ulna; shortening (excluding 64876)

25393 lengthening with autograft

25394 Osteoplasty, carpal bone, shortening

25400   Repair of nonunion or malunion, radius OR ulna; without graft (eg, compression technique)

25405   with autograft (includes obtaining graft)

25415   Repair of nonunion or malunion, radius AND ulna; without graft (eg, compression technique)

25420   with autograft (includes obtaining graft)

25425   Repair of defect with autograft; radius OR ulna

25426   radius AND ulna

25430   Insertion of vascular pedicle into carpal bone (eg, Hori procedure)

25431   Repair of nonunion of carpal bone (excluding carpal scaphoid (navicular)) (includes obtaining graft and necessary fixation), each bone

25440   Repair of nonunion, scaphoid carpal (navicular) bone, with or without radial styloidectomy (includes obtaining graft and necessary fixation)

25441   Arthroplasty with prosthetic replacement; distal radius

25442   distal ulna

25443   scaphoid carpal (navicular)

25444   lunate

25445   trapezium

25446   distal radius and partial or entire carpus (total wrist)

25447   Arthroplasty, interposition, intercarpal or carpometacarpal joints

(For wrist arthroplasty, use 25332)

25449   Revision of arthroplasty, including removal of implant, wrist joint

25450   Epiphyseal arrest by epiphysiodesis or stapling; distal radius OR ulna

25455   distal radius AND ulna

25490   Prophylactic treatment (nailing, pinning, plating or wiring) with or without methylmethacrylate; radius

25491   ulna

25492   radius AND ulna

Fracture and/or Dislocation

►(For application of external fixation in addition to internal fixation, use 20690 and the appropriate internal fixation code)◄

25500   Closed treatment of radial shaft fracture; without manipulation

25505   with manipulation

25515   Open treatment of radial shaft fracture, with or without internal or external fixation

25520   Closed treatment of radial shaft fracture and closed treatment of dislocation of distal radioulnar joint (Galeazzi fracture/dislocation)

25525   Open treatment of radial shaft fracture, with internal and/or external fixation and closed treatment of dislocation of distal radioulnar joint (Galeazzi fracture/dislocation), with or without percutaneous skeletal fixation

25526   Open treatment of radial shaft fracture, with internal and/or external fixation and open treatment, with or without internal or external fixation of distal radioulnar joint (Galeazzi fracture/dislocation), includes repair of triangular fibrocartilage complex

25530   Closed treatment of ulnar shaft fracture; without manipulation

25535   with manipulation

25545   Open treatment of ulnar shaft fracture, with or without internal or external fixation

25560   Closed treatment of radial and ulnar shaft fractures; without manipulation

25565   with manipulation

25574   Open treatment of radial AND ulnar shaft fractures, with internal or external fixation; of radius OR ulna

25575   of radius AND ulna

▲ **25600**   Closed treatment of distal radial fracture (eg, Colles or Smith type) or epiphyseal separation, includes closed treatment of fracture of ulnar styloid, when performed; without manipulation

25605   with manipulation

►(Do not report 25600, 25605 in conjunction with 25650)◄

● **25606**   Percutaneous skeletal fixation of distal radial fracture or epiphyseal separation

►(Do not report 25606 in conjunction with 25650)◄

►(For percutaneous treatment of ulnar styloid fracture, use 25651)◄

►(For open treatment of ulnar styloid fracture, use 25652)◄

● **25607**   Open treatment of distal radial extra-articular fracture or epiphyseal separation, with internal fixation

►(Do not report 25607 in conjunction with 25650)◄

►(For percutaneous treatment of ulnar styloid fracture, use 25651)◄

►(For open treatment of ulnar styloid fracture, use 25652)◄

Surgery: Musculoskeletal System

● **25608**   Open treatment of distal radial intra-articular fracture or epiphyseal separation; with internal fixation of 2 fragments

►(Do not report 25608 in conjunction with 25609)◄

● **25609**   with internal fixation of 3 or more fragments

►(Do not report 25608, 25609 in conjunction with 25650)◄

►(For percutaneous treatment of ulnar styloid fracture, use 25651)◄

►(For open treatment of ulnar styloid fracture, use 25652)◄

►(25611 has been deleted. To report, use 25606)◄

►(25620 has been deleted. To report, see 25607-25609)◄

25622   Closed treatment of carpal scaphoid (navicular) fracture; without manipulation

25624   with manipulation

25628   Open treatment of carpal scaphoid (navicular) fracture, with or without internal or external fixation

25630   Closed treatment of carpal bone fracture (excluding carpal scaphoid (navicular)); without manipulation, each bone

25635   with manipulation, each bone

25645   Open treatment of carpal bone fracture (other than carpal scaphoid (navicular)), each bone

25650   Closed treatment of ulnar styloid fracture

►(Do not report 25650 in conjunction with 25600, 25605, 25607-25609)◄

25651   Percutaneous skeletal fixation of ulnar styloid fracture

25652   Open treatment of ulnar styloid fracture

25660   Closed treatment of radiocarpal or intercarpal dislocation, one or more bones, with manipulation

25670   Open treatment of radiocarpal or intercarpal dislocation, one or more bones

25671   Percutaneous skeletal fixation of distal radioulnar dislocation

25675   Closed treatment of distal radioulnar dislocation with manipulation

25676   Open treatment of distal radioulnar dislocation, acute or chronic

25680   Closed treatment of trans-scaphoperilunar type of fracture dislocation, with manipulation

25685   Open treatment of trans-scaphoperilunar type of fracture dislocation

25690   Closed treatment of lunate dislocation, with manipulation

25695   Open treatment of lunate dislocation

Arthrodesis

25800   Arthrodesis, wrist; complete, without bone graft (includes radiocarpal and/or intercarpal and/or carpometacarpal joints)

25805   with sliding graft

25810   with iliac or other autograft (includes obtaining graft)

25820   Arthrodesis, wrist; limited, without bone graft (eg, intercarpal or radiocarpal)

25825   with autograft (includes obtaining graft)

25830   Arthrodesis, distal radioulnar joint with segmental resection of ulna, with or without bone graft (eg, Sauve-Kapandji procedure)

Amputation

25900   Amputation, forearm, through radius and ulna;

25905   open, circular (guillotine)

25907   secondary closure or scar revision

25909   re-amputation

25915   Krukenberg procedure

25920   Disarticulation through wrist;

25922   secondary closure or scar revision

25924   re-amputation

25927   Transmetacarpal amputation;

25929   secondary closure or scar revision

25931   re-amputation

Other Procedures

25999   Unlisted procedure, forearm or wrist

Hand and Fingers

Incision

26010   Drainage of finger abscess; simple

26011   complicated (eg, felon)

26020   Drainage of tendon sheath, digit and/or palm, each

26025   Drainage of palmar bursa; single, bursa

26030   multiple bursa

26034   Incision, bone cortex, hand or finger (eg, osteomyelitis or bone abscess)

26035   Decompression fingers and/or hand, injection injury (eg, grease gun)

26037   Decompressive fasciotomy, hand (excludes 26035)

(For injection injury, use 26035)

26040   Fasciotomy, palmar (eg, Dupuytren's contracture); percutaneous

26045   open, partial

            (For fasciectomy, see 26121-26125)

26055   Tendon sheath incision (eg, for trigger finger)

26060   Tenotomy, percutaneous, single, each digit

26070   Arthrotomy, with exploration, drainage, or removal of loose or foreign body; carpometacarpal joint

26075   metacarpophalangeal joint, each

26080   interphalangeal joint, each

Excision

26100   Arthrotomy with biopsy; carpometacarpal joint, each

26105   metacarpophalangeal joint, each

26110   interphalangeal joint, each

26115   Excision, tumor or vascular malformation, soft tissue of hand or finger; subcutaneous

26116   deep (subfascial or intramuscular)

26117   Radical resection of tumor (eg, malignant neoplasm), soft tissue of hand or finger

26121   Fasciectomy, palm only, with or without Z-plasty, other local tissue rearrangement, or skin grafting (includes obtaining graft)

26123   Fasciectomy, partial palmar with release of single digit including proximal interphalangeal joint, with or without Z-plasty, other local tissue rearrangement, or skin grafting (includes obtaining graft);

+ 26125   each additional digit (List separately in addition to code for primary procedure)

            (Use 26125 in conjunction with 26123)

            (For fasciotomy, see 26040, 26045)

26130   Synovectomy, carpometacarpal joint

26135   Synovectomy, metacarpophalangeal joint including intrinsic release and extensor hood reconstruction, each digit

26140   Synovectomy, proximal interphalangeal joint, including extensor reconstruction, each interphalangeal joint

26145   Synovectomy, tendon sheath, radical (tenosynovectomy), flexor tendon, palm and/or finger, each tendon

            (For tendon sheath synovectomies at wrist, see 25115, 25116)

26160   Excision of lesion of tendon sheath or joint capsule (eg, cyst, mucous cyst, or ganglion), hand or finger

            (For wrist ganglion, see 25111, 25112)

            (For trigger digit, use 26055)

▲ 26170   Excision of tendon, palm, flexor or extensor, single, each tendon

            ▶(Do not report 26170 in conjunction with 26390, 26415)◀

▲ 26180   Excision of tendon, finger, flexor or extensor, each tendon

            ▶(Do not report 26180 in conjunction with 26390, 26415)◀

26185   Sesamoidectomy, thumb or finger (separate procedure)

26200   Excision or curettage of bone cyst or benign tumor of metacarpal;

26205   with autograft (includes obtaining graft)

26210   Excision or curettage of bone cyst or benign tumor of proximal, middle, or distal phalanx of finger;

26215   with autograft (includes obtaining graft)

26230   Partial excision (craterization, saucerization, or diaphysectomy) bone (eg, osteomyelitis); metacarpal

26235   proximal or middle phalanx of finger

26236   distal phalanx of finger

26250   Radical resection, metacarpal (eg, tumor);

26255   with autograft (includes obtaining graft)

26260   Radical resection, proximal or middle phalanx of finger (eg, tumor);

26261   with autograft (includes obtaining graft)

26262   Radical resection, distal phalanx of finger (eg, tumor)

Introduction or Removal

26320   Removal of implant from finger or hand

            (For removal of foreign body in hand or finger, see 20520, 20525)

Repair, Revision, and/or Reconstruction

26340   Manipulation, finger joint, under anesthesia, each joint

            (For application of external fixation, see 20690 or 20692)

26350   Repair or advancement, flexor tendon, not in zone 2 digital flexor tendon sheath (eg, no man's land); primary or secondary without free graft, each tendon

26352   secondary with free graft (includes obtaining graft), each tendon

26356   Repair or advancement, flexor tendon, in zone 2 digital flexor tendon sheath (eg, no man's land); primary, without free graft, each tendon

26357   secondary, without free graft, each tendon

26358   secondary, with free graft (includes obtaining graft), each tendon

26370   Repair or advancement of profundus tendon, with intact superficialis tendon; primary, each tendon

26372   secondary with free graft (includes obtaining graft), each tendon

26373   secondary without free graft, each tendon

26390   Excision flexor tendon, with implantation of synthetic rod for delayed tendon graft, hand or finger, each rod

26392   Removal of synthetic rod and insertion of flexor tendon graft, hand or finger (includes obtaining graft), each rod

26410   Repair, extensor tendon, hand, primary or secondary; without free graft, each tendon

26412   with free graft (includes obtaining graft), each tendon

26415   Excision of extensor tendon, with implantation of synthetic rod for delayed tendon graft, hand or finger, each rod

26416   Removal of synthetic rod and insertion of extensor tendon graft (includes obtaining graft), hand or finger, each rod

26418   Repair, extensor tendon, finger, primary or secondary; without free graft, each tendon

26420   with free graft (includes obtaining graft) each tendon

26426   Repair of extensor tendon, central slip, secondary (eg, boutonniere deformity); using local tissue(s), including lateral band(s), each finger

26428   with free graft (includes obtaining graft), each finger

26432   Closed treatment of distal extensor tendon insertion, with or without percutaneous pinning (eg, mallet finger)

26433   Repair of extensor tendon, distal insertion, primary or secondary; without graft (eg, mallet finger)

26434   with free graft (includes obtaining graft)

(For tenovaginotomy for trigger finger, use 26055)

26437   Realignment of extensor tendon, hand, each tendon

26440   Tenolysis, flexor tendon; palm OR finger, each tendon

26442   palm AND finger, each tendon

26445   Tenolysis, extensor tendon, hand OR finger, each tendon

26449   Tenolysis, complex, extensor tendon, finger, including forearm, each tendon

26450   Tenotomy, flexor, palm, open, each tendon

26455   Tenotomy, flexor, finger, open, each tendon

26460   Tenotomy, extensor, hand or finger, open, each tendon

26471   Tenodesis; of proximal interphalangeal joint, each joint

26474   of distal joint, each joint

26476   Lengthening of tendon, extensor, hand or finger, each tendon

26477   Shortening of tendon, extensor, hand or finger, each tendon

26478   Lengthening of tendon, flexor, hand or finger, each tendon

26479   Shortening of tendon, flexor, hand or finger, each tendon

26480   Transfer or transplant of tendon, carpometacarpal area or dorsum of hand; without free graft, each tendon

26483   with free tendon graft (includes obtaining graft), each tendon

26485   Transfer or transplant of tendon, palmar; without free tendon graft, each tendon

26489   with free tendon graft (includes obtaining graft), each tendon

26490   Opponensplasty; superficialis tendon transfer type, each tendon

26492   tendon transfer with graft (includes obtaining graft), each tendon

26494   hypothenar muscle transfer

26496   other methods

(For thumb fusion in opposition, use 26820)

26497   Transfer of tendon to restore intrinsic function; ring and small finger

26498   all four fingers

26499   Correction claw finger, other methods

26500   Reconstruction of tendon pulley, each tendon; with local tissues (separate procedure)

26502   with tendon or fascial graft (includes obtaining graft) (separate procedure)

►(26504 has been deleted. To report, use 26390)◄

26508   Release of thenar muscle(s) (eg, thumb contracture)

26510   Cross intrinsic transfer, each tendon

26516   Capsulodesis, metacarpophalangeal joint; single digit

26517   two digits

26518   three or four digits

26520   Capsulectomy or capsulotomy; metacarpophalangeal joint, each joint

26525   interphalangeal joint, each joint

(To report carpometacarpal joint arthroplasty, use 25447)

26530   Arthroplasty, metacarpophalangeal joint; each joint

26531   with prosthetic implant, each joint

26535   Arthroplasty, interphalangeal joint; each joint

26536   with prosthetic implant, each joint

26540   Repair of collateral ligament, metacarpophalangeal or interphalangeal joint

Surgery: Musculoskeletal System

26541 Reconstruction, collateral ligament, metacarpophalangeal joint, single; with tendon or fascial graft (includes obtaining graft)

26542 with local tissue (eg, adductor advancement)

26545 Reconstruction, collateral ligament, interphalangeal joint, single, including graft, each joint

26546 Repair non-union, metacarpal or phalanx, (includes obtaining bone graft with or without external or internal fixation)

26548 Repair and reconstruction, finger, volar plate, interphalangeal joint

26550 Pollicization of a digit

26551 Transfer, toe-to-hand with microvascular anastomosis; great toe wrap-around with bone graft

(For great toe with web space, use 20973)

26553 other than great toe, single

26554 other than great toe, double

(Do not report code 69990 in addition to codes 26551-26554)

26555 Transfer, finger to another position without microvascular anastomosis

26556 Transfer, free toe joint, with microvascular anastomosis

(Do not report code 69990 in addition to code 26556)

(To report great toe-to-hand transfer, use 20973)

26560 Repair of syndactyly (web finger) each web space; with skin flaps

26561 with skin flaps and grafts

26562 complex (eg, involving bone, nails)

26565 Osteotomy; metacarpal, each

26567 phalanx of finger, each

26568 Osteoplasty, lengthening, metacarpal or phalanx

26580 Repair cleft hand

26587 Reconstruction of polydactylous digit, soft tissue and bone

(For excision of polydactylous digit, soft tissue only, use 11200)

26590 Repair macrodactylia, each digit

26591 Repair, intrinsic muscles of hand, each muscle

26593 Release, intrinsic muscles of hand, each muscle

26596 Excision of constricting ring of finger, with multiple Z-plasties

(To report release of scar contracture or graft repairs see 11041-11042, 14040-14041, or 15120, 15240)

Fracture and/or Dislocation

26600 Closed treatment of metacarpal fracture, single; without manipulation, each bone

26605 with manipulation, each bone

26607 Closed treatment of metacarpal fracture, with manipulation, with external fixation, each bone

26608 Percutaneous skeletal fixation of metacarpal fracture, each bone

26615 Open treatment of metacarpal fracture, single, with or without internal or external fixation, each bone

26641 Closed treatment of carpometacarpal dislocation, thumb, with manipulation

26645 Closed treatment of carpometacarpal fracture dislocation, thumb (Bennett fracture), with manipulation

26650 Percutaneous skeletal fixation of carpometacarpal fracture dislocation, thumb (Bennett fracture), with manipulation, with or without external fixation

26665 Open treatment of carpometacarpal fracture dislocation, thumb (Bennett fracture), with or without internal or external fixation

26670 Closed treatment of carpometacarpal dislocation, other than thumb, with manipulation, each joint; without anesthesia

26675 requiring anesthesia

26676 Percutaneous skeletal fixation of carpometacarpal dislocation, other than thumb, with manipulation, each joint

26685 Open treatment of carpometacarpal dislocation, other than thumb; with or without internal or external fixation, each joint

26686 complex, multiple or delayed reduction

26700 Closed treatment of metacarpophalangeal dislocation, single, with manipulation; without anesthesia

26705 requiring anesthesia

26706 Percutaneous skeletal fixation of metacarpophalangeal dislocation, single, with manipulation

26715 Open treatment of metacarpophalangeal dislocation, single, with or without internal or external fixation

26720 Closed treatment of phalangeal shaft fracture, proximal or middle phalanx, finger or thumb; without manipulation, each

26725 with manipulation, with or without skin or skeletal traction, each

26727 Percutaneous skeletal fixation of unstable phalangeal shaft fracture, proximal or middle phalanx, finger or thumb, with manipulation, each

26735 Open treatment of phalangeal shaft fracture, proximal or middle phalanx, finger or thumb, with or without internal or external fixation, each

Surgery: Musculoskeletal System

26740 Closed treatment of articular fracture, involving metacarpophalangeal or interphalangeal joint; without manipulation, each

26742   with manipulation, each

26746 Open treatment of articular fracture, involving metacarpophalangeal or interphalangeal joint, with or without internal or external fixation, each

26750 Closed treatment of distal phalangeal fracture, finger or thumb; without manipulation, each

26755   with manipulation, each

26756 Percutaneous skeletal fixation of distal phalangeal fracture, finger or thumb, each

26765 Open treatment of distal phalangeal fracture, finger or thumb, with or without internal or external fixation, each

26770 Closed treatment of interphalangeal joint dislocation, single, with manipulation; without anesthesia

26775   requiring anesthesia

26776 Percutaneous skeletal fixation of interphalangeal joint dislocation, single, with manipulation

26785 Open treatment of interphalangeal joint dislocation, with or without internal or external fixation, single

Arthrodesis

26820 Fusion in opposition, thumb, with autogenous graft (includes obtaining graft)

26841 Arthrodesis, carpometacarpal joint, thumb, with or without internal fixation;

26842   with autograft (includes obtaining graft)

26843 Arthrodesis, carpometacarpal joint, digit, other than thumb, each;

26844   with autograft (includes obtaining graft)

26850 Arthrodesis, metacarpophalangeal joint, with or without internal fixation;

26852   with autograft (includes obtaining graft)

26860 Arthrodesis, interphalangeal joint, with or without internal fixation;

+ 26861   each additional interphalangeal joint (List separately in addition to code for primary procedure)

(Use 26861 in conjunction with 26860)

26862   with autograft (includes obtaining graft)

+ 26863   with autograft (includes obtaining graft), each additional joint (List separately in addition to code for primary procedure)

(Use 26863 in conjunction with 26862)

Amputation

(For hand through metacarpal bones, use 25927)

26910 Amputation, metacarpal, with finger or thumb (ray amputation), single, with or without interosseous transfer

(For repositioning, see 26550, 26555)

26951 Amputation, finger or thumb, primary or secondary, any joint or phalanx, single, including neurectomies; with direct closure

26952   with local advancement flaps (V-Y, hood)

(For repair of soft tissue defect requiring split or full thickness graft or other pedicle flaps, see 15050-15758)

Other Procedures

26989 Unlisted procedure, hands or fingers

Pelvis and Hip Joint

Including head and neck of femur.

Incision

(For incision and drainage procedures, superficial, see 10040-10160)

26990 Incision and drainage, pelvis or hip joint area; deep abscess or hematoma

26991   infected bursa

26992 Incision, bone cortex, pelvis and/or hip joint (eg, osteomyelitis or bone abscess)

27000 Tenotomy, adductor of hip, percutaneous (separate procedure)

27001 Tenotomy, adductor of hip, open

(To report bilateral procedures, report 27001 with modifier 50)

27003 Tenotomy, adductor, subcutaneous, open, with obturator neurectomy

(To report bilateral procedures, report 27003 with modifier 50)

27005 Tenotomy, hip flexor(s), open (separate procedure)

27006 Tenotomy, abductors and/or extensor(s) of hip, open (separate procedure)

27025 Fasciotomy, hip or thigh, any type

(To report bilateral procedures, report 27025 with modifier 50)

27030 Arthrotomy, hip, with drainage (eg, infection)

27033 Arthrotomy, hip, including exploration or removal of loose or foreign body

27035   Denervation, hip joint, intrapelvic or extrapelvic intra-articular branches of sciatic, femoral, or obturator nerves

(For obturator neurectomy, see 64763, 64766)

27036   Capsulectomy or capsulotomy, hip, with or without excision of heterotopic bone, with release of hip flexor muscles (ie, gluteus medius, gluteus minimus, tensor fascia latae, rectus femoris, sartorius, iliopsoas)

Excision

27040   Biopsy, soft tissue of pelvis and hip area; superficial

27041   deep, subfascial or intramuscular

(For needle biopsy of soft tissue, use 20206)

27047   Excision, tumor, pelvis and hip area; subcutaneous tissue

27048   deep, subfascial, intramuscular

27049   Radical resection of tumor, soft tissue of pelvis and hip area (eg, malignant neoplasm)

27050   Arthrotomy, with biopsy; sacroiliac joint

27052   hip joint

27054   Arthrotomy with synovectomy, hip joint

27060   Excision; ischial bursa

27062   trochanteric bursa or calcification

(For arthrocentesis or needling of bursa, use 20610)

27065   Excision of bone cyst or benign tumor; superficial (wing of ilium, symphysis pubis, or greater trochanter of femur) with or without autograft

27066   deep, with or without autograft

27067   with autograft requiring separate incision

27070   Partial excision (craterization, saucerization) (eg, osteomyelitis or bone abscess); superficial (eg, wing of ilium, symphysis pubis, or greater trochanter of femur)

27071   deep (subfascial or intramuscular)

27075   Radical resection of tumor or infection; wing of ilium, one pubic or ischial ramus or symphysis pubis

27076   ilium, including acetabulum, both pubic rami, or ischium and acetabulum

27077   innominate bone, total

27078   ischial tuberosity and greater trochanter of femur

27079   ischial tuberosity and greater trochanter of femur, with skin flaps

27080   Coccygectomy, primary

(For pressure (decubitus) ulcer, see 15920, 15922 and 15931-15958)

Introduction or Removal

27086   Removal of foreign body, pelvis or hip; subcutaneous tissue

27087   deep (subfascial or intramuscular)

27090   Removal of hip prosthesis; (separate procedure)

27091   complicated, including total hip prosthesis, methylmethacrylate with or without insertion of spacer

27093   Injection procedure for hip arthrography; without anesthesia

▶(For radiological supervision and interpretation, use 73525. Do not report 77002 in conjunction with 73525)◀

27095   with anesthesia

▶(For radiological supervision and interpretation, use 73525. Do not report 77002 in conjunction with 73525)◀

27096   Injection procedure for sacroiliac joint, arthrography and/or anesthetic/steroid

(27096 is to be used only with imaging confirmation of intra-articular needle positioning)

(For radiological supervision and interpretation of sacroiliac joint arthrography, use 73542)

▶(For fluoroscopic guidance without formal arthrography, use 77003)◀

(Code 27096 is a unilateral procedure. For bilateral procedure, use modifier 50)

Repair, Revision, and/or Reconstruction

27097   Release or recession, hamstring, proximal

27098   Transfer, adductor to ischium

27100   Transfer external oblique muscle to greater trochanter including fascial or tendon extension (graft)

27105   Transfer paraspinal muscle to hip (includes fascial or tendon extension graft)

27110   Transfer iliopsoas; to greater trochanter of femur

27111   to femoral neck

27120   Acetabuloplasty; (eg, Whitman, Colonna, Haygroves, or cup type)

27122   resection, femoral head (eg, Girldestone procedure)

27125   Hemiarthroplasty, hip, partial (eg, femoral stem prosthesis, bipolar arthroplasty)

(For prosthetic replacement following fracture of the hip, use 27236)

27130   Arthroplasty, acetabular and proximal femoral prosthetic replacement (total hip arthroplasty), with or without autograft or allograft

27132   Conversion of previous hip surgery to total hip arthroplasty, with or without autograft or allograft

Surgery: Musculoskeletal System

27134 Revision of total hip arthroplasty; both components, with or without autograft or allograft

27137 acetabular component only, with or without autograft or allograft

27138 femoral component only, with or without allograft

27140 Osteotomy and transfer of greater trochanter of femur (separate procedure)

27146 Osteotomy, iliac, acetabular or innominate bone;

27147 with open reduction of hip

27151 with femoral osteotomy

27156 with femoral osteotomy and with open reduction of hip

27158 Osteotomy, pelvis, bilateral (eg, congenital malformation)

27161 Osteotomy, femoral neck (separate procedure)

27165 Osteotomy, intertrochanteric or subtrochanteric including internal or external fixation and/or cast

27170 Bone graft, femoral head, neck, intertrochanteric or subtrochanteric area (includes obtaining bone graft)

27175 Treatment of slipped femoral epiphysis; by traction, without reduction

27176 by single or multiple pinning, in situ

27177 Open treatment of slipped femoral epiphysis; single or multiple pinning or bone graft (includes obtaining graft)

27178 closed manipulation with single or multiple pinning

27179 osteoplasty of femoral neck (Heyman type procedure)

27181 osteotomy and internal fixation

27185 Epiphyseal arrest by epiphysiodesis or stapling, greater trochanter of femur

27187 Prophylactic treatment (nailing, pinning, plating or wiring) with or without methylmethacrylate, femoral neck and proximal femur

Fracture and/or Dislocation

27193 Closed treatment of pelvic ring fracture, dislocation, diastasis or subluxation; without manipulation

27194 with manipulation, requiring more than local anesthesia

27200 Closed treatment of coccygeal fracture

27202 Open treatment of coccygeal fracture

27215 Open treatment of iliac spine(s), tuberosity avulsion, or iliac wing fracture(s) (eg, pelvic fracture(s) which do not disrupt the pelvic ring), with internal fixation

27216 Percutaneous skeletal fixation of posterior pelvic ring fracture and/or dislocation (includes ilium, sacroiliac joint and/or sacrum)

27217 Open treatment of anterior ring fracture and/or dislocation with internal fixation (includes pubic symphysis and/or rami)

27218 Open treatment of posterior ring fracture and/or dislocation with internal fixation (includes ilium, sacroiliac joint and/or sacrum)

27220 Closed treatment of acetabulum (hip socket) fracture(s); without manipulation

27222 with manipulation, with or without skeletal traction

27226 Open treatment of posterior or anterior acetabular wall fracture, with internal fixation

27227 Open treatment of acetabular fracture(s) involving anterior or posterior (one) column, or a fracture running transversely across the acetabulum, with internal fixation

27228 Open treatment of acetabular fracture(s) involving anterior and posterior (two) columns, includes T-fracture and both column fracture with complete articular detachment, or single column or transverse fracture with associated acetabular wall fracture, with internal fixation

27230 Closed treatment of femoral fracture, proximal end, neck; without manipulation

27232 with manipulation, with or without skeletal traction

27235 Percutaneous skeletal fixation of femoral fracture, proximal end, neck

27236 Open treatment of femoral fracture, proximal end, neck, internal fixation or prosthetic replacement

27238 Closed treatment of intertrochanteric, peritrochanteric, or subtrochanteric femoral fracture; without manipulation

27240 with manipulation, with or without skin or skeletal traction

27244 Treatment of intertrochanteric, peritrochanteric, or subtrochanteric femoral fracture; with plate/screw type implant, with or without cerclage

27245 with intramedullary implant, with or without interlocking screws and/or cerclage

27246 Closed treatment of greater trochanteric fracture, without manipulation

27248 Open treatment of greater trochanteric fracture, with or without internal or external fixation

27250 Closed treatment of hip dislocation, traumatic; without anesthesia

27252 requiring anesthesia

27253 Open treatment of hip dislocation, traumatic, without internal fixation

27254 Open treatment of hip dislocation, traumatic, with acetabular wall and femoral head fracture, with or without internal or external fixation

(For treatment of acetabular fracture with fixation, see 27226, 27227)

27256   Treatment of spontaneous hip dislocation (developmental, including congenital or pathological), by abduction, splint or traction; without anesthesia, without manipulation

27257   with manipulation, requiring anesthesia

27258   Open treatment of spontaneous hip dislocation (developmental, including congenital or pathological), replacement of femoral head in acetabulum (including tenotomy, etc);

27259   with femoral shaft shortening

27265   Closed treatment of post hip arthroplasty dislocation; without anesthesia

27266   requiring regional or general anesthesia

Manipulation

27275   Manipulation, hip joint, requiring general anesthesia

Arthrodesis

27280   Arthrodesis, sacroiliac joint (including obtaining graft)

(To report bilateral procedures, report 27280 with modifier 50)

27282   Arthrodesis, symphysis pubis (including obtaining graft)

27284   Arthrodesis, hip joint (including obtaining graft);

27286   with subtrochanteric osteotomy

Amputation

27290   Interpelviabdominal amputation (hindquarter amputation)

27295   Disarticulation of hip

Other Procedures

27299   Unlisted procedure, pelvis or hip joint

Femur (Thigh Region) and Knee Joint

Including tibial plateaus.

Incision

(For incision and drainage of abscess or hematoma, superficial, see 10040-10160)

27301   Incision and drainage, deep abscess, bursa, or hematoma, thigh or knee region

27303   Incision, deep, with opening of bone cortex, femur or knee (eg, osteomyelitis or bone abscess)

27305   Fasciotomy, iliotibial (tenotomy), open

(For combined Ober-Yount fasciotomy, use 27025)

27306   Tenotomy, percutaneous, adductor or hamstring; single tendon (separate procedure)

27307   multiple tendons

27310   Arthrotomy, knee, with exploration, drainage, or removal of foreign body (eg, infection)

►(27315 has been deleted. To report, see 27325)◄

►(27320 has been deleted. To report, see 27326)◄

Excision

27323   Biopsy, soft tissue of thigh or knee area; superficial

27324   deep (subfascial or intramuscular)

(For needle biopsy of soft tissue, use 20206)

● 27325   Neurectomy, hamstring muscle

● 27326   Neurectomy, popliteal (gastrocnemius)

27327   Excision, tumor, thigh or knee area; subcutaneous

27328   deep, subfascial, or intramuscular

27329   Radical resection of tumor (eg, malignant neoplasm), soft tissue of thigh or knee area

27330   Arthrotomy, knee; with synovial biopsy only

27331   including joint exploration, biopsy, or removal of loose or foreign bodies

27332   Arthrotomy, with excision of semilunar cartilage (meniscectomy) knee; medial OR lateral

27333   medial AND lateral

27334   Arthrotomy, with synovectomy, knee; anterior OR posterior

27335   anterior AND posterior including popliteal area

27340   Excision, prepatellar bursa

27345   Excision of synovial cyst of popliteal space (eg, Baker's cyst)

27347   Excision of lesion of meniscus or capsule (eg, cyst, ganglion), knee

27350   Patellectomy or hemipatellectomy

27355   Excision or curettage of bone cyst or benign tumor of femur;

27356   with allograft

27357   with autograft (includes obtaining graft)

+ 27358   with internal fixation (List in addition to code for primary procedure)

(Use 27358 in conjunction with 27355, 27356, or 27357)

27360   Partial excision (craterization, saucerization, or diaphysectomy) bone, femur, proximal tibia and/or fibula (eg, osteomyelitis or bone abscess)

27365   Radical resection of tumor, bone, femur or knee

(For radical resection of tumor, soft tissue, use 27329)

Introduction or Removal

27370 Injection procedure for knee arthrography

▶(For radiological supervision and interpretation, use 73580. Do not report 77002 in conjunction with 73580)◀

27372 Removal of foreign body, deep, thigh region or knee area

(For removal of knee prosthesis including "total knee," use 27488)

(For surgical arthroscopic knee procedures, see 29870-29887)

Repair, Revision, and/or Reconstruction

27380 Suture of infrapatellar tendon; primary

27381 secondary reconstruction, including fascial or tendon graft

27385 Suture of quadriceps or hamstring muscle rupture; primary

27386 secondary reconstruction, including fascial or tendon graft

27390 Tenotomy, open, hamstring, knee to hip; single tendon

27391 multiple tendons, one leg

27392 multiple tendons, bilateral

27393 Lengthening of hamstring tendon; single tendon

27394 multiple tendons, one leg

27395 multiple tendons, bilateral

27396 Transplant, hamstring tendon to patella; single tendon

27397 multiple tendons

27400 Transfer, tendon or muscle, hamstrings to femur (eg, Egger's type procedure)

27403 Arthrotomy with meniscus repair, knee

(For arthroscopic repair, use 29882)

27405 Repair, primary, torn ligament and/or capsule, knee; collateral

27407 cruciate

(For cruciate ligament reconstruction, use 27427)

27409 collateral and cruciate ligaments

(For ligament reconstruction, see 27427-27429)

27412 Autologous chondrocyte implantation, knee

(Do not report 27412 in conjunction with 20926, 27331, 27570)

(For harvesting of chondrocytes, use 29870)

27415 Osteochondral allograft, knee, open

(For arthroscopic implant of osteochondral allograft, use 29867)

27418 Anterior tibial tubercleplasty (eg, Maquet type procedure)

27420 Reconstruction of dislocating patella; (eg, Hauser type procedure)

27422 with extensor realignment and/or muscle advancement or release (eg, Campbell, Goldwaite type procedure)

27424 with patellectomy

27425 Lateral retinacular release, open

(For arthroscopic lateral release, use 29873)

27427 Ligamentous reconstruction (augmentation), knee; extra-articular

27428 intra-articular (open)

27429 intra-articular (open) and extra-articular

(For primary repair of ligament(s) performed in conjunction with reconstruction, report 27405, 27407 or 27409 in conjunction with 27427, 27428 or 27429)

27430 Quadricepsplasty (eg, Bennett or Thompson type)

27435 Capsulotomy, posterior capsular release, knee

27437 Arthroplasty, patella; without prosthesis

27438 with prosthesis

27440 Arthroplasty, knee, tibial plateau;

27441 with debridement and partial synovectomy

27442 Arthroplasty, femoral condyles or tibial plateau(s), knee;

27443 with debridement and partial synovectomy

27445 Arthroplasty, knee, hinge prosthesis (eg, Walldius type)

27446 Arthroplasty, knee, condyle and plateau; medial OR lateral compartment

27447 medial AND lateral compartments with or without patella resurfacing (total knee arthroplasty)

(For revision of total knee arthroplasty, use 27487)

(For removal of total knee prosthesis, use 27488)

27448 Osteotomy, femur, shaft or supracondylar; without fixation

(To report bilateral procedures, report 27448 with modifier 50)

27450 with fixation

(To report bilateral procedures, report 27450 with modifier 50)

27454 Osteotomy, multiple, with realignment on intramedullary rod, femoral shaft (eg, Sofield type procedure)

27455 Osteotomy, proximal tibia, including fibular excision or osteotomy (includes correction of genu varus (bowleg) or genu valgus (knock-knee)); before epiphyseal closure

(To report bilateral procedures, report 27455 with modifier 50)

27457 after epiphyseal closure

(To report bilateral procedures, report 27457 with modifier 50)

27465	Osteoplasty, femur; shortening (excluding 64876)
27466	lengthening
27468	combined, lengthening and shortening with femoral segment transfer
27470	Repair, nonunion or malunion, femur, distal to head and neck; without graft (eg, compression technique)
27472	with iliac or other autogenous bone graft (includes obtaining graft)
27475	Arrest, epiphyseal, any method (eg, epiphysiodesis); distal femur
27477	tibia and fibula, proximal
27479	combined distal femur, proximal tibia and fibula
27485	Arrest, hemiepiphyseal, distal femur or proximal tibia or fibula (eg, genu varus or valgus)
27486	Revision of total knee arthroplasty, with or without allograft; one component
27487	femoral and entire tibial component
27488	Removal of prosthesis, including total knee prosthesis, methylmethacrylate with or without insertion of spacer, knee
27495	Prophylactic treatment (nailing, pinning, plating or wiring) with or without methylmethacrylate, femur
27496	Decompression fasciotomy, thigh and/or knee, one compartment (flexor or extensor or adductor);
27497	with debridement of nonviable muscle and/or nerve
27498	Decompression fasciotomy, thigh and/or knee, multiple compartments;
27499	with debridement of nonviable muscle and/or nerve

Fracture and/or Dislocation

(For arthroscopic treatment of intercondylar spine(s) and tuberosity fracture(s) of the knee, see 29850, 29851)

(For arthroscopic treatment of tibial fracture, see 29855, 29856)

27500	Closed treatment of femoral shaft fracture, without manipulation
27501	Closed treatment of supracondylar or transcondylar femoral fracture with or without intercondylar extension, without manipulation
27502	Closed treatment of femoral shaft fracture, with manipulation, with or without skin or skeletal traction
27503	Closed treatment of supracondylar or transcondylar femoral fracture with or without intercondylar extension, with manipulation, with or without skin or skeletal traction
27506	Open treatment of femoral shaft fracture, with or without external fixation, with insertion of intramedullary implant, with or without cerclage and/or locking screws

27507	Open treatment of femoral shaft fracture with plate/screws, with or without cerclage
27508	Closed treatment of femoral fracture, distal end, medial or lateral condyle, without manipulation
27509	Percutaneous skeletal fixation of femoral fracture, distal end, medial or lateral condyle, or supracondylar or transcondylar, with or without intercondylar extension, or distal femoral epiphyseal separation
27510	Closed treatment of femoral fracture, distal end, medial or lateral condyle, with manipulation
27511	Open treatment of femoral supracondylar or transcondylar fracture without intercondylar extension, with or without internal or external fixation
27513	Open treatment of femoral supracondylar or transcondylar fracture with intercondylar extension, with or without internal or external fixation
27514	Open treatment of femoral fracture, distal end, medial or lateral condyle, with or without internal or external fixation
27516	Closed treatment of distal femoral epiphyseal separation; without manipulation
27517	with manipulation, with or without skin or skeletal traction
27519	Open treatment of distal femoral epiphyseal separation, with or without internal or external fixation
27520	Closed treatment of patellar fracture, without manipulation
27524	Open treatment of patellar fracture, with internal fixation and/or partial or complete patellectomy and soft tissue repair
27530	Closed treatment of tibial fracture, proximal (plateau); without manipulation
27532	with or without manipulation, with skeletal traction
	(For arthroscopic treatment, see 29855, 29856)
27535	Open treatment of tibial fracture, proximal (plateau); unicondylar, with or without internal or external fixation
27536	bicondylar, with or without internal fixation
	(For arthroscopic treatment, see 29855, 29856)
27538	Closed treatment of intercondylar spine(s) and/or tuberosity fracture(s) of knee, with or without manipulation
	(For arthroscopic treatment, see 29850, 29851)
27540	Open treatment of intercondylar spine(s) and/or tuberosity fracture(s) of the knee, with or without internal or external fixation
27550	Closed treatment of knee dislocation; without anesthesia
27552	requiring anesthesia

Surgery: Musculoskeletal System

Surgery: Musculoskeletal System

27556   Open treatment of knee dislocation, with or without internal or external fixation; without primary ligamentous repair or augmentation/reconstruction

27557   with primary ligamentous repair

27558   with primary ligamentous repair, with augmentation/reconstruction

27560   Closed treatment of patellar dislocation; without anesthesia

(For recurrent dislocation, see 27420-27424)

27562   requiring anesthesia

27566   Open treatment of patellar dislocation, with or without partial or total patellectomy

Manipulation

27570   Manipulation of knee joint under general anesthesia (includes application of traction or other fixation devices)

Arthrodesis

27580   Arthrodesis, knee, any technique

Amputation

27590   Amputation, thigh, through femur, any level;

27591   immediate fitting technique including first cast

27592   open, circular (guillotine)

27594   secondary closure or scar revision

27596   re-amputation

27598   Disarticulation at knee

Other Procedures

27599   Unlisted procedure, femur or knee

Leg (Tibia and Fibula) and Ankle Joint

Incision

27600   Decompression fasciotomy, leg; anterior and/or lateral compartments only

27601   posterior compartment(s) only

27602   anterior and/or lateral, and posterior compartment(s)

(For incision and drainage procedures, superficial, see 10040-10160)

(For decompression fasciotomy with debridement, see 27892-27894)

27603   Incision and drainage, leg or ankle; deep abscess or hematoma

27604   infected bursa

27605   Tenotomy, percutaneous, Achilles tendon (separate procedure); local anesthesia

27606   general anesthesia

27607   Incision (eg, osteomyelitis or bone abscess), leg or ankle

27610   Arthrotomy, ankle, including exploration, drainage, or removal of foreign body

27612   Arthrotomy, posterior capsular release, ankle, with or without Achilles tendon lengthening

(See also 27685)

Excision

27613   Biopsy, soft tissue of leg or ankle area; superficial

27614   deep (subfascial or intramuscular)

(For needle biopsy of soft tissue, use 20206)

27615   Radical resection of tumor (eg, malignant neoplasm), soft tissue of leg or ankle area

27618   Excision, tumor, leg or ankle area; subcutaneous tissue

27619   deep (subfascial or intramuscular)

27620   Arthrotomy, ankle, with joint exploration, with or without biopsy, with or without removal of loose or foreign body

27625   Arthrotomy, with synovectomy, ankle;

27626   including tenosynovectomy

27630   Excision of lesion of tendon sheath or capsule (eg, cyst or ganglion), leg and/or ankle

27635   Excision or curettage of bone cyst or benign tumor, tibia or fibula;

27637   with autograft (includes obtaining graft)

27638   with allograft

27640   Partial excision (craterization, saucerization, or diaphysectomy) bone (eg, osteomyelitis or exostosis); tibia

27641   fibula

27645   Radical resection of tumor, bone; tibia

27646   fibula

27647   talus or calcaneus

Introduction or Removal

27648   Injection procedure for ankle arthrography

▶(For radiological supervision and interpretation, use 73615. Do not report 77002 in conjunction with 73615)◀

(For ankle arthroscopy, see 29894-29898)

Repair, Revision, and/or Reconstruction

27650   Repair, primary, open or percutaneous, ruptured Achilles tendon;

27652   with graft (includes obtaining graft)

27654   Repair, secondary, Achilles tendon, with or without graft

27656   Repair, fascial defect of leg

27658   Repair, flexor tendon, leg; primary, without graft, each tendon

27659   secondary, with or without graft, each tendon

27664   Repair, extensor tendon, leg; primary, without graft, each tendon

27665   secondary, with or without graft, each tendon

27675   Repair, dislocating peroneal tendons; without fibular osteotomy

27676   with fibular osteotomy

27680   Tenolysis, flexor or extensor tendon, leg and/or ankle; single, each tendon

27681   multiple tendons (through separate incision(s))

27685   Lengthening or shortening of tendon, leg or ankle; single tendon (separate procedure)

27686   multiple tendons (through same incision), each

27687   Gastrocnemius recession (eg, Strayer procedure)

(Toe extensors are considered as a group to be a single tendon when transplanted into midfoot)

27690   Transfer or transplant of single tendon (with muscle redirection or rerouting); superficial (eg, anterior tibial extensors into midfoot)

27691   deep (eg, anterior tibial or posterior tibial through interosseous space, flexor digitorum longus, flexor hallucis longus, or peroneal tendon to midfoot or hindfoot)

+ 27692   each additional tendon (List separately in addition to code for primary procedure)

(Use 27692 in conjunction with 27690, 27691)

27695   Repair, primary, disrupted ligament, ankle; collateral

27696   both collateral ligaments

27698   Repair, secondary, disrupted ligament, ankle, collateral (eg, Watson-Jones procedure)

27700   Arthroplasty, ankle;

27702   with implant (total ankle)

27703   revision, total ankle

27704   Removal of ankle implant

27705   Osteotomy; tibia

27707   fibula

27709   tibia and fibula

27712   multiple, with realignment on intramedullary rod (eg, Sofield type procedure)

(For osteotomy to correct genu varus (bowleg) or genu valgus (knock-knee), see 27455-27457)

27715   Osteoplasty, tibia and fibula, lengthening or shortening

27720   Repair of nonunion or malunion, tibia; without graft, (eg, compression technique)

27722   with sliding graft

27724   with iliac or other autograft (includes obtaining graft)

27725   by synostosis, with fibula, any method

27727   Repair of congenital pseudarthrosis, tibia

27730   Arrest, epiphyseal (epiphysiodesis), open; distal tibia

27732   distal fibula

27734   distal tibia and fibula

27740   Arrest, epiphyseal (epiphysiodesis), any method, combined, proximal and distal tibia and fibula;

27742   and distal femur

(For epiphyseal arrest of proximal tibia and fibula, use 27477)

27745   Prophylactic treatment (nailing, pinning, plating or wiring) with or without methylmethacrylate, tibia

Fracture and/or Dislocation

27750   Closed treatment of tibial shaft fracture (with or without fibular fracture); without manipulation

27752   with manipulation, with or without skeletal traction

27756   Percutaneous skeletal fixation of tibial shaft fracture (with or without fibular fracture) (eg, pins or screws)

27758   Open treatment of tibial shaft fracture, (with or without fibular fracture) with plate/screws, with or without cerclage

27759   Treatment of tibial shaft fracture (with or without fibular fracture) by intramedullary implant, with or without interlocking screws and/or cerclage

27760   Closed treatment of medial malleolus fracture; without manipulation

27762   with manipulation, with or without skin or skeletal traction

27766   Open treatment of medial malleolus fracture, with or without internal or external fixation

27780   Closed treatment of proximal fibula or shaft fracture; without manipulation

27781   with manipulation

Surgery: Musculoskeletal System

27784 Open treatment of proximal fibula or shaft fracture, with or without internal or external fixation

27786 Closed treatment of distal fibular fracture (lateral malleolus); without manipulation

27788 with manipulation

27792 Open treatment of distal fibular fracture (lateral malleolus), with or without internal or external fixation

(For treatment of tibia and fibula shaft fractures, see 27750-27759)

27808 Closed treatment of bimalleolar ankle fracture, (including Potts); without manipulation

27810 with manipulation

27814 Open treatment of bimalleolar ankle fracture, with or without internal or external fixation

27816 Closed treatment of trimalleolar ankle fracture; without manipulation

27818 with manipulation

27822 Open treatment of trimalleolar ankle fracture, with or without internal or external fixation, medial and/or lateral malleolus; without fixation of posterior lip

27823 with fixation of posterior lip

27824 Closed treatment of fracture of weight bearing articular portion of distal tibia (eg, pilon or tibial plafond), with or without anesthesia; without manipulation

27825 with skeletal traction and/or requiring manipulation

27826 Open treatment of fracture of weight bearing articular surface/portion of distal tibia (eg, pilon or tibial plafond), with internal or external fixation; of fibula only

27827 of tibia only

27828 of both tibia and fibula

27829 Open treatment of distal tibiofibular joint (syndesmosis) disruption, with or without internal or external fixation

27830 Closed treatment of proximal tibiofibular joint dislocation; without anesthesia

27831 requiring anesthesia

27832 Open treatment of proximal tibiofibular joint dislocation, with or without internal or external fixation, or with excision of proximal fibula

27840 Closed treatment of ankle dislocation; without anesthesia

27842 requiring anesthesia, with or without percutaneous skeletal fixation

27846 Open treatment of ankle dislocation, with or without percutaneous skeletal fixation; without repair or internal fixation

27848 with repair or internal or external fixation

(For surgical or diagnostic arthroscopic procedures, see 29894-29898)

Manipulation

27860 Manipulation of ankle under general anesthesia (includes application of traction or other fixation apparatus)

Arthrodesis

27870 Arthrodesis, ankle, open

(For arthroscopic ankle arthrodesis, use 29899)

27871 Arthrodesis, tibiofibular joint, proximal or distal

Amputation

27880 Amputation, leg, through tibia and fibula;

27881 with immediate fitting technique including application of first cast

27882 open, circular (guillotine)

27884 secondary closure or scar revision

27886 re-amputation

27888 Amputation, ankle, through malleoli of tibia and fibula (eg, Syme, Pirogoff type procedures), with plastic closure and resection of nerves

27889 Ankle disarticulation

Other Procedures

27892 Decompression fasciotomy, leg; anterior and/or lateral compartments only, with debridement of nonviable muscle and/or nerve

(For decompression fasciotomy of the leg without debridement, use 27600)

27893 posterior compartment(s) only, with debridement of nonviable muscle and/or nerve

(For decompression fasciotomy of the leg without debridement, use 27601)

27894 anterior and/or lateral, and posterior compartment(s), with debridement of nonviable muscle and/or nerve

(For decompression fasciotomy of the leg without debridement, use 27602)

27899 Unlisted procedure, leg or ankle

Foot and Toes

Incision

(For incision and drainage procedures, superficial, see 10040-10160)

28001 Incision and drainage, bursa, foot

28002 Incision and drainage below fascia, with or without tendon sheath involvement, foot; single bursal space

28003 multiple areas

28005	Incision, bone cortex (eg, osteomyelitis or bone abscess), foot
28008	Fasciotomy, foot and/or toe
	(See also 28060, 28062, 28250)
28010	Tenotomy, percutaneous, toe; single tendon
28011	multiple tendons
	(For open tenotomy, see 28230-28234)
28020	Arthrotomy, including exploration, drainage, or removal of loose or foreign body; intertarsal or tarsometatarsal joint
28022	metatarsophalangeal joint
28024	interphalangeal joint
	▶(28030 has been deleted. To report, use 28055)◀
28035	Release, tarsal tunnel (posterior tibial nerve decompression)
	(For other nerve entrapments, see 64704, 64722)

Excision

28043	Excision, tumor, foot; subcutaneous tissue
28045	deep, subfascial, intramuscular
28046	Radical resection of tumor (eg, malignant neoplasm), soft tissue of foot
28050	Arthrotomy with biopsy; intertarsal or tarsometatarsal joint
28052	metatarsophalangeal joint
28054	interphalangeal joint
● 28055	Neurectomy, intrinsic musculature of foot
28060	Fasciectomy, plantar fascia; partial (separate procedure)
28062	radical (separate procedure)
	(For plantar fasciotomy, see 28008, 28250)
28070	Synovectomy; intertarsal or tarsometatarsal joint, each
28072	metatarsophalangeal joint, each
28080	Excision, interdigital (Morton) neuroma, single, each
28086	Synovectomy, tendon sheath, foot; flexor
28088	extensor
28090	Excision of lesion, tendon, tendon sheath, or capsule (including synovectomy) (eg, cyst or ganglion); foot
28092	toe(s), each
28100	Excision or curettage of bone cyst or benign tumor, talus or calcaneus;
28102	with iliac or other autograft (includes obtaining graft)
28103	with allograft

28104	Excision or curettage of bone cyst or benign tumor, tarsal or metatarsal, except talus or calcaneus;
28106	with iliac or other autograft (includes obtaining graft)
28107	with allograft
28108	Excision or curettage of bone cyst or benign tumor, phalanges of foot
	(For ostectomy, partial (eg, hallux valgus, Silver type procedure), use 28290)
28110	Ostectomy, partial excision, fifth metatarsal head (bunionette) (separate procedure)
28111	Ostectomy, complete excision; first metatarsal head
28112	other metatarsal head (second, third or fourth)
28113	fifth metatarsal head
28114	all metatarsal heads, with partial proximal phalangectomy, excluding first metatarsal (eg, Clayton type procedure)
28116	Ostectomy, excision of tarsal coalition
28118	Ostectomy, calcaneus;
28119	for spur, with or without plantar fascial release
28120	Partial excision (craterization, saucerization, sequestrectomy, or diaphysectomy) bone (eg, osteomyelitis or bossing); talus or calcaneus
28122	tarsal or metatarsal bone, except talus or calcaneus
	(For partial excision of talus or calcaneus, use 28120)
	(For cheilectomy for hallux rigidus, use 28289)
28124	phalanx of toe
28126	Resection, partial or complete, phalangeal base, each toe
28130	Talectomy (astragalectomy)
	(For calcanectomy, use 28118)
28140	Metatarsectomy
28150	Phalangectomy, toe, each toe
28153	Resection, condyle(s), distal end of phalanx, each toe
28160	Hemiphalangectomy or interphalangeal joint excision, toe, proximal end of phalanx, each
28171	Radical resection of tumor, bone; tarsal (except talus or calcaneus)
28173	metatarsal
28175	phalanx of toe
	(For talus or calcaneus, use 27647)

Introduction or Removal

28190	Removal of foreign body, foot; subcutaneous
28192	deep
28193	complicated

Repair, Revision, and/or Reconstruction

28200   Repair, tendon, flexor, foot; primary or secondary, without free graft, each tendon

28202   secondary with free graft, each tendon (includes obtaining graft)

28208   Repair, tendon, extensor, foot; primary or secondary, each tendon

28210   secondary with free graft, each tendon (includes obtaining graft)

28220   Tenolysis, flexor, foot; single tendon

28222   multiple tendons

28225   Tenolysis, extensor, foot; single tendon

28226   multiple tendons

28230   Tenotomy, open, tendon flexor; foot, single or multiple tendon(s) (separate procedure)

28232   toe, single tendon (separate procedure)

28234   Tenotomy, open, extensor, foot or toe, each tendon

(For tendon transfer to midfoot or hindfoot, see 27690, 27691)

28238   Reconstruction (advancement), posterior tibial tendon with excision of accessory tarsal navicular bone (eg, Kidner type procedure)

(For subcutaneous tenotomy, see 28010, 28011)

(For transfer or transplant of tendon with muscle redirection or rerouting, see 27690-27692)

(For extensor hallucis longus transfer with great toe IP fusion (Jones procedure), use 28760)

28240   Tenotomy, lengthening, or release, abductor hallucis muscle

28250   Division of plantar fascia and muscle (eg, Steindler stripping) (separate procedure)

28260   Capsulotomy, midfoot; medial release only (separate procedure)

28261   with tendon lengthening

28262   extensive, including posterior talotibial capsulotomy and tendon(s) lengthening (eg, resistant clubfoot deformity)

28264   Capsulotomy, midtarsal (eg, Heyman type procedure)

28270   Capsulotomy; metatarsophalangeal joint, with or without tenorrhaphy, each joint (separate procedure)

28272   interphalangeal joint, each joint (separate procedure)

28280   Syndactylization, toes (eg, webbing or Kelikian type procedure)

28285   Correction, hammertoe (eg, interphalangeal fusion, partial or total phalangectomy)

28286   Correction, cock-up fifth toe, with plastic skin closure (eg, Ruiz-Mora type procedure)

28288   Ostectomy, partial, exostectomy or condylectomy, metatarsal head, each metatarsal head

28289   Hallux rigidus correction with cheilectomy, debridement and capsular release of the first metatarsophalangeal joint

28290   Correction, hallux valgus (bunion), with or without sesamoidectomy; simple exostectomy (eg, Silver type procedure)

28292   Keller, McBride, or Mayo type procedure

28293   resection of joint with implant

28294   with tendon transplants (eg, Joplin type procedure)

28296   with metatarsal osteotomy (eg, Mitchell, Chevron, or concentric type procedures)

28297   Lapidus-type procedure

28298   by phalanx osteotomy

28299   by double osteotomy

28300   Osteotomy; calcaneus (eg, Dwyer or Chambers type procedure), with or without internal fixation

28302   talus

28304   Osteotomy, tarsal bones, other than calcaneus or talus;

28305   with autograft (includes obtaining graft) (eg, Fowler type)

28306   Osteotomy, with or without lengthening, shortening or angular correction, metatarsal; first metatarsal

28307   first metatarsal with autograft (other than first toe)

28308   other than first metatarsal, each

28309   multiple (eg, Swanson type cavus foot procedure)

28310   Osteotomy, shortening, angular or rotational correction; proximal phalanx, first toe (separate procedure)

28312   other phalanges, any toe

28313   Reconstruction, angular deformity of toe, soft tissue procedures only (eg, overlapping second toe, fifth toe, curly toes)

28315   Sesamoidectomy, first toe (separate procedure)

28320   Repair, nonunion or malunion; tarsal bones

28322   metatarsal, with or without bone graft (includes obtaining graft)

28340   Reconstruction, toe, macrodactyly; soft tissue resection

28341   requiring bone resection

28344   Reconstruction, toe(s); polydactyly

28345   syndactyly, with or without skin graft(s), each web

28360   Reconstruction, cleft foot

Fracture and/or Dislocation

28400 Closed treatment of calcaneal fracture; without manipulation

28405   with manipulation

28406 Percutaneous skeletal fixation of calcaneal fracture, with manipulation

28415 Open treatment of calcaneal fracture, with or without internal or external fixation;

28420   with primary iliac or other autogenous bone graft (includes obtaining graft)

28430 Closed treatment of talus fracture; without manipulation

28435   with manipulation

28436 Percutaneous skeletal fixation of talus fracture, with manipulation

28445 Open treatment of talus fracture, with or without internal or external fixation

28450 Treatment of tarsal bone fracture (except talus and calcaneus); without manipulation, each

28455   with manipulation, each

28456 Percutaneous skeletal fixation of tarsal bone fracture (except talus and calcaneus), with manipulation, each

28465 Open treatment of tarsal bone fracture (except talus and calcaneus), with or without internal or external fixation, each

28470 Closed treatment of metatarsal fracture; without manipulation, each

28475   with manipulation, each

28476 Percutaneous skeletal fixation of metatarsal fracture, with manipulation, each

28485 Open treatment of metatarsal fracture, with or without internal or external fixation, each

28490 Closed treatment of fracture great toe, phalanx or phalanges; without manipulation

28495   with manipulation

28496 Percutaneous skeletal fixation of fracture great toe, phalanx or phalanges, with manipulation

28505 Open treatment of fracture great toe, phalanx or phalanges, with or without internal or external fixation

28510 Closed treatment of fracture, phalanx or phalanges, other than great toe; without manipulation, each

28515   with manipulation, each

28525 Open treatment of fracture, phalanx or phalanges, other than great toe, with or without internal or external fixation, each

28530 Closed treatment of sesamoid fracture

28531 Open treatment of sesamoid fracture, with or without internal fixation

28540 Closed treatment of tarsal bone dislocation, other than talotarsal; without anesthesia

28545   requiring anesthesia

28546 Percutaneous skeletal fixation of tarsal bone dislocation, other than talotarsal, with manipulation

28555 Open treatment of tarsal bone dislocation, with or without internal or external fixation

28570 Closed treatment of talotarsal joint dislocation; without anesthesia

28575   requiring anesthesia

28576 Percutaneous skeletal fixation of talotarsal joint dislocation, with manipulation

28585 Open treatment of talotarsal joint dislocation, with or without internal or external fixation

28600 Closed treatment of tarsometatarsal joint dislocation; without anesthesia

28605   requiring anesthesia

28606 Percutaneous skeletal fixation of tarsometatarsal joint dislocation, with manipulation

28615 Open treatment of tarsometatarsal joint dislocation, with or without internal or external fixation

28630 Closed treatment of metatarsophalangeal joint dislocation; without anesthesia

28635   requiring anesthesia

28636 Percutaneous skeletal fixation of metatarsophalangeal joint dislocation, with manipulation

28645 Open treatment of metatarsophalangeal joint dislocation, with or without internal or external fixation

28660 Closed treatment of interphalangeal joint dislocation; without anesthesia

28665   requiring anesthesia

28666 Percutaneous skeletal fixation of interphalangeal joint dislocation, with manipulation

28675 Open treatment of interphalangeal joint dislocation, with or without internal or external fixation

Arthrodesis

28705 Arthrodesis; pantalar

28715   triple

28725   subtalar

28730 Arthrodesis, midtarsal or tarsometatarsal, multiple or transverse;

28735   with osteotomy (eg, flatfoot correction)

28737 Arthrodesis, with tendon lengthening and advancement, midtarsal, tarsal navicular-cuneiform (eg, Miller type procedure)

28740 Arthrodesis, midtarsal or tarsometatarsal, single joint

Surgery: Musculoskeletal System

28750	Arthrodesis, great toe; metatarsophalangeal joint
28755	interphalangeal joint
28760	Arthrodesis, with extensor hallucis longus transfer to first metatarsal neck, great toe, interphalangeal joint (eg, Jones type procedure)

(For hammertoe operation or interphalangeal fusion, use 28285)

Amputation

28800	Amputation, foot; midtarsal (eg, Chopart type procedure)
28805	transmetatarsal
28810	Amputation, metatarsal, with toe, single
28820	Amputation, toe; metatarsophalangeal joint
28825	interphalangeal joint

(For amputation of tuft of distal phalanx, use 11752)

Other Procedures

28890	Extracorporeal shock wave, high energy, performed by a physician, requiring anesthesia other than local, including ultrasound guidance, involving the plantar fascia

(For extracorporeal shock wave therapy involving musculoskeletal system not otherwise specified, see Category III codes 0019T, 0101T, 0102T)

28899	Unlisted procedure, foot or toes

Application of Casts and Strapping

The listed procedures apply when the cast application or strapping is a replacement procedure used during or after the period of follow-up care, or when the cast application or strapping is an initial service performed without a restorative treatment or procedure(s) to stabilize or protect a fracture, injury, or dislocation and/or to afford comfort to a patient. Restorative treatment or procedure(s) rendered by another physician following the application of the initial cast/splint/strap may be reported with a treatment of fracture and/or dislocation code.

A physician who applies the initial cast, strap or splint and also assumes all of the subsequent fracture, dislocation, or injury care cannot use the application of casts and strapping codes as an initial service, since the first cast/splint or strap application is included in the treatment of fracture and/or dislocation codes. (See notes under Musculoskeletal System, page 63.) A temporary cast/splint/strap is not considered to be part of the preoperative care, and the use of the modifier 56 is not applicable. Additional evaluation and management services are reportable only if significant identifiable further services are provided at the time of the cast application or strapping.

If cast application or strapping is provided as an initial service (eg, casting of a sprained ankle or knee) in which no other procedure or treatment (eg, surgical repair, reduction of a fracture or joint dislocation) is performed or is expected to be performed by a physician rendering the initial care only, use the casting, strapping and/or supply code (99070) in addition to an evaluation and management code as appropriate.

Listed procedures include removal of cast or strapping.

(For orthotics management and training, see 97760-97762)

Body and Upper Extremity

Casts

29000	Application of halo type body cast (see 20661-20663 for insertion)
29010	Application of Risser jacket, localizer, body; only
29015	including head
29020	Application of turnbuckle jacket, body; only
29025	including head
29035	Application of body cast, shoulder to hips;
29040	including head, Minerva type
29044	including one thigh
29046	including both thighs
29049	Application, cast; figure-of-eight
29055	shoulder spica
29058	plaster Velpeau
29065	shoulder to hand (long arm)
29075	elbow to finger (short arm)
29085	hand and lower forearm (gauntlet)
29086	finger (eg, contracture)

Splints

29105	Application of long arm splint (shoulder to hand)
29125	Application of short arm splint (forearm to hand); static
29126	dynamic
29130	Application of finger splint; static
29131	dynamic

Strapping—Any Age

29200	Strapping; thorax
29220	low back
29240	shoulder (eg, Velpeau)
29260	elbow or wrist
29280	hand or finger

Lower Extremity

Casts

29305 Application of hip spica cast; one leg

29325   one and one-half spica or both legs

(For hip spica (body) cast, including thighs only, use 29046)

29345 Application of long leg cast (thigh to toes);

29355   walker or ambulatory type

29358 Application of long leg cast brace

29365 Application of cylinder cast (thigh to ankle)

29405 Application of short leg cast (below knee to toes);

29425   walking or ambulatory type

29435 Application of patellar tendon bearing (PTB) cast

29440 Adding walker to previously applied cast

29445 Application of rigid total contact leg cast

29450 Application of clubfoot cast with molding or manipulation, long or short leg

(To report bilateral procedure, use 29450 with modifier 50)

Splints

29505 Application of long leg splint (thigh to ankle or toes)

29515 Application of short leg splint (calf to foot)

Strapping—Any Age

29520 Strapping; hip

29530   knee

29540   ankle and/or foot

29550   toes

29580   Unna boot

29590 Denis-Browne splint strapping

Removal or Repair

Codes for cast removals should be employed only for casts applied by another physician.

29700 Removal or bivalving; gauntlet, boot or body cast

29705   full arm or full leg cast

29710   shoulder or hip spica, Minerva, or Risser jacket, etc.

29715   turnbuckle jacket

29720 Repair of spica, body cast or jacket

29730 Windowing of cast

29740 Wedging of cast (except clubfoot casts)

29750 Wedging of clubfoot cast

(To report bilateral procedure, use 29750 with modifier 50)

Other Procedures

29799 Unlisted procedure, casting or strapping

Endoscopy/Arthroscopy

Surgical endoscopy/arthroscopy always includes a diagnostic endoscopy/arthroscopy.

When arthroscopy is performed in conjunction with arthrotomy, add modifier 51.

29800 Arthroscopy, temporomandibular joint, diagnostic, with or without synovial biopsy (separate procedure)

29804 Arthroscopy, temporomandibular joint, surgical

(For open procedure, use 21010)

29805 Arthroscopy, shoulder, diagnostic, with or without synovial biopsy (separate procedure)

(For open procedure, see 23065-23066, 23100-23101)

29806 Arthroscopy, shoulder, surgical; capsulorrhaphy

(For open procedure, see 23450-23466)

(To report thermal capsulorrhaphy, use 29999)

29807   repair of SLAP lesion

29819   with removal of loose body or foreign body

(For open procedure, see 23040-23044, 23107)

29820   synovectomy, partial

(For open procedure, see 23105)

29821   synovectomy, complete

(For open procedure, see 23105)

29822   debridement, limited

(For open procedure, see specific open shoulder procedure performed)

29823   debridement, extensive

(For open procedure, see specific open shoulder procedure performed)

29824   distal claviculectomy including distal articular surface (Mumford procedure)

(For open procedure, use 23120)

29825   with lysis and resection of adhesions, with or without manipulation

(For open procedure, see specific open shoulder procedure performed)

Surgery: Musculoskeletal System

29826   decompression of subacromial space with partial acromioplasty, with or without coracoacromial release

(For open procedure, use 23130 or 23415)

29827   with rotator cuff repair

(For open or mini-open rotator cuff repair, use 23412)

(When arthroscopic subacromial decompression is performed at the same setting, use 29826 and append modifier 51)

(When arthroscopic distal clavicle resection is performed at the same setting, use 29824 and append modifier 51)

29830   Arthroscopy, elbow, diagnostic, with or without synovial biopsy (separate procedure)

29834   Arthroscopy, elbow, surgical; with removal of loose body or foreign body

29835   synovectomy, partial

29836   synovectomy, complete

29837   debridement, limited

29838   debridement, extensive

29840   Arthroscopy, wrist, diagnostic, with or without synovial biopsy (separate procedure)

29843   Arthroscopy, wrist, surgical; for infection, lavage and drainage

29844   synovectomy, partial

29845   synovectomy, complete

29846   excision and/or repair of triangular fibrocartilage and/or joint debridement

29847   internal fixation for fracture or instability

29848   Endoscopy, wrist, surgical, with release of transverse carpal ligament

(For open procedure, use 64721)

29850   Arthroscopically aided treatment of intercondylar spine(s) and/or tuberosity fracture(s) of the knee, with or without manipulation; without internal or external fixation (includes arthroscopy)

29851   with internal or external fixation (includes arthroscopy)

(For bone graft, use 20900, 20902)

29855   Arthroscopically aided treatment of tibial fracture, proximal (plateau); unicondylar, with or without internal or external fixation (includes arthroscopy)

29856   bicondylar, with or without internal or external fixation (includes arthroscopy)

(For bone graft, use 20900, 20902)

29860   Arthroscopy, hip, diagnostic with or without synovial biopsy (separate procedure)

29861   Arthroscopy, hip, surgical; with removal of loose body or foreign body

29862   with debridement/shaving of articular cartilage (chondroplasty), abrasion arthroplasty, and/or resection of labrum

29863   with synovectomy

29866   Arthroscopy, knee, surgical; osteochondral autograft(s) (eg, mosaicplasty) (includes harvesting of the autograft)

(Do not report 29866 in conjunction with 29870, 29871, 29875, 29884 when performed at the same session and/or 29874, 29877, 29879, 29885-29887 when performed in the same compartment)

29867   osteochondral allograft (eg, mosaicplasty)

(Do not report 29867 in conjunction with 27570, 29870, 29871, 29875, 29884 when performed at the same session and/or 29874, 29877, 29879, 29885-29887 when performed in the same compartment)

(Do not report 29867 in conjunction with 27415)

29868   meniscal transplantation (includes arthrotomy for meniscal insertion), medial or lateral

(Do not report 29868 in conjunction with 29870, 29871, 29875, 29880, 29883, 29884 when performed at the same session or 29874, 29877, 29881, 29882 when performed in the same compartment)

29870   Arthroscopy, knee, diagnostic, with or without synovial biopsy (separate procedure)

(For open autologous chondrocyte implantation of the knee, use 27412)

29871   Arthroscopy, knee, surgical; for infection, lavage and drainage

(For implantation of osteochondral graft for treatment of articular surface defect, see 27412, 27415, 29866, 29867)

29873   with lateral release

(For open lateral release, use 27425)

29874   for removal of loose body or foreign body (eg, osteochondritis dissecans fragmentation, chondral fragmentation)

29875   synovectomy, limited (eg, plica or shelf resection) (separate procedure)

29876   synovectomy, major, two or more compartments (eg, medial or lateral)

29877   debridement/shaving of articular cartilage (chondroplasty)

29879   abrasion arthroplasty (includes chondroplasty where necessary) or multiple drilling or microfracture

29880   with meniscectomy (medial AND lateral, including any meniscal shaving)

29881   with meniscectomy (medial OR lateral, including any meniscal shaving)

29882   with meniscus repair (medial OR lateral)

29883   with meniscus repair (medial AND lateral)

(For meniscal transplantation, medial or lateral, knee, use 29868)

29884   with lysis of adhesions, with or without manipulation (separate procedure)

29885   drilling for osteochondritis dissecans with bone grafting, with or without internal fixation (including debridement of base of lesion)

29886   drilling for intact osteochondritis dissecans lesion

29887   drilling for intact osteochondritis dissecans lesion with internal fixation

29888   Arthroscopically aided anterior cruciate ligament repair/augmentation or reconstruction

29889   Arthroscopically aided posterior cruciate ligament repair/augmentation or reconstruction

(Procedures 29888 and 29889 should not be used with reconstruction procedures 27427-27429)

29891   Arthroscopy, ankle, surgical, excision of osteochondral defect of talus and/or tibia, including drilling of the defect

29892   Arthroscopically aided repair of large osteochondritis dissecans lesion, talar dome fracture, or tibial plafond fracture, with or without internal fixation (includes arthroscopy)

29893   Endoscopic plantar fasciotomy

29894   Arthroscopy, ankle (tibiotalar and fibulotalar joints), surgical; with removal of loose body or foreign body

29895   synovectomy, partial

29897   debridement, limited

29898   debridement, extensive

29899   with ankle arthrodesis

(For open ankle arthrodesis, use 27870)

29900   Arthroscopy, metacarpophalangeal joint, diagnostic, includes synovial biopsy

(Do not report 29900 with 29901, 29902)

29901   Arthroscopy, metacarpophalangeal joint, surgical; with debridement

29902   with reduction of displaced ulnar collateral ligament (eg, Stenar lesion)

29999   Unlisted procedure, arthroscopy

Surgery: Musculoskeletal System

Notes

Respiratory System

Nose

Incision

30000   Drainage abscess or hematoma, nasal, internal approach

(For external approach, see 10060, 10140)

30020   Drainage abscess or hematoma, nasal septum

(For lateral rhinotomy, see specific application (eg, 30118, 30320))

Excision

30100   Biopsy, intranasal

(For biopsy skin of nose, see 11100, 11101)

30110   Excision, nasal polyp(s), simple

(30110 would normally be completed in an office setting)

(To report bilateral procedure, use 30110 with modifier 50)

30115   Excision, nasal polyp(s), extensive

(30115 would normally require the facilities available in a hospital setting)

(To report bilateral procedure, use 30115 with modifier 50)

30117   Excision or destruction (eg, laser), intranasal lesion; internal approach

30118   external approach (lateral rhinotomy)

30120   Excision or surgical planing of skin of nose for rhinophyma

30124   Excision dermoid cyst, nose; simple, skin, subcutaneous

30125   complex, under bone or cartilage

30130   Excision inferior turbinate, partial or complete, any method

(For excision of superior or middle turbinate, use 30999)

30140   Submucous resection inferior turbinate, partial or complete, any method

(Do not report 30130 or 30140 in conjunction with 30801, 30802, 30930)

(For submucous resection of superior or middle turbinate, use 30999)

(For endoscopic resection of concha bullosa of middle turbinate, use 31240)

(For submucous resection of nasal septum, use 30520)

(For reduction of turbinates, use 30140 with modifier 52)

30150   Rhinectomy; partial

30160   total

(For closure and/or reconstruction, primary or delayed, see **Integumentary System**, 13150-13160, 14060-14300, 15120, 15121, 15260, 15261, 15760, 20900-20912)

Introduction

30200   Injection into turbinate(s), therapeutic

30210   Displacement therapy (Proetz type)

30220   Insertion, nasal septal prosthesis (button)

Removal of Foreign Body

30300   Removal foreign body, intranasal; office type procedure

30310   requiring general anesthesia

30320   by lateral rhinotomy

Repair

(For obtaining tissues for graft, see 20900-20926, 21210)

30400   Rhinoplasty, primary; lateral and alar cartilages and/or elevation of nasal tip

(For columellar reconstruction, see 13150 et seq)

30410   complete, external parts including bony pyramid, lateral and alar cartilages, and/or elevation of nasal tip

30420   including major septal repair

30430   Rhinoplasty, secondary; minor revision (small amount of nasal tip work)

30435   intermediate revision (bony work with osteotomies)

30450   major revision (nasal tip work and osteotomies)

30460   Rhinoplasty for nasal deformity secondary to congenital cleft lip and/or palate, including columellar lengthening; tip only

30462   tip, septum, osteotomies

30465   Repair of nasal vestibular stenosis (eg, spreader grafting, lateral nasal wall reconstruction)

(30465 excludes obtaining graft. For graft procedure, see 20900-20926, 21210)

(30465 is used to report a bilateral procedure. For unilateral procedure, use modifier 52)

30520   Septoplasty or submucous resection, with or without cartilage scoring, contouring or replacement with graft

(For submucous resection of turbinates, use 30140)

Surgery: Respiratory System

Surgery: Respiratory System

30540 Repair choanal atresia; intranasal

30545   transpalatine

(Do not report modifier 63 in conjunction with 30540, 30545)

30560 Lysis intranasal synechia

30580 Repair fistula; oromaxillary (combine with 31030 if antrotomy is included)

30600   oronasal

30620 Septal or other intranasal dermatoplasty (does not include obtaining graft)

30630 Repair nasal septal perforations

Destruction

30801 Cautery and/or ablation, mucosa of inferior turbinates, unilateral or bilateral, any method; superficial

(For cautery and ablation of superior or middle turbinates, use 30999)

30802   intramural

(Do not report 30801, 30802, 30930 in conjunction with 30130 or 30140)

(For cautery performed for control of nasal hemorrhage, see 30901-30906)

Other Procedures

30901 Control nasal hemorrhage, anterior, simple (limited cautery and/or packing) any method

(To report bilateral procedure, use 30901 with modifier 50)

30903 Control nasal hemorrhage, anterior, complex (extensive cautery and/or packing) any method

(To report bilateral procedure, use 30903 with modifier 50)

30905 Control nasal hemorrhage, posterior, with posterior nasal packs and/or cautery, any method; initial

30906   subsequent

30915 Ligation arteries; ethmoidal

30920   internal maxillary artery, transantral

(For ligation external carotid artery, use 37600)

30930 Fracture nasal inferior turbinate(s), therapeutic

(Do not report 30801, 30802, 30930 in conjunction with 30130 or 30140)

(For fracture of superior or middle turbinate(s), use 30999)

30999 Unlisted procedure, nose

Accessory Sinuses

Incision

31000 Lavage by cannulation; maxillary sinus (antrum puncture or natural ostium)

(To report bilateral procedure, use 31000 with modifier 50)

31002   sphenoid sinus

31020 Sinusotomy, maxillary (antrotomy); intranasal

(To report bilateral procedure, use 31020 with modifier 50)

31030   radical (Caldwell-Luc) without removal of antrochoanal polyps

(To report bilateral procedure, use 31030 with modifier 50)

31032   radical (Caldwell-Luc) with removal of antrochoanal polyps

(To report bilateral procedure, use 31032 with modifier 50)

31040 Pterygomaxillary fossa surgery, any approach

(For transantral ligation of internal maxillary artery, use 30920)

31050 Sinusotomy, sphenoid, with or without biopsy;

31051   with mucosal stripping or removal of polyp(s)

31070 Sinusotomy frontal; external, simple (trephine operation)

(For frontal intranasal sinusotomy, use 31276)

31075   transorbital, unilateral (for mucocele or osteoma, Lynch type)

31080   obliterative without osteoplastic flap, brow incision (includes ablation)

31081   obliterative, without osteoplastic flap, coronal incision (includes ablation)

31084   obliterative, with osteoplastic flap, brow incision

31085   obliterative, with osteoplastic flap, coronal incision

31086   nonobliterative, with osteoplastic flap, brow incision

31087   nonobliterative, with osteoplastic flap, coronal incision

31090 Sinusotomy, unilateral, three or more paranasal sinuses (frontal, maxillary, ethmoid, sphenoid)

Excision

31200 Ethmoidectomy; intranasal, anterior

31201   intranasal, total

31205   extranasal, total

31225   Maxillectomy; without orbital exenteration

31230   with orbital exenteration (en bloc)

(For orbital exenteration only, see 65110 et seq)

(For skin grafts, see 15120 et seq)

Endoscopy

A surgical sinus endoscopy includes a sinusotomy (when appropriate) and diagnostic endoscopy.

Codes 31231-31294 are used to report unilateral procedures unless otherwise specified.

The codes 31231-31235 for diagnostic evaluation refer to employing a nasal/sinus endoscope to inspect the interior of the nasal cavity and the middle and superior meatus, the turbinates, and the spheno-ethmoid recess. Any time a diagnostic evaluation is performed all these areas would be inspected and a separate code is not reported for each area.

31231   Nasal endoscopy, diagnostic, unilateral or bilateral (separate procedure)

31233   Nasal/sinus endoscopy, diagnostic with maxillary sinusoscopy (via inferior meatus or canine fossa puncture)

31235   Nasal/sinus endoscopy, diagnostic with sphenoid sinusoscopy (via puncture of sphenoidal face or cannulation of ostium)

31237   Nasal/sinus endoscopy, surgical; with biopsy, polypectomy or debridement (separate procedure)

31238   with control of nasal hemorrhage

31239   with dacryocystorhinostomy

31240   with concha bullosa resection

(For endoscopic osteomeatal complex (OMC) resection with antrostomy and/or anterior ethmoidectomy, with or without removal of polyp(s), use 31254 and 31256)

(For endoscopic osteomeatal complex (OMC) resection with antrostomy, removal of antral mucosal disease, and/or anterior ethmoidectomy, with or without removal of polyp(s), use 31254 and 31267)

(For endoscopic frontal sinus exploration, osteomeatal complex (OMC) resection and/or anterior ethmoidectomy, with or without removal of polyp(s), use 31254 and 31276)

(For endoscopic frontal sinus exploration, osteomeatal complex (OMC) resection, antrostomy, and/or anterior ethmoidectomy, with or without removal of polyp(s), use 31254, 31256, and 31276)

(For endoscopic nasal diagnostic endoscopy, see 31231-31235)

(For endoscopic osteomeatal complex (OMC) resection, frontal sinus exploration, antrostomy, removal of antral mucosal disease, and/or anterior ethmoidectomy, with or without removal of polyp(s), use 31254, 31267, and 31276)

31254   Nasal/sinus endoscopy, surgical; with ethmoidectomy, partial (anterior)

31255   with ethmoidectomy, total (anterior and posterior)

31256   Nasal/sinus endoscopy, surgical, with maxillary antrostomy;

(For endoscopic anterior and posterior ethmoidectomy (APE) and antrostomy, with or without removal of polyp(s), use 31255 and 31256)

(For endoscopic anterior and posterior ethmoidectomy (APE), antrostomy and removal of antral mucosal disease, with or without removal of polyp(s), use 31255 and 31267)

(For endoscopic anterior and posterior ethmoidectomy (APE), and frontal sinus exploration, with or without removal of polyp(s), use 31255 and 31276)

31267   with removal of tissue from maxillary sinus

(For endoscopic anterior and posterior ethmoidectomy (APE), and frontal sinus exploration and antrostomy, with or without removal of polyp(s), use 31255, 31256, and 31276)

(For endoscopic anterior and posterior ethmoidectomy (APE), frontal sinus exploration, antrostomy, and removal of antral mucosal disease, with or without removal of polyp(s), use 31255, 31267, and 31276)

31276   Nasal/sinus endoscopy, surgical with frontal sinus exploration, with or without removal of tissue from frontal sinus

(For endoscopic anterior and posterior ethmoidectomy and sphenoidotomy (APS), with or without removal of polyp(s), use 31255, 31287 or 31288)

(For endoscopic anterior and posterior ethmoidectomy and sphenoidotomy (APS), and antrostomy, with or without removal of polyp(s), use 31255, 31256, and 31287 or 31288)

(For endoscopic anterior and posterior ethmoidectomy and sphenoidotomy (APS), antrostomy and removal of antral mucosal disease, with or without removal of polyp(s), use 31255, 31267, and 31287 or 31288)

(For endoscopic anterior and posterior ethmoidectomy and sphenoidotomy (APS), and frontal sinus exploration with or without removal of polyp(s), use 31255, 31287 or 31288, and 31276)

(For endoscopic anterior and posterior ethmoidectomy and sphenoidotomy (APS), with or without removal of polyp(s), with frontal sinus exploration and antrostomy, use 31255, 31256, 31287 or 31288, and 31276)

(For unilateral endoscopy of two or more sinuses, see 31231-31235)

(For endoscopic anterior and posterior ethmoidectomy and sphenoidotomy (APS), frontal sinus exploration, antrostomy and removal of antral mucosal disease, with or without removal of polyp(s), see 31255, 31267, 31287 or 31288 and 31276)

Surgery: Respiratory System

31287 Nasal/sinus endoscopy, surgical, with sphenoidotomy;

31288 with removal of tissue from the sphenoid sinus

31290 Nasal/sinus endoscopy, surgical, with repair of cerebrospinal fluid leak; ethmoid region

31291 sphenoid region

31292 Nasal/sinus endoscopy, surgical; with medial or inferior orbital wall decompression

31293 with medial orbital wall and inferior orbital wall decompression

31294 with optic nerve decompression

Other Procedures

(For hypophysectomy, transantral or transeptal approach, use 61548)

(For transcranial hypophysectomy, use 61546)

31299 Unlisted procedure, accessory sinuses

Larynx

Excision

31300 Laryngotomy (thyrotomy, laryngofissure); with removal of tumor or laryngocele, cordectomy

31320 diagnostic

31360 Laryngectomy; total, without radical neck dissection

31365 total, with radical neck dissection

31367 subtotal supraglottic, without radical neck dissection

31368 subtotal supraglottic, with radical neck dissection

31370 Partial laryngectomy (hemilaryngectomy); horizontal

31375 laterovertical

31380 anterovertical

31382 antero-latero-vertical

31390 Pharyngolaryngectomy, with radical neck dissection; without reconstruction

31395 with reconstruction

31400 Arytenoidectomy or arytenoidopexy, external approach

(For endoscopic arytenoidectomy, use 31560)

31420 Epiglottidectomy

Introduction

⊘ **31500** Intubation, endotracheal, emergency procedure

►(For injection procedure for segmental bronchography, use 31656)◄

31502 Tracheotomy tube change prior to establishment of fistula tract

Endoscopy

For endoscopic procedures, code appropriate endoscopy of each anatomic site examined. If using operating microscope, telescope, or both, use the applicable code only once per operative session.

31505 Laryngoscopy, indirect; diagnostic (separate procedure)

31510 with biopsy

31511 with removal of foreign body

31512 with removal of lesion

31513 with vocal cord injection

31515 Laryngoscopy direct, with or without tracheoscopy; for aspiration

31520 diagnostic, newborn

(Do not report modifier 63 in conjunction with 31520)

31525 diagnostic, except newborn

31526 diagnostic, with operating microscope or telescope

(Do not report code 69990 in addition to code 31526)

31527 with insertion of obturator

31528 with dilation, initial

31529 with dilation, subsequent

31530 Laryngoscopy, direct, operative, with foreign body removal;

31531 with operating microscope or telescope

(Do not report code 69990 in addition to code 31531)

31535 Laryngoscopy, direct, operative, with biopsy;

31536 with operating microscope or telescope

(Do not report code 69990 in addition to code 31536)

31540 Laryngoscopy, direct, operative, with excision of tumor and/or stripping of vocal cords or epiglottis;

31541 with operating microscope or telescope

(Do not report code 69990 in addition to code 31541)

31545 Laryngoscopy, direct, operative, with operating microscope or telescope, with submucosal removal of non-neoplastic lesion(s) of vocal cord; reconstruction with local tissue flap(s)

31546 reconstruction with graft(s) (includes obtaining autograft)

(Do not report 31546 in addition to 20926 for graft harvest)

(For reconstruction of vocal cord with allograft, use 31599)

(Do not report 31545 or 31546 in conjunction with 31540, 31541, 69990)

31560   Laryngoscopy, direct, operative, with arytenoidectomy;

31561   with operating microscope or telescope

           (Do not report code 69990 in addition to code 31561)

31570   Laryngoscopy, direct, with injection into vocal cord(s), therapeutic;

31571   with operating microscope or telescope

           (Do not report code 69990 in addition to code 31571)

31575   Laryngoscopy, flexible fiberoptic; diagnostic

31576   with biopsy

31577   with removal of foreign body

31578   with removal of lesion

           (To report flexible fiberoptic endoscopic evaluation of swallowing, see 92612-92613)

           (To report flexible fiberoptic endoscopic evaluation with sensory testing, see 92614-92615)

           (To report flexible fiberoptic endoscopic evaluation of swallowing with sensory testing, see 92616-92617)

           (For flexible fiberoptic laryngoscopy as part of flexible fiberoptic endoscopic evaluation of swallowing and/or laryngeal sensory testing by cine or video recording, see 92612-92617)

31579   Laryngoscopy, flexible or rigid fiberoptic, with stroboscopy

Repair

31580   Laryngoplasty; for laryngeal web, two stage, with keel insertion and removal

31582   for laryngeal stenosis, with graft or core mold, including tracheotomy

31584   with open reduction of fracture

           (31585 and 31586 have been deleted. To report, use the appropriate Evaluation and Management codes)

31587   Laryngoplasty, cricoid split

31588   Laryngoplasty, not otherwise specified (eg, for burns, reconstruction after partial laryngectomy)

31590   Laryngeal reinnervation by neuromuscular pedicle

Destruction

31595   Section recurrent laryngeal nerve, therapeutic (separate procedure), unilateral

Other Procedures

31599   Unlisted procedure, larynx

Trachea and Bronchi

Incision

31600   Tracheostomy, planned (separate procedure);

31601   younger than two years

31603   Tracheostomy, emergency procedure; transtracheal

31605   cricothyroid membrane

31610   Tracheostomy, fenestration procedure with skin flaps

           (For endotracheal intubation, use 31500)

           (For tracheal aspiration under direct vision, use 31515)

31611   Construction of tracheoesophageal fistula and subsequent insertion of an alaryngeal speech prosthesis (eg, voice button, Blom-Singer prosthesis)

31612   Tracheal puncture, percutaneous with transtracheal aspiration and/or injection

31613   Tracheostoma revision; simple, without flap rotation

31614   complex, with flap rotation

Endoscopy

For endoscopy procedures, code appropriate endoscopy of each anatomic site examined. Surgical bronchoscopy always includes diagnostic bronchoscopy when performed by the same physician. Codes 31622-31646 include fluoroscopic guidance, when performed.

           (For tracheoscopy, see laryngoscopy codes 31515-31578)

⊙ **31615**   Tracheobronchoscopy through established tracheostomy incision

⊙✛ **31620**   Endobronchial ultrasound (EBUS) during bronchoscopic diagnostic or therapeutic intervention(s) (List separately in addition to code for primary procedure(s))

           (Use 31620 in conjunction with 31622-31646)

⊙ **31622**   Bronchoscopy, rigid or flexible, with or without fluoroscopic guidance; diagnostic, with or without cell washing (separate procedure)

⊙ **31623**   with brushing or protected brushings

⊙ **31624**   with bronchial alveolar lavage

⊙ **31625**   with bronchial or endobronchial biopsy(s), single or multiple sites

⊙ **31628**   with transbronchial lung biopsy(s), single lobe

           (31628 should be reported only once regardless of how many transbronchial lung biopsies are performed in a lobe)

           (To report transbronchial lung biopsies performed on additional lobe, use 31632)

⊙ **31629**   with transbronchial needle aspiration biopsy(s), trachea, main stem and/or lobar bronchus(i)

(31629 should be reported only once for upper airway biopsies regardless of how many transbronchial needle aspiration biopsies are performed in the upper airway or in a lobe)

(To report transbronchial needle aspiration biopsies performed on additional lobe(s), use 31633)

31630   with tracheal/bronchial dilation or closed reduction of fracture

31631   with placement of tracheal stent(s) (includes tracheal/bronchial dilation as required)

(For placement of bronchial stent, see 31636, 31637)

(For revision of tracheal/bronchial stent, use 31638)

+ **31632**   with transbronchial lung biopsy(s), each additional lobe (List separately in addition to code for primary procedure)

(Use 31632 in conjunction with 31628)

(31632 should be reported only once regardless of how many transbronchial lung biopsies are performed in a lobe)

+ **31633**   with transbronchial needle aspiration biopsy(s), each additional lobe (List separately in addition to code for primary procedure)

(Use 31633 in conjunction with 31629)

(31633 should be reported only once regardless of how many transbronchial needle aspiration biopsies are performed in the trachea or the additional lobe)

⊙ **31635**   with removal of foreign body

31636   with placement of bronchial stent(s) (includes tracheal/bronchial dilation as required), initial bronchus

+ **31637**   each additional major bronchus stented (List separately in addition to code for primary procedure)

(Use 31637 in conjunction with 31636)

31638   with revision of tracheal or bronchial stent inserted at previous session (includes tracheal/bronchial dilation as required)

31640   with excision of tumor

31641   Bronchoscopy, (rigid or flexible); with destruction of tumor or relief of stenosis by any method other than excision (eg, laser therapy, cryotherapy)

(For bronchoscopic photodynamic therapy, report 31641 in addition to 96570, 96571 as appropriate)

31643   with placement of catheter(s) for intracavitary radioelement application

(For intracavitary radioelement application, see 77761-77763, 77781-77784)

⊙ **31645**   with therapeutic aspiration of tracheobronchial tree, initial (eg, drainage of lung abscess)

⊙ **31646**   with therapeutic aspiration of tracheobronchial tree, subsequent

(For catheter aspiration of tracheobronchial tree at bedside, use 31725)

⊙ **31656**   with injection of contrast material for segmental bronchography (fiberscope only)

(For radiological supervision and interpretation, see 71040, 71060)

Introduction

(For endotracheal intubation, use 31500)

(For tracheal aspiration under direct vision, see 31515)

▶(31700, 31708, 31710 have been deleted)◀

31715   Transtracheal injection for bronchography

(For radiological supervision and interpretation, see 71040, 71060)

(For prolonged services, see 99354-99360)

31717   Catheterization with bronchial brush biopsy

31720   Catheter aspiration (separate procedure); nasotracheal

⊙ **31725**   tracheobronchial with fiberscope, bedside

31730   Transtracheal (percutaneous) introduction of needle wire dilator/stent or indwelling tube for oxygen therapy

▶Excision, Repair◀

31750   Tracheoplasty; cervical

31755   tracheopharyngeal fistulization, each stage

31760   intrathoracic

31766   Carinal reconstruction

31770   Bronchoplasty; graft repair

31775   excision stenosis and anastomosis

(For lobectomy and bronchoplasty, use 32501)

31780   Excision tracheal stenosis and anastomosis; cervical

31781   cervicothoracic

31785   Excision of tracheal tumor or carcinoma; cervical

31786   thoracic

31800   Suture of tracheal wound or injury; cervical

31805   intrathoracic

31820   Surgical closure tracheostomy or fistula; without plastic repair

31825   with plastic repair

(For repair tracheoesophageal fistula, see 43305, 43312)

31830   Revision of tracheostomy scar

Other Procedures

31899   Unlisted procedure, trachea, bronchi

Lungs and Pleura

Incision

⊘ **32000**   Thoracentesis, puncture of pleural cavity for aspiration, initial or subsequent

         ►(If imaging guidance is performed, see 76942, 77002, 77012)◄

         (For total lung lavage, use 32997)

⊘ **32002**   Thoracentesis with insertion of tube with or without water seal (eg, for pneumothorax) (separate procedure)

         (Do not report 32002 in conjunction with 19260, 19271, 19272, 32503, 32504)

         ►(If imaging guidance is performed, see 76942, 77002, 77012)◄

32005   Chemical pleurodesis (eg, for recurrent or persistent pneumothorax)

⊙ **32019**   Insertion of indwelling tunneled pleural catheter with cuff

         (Do not report 32019 in conjunction with 32000-32005, 32020, 36000, 36410, 62318, 62319, 64450, 64470, 64475)

         (If imaging guidance is performed, use 75989)

⊙⊘ **32020**   Tube thoracostomy with or without water seal (eg, for abscess, hemothorax, empyema) (separate procedure)

         (Do not report 32020 in conjunction with 19260, 19271, 19272, 32503, 32504)

         (If imaging guidance is performed, use 75989)

32035   Thoracostomy; with rib resection for empyema

32036   with open flap drainage for empyema

32095   Thoracotomy, limited, for biopsy of lung or pleura

         (To report wound exploration due to penetrating trauma without thoractomy, use 20102)

32100   Thoracotomy, major; with exploration and biopsy

         (Do not report 32100 in conjunction with 19260, 19271, 19272, 32503, 32504)

32110   with control of traumatic hemorrhage and/or repair of lung tear

32120   for postoperative complications

32124   with open intrapleural pneumonolysis

32140   with cyst(s) removal, with or without a pleural procedure

32141   with excision-plication of bullae, with or without any pleural procedure

         (For lung volume reduction, use 32491)

32150   with removal of intrapleural foreign body or fibrin deposit

32151   with removal of intrapulmonary foreign body

32160   with cardiac massage

         (For segmental or other resections of lung, see 32480-32504)

32200   Pneumonostomy; with open drainage of abscess or cyst

⊙ **32201**   with percutaneous drainage of abscess or cyst

         (For radiological supervision and interpretation, use 75989)

32215   Pleural scarification for repeat pneumothorax

32220   Decortication, pulmonary (separate procedure); total

32225   partial

Excision

32310   Pleurectomy, parietal (separate procedure)

32320   Decortication and parietal pleurectomy

32400   Biopsy, pleura; percutaneous needle

         ►(If imaging guidance is performed, see 76942, 77002, 77012, 77021)◄

         (For fine needle aspiration, use 10021 or 10022)

         (For evaluation of fine needle aspirate, see 88172, 88173)

32402   open

32405   Biopsy, lung or mediastinum, percutaneous needle

         ►(For radiological supervision and interpretation, see 76942, 77002, 77012, 77021)◄

         (For fine needle aspiration, use 10022)

         (For evaluation of fine needle aspirate, see 88172, 88173)

►Removal◄

32420   Pneumocentesis, puncture of lung for aspiration

32440   Removal of lung, total pneumonectomy;

32442   with resection of segment of trachea followed by broncho-tracheal anastomosis (sleeve pneumonectomy)

32445   extrapleural

         (For extrapleural pneumonectomy, with empyemectomy, use 32445 and 32540)

         (If lung resection is performed with chest wall tumor resection, report the appropriate chest wall tumor resection code, 19260-19272, in addition to lung resection code 32440-32445)

Surgery: Respiratory System

Surgery: Respiratory System

32480   Removal of lung, other than total pneumonectomy; single lobe (lobectomy)

32482   two lobes (bilobectomy)

32484   single segment (segmentectomy)

(For removal of lung with bronchoplasty, use 32501)

32486   with circumferential resection of segment of bronchus followed by broncho-bronchial anastomosis (sleeve lobectomy)

32488   all remaining lung following previous removal of a portion of lung (completion pneumonectomy)

(For total or segmental lobectomy, with concomitant decortication, use 32320 and the appropriate removal of lung code)

32491   excision-plication of emphysematous lung(s) (bullous or non-bullous) for lung volume reduction, sternal split or transthoracic approach, with or without any pleural procedure

32500   wedge resection, single or multiple

(If lung resection is performed with chest wall tumor resection, report the appropriate chest wall tumor resection code, 19260-19272, in addition to lung resection code 32480-32500)

+ 32501   Resection and repair of portion of bronchus (bronchoplasty) when performed at time of lobectomy or segmentectomy (List separately in addition to code for primary procedure)

(Use 32501 in conjunction with 32480, 32482, 32484)

(32501 is to be used when a portion of the bronchus to preserved lung is removed and requires plastic closure to preserve function of that preserved lung. It is not to be used for closure for the proximal end of a resected bronchus)

32503   Resection of apical lung tumor (eg, Pancoast tumor), including chest wall resection, rib(s) resection(s), neurovascular dissection, when performed; without chest wall reconstruction(s)

32504   with chest wall reconstruction

(Do not report 32503, 32504 in conjunction with 19260, 19271, 19272, 32002, 32020, 32100)

(32520, 32522, and 32525 have been deleted)

(For performance of lung resection in conjunction with chest wall resection, see 19260, 19271, 19272 and 32480-32500, 32503, 32504)

32540   Extrapleural enucleation of empyema (empyemectomy)

(For extrapleural enucleation of empyema (empyemectomy) with lobectomy, use 32540 and the appropriate removal of lung code)

Endoscopy

Surgical thoracoscopy always includes diagnostic thoracoscopy.

For endoscopic procedures, code appropriate endoscopy of each anatomic site examined.

32601   Thoracoscopy, diagnostic (separate procedure); lungs and pleural space, without biopsy

32602   lungs and pleural space, with biopsy

32603   pericardial sac, without biopsy

32604   pericardial sac, with biopsy

32605   mediastinal space, without biopsy

32606   mediastinal space, with biopsy

(Surgical thoracoscopy always includes diagnostic thoracoscopy)

32650   Thoracoscopy, surgical; with pleurodesis (eg, mechanical or chemical)

32651   with partial pulmonary decortication

32652   with total pulmonary decortication, including intrapleural pneumonolysis

32653   with removal of intrapleural foreign body or fibrin deposit

32654   with control of traumatic hemorrhage

32655   with excision-plication of bullae, including any pleural procedure

32656   with parietal pleurectomy

32657   with wedge resection of lung, single or multiple

32658   with removal of clot or foreign body from pericardial sac

32659   with creation of pericardial window or partial resection of pericardial sac for drainage

32660   with total pericardiectomy

32661   with excision of pericardial cyst, tumor, or mass

32662   with excision of mediastinal cyst, tumor, or mass

32663   with lobectomy, total or segmental

32664   with thoracic sympathectomy

32665   with esophagomyotomy (Heller type)

(For exploratory thoracoscopy, and exploratory thoracoscopy with biopsy, see 32601-32606)

Repair

32800   Repair lung hernia through chest wall

32810   Closure of chest wall following open flap drainage for empyema (Clagett type procedure)

32815   Open closure of major bronchial fistula

32820   Major reconstruction, chest wall (posttraumatic)

Lung Transplantation

Lung allotransplantation involves three distinct components of physician work:

1) *Cadaver donor pneumonectomy(s)*, which include(s) harvesting the allograft and cold preservation of the allograft (perfusing with cold preservation solution and cold maintenance) (use 32850).

2) *Backbench work*:

Preparation of a cadaver donor single lung allograft prior to transplantation, including dissection of the allograft from surrounding soft tissues to prepare the pulmonary venous/atrial cuff, pulmonary artery, and bronchus unilaterally (use 32855).

Preparation of a cadaver donor double lung allograft prior to transplantation, including dissection of the allograft from surrounding soft tissues to prepare the pulmonary venous/atrial cuff, pulmonary artery, and bronchus bilaterally (use 32856).

3) *Recipient lung allotransplantation*, which includes transplantation of a single or double lung allograft and care of the recipient (see 32851-32854).

32850   Donor pneumonectomy(s) (including cold preservation), from cadaver donor

32851   Lung transplant, single; without cardiopulmonary bypass

32852   with cardiopulmonary bypass

32853   Lung transplant, double (bilateral sequential or en bloc); without cardiopulmonary bypass

32854   with cardiopulmonary bypass

32855   Backbench standard preparation of cadaver donor lung allograft prior to transplantation, including dissection of allograft from surrounding soft tissues to prepare pulmonary venous/atrial cuff, pulmonary artery, and bronchus; unilateral

32856   bilateral

(For repair or resection procedures on the donor lung, see 32491, 32500, 35216, or 35276)

Surgical Collapse Therapy; Thoracoplasty

(See also 32503, 32504)

32900   Resection of ribs, extrapleural, all stages

32905   Thoracoplasty, Schede type or extrapleural (all stages);

32906   with closure of bronchopleural fistula

(For open closure of major bronchial fistula, use 32815)

(For resection of first rib for thoracic outlet compression, see 21615, 21616)

32940   Pneumonolysis, extraperiosteal, including filling or packing procedures

32960   Pneumothorax, therapeutic, intrapleural injection of air

Other Procedures

32997   Total lung lavage (unilateral)

(For bronchoscopic bronchial alveolar lavage, use 31624)

● **32998**   Ablation therapy for reduction or eradication of one or more pulmonary tumor(s) including pleura or chest wall when involved by tumor extension, percutaneous, radiofrequency, unilateral

▶(For imaging guidance and monitoring, see 76940, 77013, 77022)◀

32999   Unlisted procedure, lungs and pleura

Surgery: Respiratory System

Notes

⊙=Moderate sedation   ✚=Add-on code   ✗=FDA approval pending

Cardiovascular System

Selective vascular catheterizations should be coded to include introduction and all lesser order selective catheterizations used in the approach (eg, the description for a selective right middle cerebral artery catheterization includes the introduction and placement catheterization of the right common and internal carotid arteries).

Additional second and/or third order arterial catheterizations within the same family of arteries supplied by a single first order artery should be expressed by 36218 or 36248. Additional first order or higher catheterizations in vascular families supplied by a first order vessel different from a previously selected and coded family should be separately coded using the conventions described above.

> (For monitoring, operation of pump and other nonsurgical services, see 99190-99192, 99291, 99292, 99354-99360)

> (For other medical or laboratory related services, see appropriate section)

> (For radiological supervision and interpretation, see 75600-75978)

Heart and Pericardium

Pericardium

⊙ **33010**   Pericardiocentesis; initial

> (For radiological supervision and interpretation, use 76930)

⊙ **33011**   subsequent

> (For radiological supervision and interpretation, use 76930)

33015   Tube pericardiostomy

33020   Pericardiotomy for removal of clot or foreign body (primary procedure)

33025   Creation of pericardial window or partial resection for drainage

33030   Pericardiectomy, subtotal or complete; without cardiopulmonary bypass

33031   with cardiopulmonary bypass

33050   Excision of pericardial cyst or tumor

Cardiac Tumor

33120   Excision of intracardiac tumor, resection with cardiopulmonary bypass

33130   Resection of external cardiac tumor

Transmyocardial Revascularization

33140   Transmyocardial laser revascularization, by thoracotomy; (separate procedure)

+ 33141   performed at the time of other open cardiac procedure(s) (List separately in addition to code for primary procedure)

> (Use 33141 in conjunction with 33400-33496, 33510-33536, 33542)

Pacemaker or Pacing Cardioverter-Defibrillator

A pacemaker system includes a pulse generator containing electronics, a battery, and one or more electrodes (leads). Pulse generators are placed in a subcutaneous "pocket" created in either a subclavicular site or underneath the abdominal muscles just below the ribcage. Electrodes may be inserted through a vein (transvenous) or they may be placed on the surface of the heart (epicardial). The epicardial location of electrodes requires a thoracotomy for electrode insertion.

►A single chamber pacemaker system includes a pulse generator and one electrode inserted in either the atrium or ventricle. A dual chamber pacemaker system includes a pulse generator and one electrode inserted in the right atrium and one electrode inserted in the right ventricle. In certain circumstances, an additional electrode may be required to achieve pacing of the left ventricle (bi-ventricular pacing). In this event, transvenous (cardiac vein) placement of the electrode should be separately reported using code 33224 or 33225. Epicardial placement of the electrode should be separately reported using 33202-33203.◄

Like a pacemaker system, a pacing cardioverter-defibrillator system includes a pulse generator and electrodes, although pacing cardioverter-defibrillators may require multiple leads, even when only a single chamber is being paced. A pacing cardioverter-defibrillator system may be inserted in a single chamber (pacing in the ventricle) or in dual chambers (pacing in atrium and ventricle). These devices use a combination of antitachycardia pacing, low-energy cardioversion or defibrillating shocks to treat ventricular tachycardia or ventricular fibrillation.

Pacing cardioverter-defibrillator pulse generators may be implanted in a subcutaneous infraclavicular pocket or in an abdominal pocket. Removal of a pacing cardioverter-defibrillator pulse generator requires opening of the existing subcutaneous pocket and disconnection of the pulse generator from its electrode(s). A thoracotomy (or laparotomy in the case of abdominally placed pulse generators) is not required to remove the pulse generator.

Surgery: Cardiovascular System

►The electrodes (leads) of a pacing cardioverter-defibrillator system are positioned in the heart via the venous system (transvenously), in most circumstances. In certain circumstances, an additional electrode may be required to achieve pacing of the left ventricle (bi-ventricular pacing). In this event, transvenous (cardiac vein) placement of the electrode should be separately reported using code 33224 or 33225. Epicardial placement of the electrode should be separately reported using 33202-33203.

Electrode positioning on the epicardial surface of the heart requires thoracotomy, or thoracoscopic placement of the leads. Removal of electrode(s) may first be attempted by transvenous extraction (code 33244). However, if transvenous extraction is unsuccessful, a thoracotomy may be required to remove the electrodes (code 33243). Use codes 33212, 33213, 33240 as appropriate in addition to the thoracotomy or endoscopic epicardial lead placement codes to report the insertion of the generator if done by the same physician during the same session.◄

When the "battery" of a pacemaker or pacing cardioverter-defibrillator is changed, it is actually the pulse generator that is changed. Replacement of a pulse generator should be reported with a code for removal of the pulse generator and another code for insertion of a pulse generator.

Repositioning of a pacemaker electrode, pacing cardioverter-defibrillator electrode(s), or a left ventricular pacing electrode is reported using 33215 or 33226, as appropriate. Replacement of a pacemaker electrode, pacing cardioverter-defibrillator electrode(s), or a left ventricular pacing electrode is reported using 33206-33208, 33210-33213, or 33224, as appropriate.

(For electronic, telephonic analysis of internal pacemaker system, see 93731-93736)

(For radiological supervision and interpretation with insertion of pacemaker, use 71090)

►(33200, 33201 have been deleted)◄

● **33202** Insertion of epicardial electrode(s); open incision (eg, thoracotomy, median sternotomy, subxiphoid approach)

● **33203** endoscopic approach (eg, thoracoscopy, pericardioscopy)

►(When epicardial lead placement is performed by the same physician at the same session as insertion of the generator, report 33202, 33203 in conjunction with 33212, 33213, as appropriate)◄

⊙ **33206** Insertion or replacement of permanent pacemaker with transvenous electrode(s); atrial

⊙ **33207** ventricular

⊙ **33208** atrial and ventricular

(Codes 33206-33208 include subcutaneous insertion of the pulse generator and transvenous placement of electrode(s))

⊙ **33210** Insertion or replacement of temporary transvenous single chamber cardiac electrode or pacemaker catheter (separate procedure)

⊙ **33211** Insertion or replacement of temporary transvenous dual chamber pacing electrodes (separate procedure)

⊙ **33212** Insertion or replacement of pacemaker pulse generator only; single chamber, atrial or ventricular

⊙ **33213** dual chamber

►(Use 33212, 33213, as appropriate, in conjunction with the epicardial lead placement codes 33202, 33203 to report the insertion of the generator when done by the same physician during the same session)◄

⊙ **33214** Upgrade of implanted pacemaker system, conversion of single chamber system to dual chamber system (includes removal of previously placed pulse generator, testing of existing lead, insertion of new lead, insertion of new pulse generator)

►(When epicardial electrode placement is performed, report 33214 in conjunction with 33202, 33203)◄

33215 Repositioning of previously implanted transvenous pacemaker or pacing cardioverter-defibrillator (right atrial or right ventricular) electrode

⊙ **33216** Insertion of a transvenous electrode; single chamber (one electrode) permanent pacemaker or single chamber pacing cardioverter-defibrillator

⊙ **33217** dual chamber (two electrodes) permanent pacemaker or dual chamber pacing cardioverter-defibrillator

(Do not report 33216-33217 in conjunction with 33214)

⊙ **33218** Repair of single transvenous electrode for a single chamber, permanent pacemaker or single chamber pacing cardioverter-defibrillator

(For atrial or ventricular single chamber repair of pacemaker electrode(s) with replacement of pulse generator, see 33212 or 33213 and 33218 or 33220)

⊙ **33220** Repair of two transvenous electrodes for a dual chamber permanent pacemaker or dual chamber pacing cardioverter-defibrillator

⊙ **33222** Revision or relocation of skin pocket for pacemaker

⊙ **33223** Revision of skin pocket for single or dual chamber pacing cardioverter-defibrillator

33224 Insertion of pacing electrode, cardiac venous system, for left ventricular pacing, with attachment to previously placed pacemaker or pacing cardioverter-defibrillator pulse generator (including revision of pocket, removal, insertion, and/or replacement of generator)

►(When epicardial electrode placement is performed, report 33224 in conjunction with 33202, 33203)◄

+ 33225   Insertion of pacing electrode, cardiac venous system, for left ventricular pacing, at time of insertion of pacing cardioverter-defibrillator or pacemaker pulse generator (including upgrade to dual chamber system) (List separately in addition to code for primary procedure)

(Use 33225 in conjunction with 33206, 33207, 33208, 33212, 33213, 33214, 33216, 33217, 33222, 33233, 33234, 33235, 33240, 33249)

33226   Repositioning of previously implanted cardiac venous system (left ventricular) electrode (including removal, insertion and/or replacement of generator)

⊙ **33233**   Removal of permanent pacemaker pulse generator

⊙ **33234**   Removal of transvenous pacemaker electrode(s); single lead system, atrial or ventricular

⊙ **33235**   dual lead system

33236   Removal of permanent epicardial pacemaker and electrodes by thoracotomy; single lead system, atrial or ventricular

33237   dual lead system

33238   Removal of permanent transvenous electrode(s) by thoracotomy

⊙ **33240**   Insertion of single or dual chamber pacing cardioverter-defibrillator pulse generator

►(Use 33240, as appropriate, in addition to the epicardial lead placement codes to report the insertion of the generator when done by the same physician during the same session)◄

⊙ **33241**   Subcutaneous removal of single or dual chamber pacing cardioverter-defibrillator pulse generator

(For removal of electrode(s) by thoracotomy, use 33243 in conjunction with 33241)

(For removal of electrode(s) by transvenous extraction, use 33244 in conjunction with 33241)

(For removal and reinsertion of a pacing cardioverter-defibrillator system (pulse generator and electrodes), report 33241 and 33243 or 33244 and 33249)

(For repair of implantable cardioverter-defibrillator pulse generator and/or leads, see 33218, 33220)

33243   Removal of single or dual chamber pacing cardioverter-defibrillator electrode(s); by thoracotomy

⊙ **33244**   by transvenous extraction

(For subcutaneous removal of the pulse generator, use 33241 in conjunction with 33243 or 33244)

►(33245, 33246 have been deleted)◄

⊙ **33249**   Insertion or repositioning of electrode lead(s) for single or dual chamber pacing cardioverter-defibrillator and insertion of pulse generator

(For removal and reinsertion of a pacing cardioverter-defibrillator system (pulse generator and electrodes), report 33241 and 33243 or 33244 and 33249)

(For insertion of implantable cardioverter-defibrillator lead(s), without thoracotomy, use 33216)

Electrophysiologic Operative Procedures

►This family of codes describes the surgical treatment of supraventricular dysrhythmias. Tissue ablation, disruption and reconstruction can be accomplished by many methods including surgical incision or through the use of a variety of energy sources (eg, radiofrequency, cryotherapy, microwave, ultrasound, laser). If excision or isolation of the left atrial appendage by any method, including stapling, oversewing, ligation, or plication, is performed in conjunction with any of the atrial tissue ablation and reconstruction (maze) procedures (33254-33256, 33265-33266), it is considered part of the procedure. Codes 33254-33256 are only to be reported when there is no concurrently performed procedure that requires median sternotomy or cardiopulmonary bypass. When 33254-33256 are performed with a concurrent procedure that requires a median sternotomy or cardiopulmonary bypass, report the operative (nonthoracoscopic) electrophysiologic procedure with unlisted procedure code 33999.

Definitions

Limited operative ablation and reconstruction includes:

Surgical isolation of triggers of supraventricular dysrhythmias by operative ablation that isolates the pulmonary veins or other anatomically defined triggers in the left or right atrium.

Extensive operative ablation and reconstruction includes:

1. The services included in "*limited*"

2. Additional ablation of atrial tissue to eliminate sustained supraventricular dysrhythmias. This must include operative ablation that involves either the right atrium, the atrial septum, or left atrium in continuity with the atrioventricular annulus.◄

►Incision◄

33250   Operative ablation of supraventricular arrhythmogenic focus or pathway (eg, Wolff-Parkinson-White, atrioventricular node re-entry), tract(s) and/or focus (foci); without cardiopulmonary bypass

33251   with cardiopulmonary bypass

►(33253 has been deleted. To report, use 33254–33256)◄

● **33254** Operative tissue ablation and reconstruction of atria, limited (eg, modified maze procedure)

● **33255** Operative tissue ablation and reconstruction of atria, extensive (eg, maze procedure); without cardiopulmonary bypass

● **33256**   with cardiopulmonary bypass

►(Do not report 33254-33256 in conjunction with 32020, 32100, 33120, 33130, 33210, 33211, 33400-33507, 33510-33523, 33533-33548, 33600-33853, 33860-33863, 33910-33920)◄

33261 Operative ablation of ventricular arrhythmogenic focus with cardiopulmonary bypass

►Endoscopy◄

● **33265** Endoscopy, surgical; operative tissue ablation and reconstruction of atria, limited (eg, modified maze procedure), without cardiopulmonary bypass

● **33266**   operative tissue ablation and reconstruction of atria, extensive (eg, maze procedure), without cardiopulmonary bypass

►(Do not report 33265-33266 in conjunction with 32020, 33210, 33211)◄

Patient-Activated Event Recorder

33282 Implantation of patient-activated cardiac event recorder

(Initial implantation includes programming. For subsequent electronic analysis and/or reprogramming, use 93727)

33284 Removal of an implantable, patient-activated cardiac event recorder

Wounds of the Heart and Great Vessels

33300 Repair of cardiac wound; without bypass

33305   with cardiopulmonary bypass

33310 Cardiotomy, exploratory (includes removal of foreign body, atrial or ventricular thrombus); without bypass

33315   with cardiopulmonary bypass

(Do not report removal of thrombus (33310-33315) in conjunction with other cardiac procedures unless a separate incision in the heart is required to remove the atrial or ventricular thrombus)

(If removal of thrombus with cardiopulmonary bypass (33315) is reported in conjunction with 33120, 33130, 33420-33430, 33460-33468, 33496, 33542, 33545, 33641-33647, 33670, 33681, 33975-33980 which requires a separate heart incision, report 33315 with modifier 59)

33320 Suture repair of aorta or great vessels; without shunt or cardiopulmonary bypass

33321   with shunt bypass

33322   with cardiopulmonary bypass

33330 Insertion of graft, aorta or great vessels; without shunt, or cardiopulmonary bypass

33332   with shunt bypass

33335   with cardiopulmonary bypass

Cardiac Valves

(For multiple valve procedures, see 33400-33478 and add modifier 51 to the secondary valve procedure code)

Aortic Valve

33400 Valvuloplasty, aortic valve; open, with cardiopulmonary bypass

33401   open, with inflow occlusion

33403   using transventricular dilation, with cardiopulmonary bypass

(Do not report modifier 63 in conjunction with 33401, 33403)

33404 Construction of apical-aortic conduit

33405 Replacement, aortic valve, with cardiopulmonary bypass; with prosthetic valve other than homograft or stentless valve

33406   with allograft valve (freehand)

(For aortic valve valvotomy, (commissurotomy) with inflow occlusion, use 33401)

(For aortic valve valvotomy, (commissurotomy) with cardiopulmonary bypass, use 33403)

33410   with stentless tissue valve

33411 Replacement, aortic valve; with aortic annulus enlargement, noncoronary cusp

33412   with transventricular aortic annulus enlargement (Konno procedure)

33413   by translocation of autologous pulmonary valve with allograft replacement of pulmonary valve (Ross procedure)

33414 Repair of left ventricular outflow tract obstruction by patch enlargement of the outflow tract

33415 Resection or incision of subvalvular tissue for discrete subvalvular aortic stenosis

33416 Ventriculomyotomy (-myectomy) for idiopathic hypertrophic subaortic stenosis (eg, asymmetric septal hypertrophy)

33417 Aortoplasty (gusset) for supravalvular stenosis

Mitral Valve

33420   Valvotomy, mitral valve; closed heart

33422   open heart, with cardiopulmonary bypass

33425   Valvuloplasty, mitral valve, with cardiopulmonary bypass;

33426   with prosthetic ring

33427   radical reconstruction, with or without ring

33430   Replacement, mitral valve, with cardiopulmonary bypass

Tricuspid Valve

33460   Valvectomy, tricuspid valve, with cardiopulmonary bypass

33463   Valvuloplasty, tricuspid valve; without ring insertion

33464   with ring insertion

33465   Replacement, tricuspid valve, with cardiopulmonary bypass

33468   Tricuspid valve repositioning and plication for Ebstein anomaly

Pulmonary Valve

33470   Valvotomy, pulmonary valve, closed heart; transventricular

         (Do not report modifier 63 in conjunction with 33470)

33471   via pulmonary artery

         (To report percutaneous valvuloplasty of pulmonary valve, use 92990)

33472   Valvotomy, pulmonary valve, open heart; with inflow occlusion

         (Do not report modifier 63 in conjunction with 33472)

33474   with cardiopulmonary bypass

33475   Replacement, pulmonary valve

33476   Right ventricular resection for infundibular stenosis, with or without commissurotomy

33478   Outflow tract augmentation (gusset), with or without commissurotomy or infundibular resection

         (Use 33478 in conjunction with 33768 when a cavopulmonary anastomosis to a second superior vena cava is performed)

Other Valvular Procedures

33496   Repair of non-structural prosthetic valve dysfunction with cardiopulmonary bypass (separate procedure)

         (For reoperation, use 33530 in addition to 33496)

Coronary Artery Anomalies

Basic procedures include endarterectomy or angioplasty.

33500   Repair of coronary arteriovenous or arteriocardiac chamber fistula; with cardiopulmonary bypass

33501   without cardiopulmonary bypass

33502   Repair of anomalous coronary artery from pulmonary artery origin; by ligation

33503   by graft, without cardiopulmonary bypass

         (Do not report modifier 63 in conjunction with 33502, 33503)

33504   by graft, with cardiopulmonary bypass

33505   with construction of intrapulmonary artery tunnel (Takeuchi procedure)

33506   by translocation from pulmonary artery to aorta

         (Do not report modifier 63 in conjunction with 33505, 33506)

33507   Repair of anomalous (eg, intramural) aortic origin of coronary artery by unroofing or translocation

Endoscopy

Surgical vascular endoscopy always includes diagnostic endoscopy.

+ 33508   Endoscopy, surgical, including video-assisted harvest of vein(s) for coronary artery bypass procedure (List separately in addition to code for primary procedure)

         (Use 33508 in conjunction with 33510-33523)

         (For open harvest of upper extremity vein procedure, use 35500)

Venous Grafting Only for Coronary Artery Bypass

The following codes are used to report coronary artery bypass procedures using venous grafts only. These codes should NOT be used to report the performance of coronary artery bypass procedures using arterial grafts and venous grafts during the same procedure. See 33517-33523 and 33533-33536 for reporting combined arterial-venous grafts.

Procurement of the saphenous vein graft is included in the description of the work for 33510-33516 and should not be reported as a separate service or co-surgery. To report harvesting of an upper extremity vein, use 35500 in addition to the bypass procedure. To report harvesting of a femoropopliteal vein segment, report 35572 in addition to the bypass procedure. When surgical assistant performs graft procurement, add modifier 80 to 33510-33516.

Surgery: Cardiovascular System

33510   Coronary artery bypass, vein only; single coronary venous graft

33511   two coronary venous grafts

33512   three coronary venous grafts

33513   four coronary venous grafts

33514   five coronary venous grafts

33516   six or more coronary venous grafts

Combined Arterial-Venous Grafting for Coronary Bypass

The following codes are used to report coronary artery bypass procedures using venous grafts and arterial grafts during the same procedure. These codes may NOT be used alone.

To report combined arterial-venous grafts it is necessary to report two codes: 1) the appropriate combined arterial-venous graft code (33517-33523); and 2) the appropriate arterial graft code (33533-33536).

Procurement of the saphenous vein graft is included in the description of the work for 33517-33523 and should not be reported as a separate service or co-surgery. Procurement of the artery for grafting is included in the description of the work for 33533-33536 and should not be reported as a separate service or co-surgery, except when an upper extremity artery (eg, radial artery) is procured. To report harvesting of an upper extremity artery, use 35600 in addition to the bypass procedure. To report harvesting of an upper extremity vein, use 35500 in addition to the bypass procedure. To report harvesting of a femoropopliteal vein segment, report 35572 in addition to the bypass procedure. When surgical assistant performs arterial and/or venous graft procurement, add modifier 80 to 33517-33523, 33533-33536, as appropriate.

⊘ 33517   Coronary artery bypass, using venous graft(s) and arterial graft(s); single vein graft (List separately in addition to code for arterial graft)

⊘ 33518   two venous grafts (List separately in addition to code for arterial graft)

⊘ 33519   three venous grafts (List separately in addition to code for arterial graft)

⊘ 33521   four venous grafts (List separately in addition to code for arterial graft)

⊘ 33522   five venous grafts (List separately in addition to code for arterial graft)

⊘ 33523   six or more venous grafts (List separately in addition to code for arterial graft)

+ 33530   Reoperation, coronary artery bypass procedure or valve procedure, more than one month after original operation (List separately in addition to code for primary procedure)

(Use 33530 in conjunction with 33400-33496; 33510-33536, 33863)

Arterial Grafting for Coronary Artery Bypass

The following codes are used to report coronary artery bypass procedures using either arterial grafts only or a combination of arterial-venous grafts. The codes include the use of the internal mammary artery, gastroepiploic artery, epigastric artery, radial artery, and arterial conduits procured from other sites.

To report combined arterial-venous grafts it is necessary to report two codes: 1) the appropriate arterial graft code (33533-33536); and 2) the appropriate combined arterial-venous graft code (33517-33523).

Procurement of the artery for grafting is included in the description of the work for 33533-33536 and should not be reported as a separate service or co-surgery, except when an upper extremity artery (eg, radial artery) is procured. To report harvesting of an upper extremity artery, use 35600 in addition to the bypass procedure. To report harvesting of an upper extremity vein, use 35500 in addition to the bypass procedure. To report harvesting of a femoropopliteal vein segment, report 35572 in addition to the bypass procedure. When surgical assistant performs arterial and/or venous graft procurement, add modifier 80 to 33517-33523, 33533-33536, as appropriate.

33533   Coronary artery bypass, using arterial graft(s); single arterial graft

33534   two coronary arterial grafts

33535   three coronary arterial grafts

33536   four or more coronary arterial grafts

33542   Myocardial resection (eg, ventricular aneurysmectomy)

33545   Repair of postinfarction ventricular septal defect, with or without myocardial resection

33548   Surgical ventricular restoration procedure, includes prosthetic patch, when performed (eg, ventricular remodeling, SVR, SAVER, DOR procedures)

(Do not report 33548 in conjunction with 32020, 33210, 33211, 33310, 33315)

(For Batista procedure or pachopexy, use 33999)

Coronary Endarterectomy

+ 33572   Coronary endarterectomy, open, any method, of left anterior descending, circumflex, or right coronary artery performed in conjunction with coronary artery bypass graft procedure, each vessel (List separately in addition to primary procedure)

(Use 33572 in conjunction with 33510-33516, 33533-33536)

Surgery: Cardiovascular System

Single Ventricle and Other Complex Cardiac Anomalies

33600   Closure of atrioventricular valve (mitral or tricuspid) by suture or patch

33602   Closure of semilunar valve (aortic or pulmonary) by suture or patch

33606   Anastomosis of pulmonary artery to aorta (Damus-Kaye-Stansel procedure)

33608   Repair of complex cardiac anomaly other than pulmonary atresia with ventricular septal defect by construction or replacement of conduit from right or left ventricle to pulmonary artery

(For repair of pulmonary artery arborization anomalies by unifocalization, see 33925-33926)

33610   Repair of complex cardiac anomalies (eg, single ventricle with subaortic obstruction) by surgical enlargement of ventricular septal defect

(Do not report modifier 63 in conjunction with 33610)

33611   Repair of double outlet right ventricle with intraventricular tunnel repair;

(Do not report modifier 63 in conjunction with 33611)

33612   with repair of right ventricular outflow tract obstruction

33615   Repair of complex cardiac anomalies (eg, tricuspid atresia) by closure of atrial septal defect and anastomosis of atria or vena cava to pulmonary artery (simple Fontan procedure)

33617   Repair of complex cardiac anomalies (eg, single ventricle) by modified Fontan procedure

(Use 33617 in conjunction with 33768 when a cavopulmonary anastomosis to a second superior vena cava is performed)

33619   Repair of single ventricle with aortic outflow obstruction and aortic arch hypoplasia (hypoplastic left heart syndrome) (eg, Norwood procedure)

(Do not report modifier 63 in conjunction with 33619)

Septal Defect

33641   Repair atrial septal defect, secundum, with cardiopulmonary bypass, with or without patch

33645   Direct or patch closure, sinus venosus, with or without anomalous pulmonary venous drainage

►(Do not report 33645 in conjunction with 33724, 33726)◄

33647   Repair of atrial septal defect and ventricular septal defect, with direct or patch closure

(Do not report modifier 63 in conjunction with 33647)

(For repair of tricuspid atresia (eg, Fontan, Gago procedures), use 33615)

33660   Repair of incomplete or partial atrioventricular canal (ostium primum atrial septal defect), with or without atrioventricular valve repair

33665   Repair of intermediate or transitional atrioventricular canal, with or without atrioventricular valve repair

33670   Repair of complete atrioventricular canal, with or without prosthetic valve

(Do not report modifier 63 in conjunction with 33670)

● **33675**   Closure of multiple ventricular septal defects;

● **33676**   with pulmonary valvotomy or infundibular resection (acyanotic)

● **33677**   with removal of pulmonary artery band, with or without gusset

►(Do not report 33675-33677 in conjunction with 32002, 32020, 32100, 33210, 33681, 33684, 33688)◄

►(For transmyocardial closure, see Category III codes 0166T and 0167T)◄

►(For percutaneous closure, use 93581)◄

▲ **33681**   Closure of single ventricular septal defect, with or without patch;

33684   with pulmonary valvotomy or infundibular resection (acyanotic)

33688   with removal of pulmonary artery band, with or without gusset

►(For pulmonary vein repair requiring creation of atrial septal defect, use 33724)◄

33690   Banding of pulmonary artery

(Do not report modifier 63 in conjunction with 33690)

33692   Complete repair tetralogy of Fallot without pulmonary atresia;

33694   with transannular patch

(Do not report modifier 63 in conjunction with 33694)

(For ligation and takedown of a systemic-to-pulmonary artery shunt, performed in conjunction with a congenital heart procedure; see 33924)

33697   Complete repair tetralogy of Fallot with pulmonary atresia including construction of conduit from right ventricle to pulmonary artery and closure of ventricular septal defect

(For ligation and takedown of a systemic-to-pulmonary artery shunt, performed in conjunction with a congenital heart procedure; see 33924)

Surgery: Cardiovascular System

Sinus of Valsalva

33702   Repair sinus of Valsalva fistula, with cardiopulmonary bypass;

33710   with repair of ventricular septal defect

33720   Repair sinus of Valsalva aneurysm, with cardiopulmonary bypass

33722   Closure of aortico-left ventricular tunnel

▶Venous Anomalies◀

● **33724**   Repair of isolated partial anomalous pulmonary venous return (eg, Scimitar Syndrome)

   ▶(Do not report 33724 in conjunction with 32020, 33210, 33211)◀

● **33726**   Repair of pulmonary venous stenosis

   ▶(Do not report 33726 in conjunction with 32020, 33210, 33211)◀

33730   Complete repair of anomalous pulmonary venous return (supracardiac, intracardiac, or infracardiac types)

   (Do not report modifier 63 in conjunction with 33730)

   ▶(For partial anomalous pulmonary venous return, use 33724; for repair of pulmonary venous stenosis, use 33726)◀

33732   Repair of cor triatriatum or supravalvular mitral ring by resection of left atrial membrane

   (Do not report modifier 63 in conjunction with 33732)

Shunting Procedures

33735   Atrial septectomy or septostomy; closed heart (Blalock-Hanlon type operation)

33736   open heart with cardiopulmonary bypass

   (Do not report modifier 63 in conjunction with 33735, 33736)

33737   open heart, with inflow occlusion

   (For transvenous method cardiac catheterization balloon atrial septectomy or septostomy (Rashkind type), use 92992)

   (For blade method cardiac catheterization atrial septectomy or septostomy (Sang-Park septostomy), use 92993)

33750   Shunt; subclavian to pulmonary artery (Blalock-Taussig type operation)

33755   ascending aorta to pulmonary artery (Waterston type operation)

33762   descending aorta to pulmonary artery (Potts-Smith type operation)

   (Do not report modifier 63 in conjunction with 33750, 33755, 33762)

33764   central, with prosthetic graft

33766   superior vena cava to pulmonary artery for flow to one lung (classical Glenn procedure)

33767   superior vena cava to pulmonary artery for flow to both lungs (bidirectional Glenn procedure)

+ **33768**   Anastomosis, cavopulmonary, second superior vena cava (List separately in addition to primary procedure)

   (Use 33768 in conjunction with 33478, 33617, 33767)

   (Do not report 33768 in conjunction with 32020, 33210, 33211)

Transposition of the Great Vessels

33770   Repair of transposition of the great arteries with ventricular septal defect and subpulmonary stenosis; without surgical enlargement of ventricular septal defect

33771   with surgical enlargement of ventricular septal defect

33774   Repair of transposition of the great arteries, atrial baffle procedure (eg, Mustard or Senning type) with cardiopulmonary bypass;

33775   with removal of pulmonary band

33776   with closure of ventricular septal defect

33777   with repair of subpulmonic obstruction

33778   Repair of transposition of the great arteries, aortic pulmonary artery reconstruction (eg, Jatene type);

   (Do not report modifier 63 in conjunction with 33778)

33779   with removal of pulmonary band

33780   with closure of ventricular septal defect

33781   with repair of subpulmonic obstruction

Truncus Arteriosus

33786   Total repair, truncus arteriosus (Rastelli type operation)

   (Do not report modifier 63 in conjunction with 33786)

33788   Reimplantation of an anomalous pulmonary artery

   (For pulmonary artery band, use 33690)

Aortic Anomalies

33800   Aortic suspension (aortopexy) for tracheal decompression (eg, for tracheomalacia) (separate procedure)

33802   Division of aberrant vessel (vascular ring);

33803   with reanastomosis

33813   Obliteration of aortopulmonary septal defect; without cardiopulmonary bypass

33814   with cardiopulmonary bypass

33820   Repair of patent ductus arteriosus; by ligation

33822   by division, younger than 18 years

33824   by division, 18 years and older

33840   Excision of coarctation of aorta, with or without associated patent ductus arteriosus; with direct anastomosis

33845   with graft

33851   repair using either left subclavian artery or prosthetic material as gusset for enlargement

33852   Repair of hypoplastic or interrupted aortic arch using autogenous or prosthetic material; without cardiopulmonary bypass

33853   with cardiopulmonary bypass

(For repair of hypoplastic left heart syndrome (eg, Norwood type), via excision of coarctation of aorta, use 33619)

Thoracic Aortic Aneurysm

33860   Ascending aorta graft, with cardiopulmonary bypass, with or without valve suspension;

33861   with coronary reconstruction

33863   with aortic root replacement using composite prosthesis and coronary reconstruction

(For graft of ascending aorta, with cardiopulmonary bypass and valve replacement, with or without coronary implant or valve suspension; use 33860 or 33861 and 33405 or 33406)

33870   Transverse arch graft, with cardiopulmonary bypass

33875   Descending thoracic aorta graft, with or without bypass

33877   Repair of thoracoabdominal aortic aneurysm with graft, with or without cardiopulmonary bypass

Endovascular Repair of Descending Thoracic Aorta

Codes 33880-33891 represent a family of procedures to report placement of an endovascular graft for repair of the descending thoracic aorta. These codes include all device introduction, manipulation, positioning, and deployment. All balloon angioplasty and/or stent deployment within the target treatment zone for the endoprosthesis, either before or after endograft deployment, are not separately reportable. Open arterial exposure and associated closure of the arteriotomy sites (eg, 34812, 34820, 34833, 34834), introduction of guidewires and catheters (eg, 36140, 36200-36218), and extensive repair or replacement of an artery (eg, 35226, 35286) should be additionally reported. Transposition of subclavian artery to carotid, and carotid-carotid bypass performed in conjunction with endovascular repair of the descending thoracic aorta (eg, 33889, 33891) should be separately reported. The primary codes, 33880 and 33881, include placement of all distal extensions, if required, in the distal thoracic aorta, while proximal extensions, if needed, are reported separately.

For fluoroscopic guidance in conjunction with endovascular repair of the thoracic aorta, see codes 75956-75959 as appropriate. Codes 75956 and 75957 include all angiography of the thoracic aorta and its branches for diagnostic imaging prior to deployment of the primary endovascular devices (including all routine components of modular devices), fluoroscopic guidance in the delivery of the endovascular components, and intraprocedural arterial angiography (eg, confirm position, detect endoleak, evaluate runoff). Code 75958 includes the analogous services for placement of each proximal thoracic endovascular extension. Code 75959 includes the analogous services for placement of a distal thoracic endovascular extension(s) placed during a procedure after the primary repair.

Other interventional procedures performed at the time of endovascular repair of the descending thoracic aorta should be additionally reported (eg, innominate, carotid, subclavian, visceral, or iliac artery transluminal angioplasty or stenting, arterial embolization, intravascular ultrasound) when performed before or after deployment of the aortic prostheses.

33880   Endovascular repair of descending thoracic aorta (eg, aneurysm, pseudoaneurysm, dissection, penetrating ulcer, intramural hematoma, or traumatic disruption); involving coverage of left subclavian artery origin, initial endoprosthesis plus descending thoracic aortic extension(s), if required, to level of celiac artery origin

(For radiological supervision and interpretation, use 75956 in conjunction with 33880)

33881   not involving coverage of left subclavian artery origin, initial endoprosthesis plus descending thoracic aortic extension(s), if required, to level of celiac artery origin

(For radiological supervision and interpretation, use 75957 in conjunction with 33881)

33883   Placement of proximal extension prosthesis for endovascular repair of descending thoracic aorta (eg, aneurysm, pseudoaneurysm, dissection, penetrating ulcer, intramural hematoma, or traumatic disruption); initial extension

(For radiological supervision and interpretation, use 75958 in conjunction with 33883)

(Do not report 33881, 33883 when extension placement converts repair to cover left subclavian origin. Use only 33880)

+ 33884   each additional proximal extension (List separately in addition to code for primary procedure)

(Use 33884 in conjunction with 33883)

(For radiological supervision and interpretation, use 75958 in conjunction with 33884)

33886 Placement of distal extension prosthesis(s) delayed after endovascular repair of descending thoracic aorta

(Do not report 33886 in conjunction with 33880, 33881)

(Report 33886 once, regardless of number of modules deployed)

(For radiological supervision and interpretation, use 75959 in conjunction with 33886)

33889 Open subclavian to carotid artery transposition performed in conjunction with endovascular repair of descending thoracic aorta, by neck incision, unilateral

(Do not report 33889 in conjunction with 35694)

33891 Bypass graft, with other than vein, transcervical retropharyngeal carotid-carotid, performed in conjunction with endovascular repair of descending thoracic aorta, by neck incision

(Do not report 33891 in conjunction with 35509, 35601)

Pulmonary Artery

33910 Pulmonary artery embolectomy; with cardiopulmonary bypass

33915 without cardiopulmonary bypass

33916 Pulmonary endarterectomy, with or without embolectomy, with cardiopulmonary bypass

33917 Repair of pulmonary artery stenosis by reconstruction with patch or graft

(33918, 33919 have been deleted. To report, see 33925, 33926)

33920 Repair of pulmonary atresia with ventricular septal defect, by construction or replacement of conduit from right or left ventricle to pulmonary artery

(For repair of other complex cardiac anomalies by construction or replacement of right or left ventricle to pulmonary artery conduit, use 33608)

33922 Transection of pulmonary artery with cardiopulmonary bypass

(Do not report modifier 63 in conjunction with 33922)

+ 33924 Ligation and takedown of a systemic-to-pulmonary artery shunt, performed in conjunction with a congenital heart procedure (List separately in addition to code for primary procedure)

(Use 33924 in conjunction with 33470-33475, 33600-33619, 33684-33688, 33692-33697, 33735-33767, 33770-33781, 33786, 33920-33922)

33925 Repair of pulmonary artery arborization anomalies by unifocalization; without cardiopulmonary bypass

33926 with cardiopulmonary bypass

Heart/Lung Transplantation

Heart with or without lung allotransplantation involves three distinct components of physician work:

1) *Cadaver donor cardiectomy with or without pneumonectomy*, which includes harvesting the allograft and cold preservation of the allograft (perfusing with cold preservation solution and cold maintenance) (see 33930, 33940).

2) *Backbench work*:

Preparation of a cadaver donor heart and lung allograft prior to transplantation, including dissection of the allograft from surrounding soft tissues to prepare the aorta, superior vena cava, inferior vena cava, and trachea for implantation (use 33933).

Preparation of a cadaver donor heart allograft prior to transplantation, including dissection of the allograft from surrounding soft tissues to prepare aorta, superior vena cava, inferior vena cava, pulmonary artery, and left atrium for implantation (use 33944).

3) *Recipient heart with or without lung allotransplantation*, which includes transplantation of allograft and care of the recipient (see 33935, 33945).

(For implantation of a total replacement heart system (artificial heart) with recipient cardiectomy or heart replacement system components, see Category III codes 0051T-0053T)

33930 Donor cardiectomy-pneumonectomy (including cold preservation)

33933 Backbench standard preparation of cadaver donor heart/lung allograft prior to transplantation, including dissection of allograft from surrounding soft tissues to prepare aorta, superior vena cava, inferior vena cava, and trachea for implantation

33935 Heart-lung transplant with recipient cardiectomy-pneumonectomy

33940 Donor cardiectomy (including cold preservation)

33944 Backbench standard preparation of cadaver donor heart allograft prior to transplantation, including dissection of allograft from surrounding soft tissues to prepare aorta, superior vena cava, inferior vena cava, pulmonary artery, and left atrium for implantation

(For repair or resection procedures on the donor heart, see 33300, 33310, 33320, 33400, 33463, 33464, 33510, 33641, 35216, 35276 or 35685)

33945 Heart transplant, with or without recipient cardiectomy

Cardiac Assist

(For percutaneous implantation of extracorporeal ventricular assist device or for removal of percutaneously implanted extracorporeal ventricular assist device, see Category III codes 0048T-0050T)

33960   Prolonged extracorporeal circulation for cardiopulmonary insufficiency; initial 24 hours

+ 33961   each additional 24 hours (List separately in addition to code for primary procedure)

(Do not report modifier 63 in conjunction with 33960, 33961)

(Use 33961 in conjunction with 33960)

(For insertion of cannula for prolonged extracorporeal circulation, use 36822)

33967   Insertion of intra-aortic balloon assist device, percutaneous

33968   Removal of intra-aortic balloon assist device, percutaneous

33970   Insertion of intra-aortic balloon assist device through the femoral artery, open approach

33971   Removal of intra-aortic balloon assist device including repair of femoral artery, with or without graft

33973   Insertion of intra-aortic balloon assist device through the ascending aorta

33974   Removal of intra-aortic balloon assist device from the ascending aorta, including repair of the ascending aorta, with or without graft

33975   Insertion of ventricular assist device; extracorporeal, single ventricle

33976   extracorporeal, biventricular

33977   Removal of ventricular assist device; extracorporeal, single ventricle

33978   extracorporeal, biventricular

33979   Insertion of ventricular assist device, implantable intracorporeal, single ventricle

33980   Removal of ventricular assist device, implantable intracorporeal, single ventricle

Other Procedures

33999   Unlisted procedure, cardiac surgery

Arteries and Veins

Primary vascular procedure listings include establishing both inflow and outflow by whatever procedures necessary. Also included is that portion of the operative arteriogram performed by the surgeon, as indicated. Sympathectomy, when done, is included in the listed aortic procedures. For unlisted vascular procedure, use 37799.

Embolectomy/Thrombectomy

Arterial, With or Without Catheter

34001   Embolectomy or thrombectomy, with or without catheter; carotid, subclavian or innominate artery, by neck incision

34051   innominate, subclavian artery, by thoracic incision

34101   axillary, brachial, innominate, subclavian artery, by arm incision

34111   radial or ulnar artery, by arm incision

34151   renal, celiac, mesentery, aortoiliac artery, by abdominal incision

34201   femoropopliteal, aortoiliac artery, by leg incision

34203   popliteal-tibio-peroneal artery, by leg incision

Venous, Direct or With Catheter

34401   Thrombectomy, direct or with catheter; vena cava, iliac vein, by abdominal incision

34421   vena cava, iliac, femoropopliteal vein, by leg incision

34451   vena cava, iliac, femoropopliteal vein, by abdominal and leg incision

34471   subclavian vein, by neck incision

34490   axillary and subclavian vein, by arm incision

Venous Reconstruction

34501   Valvuloplasty, femoral vein

34502   Reconstruction of vena cava, any method

34510   Venous valve transposition, any vein donor

34520   Cross-over vein graft to venous system

34530   Saphenopopliteal vein anastomosis

Endovascular Repair of Abdominal Aortic Aneurysm

Codes 34800-34826 represent a family of component procedures to report placement of an endovascular graft for abdominal aortic aneurysm repair. These codes describe open femoral or iliac artery exposure, device manipulation and deployment, and closure of the arteriotomy sites. Balloon angioplasty and/or stent deployment within the target treatment zone for the endoprosthesis, either before or after endograft deployment, are not separately reportable. Introduction of guidewires and catheters should be reported separately (eg, 36200, 36245-36248, 36140). Extensive repair or replacement of an artery should be additionally reported (eg, 35226 or 35286).

Surgery: Cardiovascular System

For fluoroscopic guidance in conjunction with endovascular aneurysm repair, see code 75952 or 75953, as appropriate. Code 75952 includes angiography of the aorta and its branches for diagnostic imaging prior to deployment of the endovascular device (including all routine components of modular devices), fluoroscopic guidance in the delivery of the endovascular components, and intraprocedural arterial angiography (eg, confirm position, detect endoleak, evaluate runoff). Code 75953 includes the analogous services for placement of additional extension prostheses (not for routine components of modular devices).

Other interventional procedures performed at the time of endovascular abdominal aortic aneurysm repair should be additionally reported (eg, renal transluminal angioplasty, arterial embolization, intravascular ultrasound, balloon angioplasty or stenting of native artery(s) outside the endoprosthesis target zone, when done before or after deployment of graft).

34800   Endovascular repair of infrarenal abdominal aortic aneurysm or dissection; using aorto-aortic tube prosthesis

34802   using modular bifurcated prosthesis (one docking limb)

34803   using modular bifurcated prosthesis (two docking limbs)

(For endovascular repair of abdominal aortic aneurysm or dissection involving visceral vessels using a fenestrated modular bifurcated prosthesis (two docking limbs), use Category III codes 0078T, 0079T)

34804   using unibody bifurcated prosthesis

34805   using aorto-uniiliac or aorto-unifemoral prosthesis

+ 34808   Endovascular placement of iliac artery occlusion device (List separately in addition to code for primary procedure)

(Use 34808 in conjunction with 34800, 34805, 34813, 34825, 34826)

(For radiological supervision and interpretation, use 75952 in conjunction with 34800-34808)

(For open arterial exposure, report 34812, 34820, 34833, 34834 as appropriate, in addition to 34800-34808)

34812   Open femoral artery exposure for delivery of endovascular prosthesis, by groin incision, unilateral

(For bilateral procedure, use modifier 50)

+ 34813   Placement of femoral-femoral prosthetic graft during endovascular aortic aneurysm repair (List separately in addition to code for primary procedure)

(Use 34813 in conjunction with 34812)

▶(For femoral artery grafting, see 35521, 35533, 35539, 35540, 35551-35558, 35566, 35621, 35646, 35651-35661, 35666, 35700)◀

34820   Open iliac artery exposure for delivery of endovascular prosthesis or iliac occlusion during endovascular therapy, by abdominal or retroperitoneal incision, unilateral

(For bilateral procedure, use modifier 50)

34825   Placement of proximal or distal extension prosthesis for endovascular repair of infrarenal abdominal aortic or iliac aneurysm, false aneurysm, or dissection; initial vessel

+ 34826   each additional vessel (List separately in addition to code for primary procedure)

(Use 34826 in conjunction with 34825)

(Use 34825, 34826 in addition to 34800-34808, 34900 as appropriate)

(For staged procedure, use modifier 58)

(For radiological supervision and interpretation, use 75953)

34830   Open repair of infrarenal aortic aneurysm or dissection, plus repair of associated arterial trauma, following unsuccessful endovascular repair; tube prosthesis

34831   aorto-bi-iliac prosthesis

34832   aorto-bifemoral prosthesis

34833   Open iliac artery exposure with creation of conduit for delivery of aortic or iliac endovascular prosthesis, by abdominal or retroperitoneal incision, unilateral

(For bilateral procedure, use modifier 50)

(Do not report 34833 in addition to 34820)

34834   Open brachial artery exposure to assist in the deployment of aortic or iliac endovascular prosthesis by arm incision, unilateral

(For bilateral procedure, use modifier 50)

Endovascular Repair of Iliac Aneurysm

Code 34900 represents a procedure to report introduction, positioning, and deployment of an endovascular graft for treatment of aneurysm, pseudoaneurysm, or arteriovenous malformation or trauma of the iliac artery (common, hypogastric, external). All balloon angioplasty and/or stent deployments within the target treatment zone for the endoprosthesis, either before or after endograft deployment, are included in the work of 34900 and are not separately reportable. Open femoral or iliac artery exposure (eg, 34812, 34820), introduction of guidewires and catheters (eg, 36200, 36215-36218), and extensive repair or replacement of an artery (eg, 35206-35286) should be additionally reported.

Surgery: Cardiovascular System

For fluoroscopic guidance in conjunction with endovascular iliac aneurysm repair, see code 75954. Code 75954 includes angiography of the aorta and iliac arteries for diagnostic imaging prior to deployment of the endovascular device (including all routine components), fluoroscopic guidance in the delivery of the endovascular components, and intraprocedural arterial angiography to confirm appropriate position of the graft, detect endoleaks, and evaluate the status of the runoff vessels (eg, evaluation for dissection, stenosis, thrombosis, distal embolization, or iatrogenic injury).

Other interventional procedures performed at the time of endovascular iliac aneurysm repair should be additionally reported (eg, transluminal angioplasty outside the aneurysm target zone, arterial embolization, intravascular ultrasound).

34900　Endovascular graft placement for repair of iliac artery (eg, aneurysm, pseudoaneurysm, arteriovenous malformation, trauma)

(For radiological supervision and interpretation, use 75954)

(For placement of extension prosthesis during endovascular iliac artery repair, use 34825)

(For bilateral procedure, use modifier 50)

Direct Repair of Aneurysm or Excision (Partial or Total) and Graft Insertion for Aneurysm, Pseudoaneurysm, Ruptured Aneurysm, and Associated Occlusive Disease

Procedures 35001-35152 include preparation of artery for anastomosis including endarterectomy.

(For direct repairs associated with occlusive disease only, see 35201-35286)

(For intracranial aneurysm, see 61700 et seq)

(For endovascular repair of abdominal aortic aneurysm, see 34800-34826)

(For endovascular repair of iliac artery aneurysm, see 34900)

(For thoracic aortic aneurysm, see 33860-33875)

(For endovascular repair of descending thoracic aorta, involving coverage of left subclavian artery origin, use 33880)

35001　Direct repair of aneurysm, pseudoaneurysm, or excision (partial or total) and graft insertion, with or without patch graft; for aneurysm and associated occlusive disease, carotid, subclavian artery, by neck incision

35002　for ruptured aneurysm, carotid, subclavian artery, by neck incision

35005　for aneurysm, pseudoaneurysm, and associated occlusive disease, vertebral artery

35011　for aneurysm and associated occlusive disease, axillary-brachial artery, by arm incision

35013　for ruptured aneurysm, axillary-brachial artery, by arm incision

35021　for aneurysm, pseudoaneurysm, and associated occlusive disease, innominate, subclavian artery, by thoracic incision

35022　for ruptured aneurysm, innominate, subclavian artery, by thoracic incision

35045　for aneurysm, pseudoaneurysm, and associated occlusive disease, radial or ulnar artery

35081　for aneurysm, pseudoaneurysm, and associated occlusive disease, abdominal aorta

35082　for ruptured aneurysm, abdominal aorta

35091　for aneurysm, pseudoaneurysm, and associated occlusive disease, abdominal aorta involving visceral vessels (mesenteric, celiac, renal)

35092　for ruptured aneurysm, abdominal aorta involving visceral vessels (mesenteric, celiac, renal)

35102　for aneurysm, pseudoaneurysm, and associated occlusive disease, abdominal aorta involving iliac vessels (common, hypogastric, external)

35103　for ruptured aneurysm, abdominal aorta involving iliac vessels (common, hypogastric, external)

35111　for aneurysm, pseudoaneurysm, and associated occlusive disease, splenic artery

35112　for ruptured aneurysm, splenic artery

35121　for aneurysm, pseudoaneurysm, and associated occlusive disease, hepatic, celiac, renal, or mesenteric artery

35122　for ruptured aneurysm, hepatic, celiac, renal, or mesenteric artery

35131　for aneurysm, pseudoaneurysm, and associated occlusive disease, iliac artery (common, hypogastric, external)

35132　for ruptured aneurysm, iliac artery (common, hypogastric, external)

35141　for aneurysm, pseudoaneurysm, and associated occlusive disease, common femoral artery (profunda femoris, superficial femoral)

35142　for ruptured aneurysm, common femoral artery (profunda femoris, superficial femoral)

35151　for aneurysm, pseudoaneurysm, and associated occlusive disease, popliteal artery

35152　for ruptured aneurysm, popliteal artery

(35161, 35162 have been deleted. To report, use 37799)

Repair Arteriovenous Fistula

35180 Repair, congenital arteriovenous fistula; head and neck

35182   thorax and abdomen

35184   extremities

35188 Repair, acquired or traumatic arteriovenous fistula; head and neck

35189   thorax and abdomen

35190   extremities

Repair Blood Vessel Other Than for Fistula, With or Without Patch Angioplasty

(For AV fistula repair, see 35180-35190)

35201 Repair blood vessel, direct; neck

35206   upper extremity

35207   hand, finger

35211   intrathoracic, with bypass

35216   intrathoracic, without bypass

35221   intra-abdominal

35226   lower extremity

35231 Repair blood vessel with vein graft; neck

35236   upper extremity

35241   intrathoracic, with bypass

35246   intrathoracic, without bypass

35251   intra-abdominal

35256   lower extremity

35261 Repair blood vessel with graft other than vein; neck

35266   upper extremity

35271   intrathoracic, with bypass

35276   intrathoracic, without bypass

35281   intra-abdominal

35286   lower extremity

Thromboendarterectomy

(For coronary artery, see 33510-33536 and 33572)

►(35301-35372 include harvest of saphenous or upper extremity vein when performed)◄

▲ **35301** Thromboendarterectomy, including patch graft, if performed; carotid, vertebral, subclavian, by neck incision

● **35302**   superficial femoral artery

● **35303**   popliteal artery

►(Do not report 35302, 35303 in conjunction with 35483, 35500)◄

● **35304**   tibioperoneal trunk artery

● **35305**   tibial or peroneal artery, initial vessel

+● **35306**   each additional tibial or peroneal artery (List separately in addition to code for primary procedure)

►(Use 35306 in conjunction with 35305)◄

►(Do not report 35304, 35305, 35306 in conjunction with 35485, 35500)◄

35311   subclavian, innominate, by thoracic incision

35321   axillary-brachial

35331   abdominal aorta

35341   mesenteric, celiac, or renal

35351   iliac

35355   iliofemoral

35361   combined aortoiliac

35363   combined aortoiliofemoral

35371   common femoral

35372   deep (profunda) femoral

►(35381 has been deleted. For thromboendarterectomy of the superficial femoral artery, use 35302; of the popliteal artery, use 35303; of the tibioperoneal trunk, use 35304; of the tibial or peroneal artery, see 35305, 35306)◄

+ **35390** Reoperation, carotid, thromboendarterectomy, more than one month after original operation (List separately in addition to code for primary procedure)

(Use 35390 in conjunction with 35301)

Angioscopy

+ **35400** Angioscopy (non-coronary vessels or grafts) during therapeutic intervention (List separately in addition to code for primary procedure)

Transluminal Angioplasty

If done as part of another operation, use modifier 51 or use modifier 52.

(For radiological supervision and interpretation, see 75962-75968 and 75978)

Open

35450 Transluminal balloon angioplasty, open; renal or other visceral artery

35452   aortic

35454   iliac

35456   femoral-popliteal

35458   brachiocephalic trunk or branches, each vessel

| 35459 | tibioperoneal trunk and branches |
| 35460 | venous |

Percutaneous

Codes for catheter placement and the radiologic supervision and interpretation should also be reported, in addition to the code(s) for the therapeutic aspect of the procedure.

⊙ **35470** Transluminal balloon angioplasty, percutaneous; tibioperoneal trunk or branches, each vessel

⊙ **35471** renal or visceral artery

⊙ **35472** aortic

⊙ **35473** iliac

⊙ **35474** femoral-popliteal

⊙ **35475** brachiocephalic trunk or branches, each vessel

⊙ **35476** venous

(For radiological supervision and interpretation, use 75978)

Transluminal Atherectomy

If done as part of another operation, use modifier 51 or use modifier 52.

(For radiological supervision and interpretation, see 75992-75996)

Open

35480	Transluminal peripheral atherectomy, open; renal or other visceral artery
35481	aortic
35482	iliac
35483	femoral-popliteal
35484	brachiocephalic trunk or branches, each vessel
35485	tibioperoneal trunk and branches

Percutaneous

Codes for catheter placement and the radiologic supervision and interpretation should also be reported, in addition to the code(s) for the therapeutic aspect of the procedure.

35490	Transluminal peripheral atherectomy, percutaneous; renal or other visceral artery
35491	aortic
35492	iliac
35493	femoral-popliteal
35494	brachiocephalic trunk or branches, each vessel
35495	tibioperoneal trunk and branches

Bypass Graft

Vein

Procurement of the saphenous vein graft is included in the description of the work for 35501-35587 and should not be reported as a separate service or co-surgery. To report harvesting of an upper extremity vein, use 35500 in addition to the bypass procedure. To report harvesting of a femoropopliteal vein segment, use 35572 in addition to the bypass procedure. To report harvesting and construction of an autogenous composite graft of two segments from two distant locations, report 35682 in addition to the bypass procedure, for autogenous composite of three or more segments from distant sites, report 35683.

+ **35500** Harvest of upper extremity vein, one segment, for lower extremity or coronary artery bypass procedure (List separately in addition to code for primary procedure)

(Use 35500 in conjunction with 33510-33536, 35556, 35566, 35571, 35583-35587)

(For harvest of more than one vein segment, see 35682, 35683)

(For endoscopic procedure, use 33508)

▲ **35501** Bypass graft, with vein; common carotid-ipsilateral internal carotid

▲ **35506** carotid-subclavian or subclavian-carotid

▶(35507 has been deleted. For subclavian-carotid bypass with vein, use 35506)◀

35508	carotid-vertebral
▲ 35509	carotid-contralateral carotid
35510	carotid-brachial
35511	subclavian-subclavian
35512	subclavian-brachial
35515	subclavian-vertebral
35516	subclavian-axillary
35518	axillary-axillary
35521	axillary-femoral

(For bypass graft performed with synthetic graft, use 35621)

35522	axillary-brachial
35525	brachial-brachial
35526	aortosubclavian or carotid

(For bypass graft performed with synthetic graft, use 35626)

| 35531 | aortoceliac or aortomesenteric |
| 35533 | axillary-femoral-femoral |

(For bypass graft performed with synthetic graft, use 35654)

Surgery: Cardiovascular System

35536   splenorenal

● 35537   aortoiliac

►(For bypass graft performed with synthetic graft, use 35637)◄

►(Do not report 35537 in conjunction with 35538)◄

● 35538   aortobi-iliac

►(For bypass graft performed with synthetic graft, use 35638)◄

►(Do not report 35538 in conjunction with 35537)◄

● 35539   aortofemoral

►(For bypass graft performed with synthetic graft, use 35647)◄

►(Do not report 35539 in conjunction with 35540)◄

● 35540   aortobifemoral

►(For bypass graft performed with synthetic graft, use 35646)◄

►(Do not report 35540 in conjunction with 35539)◄

►(35541 has been deleted. For aortoiliac graft with vein, use 35537. For aortobi-iliac graft with vein, use 35538)◄

►(35546 has been deleted. For aortofemoral graft with vein use 35539. For aortobifemoral graft with vein, use 35540)◄

35548   aortoiliofemoral, unilateral

(For bypass graft performed with synthetic graft, use 37799)

35549   aortoiliofemoral, bilateral

(For bypass graft performed with synthetic graft, use 37799)

35551   aortofemoral-popliteal

35556   femoral-popliteal

35558   femoral-femoral

35560   aortorenal

35563   ilioiliac

35565   iliofemoral

35566   femoral-anterior tibial, posterior tibial, peroneal artery or other distal vessels

35571   popliteal-tibial, -peroneal artery or other distal vessels

+ 35572   Harvest of femoropopliteal vein, one segment, for vascular reconstruction procedure (eg, aortic, vena caval, coronary, peripheral artery) (List separately in addition to code for primary procedure)

(Use 35572 in conjunction with 33510-33516, 33517-33523, 33533-33536, 34502, 34520, 35001, 35002, 35011-35022, 35102, 35103, 35121-35152, 35231-35256, 35501-35587, 35879-35907)

(For bilateral procedure, use modifier 50)

In-Situ Vein

(35582 has been deleted)

►(To report aortobifemoral bypass using synthetic conduit, and femoral-popliteal bypass with vein conduit in-situ, use 35646 and 35583. To report aorto(uni)femoral bypass with synthetic conduit, and femoral-popliteal bypass with vein conduit in-situ, use 35647 and 35583. To report aortofemoral bypass using vein conduit, and femoral-popliteal bypass with vein conduit in-situ, use 35539 and 35583)◄

35583   In-situ vein bypass; femoral-popliteal

35585   femoral-anterior tibial, posterior tibial, or peroneal artery

35587   popliteal-tibial, peroneal

Other Than Vein

(For arterial transposition and/or reimplantation, see 35691-35695)

⊘ 35600   Harvest of upper extremity artery, one segment, for coronary artery bypass procedure

▲ 35601   Bypass graft, with other than vein; common carotid-ipsilateral internal carotid

35606   carotid-subclavian

(For open transcervical common carotid-common carotid bypass performed in conjunction with endovascular repair of descending thoracic aorta, use 33891)

(For open subclavian to carotid artery transposition performed in conjunction with endovascular thoracic aneurysm repair by neck incision, use 33889)

35612   subclavian-subclavian

35616   subclavian-axillary

35621   axillary-femoral

35623   axillary-popliteal or -tibial

35626   aortosubclavian or carotid

35631   aortoceliac, aortomesenteric, aortorenal

35636   splenorenal (splenic to renal arterial anastomosis)

● 35637   aortoiliac

►(Do not report 35637 in conjunction with 35638, 35646)◄

● 35638   aortobi-iliac

►(Do not report 35638 in conjunction with 35637, 35646)◄

►(35641 has been deleted. For aortoiliac graft constructed with conduit other than vein, use 35637. For aortobi-iliac graft with other than vein, use 35638)◄

(For open placement of aorto-bi-iliac prosthesis following unsuccessful endovascular repair, use 34831)

35642	carotid-vertebral
35645	subclavian-vertebral
35646	aortobifemoral

▶(For bypass graft performed with vein graft, use 35540)◀

(For open placement of aortobifemoral prosthesis following unsuccessful endovascular repair, use 34832)

35647	aortofemoral

▶(For bypass graft performed with vein graft, use 35539)◀

35650	axillary-axillary
35651	aortofemoral-popliteal
35654	axillary-femoral-femoral
35656	femoral-popliteal
35661	femoral-femoral
35663	ilioiliac
35665	iliofemoral
35666	femoral-anterior tibial, posterior tibial, or peroneal artery
35671	popliteal-tibial or -peroneal artery

Composite Grafts

Codes 35682-35683 are used to report harvest and anastomosis of multiple vein segments from distant sites for use as arterial bypass graft conduits. These codes are intended for use when the two or more vein segments are harvested from a limb other than that undergoing bypass. Add-on codes 35682 and 35683 may be reported in addition to codes 35556, 35566, 35571, 35583-35587, as appropriate.

+ 35681 Bypass graft; composite, prosthetic and vein (List separately in addition to code for primary procedure)

(Do not report 35681 in addition to 35682, 35683)

+ 35682 autogenous composite, two segments of veins from two locations (List separately in addition to code for primary procedure)

(Do not report 35682 in addition to 35681, 35683)

+ 35683 autogenous composite, three or more segments of vein from two or more locations (List separately in addition to code for primary procedure)

(Do not report 35683 in addition to 35681, 35682)

Adjuvant Techniques

Adjuvant (additional) technique(s) may be required at the time a bypass graft is created to improve patency of the lower extremity autogenous or synthetic bypass graft (eg, femoral-popliteal, femoral-tibial, or popliteal-tibial arteries). Code 35685 should be reported in addition to the primary synthetic bypass graft procedure, when an interposition of venous tissue (vein patch or cuff) is placed at the anastomosis between the synthetic bypass conduit and the involved artery (includes harvest).

Code 35686 should be reported in addition to the primary bypass graft procedure, when autogenous vein is used to create a fistula between the tibial or peroneal artery and vein at or beyond the distal bypass anastomosis site of the involved artery.

(For composite graft(s), see 35681-35683)

+ 35685 Placement of vein patch or cuff at distal anastomosis of bypass graft, synthetic conduit (List separately in addition to code for primary procedure)

(Use 35685 in conjunction with 35656, 35666, or 35671)

+ 35686 Creation of distal arteriovenous fistula during lower extremity bypass surgery (non-hemodialysis) (List separately in addition to code for primary procedure)

(Use 35686 in conjunction with 35556, 35566, 35571, 35583-35587, 35623, 35656, 35666, 35671)

Arterial Transposition

35691	Transposition and/or reimplantation; vertebral to carotid artery
35693	vertebral to subclavian artery
35694	subclavian to carotid artery

(For open subclavian to carotid artery transposition performed in conjunction with endovascular repair of descending thoracic aorta, use 33889)

35695	carotid to subclavian artery

+ 35697 Reimplantation, visceral artery to infrarenal aortic prosthesis, each artery (List separately in addition to code for primary procedure)

(Do not report 35697 in conjunction with 33877)

▶Excision, Exploration, Repair, Revision◀

+ 35700 Reoperation, femoral-popliteal or femoral (popliteal)-anterior tibial, posterior tibial, peroneal artery, or other distal vessels, more than one month after original operation (List separately in addition to code for primary procedure)

(Use 35700 in conjunction with 35556, 35566, 35571, 35583, 35585, 35587, 35656, 35666, 35671)

35701	Exploration (not followed by surgical repair), with or without lysis of artery; carotid artery
35721	femoral artery
35741	popliteal artery
35761	other vessels

Surgery: Cardiovascular System

Surgery: Cardiovascular System

35800 Exploration for postoperative hemorrhage, thrombosis or infection; neck

35820 chest

35840 abdomen

35860 extremity

35870 Repair of graft-enteric fistula

35875 Thrombectomy of arterial or venous graft (other than hemodialysis graft or fistula);

35876 with revision of arterial or venous graft

(For thrombectomy of hemodialysis graft or fistula, see 36831, 36833)

Codes 35879 and 35881 describe open revision of graft-threatening stenoses of lower extremity arterial bypass graft(s) (previously constructed with autogenous vein conduit) using vein patch angioplasty or segmental vein interposition techniques. For thrombectomy with revision of any non-coronary arterial or venous graft, including those of the lower extremity, (other than hemodialysis graft or fistula), use 35876. For direct repair (other than for fistula) of a lower extremity blood vessel (with or without patch angioplasty), use 35226. For repair (other than for fistula) of a lower extremity blood vessel using a vein graft, use 35256.

35879 Revision, lower extremity arterial bypass, without thrombectomy, open; with vein patch angioplasty

35881 with segmental vein interposition

►(For revision of femoral anastomosis of synthetic arterial bypass graft, see 35883, 35884)◄

(For excision of infected graft, see 35901-35907 and appropriate revascularization code)

● **35883** Revision, femoral anastomosis of synthetic arterial bypass graft in groin, open; with nonautogenous patch graft (eg, Dacron, ePTFE, bovine pericardium)

►(For bilateral procedure, use modifier 50)◄

►(Do not report 35883 in conjunction with 35700, 35875, 35876, 35884)◄

● **35884** with autogenous vein patch graft

►(For bilateral procedure, use modifier 50)◄

►(Do not report 35884 in conjunction with 35700, 35875, 35876, 35883)◄

35901 Excision of infected graft; neck

35903 extremity

35905 thorax

35907 abdomen

Vascular Injection Procedures

Listed services for injection procedures include necessary local anesthesia, introduction of needles or catheter, injection of contrast media with or without automatic power injection, and/or necessary pre- and postinjection care specifically related to the injection procedure.

Catheters, drugs, and contrast media are not included in the listed service for the injection procedures.

Selective vascular catheterization should be coded to include introduction and all lesser order selective catheterization used in the approach (eg, the description for a selective right middle cerebral artery catheterization includes the introduction and placement catheterization of the right common and internal carotid arteries).

Additional second and/or third order arterial catheterization within the same family of arteries or veins supplied by a single first order vessel should be expressed by 36012, 36218 or 36248.

Additional first order or higher catheterization in vascular families supplied by a first order vessel different from a previously selected and coded family should be separately coded using the conventions described above.

(For radiological supervision and interpretation, see **Radiology**)

(For injection procedures in conjunction with cardiac catheterization, see 93541-93545)

(For chemotherapy of malignant disease, see 96401-96549)

Intravenous

An intracatheter is a sheathed combination of needle and short catheter.

36000 Introduction of needle or intracatheter, vein

36002 Injection procedures (eg, thrombin) for percutaneous treatment of extremity pseudoaneurysm

►(For imaging guidance, see 76942, 77002, 77012, 77021)◄

(For ultrasound guided compression repair of pseudoaneurysms, use 76936)

(Do not report 36002 for vascular sealant of an arteriotomy site)

36005 Injection procedure for extremity venography (including introduction of needle or intracatheter)

(For radiological supervision and interpretation, see 75820, 75822)

36010 Introduction of catheter, superior or inferior vena cava

36011 Selective catheter placement, venous system; first order branch (eg, renal vein, jugular vein)

36012 second order, or more selective, branch (eg, left adrenal vein, petrosal sinus)

36013 Introduction of catheter, right heart or main pulmonary artery

36014 Selective catheter placement, left or right pulmonary artery

36015 Selective catheter placement, segmental or subsegmental pulmonary artery

(For insertion of flow directed catheter (eg, Swan-Ganz), use 93503)

(For venous catheterization for selective organ blood sampling, use 36500)

Intra-Arterial—Intra-Aortic

(For radiological supervision and interpretation, see **Radiology**)

36100 Introduction of needle or intracatheter, carotid or vertebral artery

(For bilateral procedure, report 36100 with modifier 50)

36120 Introduction of needle or intracatheter; retrograde brachial artery

36140 extremity artery

36145 arteriovenous shunt created for dialysis (cannula, fistula, or graft)

(For insertion of arteriovenous cannula, see 36810-36821)

36160 Introduction of needle or intracatheter, aortic, translumbar

36200 Introduction of catheter, aorta

36215 Selective catheter placement, arterial system; each first order thoracic or brachiocephalic branch, within a vascular family

(For catheter placement for coronary angiography, use 93508)

36216 initial second order thoracic or brachiocephalic branch, within a vascular family

36217 initial third order or more selective thoracic or brachiocephalic branch, within a vascular family

+ 36218 additional second order, third order, and beyond, thoracic or brachiocephalic branch, within a vascular family (List in addition to code for initial second or third order vessel as appropriate)

(Use 36218 in conjunction with 36216, 36217)

(For angiography, see 75600-75790)

(For angioplasty, see 35470-35475)

(For transcatheter therapies, see 37200-37208, 61624, 61626)

(When coronary artery, arterial conduit (eg, internal mammary, inferior epigastric or free radical artery) or venous bypass graft angiography is performed in conjunction with cardiac catheterization, see the appropriate cardiac catheterization, injection procedure, and imaging supervision code(s) (93501-93556) in the **Medicine** section of the CPT codebook. When coronary artery, arterial coronary conduit or venous bypass graft angiography is performed without concomitant left heart cardiac catheterization, use 93508. When internal mammary artery angiography only is performed without a concomitant left heart cardiac catheterization, use 36216 or 36217 as appropriate.)

36245 Selective catheter placement, arterial system; each first order abdominal, pelvic, or lower extremity artery branch, within a vascular family

36246 initial second order abdominal, pelvic, or lower extremity artery branch, within a vascular family

36247 initial third order or more selective abdominal, pelvic, or lower extremity artery branch, within a vascular family

+ 36248 additional second order, third order, and beyond, abdominal, pelvic, or lower extremity artery branch, within a vascular family (List in addition to code for initial second or third order vessel as appropriate)

(Use 36248 in conjunction with 36246, 36247)

36260 Insertion of implantable intra-arterial infusion pump (eg, for chemotherapy of liver)

36261 Revision of implanted intra-arterial infusion pump

36262 Removal of implanted intra-arterial infusion pump

36299 Unlisted procedure, vascular injection

Venous

Venipuncture, needle or catheter for diagnostic study or intravenous therapy, percutaneous.

36400 Venipuncture, younger than age 3 years, necessitating physician's skill, not to be used for routine venipuncture; femoral or jugular vein

36405 scalp vein

36406 other vein

36410 Venipuncture, age 3 years or older, necessitating physician's skill (separate procedure), for diagnostic or therapeutic purposes (not to be used for routine venipuncture)

36415 Collection of venous blood by venipuncture

(Do not report modifier 63 in conjunction with 36415)

36416 Collection of capillary blood specimen (eg, finger, heel, ear stick)

36420   Venipuncture, cutdown; younger than age 1 year

(Do not report modifier 63 in conjunction with 36420)

36425   age 1 or over

36430   Transfusion, blood or blood components

36440   Push transfusion, blood, 2 years or younger

36450   Exchange transfusion, blood; newborn

(Do not report modifier 63 in conjunction with 36450)

36455   other than newborn

36460   Transfusion, intrauterine, fetal

(Do not report modifier 63 in conjunction with 36460)

(For radiological supervision and interpretation, use 76941)

36468   Single or multiple injections of sclerosing solutions, spider veins (telangiectasia); limb or trunk

36469   face

36470   Injection of sclerosing solution; single vein

36471   multiple veins, same leg

36475   Endovenous ablation therapy of incompetent vein, extremity, inclusive of all imaging guidance and monitoring, percutaneous, radiofrequency; first vein treated

+ 36476   second and subsequent veins treated in a single extremity, each through separate access sites (List separately in addition to code for primary procedure)

(Use 36476 in conjunction with 36475)

►(Do not report 36475, 36476 in conjunction with 36000-36005, 36410, 36425, 36478, 36479, 37204, 75894, 76000, 76001, 76937, 76942, 77022, 93970, 93971)◄

36478   Endovenous ablation therapy of incompetent vein, extremity, inclusive of all imaging guidance and monitoring, percutaneous, laser; first vein treated

+ 36479   second and subsequent veins treated in a single extremity, each through separate access sites (List separately in addition to code for primary procedure)

(Use 36479 in conjunction with 36478)

►(Do not report 36478, 36479 in conjunction with 36000-36005, 36410, 36425, 36475, 36476, 37204, 75894, 76000, 76001, 76937, 76942, 77022, 93970, 93971)◄

36481   Percutaneous portal vein catheterization by any method

(For radiological supervision and interpretation, see 75885, 75887)

36500   Venous catheterization for selective organ blood sampling

(For catheterization in superior or inferior vena cava, use 36010)

(For radiological supervision and interpretation, use 75893)

36510   Catheterization of umbilical vein for diagnosis or therapy, newborn

(Do not report modifier 63 in conjunction with 36510)

36511   Therapeutic apheresis; for white blood cells

36512   for red blood cells

36513   for platelets

36514   for plasma pheresis

36515   with extracorporeal immunoadsorption and plasma reinfusion

36516   with extracorporeal selective adsorption or selective filtration and plasma reinfusion

(For physician evaluation, use modifier 26)

36522   Photopheresis, extracorporeal

36540   Collection of blood specimen from a completely implantable venous access device

(Do not report 36540 in conjunction with 36415, 36416)

(For collection of venous blood specimen by venipuncture, use 36415)

(For collection of capillary blood specimen, use 36416)

36550   Declotting by thrombolytic agent of implanted vascular access device or catheter

Central Venous Access Procedures

To qualify as a central venous access catheter or device, the tip of the catheter/device must terminate in the subclavian, brachiocephalic (innominate) or iliac veins, the superior or inferior vena cava, or the right atrium. The venous access device may be either centrally inserted (jugular, subclavian, femoral vein or inferior vena cava catheter entry site) or peripherally inserted (eg, basilic or cephalic vein). The device may be accessed for use either via exposed catheter (external to the skin), via a subcutaneous port or via a subcutaneous pump.

The procedures involving these types of devices fall into five categories:

1) *Insertion* (placement of catheter through a newly established venous access)

2) *Repair* (fixing device without replacement of either catheter or port/pump, other than pharmacologic or mechanical correction of intracatheter or pericatheter occlusion (see 36595 or 36596))

3) *Partial replacement* of only the catheter component associated with a port/pump device, but not entire device

4) *Complete replacement* of entire device via same venous access site (complete exchange)

5) *Removal* of entire device.

There is no coding distinction between venous access achieved percutaneously versus by cutdown or based on catheter size.

For the repair, partial (catheter only) replacement, complete replacement, or removal of both catheters (placed from separate venous access sites) of a multi-catheter device, with or without subcutaneous ports/pumps, use the appropriate code describing the service with a frequency of two.

If an existing central venous access device is removed and a new one placed via a separate venous access site, appropriate codes for both procedures (removal of old, if code exists, and insertion of new device) should be reported.

►When imaging is used for these procedures, either for gaining access to the venous entry site or for manipulating the catheter into final central position, use 76937, 77001.◄

(For refilling and maintenance of an implantable pump or reservoir for intravenous or intra-arterial drug delivery, use 96522)

Insertion of Central Venous Access Device

⊙ **36555**   Insertion of non-tunneled centrally inserted central venous catheter; younger than 5 years of age

(For peripherally inserted non-tunneled central venous catheter, younger than 5 years of age, use 36568)

36556   age 5 years or older

(For peripherally inserted non-tunneled central venous catheter, age 5 years or older, use 36569)

⊙ **36557**   Insertion of tunneled centrally inserted central venous catheter, without subcutaneous port or pump; younger than 5 years of age

⊙ **36558**   age 5 years or older

(For peripherally inserted central venous catheter with port, 5 years or older, use 36571)

⊙ **36560**   Insertion of tunneled centrally inserted central venous access device, with subcutaneous port; younger than 5 years of age

(For peripherally inserted central venous access device with subcutaneous port, younger than 5 years of age, use 36570)

⊙ **36561**   age 5 years or older

(For peripherally inserted central venous catheter with subcutaneous port, 5 years or older, use 36571)

⊙ **36563**   Insertion of tunneled centrally inserted central venous access device with subcutaneous pump

⊙ **36565**   Insertion of tunneled centrally inserted central venous access device, requiring two catheters via two separate venous access sites; without subcutaneous port or pump (eg, Tesio type catheter)

⊙ **36566**   with subcutaneous port(s)

⊙ **36568**   Insertion of peripherally inserted central venous catheter (PICC), without subcutaneous port or pump; younger than 5 years of age

(For placement of centrally inserted non-tunneled central venous catheter, without subcutaneous port or pump, younger than 5 years of age, use 36555)

36569   age 5 years or older

(For placement of centrally inserted non-tunneled central venous catheter, without subcutaneous port or pump, age 5 years or older, use 36556)

⊙ **36570**   Insertion of peripherally inserted central venous access device, with subcutaneous port; younger than 5 years of age

(For insertion of tunneled centrally inserted central venous access device with subcutaneous port, younger than 5 years of age, use 36560)

⊙ **36571**   age 5 years or older

(For insertion of tunneled centrally inserted central venous access device with subcutaneous port, age 5 years or older, use 36561)

Repair of Central Venous Access Device

(For mechanical removal of pericatheter obstructive material, use 36595)

(For mechanical removal of intracatheter obstructive material, use 36596)

36575   Repair of tunneled or non-tunneled central venous access catheter, without subcutaneous port or pump, central or peripheral insertion site

⊙ **36576**   Repair of central venous access device, with subcutaneous port or pump, central or peripheral insertion site

Partial Replacement of Central Venous Access Device (Catheter Only)

⊙ **36578**   Replacement, catheter only, of central venous access device, with subcutaneous port or pump, central or peripheral insertion site

(For complete replacement of entire device through same venous access, use 36582 or 36583)

Surgery: Cardiovascular System

Complete Replacement of Central Venous Access Device Through Same Venous Access Site

36580 Replacement, complete, of a non-tunneled centrally inserted central venous catheter, without subcutaneous port or pump, through same venous access

⊙ **36581** Replacement, complete, of a tunneled centrally inserted central venous catheter, without subcutaneous port or pump, through same venous access

⊙ **36582** Replacement, complete, of a tunneled centrally inserted central venous access device, with subcutaneous port, through same venous access

⊙ **36583** Replacement, complete, of a tunneled centrally inserted central venous access device, with subcutaneous pump, through same venous access

36584 Replacement, complete, of a peripherally inserted central venous catheter (PICC), without subcutaneous port or pump, through same venous access

⊙ **36585** Replacement, complete, of a peripherally inserted central venous access device, with subcutaneous port, through same venous access

Removal of Central Venous Access Device

36589 Removal of tunneled central venous catheter, without subcutaneous port or pump

⊙ **36590** Removal of tunneled central venous access device, with subcutaneous port or pump, central or peripheral insertion

(Do not report 36589 or 36590 for removal of non-tunneled central venous catheters)

Mechanical Removal of Obstructive Material

36595 Mechanical removal of pericatheter obstructive material (eg, fibrin sheath) from central venous device via separate venous access

(Do not report 36595 in conjunction with 36550)

(For venous catheterization, see 36010-36012)

(For radiological supervision and interpretation, use 75901)

36596 Mechanical removal of intraluminal (intracatheter) obstructive material from central venous device through device lumen

(Do not report 36596 in conjunction with 36550)

(For venous catheterization, see 36010-36012)

(For radiological supervision and interpretation, use 75902)

Other Central Venous Access Procedures

36597 Repositioning of previously placed central venous catheter under fluoroscopic guidance

(For fluoroscopic guidance, use 76000)

36598 Contrast injection(s) for radiologic evaluation of existing central venous access device, including fluoroscopy, image documentation and report

(Do not report 36598 in conjunction with 76000)

(Do not report 36598 in conjunction with 36595, 36596)

(For complete diagnostic studies, see 75820, 75825, 75827)

Arterial

36600 Arterial puncture, withdrawal of blood for diagnosis

⊘ **36620** Arterial catheterization or cannulation for sampling, monitoring or transfusion (separate procedure); percutaneous

36625 cutdown

36640 Arterial catheterization for prolonged infusion therapy (chemotherapy), cutdown

(See also 96420-96425)

(For arterial catheterization for occlusion therapy, see 75894)

⊘ **36660** Catheterization, umbilical artery, newborn, for diagnosis or therapy

(Do not report modifier 63 in conjunction with 36660)

Intraosseous

36680 Placement of needle for intraosseous infusion

Hemodialysis Access, Intervascular Cannulation for Extracorporeal Circulation, or Shunt Insertion

36800 Insertion of cannula for hemodialysis, other purpose (separate procedure); vein to vein

36810 arteriovenous, external (Scribner type)

36815 arteriovenous, external revision, or closure

36818 Arteriovenous anastomosis, open; by upper arm cephalic vein transposition

(Do not report 36818 in conjunction with 36819, 36820, 36821, 36830 during a unilateral upper extremity procedure. For bilateral upper extremity open arteriovenous anastomoses performed at the same operative session, use modifier 50 or 59 as appropriate)

36819   by upper arm basilic vein transposition

(Do not report 36819 in conjunction with 36818, 36820, 36821, 36830 during a unilateral upper extremity procedure. For bilateral upper extremity open arteriovenous anastomoses performed at the same operative session, use modifier 50 or 59 as appropriate)

36820   by forearm vein transposition

36821   direct, any site (eg, Cimino type) (separate procedure)

36822   Insertion of cannula(s) for prolonged extracorporeal circulation for cardiopulmonary insufficiency (ECMO) (separate procedure)

(For maintenance of prolonged extracorporeal circulation, see 33960, 33961)

36823   Insertion of arterial and venous cannula(s) for isolated extracorporeal circulation including regional chemotherapy perfusion to an extremity, with or without hyperthermia, with removal of cannula(s) and repair of arteriotomy and venotomy sites

(36823 includes chemotherapy perfusion supported by a membrane oxygenator/perfusion pump. Do not report 96409-96425 in conjunction with 36823)

36825   Creation of arteriovenous fistula by other than direct arteriovenous anastomosis (separate procedure); autogenous graft

(For direct arteriovenous anastomosis, use 36821)

36830   nonautogenous graft (eg, biological collagen, thermoplastic graft)

(For direct arteriovenous anastomosis, use 36821)

36831   Thrombectomy, open, arteriovenous fistula without revision, autogenous or nonautogenous dialysis graft (separate procedure)

36832   Revision, open, arteriovenous fistula; without thrombectomy, autogenous or nonautogenous dialysis graft (separate procedure)

36833   with thrombectomy, autogenous or nonautogenous dialysis graft (separate procedure)

36834   Plastic repair of arteriovenous aneurysm (separate procedure)

36835   Insertion of Thomas shunt (separate procedure)

36838   Distal revascularization and interval ligation (DRIL), upper extremity hemodialysis access (steal syndrome)

(Do not report 36838 in conjunction with 35512, 35522, 36832, 37607, 37618)

36860   External cannula declotting (separate procedure); without balloon catheter

36861   with balloon catheter

(If imaging guidance is performed, use 76000)

⊙ **36870**   Thrombectomy, percutaneous, arteriovenous fistula, autogenous or nonautogenous graft (includes mechanical thrombus extraction and intra-graft thrombolysis)

(Do not report 36550 in conjunction with 36870)

(For catheterization, use 36145)

(For radiological supervision and interpretation, use 75790)

Portal Decompression Procedures

37140   Venous anastomosis, open; portocaval

(For peritoneal-venous shunt, use 49425)

37145   renoportal

37160   caval-mesenteric

37180   splenorenal, proximal

37181   splenorenal, distal (selective decompression of esophagogastric varices, any technique)

(For percutaneous procedure, use 37182)

37182   Insertion of transvenous intrahepatic portosystemic shunt(s) (TIPS) (includes venous access, hepatic and portal vein catheterization, portography with hemodynamic evaluation, intrahepatic tract formation/dilatation, stent placement and all associated imaging guidance and documentation)

(Do not report 75885 or 75887 in conjunction with 37182)

(For open procedure, use 37140)

37183   Revision of transvenous intrahepatic portosystemic shunt(s) (TIPS) (includes venous access, hepatic and portal vein catheterization, portography with hemodynamic evaluation, intrahepatic tract recanulization/dilatation, stent placement and all associated imaging guidance and documentation)

(Do not report 75885 or 75887 in conjunction with 37183)

(For repair of arteriovenous aneurysm, use 36834)

Transcatheter Procedures

Codes for catheter placement and the radiologic supervision and interpretation should also be reported, in addition to the code(s) for the therapeutic aspect of the procedure.

Mechanical Thrombectomy

Code(s) for catheter placement(s), diagnostic studies, and other percutaneous interventions (eg, transluminal balloon angioplasty, stent placement) provided are separately reportable.

Codes 37184-37188 specifically include intraprocedural fluoroscopic radiological supervision and interpretation services for guidance of the procedure.

(right margin, vertical) **Surgery: Cardiovascular System**

Intraprocedural injection(s) of a thrombolytic agent is an included service and not separately reportable in conjunction with mechanical thrombectomy. However, subsequent or prior continuous infusion of a thrombolytic is not an included service and is separately reportable (see 37201, 75896, 75898).

For coronary mechanical thrombectomy, use 92973.

For mechanical thrombectomy for dialysis fistula, use 36870.

Arterial Mechanical Thrombectomy

Arterial mechanical thrombectomy may be performed as a "primary" transcatheter procedure with pretreatment planning, performance of the procedure, and postprocedure evaluation focused on providing this service. Primary mechanical thrombectomy is reported per vascular family using 37184 for the initial vessel treated and 37185 for second or all subsequent vessel(s) within the same vascular family. To report mechanical thrombectomy of an additional vascular family treated through a separate access site, use modifier 51 in conjunction with 37184-37185.

Do NOT report 37184-37185 for mechanical thrombectomy performed for treatment of thrombus or embolus complicating other percutaneous interventional procedures. See 37186 for these procedures.

Arterial mechanical thrombectomy is considered a "secondary" transcatheter procedure for removal or retrieval of short segments of thrombus or embolus when performed either before or after another percutaneous intervention (eg, percutaneous transluminal balloon angioplasty, stent placement). Secondary mechanical thrombectomy is reported using 37186. Do NOT report 37186 in conjunction with 37184-37185.

Venous Mechanical Thrombectomy

Use 37187 to report the initial application of venous mechanical thrombectomy. To report bilateral venous mechanical thrombectomy performed through a separate access site(s), use modifier 50 in conjunction with 37187. For repeat treatment on a subsequent day during a course of thrombolytic therapy, use 37188.

Arterial Mechanical Thrombectomy

⊙ **37184**   Primary percutaneous transluminal mechanical thrombectomy, noncoronary, arterial or arterial bypass graft, including fluoroscopic guidance and intraprocedural pharmacological thrombolytic injection(s); initial vessel

(Do not report 37184 in conjunction with 76000, 76001, 90774, 99143-99150)

⊙+ **37185**   second and all subsequent vessel(s) within the same vascular family (List separately in addition to code for primary mechanical thrombectomy procedure)

(Do not report 37185 in conjunction with 76000, 76001, 90775)

⊙+ **37186**   Secondary percutaneous transluminal thrombectomy (eg, nonprimary mechanical, snare basket, suction technique), noncoronary, arterial or arterial bypass graft, including fluoroscopic guidance and intraprocedural pharmacological thrombolytic injections, provided in conjunction with another percutaneous intervention other than primary mechanical thrombectomy (List separately in addition to code for primary procedure)

(Do not report 37186 in conjunction with 76000, 76001, 90775)

Venous Mechanical Thrombectomy

⊙ **37187**   Percutaneous transluminal mechanical thrombectomy, vein(s), including intraprocedural pharmacological thrombolytic injections and fluoroscopic guidance

(Do not report 37187 in conjunction with 76000, 76001, 90775)

⊙ **37188**   Percutaneous transluminal mechanical thrombectomy, vein(s), including intraprocedural pharmacological thrombolytic injections and fluoroscopic guidance, repeat treatment on subsequent day during course of thrombolytic therapy

(Do not report 37188 in conjunction with 76000, 76001, 90775)

Other Procedures

37195   Thrombolysis, cerebral, by intravenous infusion

37200   Transcatheter biopsy

(For radiological supervision and interpretation, use 75970)

37201   Transcatheter therapy, infusion for thrombolysis other than coronary

(For radiological supervision and interpretation, use 75896)

37202   Transcatheter therapy, infusion other than for thrombolysis, any type (eg, spasmolytic, vasoconstrictive)

(For thrombolysis of coronary vessels, see 92975, 92977)

(For radiological supervision and interpretation, use 75896)

⊙ **37203**   Transcatheter retrieval, percutaneous, of intravascular foreign body (eg, fractured venous or arterial catheter)

(For radiological supervision and interpretation, use 75961)

37204   Transcatheter occlusion or embolization (eg, for tumor destruction, to achieve hemostasis, to occlude a vascular malformation), percutaneous, any method, non-central nervous system, non-head or neck

(See also 61624, 61626)

(For radiological supervision and interpretation, use 75894)

►(For uterine fibroid embolization [uterine artery embolization performed to treat uterine fibroids], use 37210)◄

►(For obstetrical and gynecologic embolization procedures other than uterine fibroid embolization [eg, embolization to treat obstetrical or postpartum hemorrhage], use 37204)◄

37205   Transcatheter placement of an intravascular stent(s), (except coronary, carotid, and vertebral vessel), percutaneous; initial vessel

(For radiological supervision and interpretation, use 75960)

(For coronary stent placement, see 92980, 92981; intracranial, use 61635)

+ 37206   each additional vessel (List separately in addition to code for primary procedure)

(Use 37206 in conjunction with 37205)

(For transcatheter placement of intravascular cervical carotid artery stent(s), see 37215, 37216)

(For transcatheter placement of extracranial vertebral or intrathoracic carotid artery stent(s), see Category III codes 0075T, 0076T)

(For radiological supervision and interpretation, use 75960)

37207   Transcatheter placement of an intravascular stent(s), (non-coronary vessel), open; initial vessel

+ 37208   each additional vessel (List separately in addition to code for primary procedure)

(Use 37208 in conjunction with 37207)

(For radiological supervision and interpretation, use 75960)

(For catheterizations, see 36215-36248)

(For transcatheter placement of intracoronary stent(s), see 92980, 92981)

37209   Exchange of a previously placed intravascular catheter during thrombolytic therapy

(For radiological supervision and interpretation, use 75900)

⊙● **37210**   Uterine fibroid embolization (UFE, embolization of the uterine arteries to treat uterine fibroids, leiomyomata), percutaneous approach inclusive of vascular access, vessel selection, embolization, and all radiological supervision and interpretation, intraprocedural roadmapping, and imaging guidance necessary to complete the procedure

►(37210 includes all catheterizations and intraprocedural imaging required for a UFE procedure to confirm the presence of previously known fibroids and to roadmap vascular anatomy to enable appropriate therapy)◄

►(Do not report 37210 in conjunction with 36200, 36245-36248, 37204, 75894, 75898)◄

►(For all other non-central nervous system (CNS) embolization procedures, use 37204)◄

⊙ **37215**   Transcatheter placement of intravascular stent(s), cervical carotid artery, percutaneous; with distal embolic protection

⊙ **37216**   without distal embolic protection

(37215 and 37216 include all ipsilateral selective carotid catheterization, all diagnostic imaging for ipsilateral, cervical and cerebral carotid arteriography, and all related radiological supervision and interpretation. When ipsilateral carotid arteriogram (including imaging and selective catheterization) confirms the need for carotid stenting, 37215 and 37216 are inclusive of these services. If carotid stenting is not indicated, then the appropriate codes for carotid catheterization and imaging should be reported in lieu of 37215 and 37216)

(Do not report 37215, 37216 in conjunction with 75671, 75680)

(For transcatheter placement of extracranial vertebral or intrathoracic carotid artery stent(s), see Category III codes 0075T, 0076T)

(For percutaneous transcatheter placement of intravascular stents other than coronary, carotid, or vertebral, see 37205, 37206)

Intravascular Ultrasound Services

Intravascular ultrasound services include all transducer manipulations and repositioning within the specific vessel being examined, both before and after therapeutic intervention (eg, stent placement).

Vascular access for intravascular ultrasound performed during a therapeutic intervention is not reported separately.

+ 37250   Intravascular ultrasound (non-coronary vessel) during diagnostic evaluation and/or therapeutic intervention; initial vessel (List separately in addition to code for primary procedure)

+ 37251   each additional vessel (List separately in addition to code for primary procedure)

(Use 37251 in conjunction with 37250)

(For catheterizations, see 36215-36248)

(For transcatheter therapies, see 37200-37208, 61624, 61626)

(For radiological supervision and interpretation see 75945, 75946)

Surgery: Cardiovascular System

Endoscopy

Surgical vascular endoscopy always includes diagnostic endoscopy.

37500 Vascular endoscopy, surgical, with ligation of perforator veins, subfascial (SEPS)

(For open procedure, use 37760)

37501 Unlisted vascular endoscopy procedure

Ligation

(For phleborraphy and arteriorraphy, see 35201-35286)

37565 Ligation, internal jugular vein

37600 Ligation; external carotid artery

37605   internal or common carotid artery

37606   internal or common carotid artery, with gradual occlusion, as with Selverstone or Crutchfield clamp

(For transcatheter permanent arterial occlusion or embolization, see 61624-61626)

(For endovascular temporary arterial balloon occlusion, use 61623)

(For ligation treatment of intracranial aneurysm, use 61703)

37607 Ligation or banding of angioaccess arteriovenous fistula

37609 Ligation or biopsy, temporal artery

37615 Ligation, major artery (eg, post-traumatic, rupture); neck

37616   chest

37617   abdomen

37618   extremity

37620 Interruption, partial or complete, of inferior vena cava by suture, ligation, plication, clip, extravascular, intravascular (umbrella device)

(For radiological supervision and interpretation, use 75940)

37650 Ligation of femoral vein

(For bilateral procedure, report 37650 with modifier 50)

37660 Ligation of common iliac vein

37700 Ligation and division of long saphenous vein at saphenofemoral junction, or distal interruptions

(Do not report 37700 in conjunction with 37718, 37722)

(For bilateral procedure, report 37700 with modifier 50)

37718 Ligation, division, and stripping, short saphenous vein

(For bilateral procedure, use modifier 50)

(Do not report 37718 in conjunction with 37735, 37780)

(37720 has been deleted)

37722 Ligation, division, and stripping, long (greater) saphenous veins from saphenofemoral junction to knee or below

(For ligation and stripping of the short saphenous vein, use 37718)

(For bilateral procedure, report 37722 with modifier 50)

(Do not report 37722 in conjunction with 37700, 37735)

(37730 has been deleted. For ligation, division, and stripping of the greater saphenous vein, use 37722. For ligation, division, and stripping of the short saphenous vein, use 37718)

37735 Ligation and division and complete stripping of long or short saphenous veins with radical excision of ulcer and skin graft and/or interruption of communicating veins of lower leg, with excision of deep fascia

(Do not report 37735 in conjunction with 37700, 37718, 37722, 37780)

(For bilateral procedure, report 37735 with modifier 50)

37760 Ligation of perforator veins, subfascial, radical (Linton type), with or without skin graft, open

(For endoscopic procedure, use 37500)

37765 Stab phlebectomy of varicose veins, one extremity; 10-20 stab incisions

(For less than 10 incisions, use 37799)

(For more than 20 incisions, use 37766)

37766   more than 20 incisions

37780 Ligation and division of short saphenous vein at saphenopopliteal junction (separate procedure)

(For bilateral procedure, report 37780 with modifier 50)

37785 Ligation, division, and/or excision of varicose vein cluster(s), one leg

(For bilateral procedure, report 37785 with modifier 50)

Other Procedures

37788 Penile revascularization, artery, with or without vein graft

37790 Penile venous occlusive procedure

37799 Unlisted procedure, vascular surgery

Hemic and Lymphatic Systems

Spleen

Excision

38100 Splenectomy; total (separate procedure)

38101   partial (separate procedure)

+ 38102   total, en bloc for extensive disease, in conjunction with other procedure (List in addition to code for primary procedure)

Repair

38115 Repair of ruptured spleen (splenorrhaphy) with or without partial splenectomy

Laparoscopy

Surgical laparoscopy always includes diagnostic laparoscopy. To report a diagnostic laparoscopy (peritoneoscopy) (separate procedure), use 49320.

38120 Laparoscopy, surgical, splenectomy

38129 Unlisted laparoscopy procedure, spleen

Introduction

38200 Injection procedure for splenoportography

(For radiological supervision and interpretation, use 75810)

General

Bone Marrow or Stem Cell Services/Procedures

Codes 38207-38215 describe various steps used to preserve, prepare and purify bone marrow/stem cells prior to transplantation or reinfusion. Each code may be reported only once per day regardless of the quantity of bone marrow/stem cells manipulated.

38204 Management of recipient hematopoietic progenitor cell donor search and cell acquisition

38205 Blood-derived hematopoietic progenitor cell harvesting for transplantation, per collection; allogenic

38206   autologous

38207 Transplant preparation of hematopoietic progenitor cells; cryopreservation and storage

(For diagnostic cryopreservation and storage, see 88240)

38208   thawing of previously frozen harvest, without washing

(For diagnostic thawing and expansion of frozen cells, see 88241)

38209   thawing of previously frozen harvest, with washing

38210   specific cell depletion within harvest, T-cell depletion

38211   tumor cell depletion

38212   red blood cell removal

38213   platelet depletion

38214   plasma (volume) depletion

38215   cell concentration in plasma, mononuclear, or buffy coat layer

(Do not report 38207-38215 in conjunction with 88182, 88184-88189)

38220 Bone marrow; aspiration only

38221   biopsy, needle or trocar

(For bone marrow biopsy interpretation, use 88305)

38230 Bone marrow harvesting for transplantation

(For autologous and allogenic blood-derived peripheral stem cell harvesting for transplantation, see 38205-38206)

38240 Bone marrow or blood-derived peripheral stem cell transplantation; allogenic

38241   autologous

38242   allogeneic donor lymphocyte infusions

(For bone marrow aspiration, use 38220)

(For modification, treatment, and processing of bone marrow or blood-derived stem cell specimens for transplantation, use 38210-38213)

(For cryopreservation, freezing and storage of blood-derived stem cells for transplantation, use 88240)

(For thawing and expansion of blood-derived stem cells for transplantation, use 88241)

(For compatibility studies, see 86812-86822)

Lymph Nodes and Lymphatic Channels

Incision

38300 Drainage of lymph node abscess or lymphadenitis; simple

38305   extensive

38308 Lymphangiotomy or other operations on lymphatic channels

38380 Suture and/or ligation of thoracic duct; cervical approach

38381   thoracic approach

38382   abdominal approach

Excision

(For injection for sentinel node identification, use 38792)

38500 Biopsy or excision of lymph node(s); open, superficial

(Do not report 38500 with 38700-38780)

38505   by needle, superficial (eg, cervical, inguinal, axillary)

▶(If imaging guidance is performed, see 76942, 77012, 77021)◀

(For fine needle aspiration, use 10021 or 10022)

(For evaluation of fine needle aspirate, see 88172, 88173)

38510   open, deep cervical node(s)

38520   open, deep cervical node(s) with excision scalene fat pad

Surgery: Cardiovascular System

Surgery: Cardiovascular System

38525   open, deep axillary node(s)

38530   open, internal mammary node(s)

(Do not report 38530 with 38720-38746)

(For percutaneous needle biopsy, retroperitoneal lymph node or mass, use 49180. For fine needle aspiration, use 10022)

38542   Dissection, deep jugular node(s)

(For radical cervical neck dissection, use 38720)

38550   Excision of cystic hygroma, axillary or cervical; without deep neurovascular dissection

38555   with deep neurovascular dissection

Limited Lymphadenectomy for Staging

38562   Limited lymphadenectomy for staging (separate procedure); pelvic and para-aortic

(When combined with prostatectomy, use 55812 or 55842)

(When combined with insertion of radioactive substance into prostate, use 55862)

38564   retroperitoneal (aortic and/or splenic)

Laparoscopy

Surgical laparoscopy always includes diagnostic laparoscopy. To report a diagnostic laparoscopy (peritoneoscopy) (separate procedure), use 49320.

38570   Laparoscopy, surgical; with retroperitoneal lymph node sampling (biopsy), single or multiple

38571   with bilateral total pelvic lymphadenectomy

38572   with bilateral total pelvic lymphadenectomy and peri-aortic lymph node sampling (biopsy), single or multiple

(For drainage of lymphocele to peritoneal cavity, use 49323)

38589   Unlisted laparoscopy procedure, lymphatic system

Radical Lymphadenectomy (Radical Resection of Lymph Nodes)

(For limited pelvic and retroperitoneal lymphadenectomies, see 38562, 38564)

38700   Suprahyoid lymphadenectomy

(For bilateral procedure, report 38700 with modifier 50)

38720   Cervical lymphadenectomy (complete)

(For bilateral procedure, report 38720 with modifier 50)

38724   Cervical lymphadenectomy (modified radical neck dissection)

38740   Axillary lymphadenectomy; superficial

38745   complete

+ 38746   Thoracic lymphadenectomy, regional, including mediastinal and peritracheal nodes (List separately in addition to code for primary procedure)

+ 38747   Abdominal lymphadenectomy, regional, including celiac, gastric, portal, peripancreatic, with or without para-aortic and vena caval nodes (List separately in addition to code for primary procedure)

38760   Inguinofemoral lymphadenectomy, superficial, including Cloquets node (separate procedure)

(For bilateral procedure, report 38760 with modifier 50)

38765   Inguinofemoral lymphadenectomy, superficial, in continuity with pelvic lymphadenectomy, including external iliac, hypogastric, and obturator nodes (separate procedure)

(For bilateral procedure, report 38765 with modifier 50)

38770   Pelvic lymphadenectomy, including external iliac, hypogastric, and obturator nodes (separate procedure)

(For bilateral procedure, report 38770 with modifier 50)

38780   Retroperitoneal transabdominal lymphadenectomy, extensive, including pelvic, aortic, and renal nodes (separate procedure)

►(For excision and repair of lymphedematous skin and subcutaneous tissue, see 15004-15005, 15570-15650)◄

Introduction

38790   Injection procedure; lymphangiography

(For bilateral procedure, report 38790 with modifier 50)

(For radiological supervision and interpretation, see 75801-75807)

⊘ 38792   for identification of sentinel node

(For excision of sentinel node, see 38500-38542)

(For nuclear medicine lymphatics and lymph gland imaging, use 78195)

38794   Cannulation, thoracic duct

Other Procedures

38999   Unlisted procedure, hemic or lymphatic system

Mediastinum and Diaphragm

Mediastinum

Incision

39000   Mediastinotomy with exploration, drainage, removal of foreign body, or biopsy; cervical approach

39010   transthoracic approach, including either transthoracic or median sternotomy

Excision

39200   Excision of mediastinal cyst

39220   Excision of mediastinal tumor

(For substernal thyroidectomy, use 60270)

(For thymectomy, use 60520)

Endoscopy

39400   Mediastinoscopy, with or without biopsy

Other Procedures

39499   Unlisted procedure, mediastinum

Diaphragm

Repair

(For transabdominal repair of diaphragmatic (esophageal hiatal) hernia, see 43324, 43325)

39501   Repair, laceration of diaphragm, any approach

39502   Repair, paraesophageal hiatus hernia, transabdominal, with or without fundoplasty, vagotomy, and/or pyloroplasty, except neonatal

39503   Repair, neonatal diaphragmatic hernia, with or without chest tube insertion and with or without creation of ventral hernia

(Do not report modifier 63 in conjunction with 39503)

39520   Repair, diaphragmatic hernia (esophageal hiatal); transthoracic

39530   combined, thoracoabdominal

39531   combined, thoracoabdominal, with dilation of stricture (with or without gastroplasty)

39540   Repair, diaphragmatic hernia (other than neonatal), traumatic; acute

39541   chronic

39545   Imbrication of diaphragm for eventration, transthoracic or transabdominal, paralytic or nonparalytic

39560   Resection, diaphragm; with simple repair (eg, primary suture)

39561   with complex repair (eg, prosthetic material, local muscle flap)

Other Procedures

39599   Unlisted procedure, diaphragm

Surgery: Cardiovascular System

Notes

Digestive System

Lips

(For procedures on skin of lips, see 10040 et seq)

Excision

40490   Biopsy of lip

40500   Vermilionectomy (lip shave), with mucosal advancement

40510   Excision of lip; transverse wedge excision with primary closure

40520   V-excision with primary direct linear closure

(For excision of mucous lesions, see 40810-40816)

40525   full thickness, reconstruction with local flap (eg, Estlander or fan)

40527   full thickness, reconstruction with cross lip flap (Abbe-Estlander)

40530   Resection of lip, more than one-fourth, without reconstruction

(For reconstruction, see 13131 et seq)

Repair (Cheiloplasty)

40650   Repair lip, full thickness; vermilion only

40652   up to half vertical height

40654   over one-half vertical height, or complex

40700   Plastic repair of cleft lip/nasal deformity; primary, partial or complete, unilateral

40701   primary bilateral, one stage procedure

40702   primary bilateral, one of two stages

40720   secondary, by recreation of defect and reclosure

(For bilateral procedure, report 40720 with modifier 50)

(To report rhinoplasty only for nasal deformity secondary to congenital cleft lip, see 30460, 30462)

(For repair of cleft lip, with cross lip pedicle flap (Abbe-Estlander type), use 40527)

40761   with cross lip pedicle flap (Abbe-Estlander type), including sectioning and inserting of pedicle

(For repair cleft palate, see 42200 et seq)

(For other reconstructive procedures, see 14060, 14061, 15120-15261, 15574, 15576, 15630)

Other Procedures

40799   Unlisted procedure, lips

Vestibule of Mouth

The vestibule is the part of the oral cavity outside the dentoalveolar structures; it includes the mucosal and submucosal tissue of lips and cheeks.

Incision

40800   Drainage of abscess, cyst, hematoma, vestibule of mouth; simple

40801   complicated

40804   Removal of embedded foreign body, vestibule of mouth; simple

40805   complicated

40806   Incision of labial frenum (frenotomy)

Excision, Destruction

40808   Biopsy, vestibule of mouth

40810   Excision of lesion of mucosa and submucosa, vestibule of mouth; without repair

40812   with simple repair

40814   with complex repair

40816   complex, with excision of underlying muscle

40818   Excision of mucosa of vestibule of mouth as donor graft

40819   Excision of frenum, labial or buccal (frenumectomy, frenulectomy, frenectomy)

40820   Destruction of lesion or scar of vestibule of mouth by physical methods (eg, laser, thermal, cryo, chemical)

Repair

40830   Closure of laceration, vestibule of mouth; 2.5 cm or less

40831   over 2.5 cm or complex

40840   Vestibuloplasty; anterior

40842   posterior, unilateral

40843   posterior, bilateral

40844   entire arch

40845   complex (including ridge extension, muscle repositioning)

▶(For skin grafts, see 15002 et seq)◀

Other Procedures

40899   Unlisted procedure, vestibule of mouth

Tongue and Floor of Mouth

Incision

41000   Intraoral incision and drainage of abscess, cyst, or hematoma of tongue or floor of mouth; lingual

41005   sublingual, superficial

41006   sublingual, deep, supramylohyoid

41007   submental space

41008   submandibular space

41009   masticator space

41010   Incision of lingual frenum (frenotomy)

41015   Extraoral incision and drainage of abscess, cyst, or hematoma of floor of mouth; sublingual

41016   submental

41017   submandibular

41018   masticator space

     (For frenoplasty, use 41520)

Excision

41100   Biopsy of tongue; anterior two-thirds

41105   posterior one-third

41108   Biopsy of floor of mouth

41110   Excision of lesion of tongue without closure

41112   Excision of lesion of tongue with closure; anterior two-thirds

41113   posterior one-third

41114   with local tongue flap

     (List 41114 in addition to code 41112 or 41113)

41115   Excision of lingual frenum (frenectomy)

41116   Excision, lesion of floor of mouth

41120   Glossectomy; less than one-half tongue

41130   hemiglossectomy

41135   partial, with unilateral radical neck dissection

41140   complete or total, with or without tracheostomy, without radical neck dissection

41145   complete or total, with or without tracheostomy, with unilateral radical neck dissection

41150   composite procedure with resection floor of mouth and mandibular resection, without radical neck dissection

41153   composite procedure with resection floor of mouth, with suprahyoid neck dissection

41155   composite procedure with resection floor of mouth, mandibular resection, and radical neck dissection (Commando type)

Repair

41250   Repair of laceration 2.5 cm or less; floor of mouth and/or anterior two-thirds of tongue

41251   posterior one-third of tongue

41252   Repair of laceration of tongue, floor of mouth, over 2.6 cm or complex

Other Procedures

41500   Fixation of tongue, mechanical, other than suture (eg, K-wire)

41510   Suture of tongue to lip for micrognathia (Douglas type procedure)

41520   Frenoplasty (surgical revision of frenum, eg, with Z-plasty)

     (For frenotomy, see 40806, 41010)

41599   Unlisted procedure, tongue, floor of mouth

Dentoalveolar Structures

Incision

41800   Drainage of abscess, cyst, hematoma from dentoalveolar structures

41805   Removal of embedded foreign body from dentoalveolar structures; soft tissues

41806   bone

Excision, Destruction

41820   Gingivectomy, excision gingiva, each quadrant

41821   Operculectomy, excision pericoronal tissues

41822   Excision of fibrous tuberosities, dentoalveolar structures

41823   Excision of osseous tuberosities, dentoalveolar structures

41825   Excision of lesion or tumor (except listed above), dentoalveolar structures; without repair

41826   with simple repair

41827   with complex repair

     (For nonexcisional destruction, use 41850)

41828   Excision of hyperplastic alveolar mucosa, each quadrant (specify)

41830   Alveolectomy, including curettage of osteitis or sequestrectomy

41850   Destruction of lesion (except excision), dentoalveolar structures

Other Procedures

41870   Periodontal mucosal grafting

41872   Gingivoplasty, each quadrant (specify)

41874	Alveoloplasty, each quadrant (specify)

(For closure of lacerations, see 40830, 40831)

(For segmental osteotomy, use 21206)

(For reduction of fractures, see 21421-21490)

41899   Unlisted procedure, dentoalveolar structures

Palate and Uvula

Incision

42000   Drainage of abscess of palate, uvula

Excision, Destruction

42100   Biopsy of palate, uvula

42104   Excision, lesion of palate, uvula; without closure

42106   with simple primary closure

42107   with local flap closure

(For skin graft, see 14040-14300)

(For mucosal graft, use 40818)

42120   Resection of palate or extensive resection of lesion

(For reconstruction of palate with extraoral tissue, see 14040-14300, 15050, 15120, 15240, 15576)

42140   Uvulectomy, excision of uvula

42145   Palatopharyngoplasty (eg, uvulopalatopharyngoplasty, uvulopharyngoplasty)

(For removal of exostosis of the bony palate, see 21031, 21032)

42160   Destruction of lesion, palate or uvula (thermal, cryo or chemical)

Repair

42180   Repair, laceration of palate; up to 2 cm

42182   over 2 cm or complex

42200   Palatoplasty for cleft palate, soft and/or hard palate only

42205   Palatoplasty for cleft palate, with closure of alveolar ridge; soft tissue only

42210   with bone graft to alveolar ridge (includes obtaining graft)

42215   Palatoplasty for cleft palate; major revision

42220   secondary lengthening procedure

42225   attachment pharyngeal flap

42226   Lengthening of palate, and pharyngeal flap

42227   Lengthening of palate, with island flap

42235   Repair of anterior palate, including vomer flap

(For repair of oronasal fistula, use 30600)

42260   Repair of nasolabial fistula

(For repair of cleft lip, see 40700 et seq)

42280   Maxillary impression for palatal prosthesis

42281   Insertion of pin-retained palatal prosthesis

Other Procedures

42299   Unlisted procedure, palate, uvula

Salivary Gland and Ducts

Incision

42300   Drainage of abscess; parotid, simple

42305   parotid, complicated

42310   Drainage of abscess; submaxillary or sublingual, intraoral

42320   submaxillary, external

(42325, 42326 have been deleted)

42330   Sialolithotomy; submandibular (submaxillary), sublingual or parotid, uncomplicated, intraoral

42335   submandibular (submaxillary), complicated, intraoral

42340   parotid, extraoral or complicated intraoral

Excision

42400   Biopsy of salivary gland; needle

(For fine needle aspiration, see 10021, 10022)

(For evaluation of fine needle aspirate, see 88172, 88173)

►(If imaging guidance is performed, see 76942, 77002, 77012, 77021)◄

42405   incisional

►(If imaging guidance is performed, see 76942, 77002, 77012, 77021)◄

42408   Excision of sublingual salivary cyst (ranula)

42409   Marsupialization of sublingual salivary cyst (ranula)

42410   Excision of parotid tumor or parotid gland; lateral lobe, without nerve dissection

42415   lateral lobe, with dissection and preservation of facial nerve

42420   total, with dissection and preservation of facial nerve

42425   total, en bloc removal with sacrifice of facial nerve

42426   total, with unilateral radical neck dissection

(For suture or grafting of facial nerve, see 64864, 64865, 69740, 69745)

42440   Excision of submandibular (submaxillary) gland

42450   Excision of sublingual gland

Surgery: Digestive System

Surgery: Digestive System

Repair

42500   Plastic repair of salivary duct, sialodochoplasty; primary or simple

42505   secondary or complicated

42507   Parotid duct diversion, bilateral (Wilke type procedure);

42508   with excision of one submandibular gland

42509   with excision of both submandibular glands

42510   with ligation of both submandibular (Wharton's) ducts

Other Procedures

42550   Injection procedure for sialography

(For radiological supervision and interpretation, use 70390)

42600   Closure salivary fistula

42650   Dilation salivary duct

42660   Dilation and catheterization of salivary duct, with or without injection

42665   Ligation salivary duct, intraoral

42699   Unlisted procedure, salivary glands or ducts

Pharynx, Adenoids, and Tonsils

Incision

42700   Incision and drainage abscess; peritonsillar

42720   retropharyngeal or parapharyngeal, intraoral approach

42725   retropharyngeal or parapharyngeal, external approach

Excision, Destruction

42800   Biopsy; oropharynx

42802   hypopharynx

42804   nasopharynx, visible lesion, simple

42806   nasopharynx, survey for unknown primary lesion

(For laryngoscopic biopsy, see 31510, 31535, 31536)

42808   Excision or destruction of lesion of pharynx, any method

42809   Removal of foreign body from pharynx

42810   Excision branchial cleft cyst or vestige, confined to skin and subcutaneous tissues

42815   Excision branchial cleft cyst, vestige, or fistula, extending beneath subcutaneous tissues and/or into pharynx

42820   Tonsillectomy and adenoidectomy; younger than age 12

42821   age 12 or over

42825   Tonsillectomy, primary or secondary; younger than age 12

42826   age 12 or over

42830   Adenoidectomy, primary; younger than age 12

42831   age 12 or over

42835   Adenoidectomy, secondary; younger than age 12

42836   age 12 or over

42842   Radical resection of tonsil, tonsillar pillars, and/or retromolar trigone; without closure

42844   closure with local flap (eg, tongue, buccal)

42845   closure with other flap

(For closure with other flap(s), use appropriate number for flap(s))

(When combined with radical neck dissection, use also 38720)

42860   Excision of tonsil tags

42870   Excision or destruction lingual tonsil, any method (separate procedure)

(For resection of the nasopharynx (eg, juvenile angiofibroma) by bicoronal and/or transzygomatic approach, see 61586 and 61600)

42890   Limited pharyngectomy

42892   Resection of lateral pharyngeal wall or pyriform sinus, direct closure by advancement of lateral and posterior pharyngeal walls

(When combined with radical neck dissection, use also 38720)

42894   Resection of pharyngeal wall requiring closure with myocutaneous flap

(When combined with radical neck dissection, use also 38720)

(For limited pharyngectomy with radical neck dissection, use 38720 with 42890)

Repair

42900   Suture pharynx for wound or injury

42950   Pharyngoplasty (plastic or reconstructive operation on pharynx)

(For pharyngeal flap, use 42225)

42953   Pharyngoesophageal repair

(For closure with myocutaneous or other flap, use appropriate number in addition)

Other Procedures

42955   Pharyngostomy (fistulization of pharynx, external for feeding)

42960   Control oropharyngeal hemorrhage, primary or secondary (eg, post-tonsillectomy); simple

42961   complicated, requiring hospitalization

42962   with secondary surgical intervention

42970　Control of nasopharyngeal hemorrhage, primary or secondary (eg, postadenoidectomy); simple, with posterior nasal packs, with or without anterior packs and/or cautery

42971　　　complicated, requiring hospitalization

42972　　　with secondary surgical intervention

42999　Unlisted procedure, pharynx, adenoids, or tonsils

Esophagus

Incision

(For esophageal intubation with laparotomy, use 43510)

43020　Esophagotomy, cervical approach, with removal of foreign body

43030　Cricopharyngeal myotomy

43045　Esophagotomy, thoracic approach, with removal of foreign body

Excision

(For gastrointestinal reconstruction for previous esophagectomy, see 43360, 43361)

43100　Excision of lesion, esophagus, with primary repair; cervical approach

43101　　　thoracic or abdominal approach

(For wide excision of malignant lesion of cervical esophagus, with total laryngectomy without radical neck dissection, see 43107, 43116, 43124, and 31360)

(For wide excision of malignant lesion of cervical esophagus, with total laryngectomy with radical neck dissection, see 43107, 43116, 43124, and 31365)

43107　Total or near total esophagectomy, without thoracotomy; with pharyngogastrostomy or cervical esophagogastrostomy, with or without pyloroplasty (transhiatal)

43108　　　with colon interposition or small intestine reconstruction, including intestine mobilization, preparation and anastomosis(es)

43112　Total or near total esophagectomy, with thoracotomy; with pharyngogastrostomy or cervical esophagogastrostomy, with or without pyloroplasty

43113　　　with colon interposition or small intestine reconstruction, including intestine mobilization, preparation, and anastomosis(es)

43116　Partial esophagectomy, cervical, with free intestinal graft, including microvascular anastomosis, obtaining the graft and intestinal reconstruction

(Do not report 43116 in conjunction with 69990)

(Report 43116 with the modifier 52 appended if intestinal or free jejunal graft with microvascular anastomosis is performed by another physician)

(For free jejunal graft with microvascular anastomosis performed by another physician, use 43496)

43117　Partial esophagectomy, distal two-thirds, with thoracotomy and separate abdominal incision, with or without proximal gastrectomy; with thoracic esophagogastrostomy, with or without pyloroplasty (Ivor Lewis)

43118　　　with colon interposition or small intestine reconstruction, including intestine mobilization, preparation, and anastomosis(es)

(For total esophagectomy with gastropharyngostomy, see 43107, 43124)

(For esophagogastrectomy (lower third) and vagotomy, use 43122)

43121　Partial esophagectomy, distal two-thirds, with thoracotomy only, with or without proximal gastrectomy, with thoracic esophagogastrostomy, with or without pyloroplasty

43122　Partial esophagectomy, thoracoabdominal or abdominal approach, with or without proximal gastrectomy; with esophagogastrostomy, with or without pyloroplasty

43123　　　with colon interposition or small intestine reconstruction, including intestine mobilization, preparation, and anastomosis(es)

43124　Total or partial esophagectomy, without reconstruction (any approach), with cervical esophagostomy

43130　Diverticulectomy of hypopharynx or esophagus, with or without myotomy; cervical approach

43135　　　thoracic approach

Endoscopy

For endoscopic procedures, code appropriate endoscopy of each anatomic site examined.

Surgical endoscopy always includes diagnostic endoscopy.

⊙ **43200**　Esophagoscopy, rigid or flexible; diagnostic, with or without collection of specimen(s) by brushing or washing (separate procedure)

⊙ **43201**　　　with directed submucosal injection(s), any substance

(For injection sclerosis of esophageal varices, use 43204)

⊙ **43202**　　　with biopsy, single or multiple

⊙ **43204**　　　with injection sclerosis of esophageal varices

⊙ **43205**　　　with band ligation of esophageal varices

⊙ **43215**　　　with removal of foreign body

(For radiological supervision and interpretation, use 74235)

Surgery: Digestive System

⊙ **43216**   with removal of tumor(s), polyp(s), or other lesion(s) by hot biopsy forceps or bipolar cautery

⊙ **43217**   with removal of tumor(s), polyp(s), or other lesion(s) by snare technique

⊙ **43219**   with insertion of plastic tube or stent

⊙ **43220**   with balloon dilation (less than 30 mm diameter)

(If imaging guidance is performed, use 74360)

(For endoscopic dilation with balloon 30 mm diameter or larger, use 43458)

(For dilation without visualization, use 43450-43453)

(For diagnostic fiberoptic esophagogastroscopy, use 43200, 43235)

(For fiberoptic esophagogastroscopy with biopsy or collection of specimen, use 43200, 43202, 43235, 43239)

(For fiberoptic esophagogastroscopy with removal of foreign body, use 43215, 43247)

(For fiberoptic esophagogastroscopy with removal of polyp(s), use 43217, 43251)

⊙ **43226**   with insertion of guide wire followed by dilation over guide wire

(For radiological supervision and interpretation, use 74360)

⊙ **43227**   with control of bleeding (eg, injection, bipolar cautery, unipolar cautery, laser, heater probe, stapler, plasma coagulator)

⊙ **43228**   with ablation of tumor(s), polyp(s), or other lesion(s), not amenable to removal by hot biopsy forceps, bipolar cautery or snare technique

(For esophagoscopic photodynamic therapy, report 43228 in addition to 96570, 96571 as appropriate)

⊙ **43231**   with endoscopic ultrasound examination

(Do not report 43231 in conjunction with 76975)

⊙ **43232**   with transendoscopic ultrasound-guided intramural or transmural fine needle aspiration/biopsy(s)

(Do not report 43232 in conjunction with 76942, 76975)

(For interpretation of specimen, see 88172-88173)

⊙ **43234**   Upper gastrointestinal endoscopy, simple primary examination (eg, with small diameter flexible endoscope) (separate procedure)

⊙ **43235**   Upper gastrointestinal endoscopy including esophagus, stomach, and either the duodenum and/or jejunum as appropriate; diagnostic, with or without collection of specimen(s) by brushing or washing (separate procedure)

⊙ **43236**   with directed submucosal injection(s), any substance

(For injection sclerosis of esophageal and/or gastric varices, use 43243)

⊙ **43237**   with endoscopic ultrasound examination limited to the esophagus

(Do not report 43237 in conjunction with 76942, 76975)

⊙ **43238**   with transendoscopic ultrasound-guided intramural or transmural fine needle aspiration/biopsy(s), esophagus (includes endoscopic ultrasound examination limited to the esophagus)

(Do not report 43238 in conjunction with 76942 or 76975)

⊙ **43239**   with biopsy, single or multiple

(For upper gastrointestinal endoscopy with suturing of the esophagogastric junction, use Category III code 0008T)

(For upper gastrointestinal endoscopy with injection of implant material into and along the muscle of the lower esophageal sphincter, use Category III code 0133T)

⊙ **43240**   with transmural drainage of pseudocyst

⊙ **43241**   with transendoscopic intraluminal tube or catheter placement

⊙ **43242**   with transendoscopic ultrasound-guided intramural or transmural fine needle aspiration/biopsy(s) (includes endoscopic ultrasound examination of the esophagus, stomach, and either the duodenum and/or jejunum as appropriate)

(Do not report 43242 in conjunction with 76942, 76975)

(For transendoscopic fine needle aspiration/biopsy limited to esophagus, use 43238)

(For interpretation of specimen, see 88172-88173)

⊙ **43243**   with injection sclerosis of esophageal and/or gastric varices

⊙ **43244**   with band ligation of esophageal and/or gastric varices

⊙ **43245**   with dilation of gastric outlet for obstruction (eg, balloon, guide wire, bougie)

(Do not report 43245 in conjunction with 43256)

⊙ **43246**   with directed placement of percutaneous gastrostomy tube

(For radiological supervision and interpretation, use 74350)

⊙ **43247**   with removal of foreign body

(For radiological supervision and interpretation, use 74235)

⊙ **43248**   with insertion of guide wire followed by dilation of esophagus over guide wire

⊙ **43249**   with balloon dilation of esophagus (less than 30 mm diameter)

⊙ **43250**   with removal of tumor(s), polyp(s), or other lesion(s) by hot biopsy forceps or bipolar cautery

⊙ **43251**   with removal of tumor(s), polyp(s), or other lesion(s) by snare technique

Surgery: Digestive System

⊙ **43255**   with control of bleeding, any method

⊙ **43256**   with transendoscopic stent placement (includes predilation)

⊙ **43257**   with delivery of thermal energy to the muscle of lower esophageal sphincter and/or gastric cardia, for treatment of gastroesophageal reflux disease

⊙ **43258**   with ablation of tumor(s), polyp(s), or other lesion(s) not amenable to removal by hot biopsy forceps, bipolar cautery or snare technique

(For injection sclerosis of esophageal varices, use 43204, 43243)

⊙ **43259**   with endoscopic ultrasound examination, including the esophagus, stomach, and either the duodenum and/or jejunum as appropriate

(Do not report 43259 in conjunction with 76975)

⊙ **43260**   Endoscopic retrograde cholangiopancreatography (ERCP); diagnostic, with or without collection of specimen(s) by brushing or washing (separate procedure)

(For radiological supervision and interpretation, see 74328, 74329, 74330)

⊙ **43261**   with biopsy, single or multiple

(For radiological supervision and interpretation, see 74328, 74329, 74330)

⊙ **43262**   with sphincterotomy/papillotomy

(For radiological supervision and interpretation, see 74328, 74329, 74330)

⊙ **43263**   with pressure measurement of sphincter of Oddi (pancreatic duct or common bile duct)

(For radiological supervision and interpretation, see 74328, 74329, 74330)

⊙ **43264**   with endoscopic retrograde removal of calculus/calculi from biliary and/or pancreatic ducts

(When done with sphincterotomy, also use 43262)

(For radiological supervision and interpretation, see 74328, 74329, 74330)

⊙ **43265**   with endoscopic retrograde destruction, lithotripsy of calculus/calculi, any method

(When done with sphincterotomy, also use 43262)

(For radiological supervision and interpretation, see 74328, 74329, 74330)

⊙ **43267**   with endoscopic retrograde insertion of nasobiliary or nasopancreatic drainage tube

(When done with sphincterotomy, also use 43262)

(For radiological supervision and interpretation, see 74328, 74329, 74330)

⊙ **43268**   with endoscopic retrograde insertion of tube or stent into bile or pancreatic duct

(When done with sphincterotomy, also use 43262)

(For radiological supervision and interpretation, see 74328, 74329, 74330)

⊙ **43269**   with endoscopic retrograde removal of foreign body and/or change of tube or stent

(When done with sphincterotomy, also use 43262)

(For radiological supervision and interpretation, see 74328, 74329, 74330)

⊙ **43271**   with endoscopic retrograde balloon dilation of ampulla, biliary and/or pancreatic duct(s)

(When done with sphincterotomy, also use 43262)

(For radiological supervision and interpretation, see 74328, 74329, 74330)

⊙ **43272**   with ablation of tumor(s), polyp(s), or other lesion(s) not amenable to removal by hot biopsy forceps, bipolar cautery or snare technique

(For radiological supervision and interpretation, see 74328, 74329, 74330)

Laparoscopy

Surgical laparoscopy always includes diagnostic laparoscopy. To report a diagnostic laparoscopy (peritoneoscopy) (separate procedure), use 49320.

43280   Laparoscopy, surgical, esophagogastric fundoplasty (eg, Nissen, Toupet procedures)

(For open approach, use 43324)

43289   Unlisted laparoscopy procedure, esophagus

Repair

43300   Esophagoplasty (plastic repair or reconstruction), cervical approach; without repair of tracheoesophageal fistula

43305   with repair of tracheoesophageal fistula

43310   Esophagoplasty (plastic repair or reconstruction), thoracic approach; without repair of tracheoesophageal fistula

43312   with repair of tracheoesophageal fistula

43313   Esophagoplasty for congenital defect (plastic repair or reconstruction), thoracic approach; without repair of congenital tracheoesophageal fistula

43314   with repair of congenital tracheoesophageal fistula

(Do not report modifier 63 in conjunction with 43313, 43314)

43320   Esophagogastrostomy (cardioplasty), with or without vagotomy and pyloroplasty, transabdominal or transthoracic approach

Surgery: Digestive System

43324 Esophagogastric fundoplasty (eg, Nissen, Belsey IV, Hill procedures)

(For laparoscopic procedure, use 43280)

43325 Esophagogastric fundoplasty; with fundic patch (Thal-Nissen procedure)

(For cricopharyngeal myotomy, use 43030)

43326 with gastroplasty (eg, Collis)

43330 Esophagomyotomy (Heller type); abdominal approach

43331 thoracic approach

(For thoracoscopic esophagomyotomy, use 32665)

43340 Esophagojejunostomy (without total gastrectomy); abdominal approach

43341 thoracic approach

43350 Esophagostomy, fistulization of esophagus, external; abdominal approach

43351 thoracic approach

43352 cervical approach

43360 Gastrointestinal reconstruction for previous esophagectomy, for obstructing esophageal lesion or fistula, or for previous esophageal exclusion; with stomach, with or without pyloroplasty

43361 with colon interposition or small intestine reconstruction, including intestine mobilization, preparation, and anastomosis(es)

43400 Ligation, direct, esophageal varices

43401 Transection of esophagus with repair, for esophageal varices

43405 Ligation or stapling at gastroesophageal junction for pre-existing esophageal perforation

43410 Suture of esophageal wound or injury; cervical approach

43415 transthoracic or transabdominal approach

43420 Closure of esophagostomy or fistula; cervical approach

43425 transthoracic or transabdominal approach

(For repair of esophageal hiatal hernia, see 39520 et seq)

Manipulation

(For associated esophagogram, use 74220)

43450 Dilation of esophagus, by unguided sound or bougie, single or multiple passes

(For radiological supervision and interpretation, use 74360)

⊙ **43453** Dilation of esophagus, over guide wire

(For dilation with direct visualization, use 43220)

(For dilation of esophagus, by balloon or dilator, see 43220, 43458, and 74360)

(For radiological supervision and interpretation, use 74360)

⊙ **43456** Dilation of esophagus, by balloon or dilator, retrograde

(For radiological supervision and interpretation, use 74360)

⊙ **43458** Dilation of esophagus with balloon (30 mm diameter or larger) for achalasia

(For dilation with balloon less than 30 mm diameter, use 43220)

(For radiological supervision and interpretation, use 74360)

43460 Esophagogastric tamponade, with balloon (Sengstaaken type)

(For removal of esophageal foreign body by balloon catheter, see 43215, 43247, 74235)

Other Procedures

43496 Free jejunum transfer with microvascular anastomosis

(Do not report code 69990 in addition to code 43496)

43499 Unlisted procedure, esophagus

Stomach

Incision

43500 Gastrotomy; with exploration or foreign body removal

43501 with suture repair of bleeding ulcer

43502 with suture repair of pre-existing esophagogastric laceration (eg, Mallory-Weiss)

43510 with esophageal dilation and insertion of permanent intraluminal tube (eg, Celestin or Mousseaux-Barbin)

43520 Pyloromyotomy, cutting of pyloric muscle (Fredet-Ramstedt type operation)

(Do not report modifier 63 in conjunction with 43520)

Excision

43600 Biopsy of stomach; by capsule, tube, peroral (one or more specimens)

43605 by laparotomy

43610 Excision, local; ulcer or benign tumor of stomach

43611 malignant tumor of stomach

43620 Gastrectomy, total; with esophagoenterostomy

43621 with Roux-en-Y reconstruction

43622 with formation of intestinal pouch, any type

43631 Gastrectomy, partial, distal; with gastroduodenostomy

43632 with gastrojejunostomy

43633 with Roux-en-Y reconstruction

43634 with formation of intestinal pouch

+ 43635   Vagotomy when performed with partial distal gastrectomy (List separately in addition to code(s) for primary procedure)

(Use 43635 in conjunction with 43631, 43632, 43633, 43634)

(43638, 43639 have been deleted)

43640   Vagotomy including pyloroplasty, with or without gastrostomy; truncal or selective

(For pyloroplasty, use 43800)

(For vagotomy, see 64752-64760)

43641   parietal cell (highly selective)

(For upper gastrointestinal endoscopy, see 43234-43259)

Laparoscopy

Surgical laparoscopy always includes diagnostic laparoscopy. To report a diagnostic laparoscopy (peritoneoscopy) (separate procedure), use 49320.

(For upper gastrointestinal endoscopy including esophagus, stomach, and either the duodenum and/or jejunum, see 43235-43259)

43644   Laparoscopy, surgical, gastric restrictive procedure; with gastric bypass and Roux-en-Y gastroenterostomy (roux limb 150 cm or less)

(Do not report 43644 in conjunction with 43846, 49320)

(Esophagogastroduodenoscopy (EGD) performed for a separate condition should be reported with modifier 59)

(For greater than 150 cm, use 43645)

(For open procedure, use 43846)

43645   with gastric bypass and small intestine reconstruction to limit absorption

(Do not report 43645 in conjunction with 49320, 43847)

● 43647   Laparoscopy, surgical; implantation or replacement of gastric neurostimulator electrodes, antrum

● 43648   revision or removal of gastric neurostimulator electrodes, antrum

▶(For open approach, see 43881, 43882)◀

▶(For insertion of gastric neurostimulator pulse generator, use 64590)◀

▶(For revision or removal of gastric neurostimulator pulse generator, use 64595)◀

▶(For electronic analysis and programming of gastric neurostimulator pulse generator, use 95999)◀

▶(For laparoscopic implantation, revision, or removal of gastric neurostimulator electrodes, lesser curvature [morbid obesity], see Category III codes 0155T, 0156T)◀

▶(For electronic analysis, programming, and reprogramming of gastric neurostimulator pulse generator, lesser curvature [morbid obesity], use Category III code 0162T)◀

43651   Laparoscopy, surgical; transection of vagus nerves, truncal

43652   transection of vagus nerves, selective or highly selective

43653   gastrostomy, without construction of gastric tube (eg, Stamm procedure) (separate procedure)

43659   Unlisted laparoscopy procedure, stomach

Introduction

⊙ 43750   Percutaneous placement of gastrostomy tube

(For radiological supervision and interpretation, use 74350)

43752   Naso- or oro-gastric tube placement, requiring physician's skill and fluoroscopic guidance (includes fluoroscopy, image documentation and report)

(For enteric tube placement, see 44500, 74340)

(Do not report 43752 in conjunction with critical care codes 99291-99292, neonatal critical care codes 99295-99296, pediatric critical care codes 99293-99294 or low birth weight intensive care service codes 99298-99299)

43760   Change of gastrostomy tube

(For endoscopic placement of gastrostomy tube, use 43246)

(For radiological supervision and interpretation, use 75984)

43761   Repositioning of the gastric feeding tube, any method, through the duodenum for enteric nutrition

(If imaging guidance is performed, use 75984)

Bariatric Surgery

Bariatric surgical procedures may involve the stomach, duodenum, jejunum, and/or the ileum.

Laparoscopy

Surgical laparoscopy always includes diagnostic laparoscopy. To report a diagnostic laparoscopy (separate procedure), use 49320.

Typical postoperative follow-up care (see Surgery Guidelines, CPT Surgical Package Definition) after gastric restriction using the adjustable gastric band technique includes subsequent band adjustment(s) through the postoperative period for the typical patient. Band adjustment refers to changing the gastric band component diameter by injection or aspiration of fluid through the subcutaneous port component.

Surgery: Digestive System

43770   Laparoscopy, surgical, gastric restrictive procedure; placement of adjustable gastric band (gastric band and subcutaneous port components)

(For individual component placement, report 43770 with modifier 52)

43771   revision of adjustable gastric band component only

43772   removal of adjustable gastric band component only

43773   removal and replacement of adjustable gastric band component only

(Do not report 43773 in conjunction with 43772)

43774   removal of adjustable gastric band and subcutaneous port components

(For removal and replacement of both gastric band and subcutaneous port components, use 43659)

Other Procedures

43800   Pyloroplasty

(For pyloroplasty and vagotomy, use 43640)

43810   Gastroduodenostomy

43820   Gastrojejunostomy; without vagotomy

43825   with vagotomy, any type

43830   Gastrostomy, open; without construction of gastric tube (eg, Stamm procedure) (separate procedure)

43831   neonatal, for feeding

(For change of gastrostomy tube, use 43760)

(Do not report modifier 63 in conjunction with 43831)

43832   with construction of gastric tube (eg, Janeway procedure)

(For percutaneous endoscopic gastrostomy, use 43246)

43840   Gastrorrhaphy, suture of perforated duodenal or gastric ulcer, wound, or injury

43842   Gastric restrictive procedure, without gastric bypass, for morbid obesity; vertical-banded gastroplasty

43843   other than vertical-banded gastroplasty

43845   Gastric restrictive procedure with partial gastrectomy, pylorus-preserving duodenoileostomy and ileoileostomy (50 to 100 cm common channel) to limit absorption (biliopancreatic diversion with duodenal switch)

(Do not report 43845 in conjunction with 43633, 43847, 44130, 49000)

43846   Gastric restrictive procedure, with gastric bypass for morbid obesity; with short limb (150 cm or less) Roux-en-Y gastroenterostomy

(For greater than 150 cm, use 43847)

(For laparoscopic procedure, use 43644)

43847   with small intestine reconstruction to limit absorption

43848   Revision, open, of gastric restrictive procedure for morbid obesity, other than adjustable gastric band (separate procedure)

(For adjustable gastric band procedures, see 43770-43774, 43886-43888)

43850   Revision of gastroduodenal anastomosis (gastroduodenostomy) with reconstruction; without vagotomy

43855   with vagotomy

43860   Revision of gastrojejunal anastomosis (gastrojejunostomy) with reconstruction, with or without partial gastrectomy or intestine resection; without vagotomy

43865   with vagotomy

43870   Closure of gastrostomy, surgical

43880   Closure of gastrocolic fistula

● **43881**   Implantation or replacement of gastric neurostimulator electrodes, antrum, open

● **43882**   Revision or removal of gastric neurostimulator electrodes, antrum, open

►(For laparoscopic approach, see 43647, 43648)◄

►(For insertion of gastric neurostimulator pulse generator, use 64590)◄

►(For revision or removal of gastric neurostimulator pulse generator, use 64595)◄

►(For electronic analysis and programming of gastric neurostimulator pulse generator, use 95999)◄

►(For open implantation, revision, or removal of gastric neurostimulator electrodes, lesser curvature [morbid obesity], see Category III codes 0157T, 0158T)◄

►(For electronic analysis, programming, and reprogramming of gastric neurostimulator pulse generator, lesser curvature [morbid obesity], use Category III code 0162T)◄

43886   Gastric restrictive procedure, open; revision of subcutaneous port component only

43887   removal of subcutaneous port component only

43888   removal and replacement of subcutaneous port component only

(Do not report 43888 in conjunction with 43774, 43887)

(For laparoscopic removal of both gastric band and subcutaneous port components, use 43774)

(For removal and replacement of both gastric band and subcutaneous port components, use 43659)

43999   Unlisted procedure, stomach

Intestines (Except Rectum)

Incision

44005   Enterolysis (freeing of intestinal adhesion) (separate procedure)

(Do not report 44005 in addition to 45136)

(For laparoscopic approach, use 44180)

44010   Duodenotomy, for exploration, biopsy(s), or foreign body removal

+ 44015   Tube or needle catheter jejunostomy for enteral alimentation, intraoperative, any method (List separately in addition to primary procedure)

44020   Enterotomy, small intestine, other than duodenum; for exploration, biopsy(s), or foreign body removal

44021   for decompression (eg, Baker tube)

44025   Colotomy, for exploration, biopsy(s), or foreign body removal

(For exteriorization of intestine (Mikulicz resection with crushing of spur), see 44602-44605)

44050   Reduction of volvulus, intussusception, internal hernia, by laparotomy

44055   Correction of malrotation by lysis of duodenal bands and/or reduction of midgut volvulus (eg, Ladd procedure)

(Do not report modifier 63 in conjunction with 44055)

Excision

Intestinal allotransplantation involves three distinct components of physician work:

1) ***Cadaver donor enterectomy***, which includes harvesting the intestine graft and cold preservation of the graft (perfusing with cold preservation solution and cold maintenance) (use 44132). ***Living donor enterectomy***, which includes harvesting the intestine graft, cold preservation of the graft (perfusing with cold preservation solution and cold maintenance), and care of the donor (use 44133).

2) ***Backbench work***:

Standard preparation of an intestine allograft prior to transplantation includes mobilization and fashioning of the superior mesenteric artery and vein (see 44715).

Additional reconstruction of an intestine allograft prior to transplantation may include venous and/or arterial anastomosis(es) (see 44720-44721).

3) ***Recipient intestinal allotransplantation with or without recipient enterectomy***, which includes transplantation of allograft and care of the recipient (see 44135, 44136).

44100   Biopsy of intestine by capsule, tube, peroral (one or more specimens)

44110   Excision of one or more lesions of small or large intestine not requiring anastomosis, exteriorization, or fistulization; single enterotomy

44111   multiple enterotomies

44120   Enterectomy, resection of small intestine; single resection and anastomosis

(Do not report 44120 in addition to 45136)

+ 44121   each additional resection and anastomosis (List separately in addition to code for primary procedure)

(Use 44121 in conjunction with 44120)

44125   with enterostomy

44126   Enterectomy, resection of small intestine for congenital atresia, single resection and anastomosis of proximal segment of intestine; without tapering

44127   with tapering

+ 44128   each additional resection and anastomosis (List separately in addition to code for primary procedure)

(Use 44128 in conjunction with 44126, 44127)

(Do not report modifier 63 in conjunction with 44126, 44127, 44128)

44130   Enteroenterostomy, anastomosis of intestine, with or without cutaneous enterostomy (separate procedure)

44132   Donor enterectomy (including cold preservation), open; from cadaver donor

44133   partial, from living donor

(For backbench intestinal graft preparation or reconstruction, see 44715, 44720, 44721)

44135   Intestinal allotransplantation; from cadaver donor

44136   from living donor

44137   Removal of transplanted intestinal allograft, complete

(For partial removal of transplant allograft, see 44120, 44121, 44140)

+ 44139   Mobilization (take-down) of splenic flexure performed in conjunction with partial colectomy (List separately in addition to primary procedure)

(Use 44139 in conjunction with 44140-44147)

44140   Colectomy, partial; with anastomosis

(For laparoscopic procedure, use 44204)

44141   with skin level cecostomy or colostomy

44143   with end colostomy and closure of distal segment (Hartmann type procedure)

(For laparoscopic procedure, use 44206)

44144   with resection, with colostomy or ileostomy and creation of mucofistula

44145   with coloproctostomy (low pelvic anastomosis)

(For laparoscopic procedure, use 44207)

Surgery: Digestive System

Surgery: Digestive System

44146   with coloproctostomy (low pelvic anastomosis), with colostomy

(For laparoscopic procedure, use 44208)

44147   abdominal and transanal approach

44150   Colectomy, total, abdominal, without proctectomy; with ileostomy or ileoproctostomy

(For laparoscopic procedure, use 44210)

44151   with continent ileostomy

▶(44152 and 44153 have been deleted. To report, use 44799)◄

44155   Colectomy, total, abdominal, with proctectomy; with ileostomy

(For laparoscopic procedure, use 44212)

44156   with continent ileostomy

● **44157**   with ileoanal anastomosis, includes loop ileostomy, and rectal mucosectomy, when performed

● **44158**   with ileoanal anastomosis, creation of ileal reservoir (S or J), includes loop ileostomy, and rectal mucosectomy, when performed

▶(For laparoscopic procedure, use 44211)◄

44160   Colectomy, partial, with removal of terminal ileum with ileocolostomy

(For laparoscopic procedure, use 44205)

Laparoscopy

Surgical laparoscopy always includes diagnostic laparoscopy. To report a diagnostic laparoscopy (peritoneoscopy) (separate procedure), use 49320.

Incision

44180   Laparoscopy, surgical, enterolysis (freeing of intestinal adhesion) (separate procedure)

(For laparoscopy with salpingolysis, ovariolysis, use 58660)

Enterostomy—External Fistulization of Intestines

44186   Laparoscopy, surgical; jejunostomy (eg, for decompression or feeding)

44187   ileostomy or jejunostomy, non-tube

(For open procedure, use 44310)

44188   Laparoscopy, surgical, colostomy or skin level cecostomy

(For open procedure, use 44320)

(Do not report 44188 in conjunction with 44970)

(44200 has been deleted. To report, use 44180)

(44201 has been deleted. To report, use 44186)

Excision

44202   Laparoscopy, surgical; enterectomy, resection of small intestine, single resection and anastomosis

+ **44203**   each additional small intestine resection and anastomosis (List separately in addition to code for primary procedure)

(Use 44203 in conjunction with 44202)

(For open procedure, see 44120, 44121)

44204   colectomy, partial, with anastomosis

(For open procedure, use 44140)

44205   colectomy, partial, with removal of terminal ileum with ileocolostomy

(For open procedure, use 44160)

44206   colectomy, partial, with end colostomy and closure of distal segment (Hartmann type procedure)

(For open procedure, use 44143)

44207   colectomy, partial, with anastomosis, with coloproctostomy (low pelvic anastomosis)

(For open procedure, use 44145)

44208   colectomy, partial, with anastomosis, with coloproctostomy (low pelvic anastomosis) with colostomy

(For open procedure, use 44146)

44210   colectomy, total, abdominal, without proctectomy, with ileostomy or ileoproctostomy

(For open procedure, use 44150)

▲ **44211**   colectomy, total, abdominal, with proctectomy, with ileoanal anastomosis, creation of ileal reservoir (S or J), with loop ileostomy, includes rectal mucosectomy, when performed

▶(For open procedure, see 44157, 44158)◄

44212   colectomy, total, abdominal, with proctectomy, with ileostomy

(For open procedure, use 44155)

+ **44213**   Laparoscopy, surgical, mobilization (take-down) of splenic flexure performed in conjunction with partial colectomy (List separately in addition to primary procedure)

(Use 44213 in conjunction with 44204-44208)

(For open procedure, use 44139)

Repair

44227   Laparoscopy, surgical, closure of enterostomy, large or small intestine, with resection and anastomosis

(For open procedure, see 44625, 44626)

Other Procedures

44238   Unlisted laparoscopy procedure, intestine (except rectum)

(44239 has been deleted. To report, use 45499)

Enterostomy—External Fistulization of Intestines

44300   Enterostomy or cecostomy, tube (eg, for decompression or feeding) (separate procedure)

44310   Ileostomy or jejunostomy, non-tube

(For laparoscopic procedure, use 44187)

(Do not report 44310 in conjunction with 44144, 44150-44151, 44155, 44156, 45113, 45119, 45136)

44312   Revision of ileostomy; simple (release of superficial scar) (separate procedure)

44314   complicated (reconstruction in-depth) (separate procedure)

44316   Continent ileostomy (Kock procedure) (separate procedure)

(For fiberoptic evaluation, use 44385)

44320   Colostomy or skin level cecostomy;

(For laparoscopic procedure, use 44188)

(Do not report 44320 in conjunction with 44141, 44144, 44146, 44605, 45110, 45119, 45126, 45563, 45805, 45825, 50810, 51597, 57307, or 58240)

44322   with multiple biopsies (eg, for congenital megacolon) (separate procedure)

44340   Revision of colostomy; simple (release of superficial scar) (separate procedure)

44345   complicated (reconstruction in-depth) (separate procedure)

44346   with repair of paracolostomy hernia (separate procedure)

Endoscopy, Small Intestine and Stomal

Surgical endoscopy always includes diagnostic endoscopy.

(For upper gastrointestinal endoscopy, see 43234-43258)

⊙ 44360   Small intestinal endoscopy, enteroscopy beyond second portion of duodenum, not including ileum; diagnostic, with or without collection of specimen(s) by brushing or washing (separate procedure)

⊙ 44361   with biopsy, single or multiple

⊙ 44363   with removal of foreign body

⊙ 44364   with removal of tumor(s), polyp(s), or other lesion(s) by snare technique

⊙ 44365   with removal of tumor(s), polyp(s), or other lesion(s) by hot biopsy forceps or bipolar cautery

⊙ 44366   with control of bleeding (eg, injection, bipolar cautery, unipolar cautery, laser, heater probe, stapler, plasma coagulator)

⊙ 44369   with ablation of tumor(s), polyp(s), or other lesion(s) not amenable to removal by hot biopsy forceps, bipolar cautery or snare technique

⊙ 44370   with transendoscopic stent placement (includes predilation)

⊙ 44372   with placement of percutaneous jejunostomy tube

⊙ 44373   with conversion of percutaneous gastrostomy tube to percutaneous jejunostomy tube

(For fiberoptic jejunostomy through stoma, use 43235)

⊙ 44376   Small intestinal endoscopy, enteroscopy beyond second portion of duodenum, including ileum; diagnostic, with or without collection of specimen(s) by brushing or washing (separate procedure)

⊙ 44377   with biopsy, single or multiple

⊙ 44378   with control of bleeding (eg, injection, bipolar cautery, unipolar cautery, laser, heater probe, stapler, plasma coagulator)

⊙ 44379   with transendoscopic stent placement (includes predilation)

⊙ 44380   Ileoscopy, through stoma; diagnostic, with or without collection of specimen(s) by brushing or washing (separate procedure)

⊙ 44382   with biopsy, single or multiple

⊙ 44383   with transendoscopic stent placement (includes predilation)

⊙ 44385   Endoscopic evaluation of small intestinal (abdominal or pelvic) pouch; diagnostic, with or without collection of specimen(s) by brushing or washing (separate procedure)

⊙ 44386   with biopsy, single or multiple

⊙ 44388   Colonoscopy through stoma; diagnostic, with or without collection of specimen(s) by brushing or washing (separate procedure)

⊙ 44389   with biopsy, single or multiple

⊙ 44390   with removal of foreign body

⊙ 44391   with control of bleeding (eg, injection, bipolar cautery, unipolar cautery, laser, heater probe, stapler, plasma coagulator)

⊙ 44392   with removal of tumor(s), polyp(s), or other lesion(s) by hot biopsy forceps or bipolar cautery

⊙ 44393   with ablation of tumor(s), polyp(s), or other lesion(s) not amenable to removal by hot biopsy forceps, bipolar cautery or snare technique

⊙ 44394   with removal of tumor(s), polyp(s), or other lesion(s) by snare technique

(For colonoscopy per rectum, see 45330-45385)

⊙ 44397   with transendoscopic stent placement (includes predilation)

Introduction

⊙⊘ **44500** Introduction of long gastrointestinal tube (eg, Miller-Abbott) (separate procedure)

(For radiological supervision and interpretation, use 74340)

(For naso- or oro-gastric tube placement, use 43752)

Repair

44602 Suture of small intestine (enterorrhaphy) for perforated ulcer, diverticulum, wound, injury or rupture; single perforation

44603   multiple perforations

44604 Suture of large intestine (colorrhaphy) for perforated ulcer, diverticulum, wound, injury or rupture (single or multiple perforations); without colostomy

44605   with colostomy

44615 Intestinal stricturoplasty (enterotomy and enterorrhaphy) with or without dilation, for intestinal obstruction

44620 Closure of enterostomy, large or small intestine;

44625   with resection and anastomosis other than colorectal

44626   with resection and colorectal anastomosis (eg, closure of Hartmann type procedure)

►(For laparoscopic procedure, use 44227)◄

44640 Closure of intestinal cutaneous fistula

44650 Closure of enteroenteric or enterocolic fistula

44660 Closure of enterovesical fistula; without intestinal or bladder resection

44661   with intestine and/or bladder resection

(For closure of renocolic fistula, see 50525, 50526)

(For closure of gastrocolic fistula, use 43880)

(For closure of rectovesical fistula, see 45800, 45805)

44680 Intestinal plication (separate procedure)

Other Procedures

44700 Exclusion of small intestine from pelvis by mesh or other prosthesis, or native tissue (eg, bladder or omentum)

(For therapeutic radiation clinical treatment, see **Radiation Oncology** section)

✚ **44701** Intraoperative colonic lavage (List separately in addition to code for primary procedure)

(Use 44701 in conjunction with 44140, 44145, 44150, or 44604 as appropriate)

(Do not report 44701 in conjunction with 44300, 44950-44960)

44715 Backbench standard preparation of cadaver or living donor intestine allograft prior to transplantation, including mobilization and fashioning of the superior mesenteric artery and vein

44720 Backbench reconstruction of cadaver or living donor intestine allograft prior to transplantation; venous anastomosis, each

44721   arterial anastomosis, each

44799 Unlisted procedure, intestine

(For unlisted laparoscopic procedure, intestine except rectum, use 44238)

Meckel's Diverticulum and the Mesentery

Excision

44800 Excision of Meckel's diverticulum (diverticulectomy) or omphalomesenteric duct

44820 Excision of lesion of mesentery (separate procedure)

(With intestine resection, see 44120 or 44140 et seq)

Suture

44850 Suture of mesentery (separate procedure)

(For reduction and repair of internal hernia, use 44050)

Other Procedures

44899 Unlisted procedure, Meckel's diverticulum and the mesentery

Appendix

Incision

44900 Incision and drainage of appendiceal abscess; open

⊙ **44901**   percutaneous

(For radiological supervision and interpretation, use 75989)

Excision

44950 Appendectomy;

(Incidental appendectomy during intra-abdominal surgery does not usually warrant a separate identification. If necessary to report, add modifier 52)

✚ **44955**   when done for indicated purpose at time of other major procedure (not as separate procedure) (List separately in addition to code for primary procedure)

44960   for ruptured appendix with abscess or generalized peritonitis

Laparoscopy

Surgical laparoscopy always includes diagnostic laparoscopy. To report a diagnostic laparoscopy (peritoneoscopy) (separate procedure), use 49320.

44970　　Laparoscopy, surgical, appendectomy

44979　　Unlisted laparoscopy procedure, appendix

Rectum

Incision

45000　　Transrectal drainage of pelvic abscess

45005　　Incision and drainage of submucosal abscess, rectum

45020　　Incision and drainage of deep supralevator, pelvirectal, or retrorectal abscess

　　　　　(See also 46050, 46060)

Excision

45100　　Biopsy of anorectal wall, anal approach (eg, congenital megacolon)

　　　　　(For endoscopic biopsy, use 45305)

45108　　Anorectal myomectomy

45110　　Proctectomy; complete, combined abdominoperineal, with colostomy

　　　　　(For laparoscopic procedure, use 45395)

45111　　　　partial resection of rectum, transabdominal approach

45112　　Proctectomy, combined abdominoperineal, pull-through procedure (eg, colo-anal anastomosis)

　　　　　(For colo-anal anastomosis with colonic reservoir or pouch, use 45119)

45113　　Proctectomy, partial, with rectal mucosectomy, ileoanal anastomosis, creation of ileal reservoir (S or J), with or without loop ileostomy

45114　　Proctectomy, partial, with anastomosis; abdominal and transsacral approach

45116　　　　transsacral approach only (Kraske type)

45119　　Proctectomy, combined abdominoperineal pull-through procedure (eg, colo-anal anastomosis), with creation of colonic reservoir (eg, J-pouch), with diverting enterostomy when performed

　　　　　(For laparoscopic procedure, use 45397)

45120　　Proctectomy, complete (for congenital megacolon), abdominal and perineal approach; with pull-through procedure and anastomosis (eg, Swenson, Duhamel, or Soave type operation)

45121　　　　with subtotal or total colectomy, with multiple biopsies

45123　　Proctectomy, partial, without anastomosis, perineal approach

45126　　Pelvic exenteration for colorectal malignancy, with proctectomy (with or without colostomy), with removal of bladder and ureteral transplantations, and/or hysterectomy, or cervicectomy, with or without removal of tube(s), with or without removal of ovary(s), or any combination thereof

45130　　Excision of rectal procidentia, with anastomosis; perineal approach

45135　　　　abdominal and perineal approach

45136　　Excision of ileoanal reservoir with ileostomy

　　　　　(Do not report 45136 in addition to 44005, 44120, 44310)

45150　　Division of stricture of rectum

45160　　Excision of rectal tumor by proctotomy, transsacral or transcoccygeal approach

45170　　Excision of rectal tumor, transanal approach

Destruction

45190　　Destruction of rectal tumor (eg, electrodessication, electrosurgery, laser ablation, laser resection, cryosurgery) transanal approach

Endoscopy

Definitions

Proctosigmoidoscopy is the examination of the rectum and sigmoid colon.

Sigmoidoscopy is the examination of the entire rectum, sigmoid colon and may include examination of a portion of the descending colon.

Colonoscopy is the examination of the entire colon, from the rectum to the cecum, and may include the examination of the terminal ileum.

For an incomplete colonoscopy, with full preparation for a colonoscopy, use a colonoscopy code with the modifier 52 and provide documentation.

Surgical endoscopy always includes diagnostic endoscopy.

45300　　Proctosigmoidoscopy, rigid; diagnostic, with or without collection of specimen(s) by brushing or washing (separate procedure)

⊙ **45303**　　　　with dilation (eg, balloon, guide wire, bougie)

　　　　　(For radiological supervision and interpretation, use 74360)

⊙ **45305**　　　　with biopsy, single or multiple

⊙ **45307**　　　　with removal of foreign body

⊙ **45308**　　　　with removal of single tumor, polyp, or other lesion by hot biopsy forceps or bipolar cautery

Surgery: Digestive System

⊙ **45309**   with removal of single tumor, polyp, or other lesion by snare technique

⊙ **45315**   with removal of multiple tumors, polyps, or other lesions by hot biopsy forceps, bipolar cautery or snare technique

⊙ **45317**   with control of bleeding (eg, injection, bipolar cautery, unipolar cautery, laser, heater probe, stapler, plasma coagulator)

⊙ **45320**   with ablation of tumor(s), polyp(s), or other lesion(s) not amenable to removal by hot biopsy forceps, bipolar cautery or snare technique (eg, laser)

⊙ **45321**   with decompression of volvulus

⊙ **45327**   with transendoscopic stent placement (includes predilation)

45330   Sigmoidoscopy, flexible; diagnostic, with or without collection of specimen(s) by brushing or washing (separate procedure)

45331   with biopsy, single or multiple

⊙ **45332**   with removal of foreign body

⊙ **45333**   with removal of tumor(s), polyp(s), or other lesion(s) by hot biopsy forceps or bipolar cautery

⊙ **45334**   with control of bleeding (eg, injection, bipolar cautery, unipolar cautery, laser, heater probe, stapler, plasma coagulator)

⊙ **45335**   with directed submucosal injection(s), any substance

⊙ **45337**   with decompression of volvulus, any method

⊙ **45338**   with removal of tumor(s), polyp(s), or other lesion(s) by snare technique

⊙ **45339**   with ablation of tumor(s), polyp(s), or other lesion(s) not amenable to removal by hot biopsy forceps, bipolar cautery or snare technique

⊙ **45340**   with dilation by balloon, 1 or more strictures

(Do not report 45340 in conjunction with 45345)

⊙ **45341**   with endoscopic ultrasound examination

⊙ **45342**   with transendoscopic ultrasound guided intramural or transmural fine needle aspiration/biopsy(s)

(Do not report 45341, 45342 in conjunction with 76942, 76975)

(For interpretation of specimen, see 88172-88173)

(For transrectal ultrasound utilizing rigid probe device, use 76872)

⊙ **45345**   with transendoscopic stent placement (includes predilation)

⊙ **45355**   Colonoscopy, rigid or flexible, transabdominal via colotomy, single or multiple

(For fiberoptic colonoscopy beyond 25cm to splenic flexure, see 45330-45345)

⊙ **45378**   Colonoscopy, flexible, proximal to splenic flexure; diagnostic, with or without collection of specimen(s) by brushing or washing, with or without colon decompression (separate procedure)

⊙ **45379**   with removal of foreign body

⊙ **45380**   with biopsy, single or multiple

⊙ **45381**   with directed submucosal injection(s), any substance

⊙ **45382**   with control of bleeding (eg, injection, bipolar cautery, unipolar cautery, laser, heater probe, stapler, plasma coagulator)

⊙ **45383**   with ablation of tumor(s), polyp(s), or other lesion(s) not amenable to removal by hot biopsy forceps, bipolar cautery or snare technique

⊙ **45384**   with removal of tumor(s), polyp(s), or other lesion(s) by hot biopsy forceps or bipolar cautery

⊙ **45385**   with removal of tumor(s), polyp(s), or other lesion(s) by snare technique

(For small intestine and stomal endoscopy, see 44360-44393)

⊙ **45386**   with dilation by balloon, 1 or more strictures

(Do not report 45386 in conjunction with 45387)

⊙ **45387**   with transendoscopic stent placement (includes predilation)

⊙ **45391**   with endoscopic ultrasound examination

(Do not report 45391 in conjunction with 45330, 45341, 45342, 45378, 76872)

⊙ **45392**   with transendoscopic ultrasound guided intramural or transmural fine needle aspiration/biopsy(s)

(Do not report 45392 in conjunction with 45330, 45341, 45342, 45378, 76872)

Laparoscopy

Surgical laparoscopy always includes diagnostic laparoscopy. To report a diagnostic laparoscopy (peritoneoscopy) (separate procedure), use 49320.

Excision

45395   Laparoscopy, surgical; proctectomy, complete, combined abdominoperineal, with colostomy

(For open procedure, use 45110)

45397   proctectomy, combined abdominoperineal pull-through procedure (eg, colo-anal anastomosis), with creation of colonic reservoir (eg, J-pouch), with diverting enterostomy, when performed

(For open procedure, use 45119)

Surgery: Digestive System

Repair

45400   Laparoscopy, surgical; proctopexy (for prolapse)

(For open procedure, use 45540, 45541)

45402   proctopexy (for prolapse), with sigmoid resection

(For open procedure, use 45550)

45499   Unlisted laparoscopy procedure, rectum

Repair

45500   Proctoplasty; for stenosis

45505   for prolapse of mucous membrane

45520   Perirectal injection of sclerosing solution for prolapse

45540   Proctopexy (eg, for prolapse); abdominal approach

(For laparoscopic procedure, use 45400)

45541   perineal approach

45550   with sigmoid resection, abdominal approach

(For laparoscopic procedure, use 45402)

45560   Repair of rectocele (separate procedure)

(For repair of rectocele with posterior colporrhaphy, use 57250)

45562   Exploration, repair, and presacral drainage for rectal injury;

45563   with colostomy

45800   Closure of rectovesical fistula;

45805   with colostomy

45820   Closure of rectourethral fistula;

45825   with colostomy

(For rectovaginal fistula closure, see 57300-57308)

Manipulation

45900   Reduction of procidentia (separate procedure) under anesthesia

45905   Dilation of anal sphincter (separate procedure) under anesthesia other than local

45910   Dilation of rectal stricture (separate procedure) under anesthesia other than local

45915   Removal of fecal impaction or foreign body (separate procedure) under anesthesia

Other Procedures

Surgical diagnostic anorectal exam (45990) includes the following elements: external perineal exam, digital rectal exam, pelvic exam (when performed), diagnostic anoscopy, and diagnostic rigid proctoscopy.

45990   Anorectal exam, surgical, requiring anesthesia (general, spinal, or epidural), diagnostic

(Do not report 45990 in conjunction with 45300- 45327, 46600, 57410, 99170)

45999   Unlisted procedure, rectum

(For unlisted laparoscopic procedure, rectum, use 45499)

Anus

Incision

(For subcutaneous fistulotomy, use 46270)

46020   Placement of seton

(Do not report 46020 in addition to 46060, 46280, 46600)

46030   Removal of anal seton, other marker

46040   Incision and drainage of ischiorectal and/or perirectal abscess (separate procedure)

46045   Incision and drainage of intramural, intramuscular, or submucosal abscess, transanal, under anesthesia

46050   Incision and drainage, perianal abscess, superficial

(See also 45020, 46060)

46060   Incision and drainage of ischiorectal or intramural abscess, with fistulectomy or fistulotomy, submuscular, with or without placement of seton

(Do not report 46060 in addition to 46020)

(See also 45020)

46070   Incision, anal septum (infant)

(For anoplasty, see 46700-46705)

(Do not report modifier 63 in conjunction with 46070)

46080   Sphincterotomy, anal, division of sphincter (separate procedure)

46083   Incision of thrombosed hemorrhoid, external

Excision

46200   Fissurectomy, with or without sphincterotomy

46210   Cryptectomy; single

46211   multiple (separate procedure)

46220   Papillectomy or excision of single tag, anus (separate procedure)

46221   Hemorrhoidectomy, by simple ligature (eg, rubber band)

Surgery: Digestive System

46230   Excision of external hemorrhoid tags and/or multiple papillae

46250   Hemorrhoidectomy, external, complete

46255   Hemorrhoidectomy, internal and external, simple;

46257   with fissurectomy

46258   with fistulectomy, with or without fissurectomy

46260   Hemorrhoidectomy, internal and external, complex or extensive;

46261   with fissurectomy

46262   with fistulectomy, with or without fissurectomy

(For injection of hemorrhoids, use 46500; for destruction, see 46934-46936; for ligation, see 46945, 46946; for hemorrhoidopexy, use 46947)

46270   Surgical treatment of anal fistula (fistulectomy/fistulotomy); subcutaneous

46275   submuscular

46280   complex or multiple, with or without placement of seton

(Do not report 46280 in addition to 46020)

46285   second stage

46288   Closure of anal fistula with rectal advancement flap

46320   Enucleation or excision of external thrombotic hemorrhoid

Introduction

46500   Injection of sclerosing solution, hemorrhoids

(For excision of hemorrhoids, see 46250-46262; for destruction, see 46934-46936; for ligation, see 46945, 46946; for hemorrhoidopexy, use 46947)

46505   Chemodenervation of internal anal sphincter

(For chemodenervation of other muscles, see 64612-64614, 64640)

(Report the specific service in conjunction with the specific substance(s) or drug(s) provided)

Endoscopy

Surgical endoscopy always includes diagnostic endoscopy.

46600   Anoscopy; diagnostic, with or without collection of specimen(s) by brushing or washing (separate procedure)

(Do not report 46600 in addition to 46020)

46604   with dilation (eg, balloon, guide wire, bougie)

46606   with biopsy, single or multiple

46608   with removal of foreign body

46610   with removal of single tumor, polyp, or other lesion by hot biopsy forceps or bipolar cautery

46611   with removal of single tumor, polyp, or other lesion by snare technique

46612   with removal of multiple tumors, polyps, or other lesions by hot biopsy forceps, bipolar cautery or snare technique

46614   with control of bleeding (eg, injection, bipolar cautery, unipolar cautery, laser, heater probe, stapler, plasma coagulator)

46615   with ablation of tumor(s), polyp(s), or other lesion(s) not amenable to removal by hot biopsy forceps, bipolar cautery or snare technique

Repair

46700   Anoplasty, plastic operation for stricture; adult

46705   infant

(For simple incision of anal septum, use 46070)

(Do not report modifier 63 in conjunction with 46705)

46706   Repair of anal fistula with fibrin glue

46710   Repair of ileoanal pouch fistula/sinus (eg, perineal or vaginal), pouch advancement; transperineal approach

46712   combined transperineal and transabdominal approach

46715   Repair of low imperforate anus; with anoperineal fistula (cut-back procedure)

46716   with transposition of anoperineal or anovestibular fistula

(Do not report modifier 63 in conjunction with 46715, 46716)

46730   Repair of high imperforate anus without fistula; perineal or sacroperineal approach

46735   combined transabdominal and sacroperineal approaches

(Do not report modifier 63 in conjunction with 46730, 46735)

46740   Repair of high imperforate anus with rectourethral or rectovaginal fistula; perineal or sacroperineal approach

46742   combined transabdominal and sacroperineal approaches

(Do not report modifier 63 in conjunction with 46740, 46742)

46744   Repair of cloacal anomaly by anorectovaginoplasty and urethroplasty, sacroperineal approach

(Do not report modifier 63 in conjunction with 46744)

46746	Repair of cloacal anomaly by anorectovaginoplasty and urethroplasty, combined abdominal and sacroperineal approach;
46748	with vaginal lengthening by intestinal graft or pedicle flaps
46750	Sphincteroplasty, anal, for incontinence or prolapse; adult
46751	child
46753	Graft (Thiersch operation) for rectal incontinence and/or prolapse
46754	Removal of Thiersch wire or suture, anal canal
46760	Sphincteroplasty, anal, for incontinence, adult; muscle transplant
46761	levator muscle imbrication (Park posterior anal repair)
46762	implantation artificial sphincter

Destruction

46900	Destruction of lesion(s), anus (eg, condyloma, papilloma, molluscum contagiosum, herpetic vesicle), simple; chemical
46910	electrodesiccation
46916	cryosurgery
46917	laser surgery
46922	surgical excision
46924	Destruction of lesion(s), anus (eg, condyloma, papilloma, molluscum contagiosum, herpetic vesicle), extensive (eg, laser surgery, electrosurgery, cryosurgery, chemosurgery)
46934	Destruction of hemorrhoids, any method; internal
46935	external
46936	internal and external

(For excision of hemorrhoids, see 46250-46262; for injection, use 46500; for ligation, see 46945, 46946; for hemorrhoidopexy, use 46947)

46937	Cryosurgery of rectal tumor; benign
46938	malignant
46940	Curettage or cautery of anal fissure, including dilation of anal sphincter (separate procedure); initial
46942	subsequent

Suture

46945	Ligation of internal hemorrhoids; single procedure
46946	multiple procedures
46947	Hemorrhoidopexy (eg, for prolapsing internal hemorrhoids) by stapling

(For excision of hemorrhoids, see 46250-46262; for injection, use 46500; for destruction, see 46934-46936)

Other Procedures

| 46999 | Unlisted procedure, anus |

Liver

Incision

| 47000 | Biopsy of liver, needle; percutaneous |

▶(If imaging guidance is performed, see 76942, 77002, 77012, 77021)◀

| + 47001 | when done for indicated purpose at time of other major procedure (List separately in addition to code for primary procedure) |

▶(If imaging guidance is performed, see 76942, 77002)◀

(For fine needle aspiration in conjunction with 47000, 47001, see 10021, 10022)

(For evaluation of fine needle aspirate in conjunction with 47000, 47001, see 88172, 88173)

| 47010 | Hepatotomy; for open drainage of abscess or cyst, one or two stages |
| ⊙ 47011 | for percutaneous drainage of abscess or cyst, one or two stages |

(For radiological supervision and interpretation, use 75989)

| 47015 | Laparotomy, with aspiration and/or injection of hepatic parasitic (eg, amoebic or echinococcal) cyst(s) or abscess(es) |

Excision

47100	Biopsy of liver, wedge
47120	Hepatectomy, resection of liver; partial lobectomy
47122	trisegmentectomy
47125	total left lobectomy
47130	total right lobectomy

Liver Transplantation

Liver allotransplantation involves three distinct components of physician work:

1) **Cadaver donor hepatectomy**, which includes harvesting the graft and cold preservation of the graft (perfusing with cold preservation solution and cold maintenance) (use 47133). **Living donor hepatectomy**, which includes harvesting the graft, cold preservation of the graft (perfusing with cold preservation solution and cold maintenance), and care of the donor (see 47140-47142).

Surgery: Digestive System

2) *Backbench work*:

Standard preparation of the whole liver graft will include one of the following:

Preparation of whole liver graft (including cholecystectomy, if necessary, and dissection and removal of surrounding soft tissues to prepare vena cava, portal vein, hepatic artery, and common bile duct for implantation) (use 47143).

Preparation as described for whole liver graft, plus trisegment split into two partial grafts (use 47144).

Preparation as described for whole liver graft, plus lobe split into two partial grafts (use 47145).

Additional reconstruction of the liver graft may include venous and/or arterial anastomosis(es) (see 47146, 47147).

3) *Recipient liver allotransplantation*, which includes recipient hepatectomy (partial or whole), transplantation of the allograft (partial or whole), and care of the recipient (see 47135, 47136).

47133   Donor hepatectomy (including cold preservation), from cadaver donor

47135   Liver allotransplantation; orthotopic, partial or whole, from cadaver or living donor, any age

47136   heterotopic, partial or whole, from cadaver or living donor, any age

47140   Donor hepatectomy (including cold preservation), from living donor; left lateral segment only (segments II and III)

47141   total left lobectomy (segments II, III and IV)

47142   total right lobectomy (segments V, VI, VII and VIII)

47143   Backbench standard preparation of cadaver donor whole liver graft prior to allotransplantation, including cholecystectomy, if necessary, and dissection and removal of surrounding soft tissues to prepare the vena cava, portal vein, hepatic artery, and common bile duct for implantation; without trisegment or lobe split

47144   with trisegment split of whole liver graft into two partial liver grafts (ie, left lateral segment (segments II and III) and right trisegment (segments I and IV through VIII))

47145   with lobe split of whole liver graft into two partial liver grafts (ie, left lobe (segments II, III, and IV) and right lobe (segments I and V through VIII))

47146   Backbench reconstruction of cadaver or living donor liver graft prior to allotransplantation; venous anastomosis, each

47147   arterial anastomosis, each

(Do not report 47143-47147 in conjunction with 47120-47125, 47600, 47610)

Repair

47300   Marsupialization of cyst or abscess of liver

47350   Management of liver hemorrhage; simple suture of liver wound or injury

47360   complex suture of liver wound or injury, with or without hepatic artery ligation

47361   exploration of hepatic wound, extensive debridement, coagulation and/or suture, with or without packing of liver

47362   re-exploration of hepatic wound for removal of packing

Laparoscopy

Surgical laparoscopy always includes diagnostic laparoscopy. To report a diagnostic laparoscopy (peritoneoscopy) (separate procedure), use 49320.

47370   Laparoscopy, surgical, ablation of one or more liver tumor(s); radiofrequency

(For imaging guidance, use 76940)

47371   cryosurgical

(For imaging guidance, use 76940)

47379   Unlisted laparoscopic procedure, liver

Other Procedures

47380   Ablation, open, of one or more liver tumor(s); radiofrequency

(For imaging guidance, use 76940)

47381   cryosurgical

(For imaging guidance, use 76940)

47382   Ablation, one or more liver tumor(s), percutaneous, radiofrequency

►(For imaging guidance and monitoring, see 76940, 77013, 77022)◄

47399   Unlisted procedure, liver

Biliary Tract

Incision

47400   Hepaticotomy or hepaticostomy with exploration, drainage, or removal of calculus

47420   Choledochotomy or choledochostomy with exploration, drainage, or removal of calculus, with or without cholecystotomy; without transduodenal sphincterotomy or sphincteroplasty

47425   with transduodenal sphincterotomy or sphincteroplasty

47460   Transduodenal sphincterotomy or sphincteroplasty, with or without transduodenal extraction of calculus (separate procedure)

47480   Cholecystotomy or cholecystostomy with exploration, drainage, or removal of calculus (separate procedure)

47490   Percutaneous cholecystostomy

      (For radiological supervision and interpretation, use 75989)

Introduction

47500   Injection procedure for percutaneous transhepatic cholangiography

      (For radiological supervision and interpretation, use 74320)

47505   Injection procedure for cholangiography through an existing catheter (eg, percutaneous transhepatic or T-tube)

      (For radiological supervision and interpretation, use 74305)

47510   Introduction of percutaneous transhepatic catheter for biliary drainage

      (For radiological supervision and interpretation, use 75980)

47511   Introduction of percutaneous transhepatic stent for internal and external biliary drainage

      (For radiological supervision and interpretation, use 75982)

47525   Change of percutaneous biliary drainage catheter

      (For radiological supervision and interpretation, use 75984)

47530   Revision and/or reinsertion of transhepatic tube

      (For radiological supervision and interpretation, use 75984)

Endoscopy

Surgical endoscopy always includes diagnostic endoscopy.

+ 47550   Biliary endoscopy, intraoperative (choledochoscopy) (List separately in addition to code for primary procedure)

47552   Biliary endoscopy, percutaneous via T-tube or other tract; diagnostic, with or without collection of specimen(s) by brushing and/or washing (separate procedure)

47553   with biopsy, single or multiple

47554   with removal of calculus/calculi

47555   with dilation of biliary duct stricture(s) without stent

47556   with dilation of biliary duct stricture(s) with stent

      (For ERCP, see 43260-43272, 74363)

      (If imaging guidance is performed, see 74363, 75982)

Laparoscopy

Surgical laparoscopy always includes diagnostic laparoscopy. To report a diagnostic laparoscopy (peritoneoscopy) (separate procedure), use 49320.

47560   Laparoscopy, surgical; with guided transhepatic cholangiography, without biopsy

47561   with guided transhepatic cholangiography with biopsy

47562   cholecystectomy

47563   cholecystectomy with cholangiography

47564   cholecystectomy with exploration of common duct

47570   cholecystoenterostomy

47579   Unlisted laparoscopy procedure, biliary tract

Excision

47600   Cholecystectomy;

47605   with cholangiography

      (For laparoscopic approach, see 47562-47564)

47610   Cholecystectomy with exploration of common duct;

      (For cholecystectomy with exploration of common duct with biliary endoscopy, use 47610 with 47550)

47612   with choledochoenterostomy

47620   with transduodenal sphincterotomy or sphincteroplasty, with or without cholangiography

47630   Biliary duct stone extraction, percutaneous via T-tube tract, basket, or snare (eg, Burhenne technique)

      (For radiological supervision and interpretation, use 74327)

47700   Exploration for congenital atresia of bile ducts, without repair, with or without liver biopsy, with or without cholangiography

      (Do not report modifier 63 in conjunction with 47700)

47701   Portoenterostomy (eg, Kasai procedure)

      (Do not report modifier 63 in conjunction with 47701)

47711   Excision of bile duct tumor, with or without primary repair of bile duct; extrahepatic

47712   intrahepatic

      (For anastomosis, see 47760-47800)

47715   Excision of choledochal cyst

      ▶(47716 has been deleted. To report, use 47719)◀

Repair

● 47719   Anastomosis, choledochal cyst, without excision

47720   Cholecystoenterostomy; direct

      (For laparoscopic approach, use 47570)

▲=Revised code   ●=New code   ▶ ◀=Contains new or revised text   ⊘=Modifier 51 exempt

47721	with gastroenterostomy
47740	Roux-en-Y
47741	Roux-en-Y with gastroenterostomy
47760	Anastomosis, of extrahepatic biliary ducts and gastrointestinal tract
47765	Anastomosis, of intrahepatic ducts and gastrointestinal tract
47780	Anastomosis, Roux-en-Y, of extrahepatic biliary ducts and gastrointestinal tract
47785	Anastomosis, Roux-en-Y, of intrahepatic biliary ducts and gastrointestinal tract
47800	Reconstruction, plastic, of extrahepatic biliary ducts with end-to-end anastomosis
47801	Placement of choledochal stent
47802	U-tube hepaticoenterostomy
47900	Suture of extrahepatic biliary duct for pre-existing injury (separate procedure)

Other Procedures

47999	Unlisted procedure, biliary tract

Pancreas

(For peroral pancreatic endoscopic procedures, see 43260-43272)

Incision

48000	Placement of drains, peripancreatic, for acute pancreatitis;
48001	with cholecystostomy, gastrostomy, and jejunostomy

▶(48005 has been deleted. To report, see 48105)◀

48020	Removal of pancreatic calculus

Excision

48100	Biopsy of pancreas, open (eg, fine needle aspiration, needle core biopsy, wedge biopsy)
48102	Biopsy of pancreas, percutaneous needle

▶(For radiological supervision and interpretation, see 76942, 77002, 77012, 77021)◀

(For fine needle aspiration, use 10022)

(For evaluation of fine needle aspirate, see 88172, 88173)

● **48105**	Resection or debridement of pancreas and peripancreatic tissue for acute necrotizing pancreatitis
48120	Excision of lesion of pancreas (eg, cyst, adenoma)
48140	Pancreatectomy, distal subtotal, with or without splenectomy; without pancreaticojejunostomy
48145	with pancreaticojejunostomy

48146	Pancreatectomy, distal, near-total with preservation of duodenum (Child-type procedure)
48148	Excision of ampulla of Vater
48150	Pancreatectomy, proximal subtotal with total duodenectomy, partial gastrectomy, choledochoenterostomy and gastrojejunostomy (Whipple-type procedure); with pancreatojejunostomy
48152	without pancreatojejunostomy
48153	Pancreatectomy, proximal subtotal with near-total duodenectomy, choledochoenterostomy and duodenojejunostomy (pylorus-sparing, Whipple-type procedure); with pancreatojejunostomy
48154	without pancreatojejunostomy
48155	Pancreatectomy, total
48160	Pancreatectomy, total or subtotal, with autologous transplantation of pancreas or pancreatic islet cells

▶(48180 has been deleted. To report, see 48548)◀

Introduction

+ **48400**	Injection procedure for intraoperative pancreatography (List separately in addition to code for primary procedure)

(For radiological supervision and interpretation, see 74300-74305)

Repair

48500	Marsupialization of pancreatic cyst
48510	External drainage, pseudocyst of pancreas; open
⊙ **48511**	percutaneous

(For radiological supervision and interpretation, use 75989)

48520	Internal anastomosis of pancreatic cyst to gastrointestinal tract; direct
48540	Roux-en-Y
48545	Pancreatorrhaphy for injury
48547	Duodenal exclusion with gastrojejunostomy for pancreatic injury
● **48548**	Pancreaticojejunostomy, side-to-side anastomosis (Puestow-type operation)

Pancreas Transplantation

Pancreas allotransplantation involves three distinct components of physician work:

1) ***Cadaver donor pancreatectomy***, which includes harvesting the pancreas graft, with or without duodenal segment, and cold preservation of the graft (perfusing with cold preservation solution and cold maintenance) (use 48550).

2) *Backbench work*:

Standard preparation of a cadaver donor pancreas allograft prior to transplantation includes dissection of the allograft from surrounding soft tissues, splenectomy, duodenotomy, ligation of bile duct, ligation of mesenteric vessels, and Y-graft arterial anastomoses from the iliac artery to the superior mesenteric artery and to the splenic artery (use 48551).

Additional reconstruction of a cadaver donor pancreas allograft prior to transplantation may include venous anastomosis(es) (use 48552).

3) *Recipient pancreas allotransplantation*, which includes transplantation of allograft, and care of the recipient (use 48554).

48550 Donor pancreatectomy (including cold preservation), with or without duodenal segment for transplantation

48551 Backbench standard preparation of cadaver donor pancreas allograft prior to transplantation, including dissection of allograft from surrounding soft tissues, splenectomy, duodenotomy, ligation of bile duct, ligation of mesenteric vessels, and Y-graft arterial anastomoses from iliac artery to superior mesenteric artery and to splenic artery

48552 Backbench reconstruction of cadaver donor pancreas allograft prior to transplantation, venous anastomosis, each

(Do not report 48551 and 48552 in conjunction with 35531, 35563, 35685, 38100-38102, 44010, 44820, 44850, 47460, 47505-47525, 47550-47556, 48100-48120, 48545)

48554 Transplantation of pancreatic allograft

48556 Removal of transplanted pancreatic allograft

Other Procedures

48999 Unlisted procedure, pancreas

Abdomen, Peritoneum, and Omentum

Incision

49000 Exploratory laparotomy, exploratory celiotomy with or without biopsy(s) (separate procedure)

(To report wound exploration due to penetrating trauma without laparotomy, use 20102)

49002 Reopening of recent laparotomy

(To report re-exploration of hepatic wound for removal of packing, use 47362)

49010 Exploration, retroperitoneal area with or without biopsy(s) (separate procedure)

(To report wound exploration due to penetrating trauma without laparotomy, use 20102)

49020 Drainage of peritoneal abscess or localized peritonitis, exclusive of appendiceal abscess; open

(For appendiceal abscess, use 44900)

⊙ **49021** percutaneous

(For radiological supervision and interpretation, use 75989)

49040 Drainage of subdiaphragmatic or subphrenic abscess; open

⊙ **49041** percutaneous

(For radiological supervision and interpretation, use 75989)

49060 Drainage of retroperitoneal abscess; open

⊙ **49061** percutaneous

(For laparoscopic drainage, use 49323)

(For radiological supervision and interpretation, use 75989)

49062 Drainage of extraperitoneal lymphocele to peritoneal cavity, open

49080 Peritoneocentesis, abdominal paracentesis, or peritoneal lavage (diagnostic or therapeutic); initial

49081 subsequent

▶(If imaging guidance is performed, see 76942, 77012)◀

▶(49085 has been deleted. To report, see 49402)◀

Excision, Destruction

▶(For lysis of intestinal adhesions, use 44005)◀

49180 Biopsy, abdominal or retroperitoneal mass, percutaneous needle

▶(If imaging guidance is performed, see 76942, 77002, 77012, 77021)◀

(For fine needle aspiration, use 10021 or 10022)

(For evaluation of fine needle aspirate, see 88172, 88173)

49200 Excision or destruction, open, intra-abdominal or retroperitoneal tumors or cysts or endometriomas;

49201 extensive

▶(For resection of recurrent ovarian, tubal, primary peritoneal, or uterine malignancy, see 58957, 58958)◀

(For open cryoablation of renal tumor, use 50250)

(For percutaneous cryotherapy ablation of renal tumors, use Category III code 0135T)

49215 Excision of presacral or sacrococcygeal tumor

(Do not report modifier 63 in conjunction with 49215)

49220 Staging laparotomy for Hodgkins disease or lymphoma (includes splenectomy, needle or open biopsies of both liver lobes, possibly also removal of abdominal nodes, abdominal node and/or bone marrow biopsies, ovarian repositioning)

Surgery: Digestive System

49250   Umbilectomy, omphalectomy, excision of umbilicus (separate procedure)

49255   Omentectomy, epiploectomy, resection of omentum (separate procedure)

Laparoscopy

Surgical laparoscopy always includes diagnostic laparoscopy. To report a diagnostic laparoscopy (peritoneoscopy), (separate procedure), use 49320.

For laparoscopic fulguration or excision of lesions of the ovary, pelvic viscera, or peritoneal surface use 58662.

49320   Laparoscopy, abdomen, peritoneum, and omentum, diagnostic, with or without collection of specimen(s) by brushing or washing (separate procedure)

49321   Laparoscopy, surgical; with biopsy (single or multiple)

49322   with aspiration of cavity or cyst (eg, ovarian cyst) (single or multiple)

49323   with drainage of lymphocele to peritoneal cavity

(For percutaneous or open drainage, see 49060, 49061)

● **49324**   with insertion of intraperitoneal cannula or catheter, permanent

▶(For subcutaneous extension of intraperitoneal catheter with remote chest exit site, use 49435 in conjunction with 49324)◀

▶(For open insertion of permanent intraperitoneal cannula or catheter, use 49421)◀

● **49325**   with revision of previously placed intraperitoneal cannula or catheter, with removal of intraluminal obstructive material if performed

+● **49326**   with omentopexy (omental tacking procedure) (List separately in addition to code for primary procedure)

▶(Use 49326 in conjunction with 49324, 49325)◀

49329   Unlisted laparoscopy procedure, abdomen, peritoneum and omentum

---

▶Introduction, Revision, Removal◀

49400   Injection of air or contrast into peritoneal cavity (separate procedure)

(For radiological supervision and interpretation, use 74190)

● **49402**   Removal of peritoneal foreign body from peritoneal cavity

▶(For lysis of intestinal adhesions, use 44005)◀

49419   Insertion of intraperitoneal cannula or catheter, with subcutaneous reservoir, permanent (ie, totally implantable)

(For removal, use 49422)

49420   Insertion of intraperitoneal cannula or catheter for drainage or dialysis; temporary

49421   permanent

▶(For laparoscopic insertion of permanent intraperitoneal cannula or catheter, use 49324)◀

▶(For subcutaneous extension of intraperitoneal catheter with remote chest exit site, use 49435 in conjunction with 49421)◀

49422   Removal of permanent intraperitoneal cannula or catheter

(For removal of a temporary catheter/cannula, use appropriate E/M code)

49423   Exchange of previously placed abscess or cyst drainage catheter under radiological guidance (separate procedure)

(For radiological supervision and interpretation, use 75984)

49424   Contrast injection for assessment of abscess or cyst via previously placed drainage catheter or tube (separate procedure)

(For radiological supervision and interpretation, use 76080)

49425   Insertion of peritoneal-venous shunt

49426   Revision of peritoneal-venous shunt

(For shunt patency test, use 78291)

49427   Injection procedure (eg, contrast media) for evaluation of previously placed peritoneal-venous shunt

(For radiological supervision and interpretation, see 75809, 78291)

49428   Ligation of peritoneal-venous shunt

49429   Removal of peritoneal-venous shunt

+● **49435**   Insertion of subcutaneous extension to intraperitoneal cannula or catheter with remote chest exit site (List separately in addition to code for primary procedure)

▶(Use 49435 in conjunction with 49324, 49421)◀

● **49436**   Delayed creation of exit site from embedded subcutaneous segment of intraperitoneal cannula or catheter

---

Repair

Hernioplasty, Herniorrhaphy, Herniotomy

The hernia repair codes in this section are categorized primarily by the type of hernia (inguinal, femoral, incisional, etc).

Some types of hernias are further categorized as "initial" or "recurrent" based on whether or not the hernia has required previous repair(s).

Additional variables accounted for by some of the codes include patient age and clinical presentation (reducible vs. incarcerated or strangulated).

With the exception of the incisional hernia repairs (see 49560-49566) the use of mesh or other prostheses is not separately reported.

The excision/repair of strangulated organs or structures such as testicle(s), intestine, ovaries are reported by using the appropriate code for the excision/repair (eg, 44120, 54520, and 58940) in addition to the appropriate code for the repair of the strangulated hernia.

(For reduction and repair of intra-abdominal hernia, use 44050)

(For debridement of abdominal wall, see 11042, 11043)

(Codes 49491-49651 are unilateral procedures. To report bilateral procedures, report modifier 50 with the appropriate procedure code)

49491　Repair, initial inguinal hernia, preterm infant (younger than 37 weeks gestation at birth), performed from birth up to 50 weeks postconception age, with or without hydrocelectomy; reducible

49492　　　incarcerated or strangulated

(Do not report modifier 63 in conjunction with 49491, 49492)

(Postconception age equals gestational age at birth plus age of infant in weeks at the time of the hernia repair. Initial inguinal hernia repairs that are performed on preterm infants who are older than 50 weeks postconception age and younger than age 6 months at the time of surgery, should be reported using codes 49495, 49496)

49495　Repair, initial inguinal hernia, full term infant younger than age 6 months, or preterm infant older than 50 weeks postconception age and younger than age 6 months at the time of surgery, with or without hydrocelectomy; reducible

49496　　　incarcerated or strangulated

(Do not report modifier 63 in conjunction with 49495, 49496)

(Postconception age equals gestational age at birth plus age in weeks at the time of the hernia repair. Initial inguinal hernia repairs that are performed on preterm infants who are younger than or up to 50 weeks postconception age but younger than 6 months of age since birth, should be reported using codes 49491, 49492. Inguinal hernia repairs on infants age 6 months to younger than 5 years should be reported using codes 49500-49501)

49500　Repair initial inguinal hernia, age 6 months to younger than 5 years, with or without hydrocelectomy; reducible

49501　　　incarcerated or strangulated

49505　Repair initial inguinal hernia, age 5 years or older; reducible

49507　　　incarcerated or strangulated

(For inguinal hernia repair, with simple orchiectomy, see 49505 or 49507 and 54520)

(For inguinal hernia repair, with excision of hydrocele or spermatocele, see 49505 or 49507 and 54840 or 55040)

49520　Repair recurrent inguinal hernia, any age; reducible

49521　　　incarcerated or strangulated

49525　Repair inguinal hernia, sliding, any age

(For incarcerated or strangulated inguinal hernia repair, see 49496, 49501, 49507, 49521)

49540　Repair lumbar hernia

49550　Repair initial femoral hernia, any age; reducible

49553　　　incarcerated or strangulated

49555　Repair recurrent femoral hernia; reducible

49557　　　incarcerated or strangulated

49560　Repair initial incisional or ventral hernia; reducible

49561　　　incarcerated or strangulated

49565　Repair recurrent incisional or ventral hernia; reducible

49566　　　incarcerated or strangulated

+ 49568　Implantation of mesh or other prosthesis for incisional or ventral hernia repair (List separately in addition to code for the incisional or ventral hernia repair)

49570　Repair epigastric hernia (eg, preperitoneal fat); reducible (separate procedure)

49572　　　incarcerated or strangulated

49580　Repair umbilical hernia, younger than age 5 years; reducible

49582　　　incarcerated or strangulated

49585　Repair umbilical hernia, age 5 years or older; reducible

49587　　　incarcerated or strangulated

49590　Repair spigelian hernia

49600　Repair of small omphalocele, with primary closure

(Do not report modifier 63 in conjunction with 49600)

49605　Repair of large omphalocele or gastroschisis; with or without prosthesis

49606　　　with removal of prosthesis, final reduction and closure, in operating room

(Do not report modifier 63 in conjunction with 49605, 49606)

Surgery: Digestive System

49610   Repair of omphalocele (Gross type operation); first stage

49611   second stage

(Do not report modifier 63 in conjunction with 49610, 49611)

(For diaphragmatic or hiatal hernia repair, see 39502-39541)

(For surgical repair of omentum, use 49999)

Laparoscopy

Surgical laparoscopy always includes diagnostic laparoscopy. To report a diagnostic laparoscopy (peritoneoscopy) (separate procedure), use 49320.

49650   Laparoscopy, surgical; repair initial inguinal hernia

49651   repair recurrent inguinal hernia

49659   Unlisted laparoscopy procedure, hernioplasty, herniorrhaphy, herniotomy

Suture

49900   Suture, secondary, of abdominal wall for evisceration or dehiscence

(For suture of ruptured diaphragm, see 39540, 39541)

(For debridement of abdominal wall, see 11042, 11043)

Other Procedures

49904   Omental flap, extra-abdominal (eg, for reconstruction of sternal and chest wall defects)

(Code 49904 includes harvest and transfer. If a second surgeon harvests the omental flap, then the two surgeons should code 49904 as co-surgeons, using modifier 62)

+ 49905   Omental flap, intra-abdominal (List separately in addition to code for primary procedure)

(Do not report 49905 in conjunction with 44700)

49906   Free omental flap with microvascular anastomosis

(Do not report code 69990 in addition to 49906)

49999   Unlisted procedure, abdomen, peritoneum and omentum

Urinary System

►(For provision of chemotherapeutic agents, report both the specific service in addition to code(s) for the specific substance(s) or drug(s) provided)◄

Kidney

Incision

(For retroperitoneal exploration, abscess, tumor, or cyst, see 49010, 49060, 49200, 49201)

50010   Renal exploration, not necessitating other specific procedures

(For laparoscopic ablation of renal mass lesion(s), use 50542)

50020   Drainage of perirenal or renal abscess; open

⊙ **50021**   percutaneous

(For radiological supervision and interpretation, use 75989)

50040   Nephrostomy, nephrotomy with drainage

50045   Nephrotomy, with exploration

(For renal endoscopy performed in conjunction with this procedure, see 50570-50580)

50060   Nephrolithotomy; removal of calculus

50065   secondary surgical operation for calculus

50070   complicated by congenital kidney abnormality

50075   removal of large staghorn calculus filling renal pelvis and calyces (including anatrophic pyelolithotomy)

50080   Percutaneous nephrostolithotomy or pyelostolithotomy, with or without dilation, endoscopy, lithotripsy, stenting, or basket extraction; up to 2 cm

50081   over 2 cm

(For establishment of nephrostomy without nephrostolithotomy, see 50040, 50395, 52334)

(For fluoroscopic guidance, see 76000, 76001)

50100   Transection or repositioning of aberrant renal vessels (separate procedure)

50120   Pyelotomy; with exploration

(For renal endoscopy performed in conjunction with this procedure, see 50570-50580)

50125   with drainage, pyelostomy

50130   with removal of calculus (pyelolithotomy, pelviolithotomy, including coagulum pyelolithotomy)

50135   complicated (eg, secondary operation, congenital kidney abnormality)

(For supply of anticarcinogenic agents, use 99070 in addition to code for primary procedure)

Excision

(For excision of retroperitoneal tumor or cyst, see 49200, 49201)

(For laparoscopic ablation of renal mass lesion(s), use 50542)

50200   Renal biopsy; percutaneous, by trocar or needle

►(For radiological supervision and interpretation, see 76942, 77002, 77012, 77021)◄

(For fine needle aspiration, use 10022)

(For evaluation of fine needle aspirate, see 88172, 88173)

50205   by surgical exposure of kidney

50220   Nephrectomy, including partial ureterectomy, any open approach including rib resection;

50225   complicated because of previous surgery on same kidney

50230   radical, with regional lymphadenectomy and/or vena caval thrombectomy

(When vena caval resection with reconstruction is necessary, use 37799)

50234   Nephrectomy with total ureterectomy and bladder cuff; through same incision

50236   through separate incision

50240   Nephrectomy, partial

(For laparoscopic partial nephrectomy, use 50543)

50250   Ablation, open, one or more renal mass lesion(s), cryosurgical, including intraoperative ultrasound, if performed

(For laparoscopic ablation of renal mass lesions, use 50542)

(For percutaneous cryotherapy ablation of renal tumors, use 0135T)

50280   Excision or unroofing of cyst(s) of kidney

(For laparoscopic ablation of renal cysts, use 50541)

50290   Excision of perinephric cyst

Renal Transplantation

Renal *auto*transplantation includes reimplantation of the autograft as the primary procedure, along with secondary extra-corporeal procedure(s) (eg, partial nephrectomy, nephrolithotomy) reported with modifier 51 (see 50380 and applicable secondary procedure(s)).

Renal *allo*transplantation involves three distinct components of physician work:

1) ***Cadaver donor nephrectomy, unilateral or bilateral,*** which includes harvesting the graft(s) and cold preservation of the graft(s) (perfusing with cold preservation solution and cold maintenance)

Surgery: Urinary System

(use 50300). *Living donor nephrectomy*, which includes harvesting the graft, cold preservation of the graft (perfusing with cold preservation solution and cold maintenance), and care of the donor (see 50320, 50547).

2) *Backbench work*:

Standard preparation of a cadaver donor renal allograft prior to transplantation including dissection and removal of perinephric fat, diaphragmatic and retroperitoneal attachments; excision of adrenal gland; and preparation of ureter(s), renal vein(s), and renal artery(s), ligating branches, as necessary (use 50323).

Standard preparation of a living donor renal allograft (open or laparoscopic) prior to transplantation including dissection and removal of perinephric fat and preparation of ureter(s), renal vein(s), and renal artery(s), ligating branches, as necessary (use 50325).

Additional reconstruction of a cadaver or living donor renal allograft prior to transplantation may include venous, arterial, and/or ureteral anastomosis(es) necessary for implantation (see 50327-50329).

3) *Recipient renal allotransplantation*, which includes transplantation of the allograft (with or without recipient nephrectomy) and care of the recipient (see 50360, 50365).

(For dialysis, see 90935-90999)

(For laparoscopic donor nephrectomy, use 50547)

(For laparoscopic drainage of lymphocele to peritoneal cavity, use 49323)

50300   Donor nephrectomy (including cold preservation); from cadaver donor, unilateral or bilateral

50320   open, from living donor

50323   Backbench standard preparation of cadaver donor renal allograft prior to transplantation, including dissection and removal of perinephric fat, diaphragmatic and retroperitoneal attachments, excision of adrenal gland, and preparation of ureter(s), renal vein(s), and renal artery(s), ligating branches, as necessary

(Do not report 50323 in conjunction with 60540, 60545)

50325   Backbench standard preparation of living donor renal allograft (open or laparoscopic) prior to transplantation, including dissection and removal of perinephric fat and preparation of ureter(s), renal vein(s), and renal artery(s), ligating branches, as necessary

50327   Backbench reconstruction of cadaver or living donor renal allograft prior to transplantation; venous anastomosis, each

50328   arterial anastomosis, each

50329   ureteral anastomosis, each

50340   Recipient nephrectomy (separate procedure)

(For bilateral procedure, report 50340 with modifier 50)

50360   Renal allotransplantation, implantation of graft; without recipient nephrectomy

50365   with recipient nephrectomy

(For bilateral procedure, report 50365 with modifier 50)

50370   Removal of transplanted renal allograft

50380   Renal autotransplantation, reimplantation of kidney

(For renal autotransplantation extra-corporeal (bench) surgery, use autotransplantation as the primary procedure and report secondary procedure(s) (eg, partial nephrectomy, nephrolithotomy) with modifier 51)

Introduction

Renal Pelvis Catheter Procedures

Internally Dwelling

⊙ 50382   Removal (via snare/capture) and replacement of internally dwelling ureteral stent via percutaneous approach, including radiological supervision and interpretation

(For bilateral procedure, use modifier 50)

⊙ 50384   Removal (via snare/capture) of internally dwelling ureteral stent via percutaneous approach, including radiological supervision and interpretation

(For bilateral procedure, use modifier 50)

(Do not report 50382, 50384 in conjunction with 50395)

Externally Accessible

⊙ 50387   Removal and replacement of externally accessible transnephric ureteral stent (eg, external/internal stent) requiring fluoroscopic guidance, including radiological supervision and interpretation

(For bilateral procedure, use modifier 50)

(For removal and replacement of externally accessible ureteral stent via ureterostomy or ilieal conduit, use 50688)

(For removal without replacement of an externally accessible ureteral stent not requiring fluoroscopic guidance, see **Evaluation and Management** services codes)

50389   Removal of nephrostomy tube, requiring fluoroscopic guidance (eg, with concurrent indwelling ureteral stent)

(Removal of nephrostomy tube not requiring fluoroscopic guidance is considered inherent to E/M services. Report the appropriate level of E/M service provided)

Surgery: Urinary System

Other Introduction Procedures

50390 Aspiration and/or injection of renal cyst or pelvis by needle, percutaneous

►(For radiological supervision and interpretation, see 74425, 74470, 76942, 77002, 77012, 77021)◄

(For evaluation of fine needle aspirate, see 88172, 88173)

50391 Instillation(s) of therapeutic agent into renal pelvis and/or ureter through established nephrostomy, pyelostomy or ureterostomy tube (eg, anticarcinogenic or antifungal agent)

50392 Introduction of intracatheter or catheter into renal pelvis for drainage and/or injection, percutaneous

►(For radiological supervision and interpretation, see 74475, 76942, 77012)◄

50393 Introduction of ureteral catheter or stent into ureter through renal pelvis for drainage and/or injection, percutaneous

►(For radiological supervision and interpretation, see 74480, 76942, 77002, 77012)◄

50394 Injection procedure for pyelography (as nephrostogram, pyelostogram, antegrade pyeloureterograms) through nephrostomy or pyelostomy tube, or indwelling ureteral catheter

(For radiological supervision and interpretation, use 74425)

50395 Introduction of guide into renal pelvis and/or ureter with dilation to establish nephrostomy tract, percutaneous

(For radiological supervision and interpretation, see 74475, 74480, 74485)

(For nephrostolithotomy, see 50080, 50081)

(For retrograde percutaneous nephrostomy, use 52334)

(For endoscopic surgery, see 50551-50561)

50396 Manometric studies through nephrostomy or pyelostomy tube, or indwelling ureteral catheter

(For radiological supervision and interpretation, see 74425, 74475, 74480)

50398 Change of nephrostomy or pyelostomy tube

(For radiological supervision and interpretation, use 75984)

Repair

50400 Pyeloplasty (Foley Y-pyeloplasty), plastic operation on renal pelvis, with or without plastic operation on ureter, nephropexy, nephrostomy, pyelostomy, or ureteral splinting; simple

50405   complicated (congenital kidney abnormality, secondary pyeloplasty, solitary kidney, calycoplasty)

(For laparoscopic approach, use 50544)

50500 Nephrorrhaphy, suture of kidney wound or injury

50520 Closure of nephrocutaneous or pyelocutaneous fistula

50525 Closure of nephrovisceral fistula (eg, renocolic), including visceral repair; abdominal approach

50526   thoracic approach

50540 Symphysiotomy for horseshoe kidney with or without pyeloplasty and/or other plastic procedure, unilateral or bilateral (one operation)

Laparoscopy

Surgical laparoscopy always includes diagnostic laparoscopy. To report a diagnostic laparoscopy (peritoneoscopy) (separate procedure), use 49320.

50541 Laparoscopy, surgical; ablation of renal cysts

50542   ablation of renal mass lesion(s)

(For open procedure, see 50220-50240)

(For open cryosurgical ablation, use 50250)

(For percutaneous cryotherapy ablation of renal tumors, use 0135T)

50543   partial nephrectomy

(For open procedure, use 50240)

50544   pyeloplasty

50545   radical nephrectomy (includes removal of Gerota's fascia and surrounding fatty tissue, removal of regional lymph nodes, and adrenalectomy)

(For open procedure, use 50230)

50546   nephrectomy, including partial ureterectomy

50547   donor nephrectomy (including cold preservation), from living donor

(For open procedure, use 50320)

(For backbench renal allograft standard preparation prior to transplantation, use 50325)

(For backbench renal allograft reconstruction prior to transplantation, see 50327-50329)

50548   nephrectomy with total ureterectomy

(For open procedure, see 50234, 50236)

50549 Unlisted laparoscopy procedure, renal

(For laparoscopic drainage of lymphocele to peritoneal cavity, use 49323)

Surgery: Urinary System

Endoscopy

(For supplies and materials, use 99070)

50551   Renal endoscopy through established nephrostomy or pyelostomy, with or without irrigation, instillation, or ureteropyelography, exclusive of radiologic service;

50553   with ureteral catheterization, with or without dilation of ureter

50555   with biopsy

50557   with fulguration and/or incision, with or without biopsy

(50559 has been deleted)

50561   with removal of foreign body or calculus

50562   with resection of tumor

(When procedures 50570-50580 provide a significant identifiable service, they may be added to 50045 and 50120)

50570   Renal endoscopy through nephrotomy or pyelotomy, with or without irrigation, instillation, or ureteropyelography, exclusive of radiologic service;

(For nephrotomy, use 50045)

(For pyelotomy, use 50120)

50572   with ureteral catheterization, with or without dilation of ureter

50574   with biopsy

50575   with endopyelotomy (includes cystoscopy, ureteroscopy, dilation of ureter and ureteral pelvic junction, incision of ureteral pelvic junction and insertion of endopyelotomy stent)

50576   with fulguration and/or incision, with or without biopsy

(50578 has been deleted)

50580   with removal of foreign body or calculus

Other Procedures

50590   Lithotripsy, extracorporeal shock wave

⊙ **50592**   Ablation, one or more renal tumor(s), percutaneous, unilateral, radiofrequency

(50592 is a unilateral procedure. For bilateral procedure, report 50592 with modifier 50)

►(For imaging guidance and monitoring, see 76940, 77013, 77022)◄

(For percutaneous cryotherapy ablation of renal tumors, use 0135T)

Ureter

Incision

50600   Ureterotomy with exploration or drainage (separate procedure)

(For ureteral endoscopy performed in conjunction with this procedure, see 50970-50980)

50605   Ureterotomy for insertion of indwelling stent, all types

50610   Ureterolithotomy; upper one-third of ureter

50620   middle one-third of ureter

50630   lower one-third of ureter

(For laparoscopic approach, use 50945)

(For transvesical ureterolithotomy, use 51060)

(For cystotomy with stone basket extraction of ureteral calculus, use 51065)

(For endoscopic extraction or manipulation of ureteral calculus, see 50080, 50081, 50561, 50961, 50980, 52320-52330, 52352, 52353)

Excision

(For ureterocele, see 51535, 52300)

50650   Ureterectomy, with bladder cuff (separate procedure)

50660   Ureterectomy, total, ectopic ureter, combination abdominal, vaginal and/or perineal approach

Introduction

50684   Injection procedure for ureterography or ureteropyelography through ureterostomy or indwelling ureteral catheter

(For radiological supervision and interpretation, use 74425)

50686   Manometric studies through ureterostomy or indwelling ureteral catheter

50688   Change of ureterostomy tube or externally accessible ureteral stent via ileal conduit

(If imaging guidance is performed, use 75984)

50690   Injection procedure for visualization of ileal conduit and/or ureteropyelography, exclusive of radiologic service

(For radiological supervision and interpretation, use 74425)

Repair

50700   Ureteroplasty, plastic operation on ureter (eg, stricture)

50715   Ureterolysis, with or without repositioning of ureter for retroperitoneal fibrosis

(For bilateral procedure, report 50715 with modifier 50)

Surgery: Urinary System

50722   Ureterolysis for ovarian vein syndrome

50725   Ureterolysis for retrocaval ureter, with reanastomosis of upper urinary tract or vena cava

50727   Revision of urinary-cutaneous anastomosis (any type urostomy);

50728   with repair of fascial defect and hernia

50740   Ureteropyelostomy, anastomosis of ureter and renal pelvis

50750   Ureterocalycostomy, anastomosis of ureter to renal calyx

50760   Ureteroureterostomy

50770   Transureteroureterostomy, anastomosis of ureter to contralateral ureter

(Codes 50780-50785 include minor procedures to prevent vesicoureteral reflux)

50780   Ureteroneocystostomy; anastomosis of single ureter to bladder

(For bilateral procedure, report 50780 with modifier 50)

(When combined with cystourethroplasty or vesical neck revision, use 51820)

50782   anastomosis of duplicated ureter to bladder

50783   with extensive ureteral tailoring

50785   with vesico-psoas hitch or bladder flap

(For bilateral procedure, report 50785 with modifier 50)

50800   Ureteroenterostomy, direct anastomosis of ureter to intestine

(For bilateral procedure, report 50800 with modifier 50)

50810   Ureterosigmoidostomy, with creation of sigmoid bladder and establishment of abdominal or perineal colostomy, including intestine anastomosis

50815   Ureterocolon conduit, including intestine anastomosis

(For bilateral procedure, report 50815 with modifier 50)

50820   Ureteroileal conduit (ileal bladder), including intestine anastomosis (Bricker operation)

(For bilateral procedure, report 50820 with modifier 50)

(For combination of 50800-50820 with cystectomy, see 51580-51595)

50825   Continent diversion, including intestine anastomosis using any segment of small and/or large intestine (Kock pouch or Camey enterocystoplasty)

50830   Urinary undiversion (eg, taking down of ureteroileal conduit, ureterosigmoidostomy or ureteroenterostomy with ureteroureterostomy or ureteroneocystostomy)

50840   Replacement of all or part of ureter by intestine segment, including intestine anastomosis

(For bilateral procedure, report 50840 with modifier 50)

50845   Cutaneous appendico-vesicostomy

50860   Ureterostomy, transplantation of ureter to skin

(For bilateral procedure, report 50860 with modifier 50)

50900   Ureterorrhaphy, suture of ureter (separate procedure)

50920   Closure of ureterocutaneous fistula

50930   Closure of ureterovisceral fistula (including visceral repair)

50940   Deligation of ureter

(For ureteroplasty, ureterolysis, see 50700-50860)

Laparoscopy

Surgical laparoscopy always includes diagnostic laparoscopy. To report a diagnostic laparoscopy (peritoneoscopy) (separate procedure), use 49320.

50945   Laparoscopy, surgical; ureterolithotomy

50947   ureteroneocystostomy with cystoscopy and ureteral stent placement

50948   ureteroneocystostomy without cystoscopy and ureteral stent placement

(For open ureteroneocystostomy, see 50780-50785)

50949   Unlisted laparoscopy procedure, ureter

Endoscopy

50951   Ureteral endoscopy through established ureterostomy, with or without irrigation, instillation, or ureteropyelography, exclusive of radiologic service;

50953   with ureteral catheterization, with or without dilation of ureter

50955   with biopsy

50957   with fulguration and/or incision, with or without biopsy

(50959 has been deleted)

50961   with removal of foreign body or calculus

(When procedures 50970-50980 provide a significant identifiable service, they may be added to 50600)

50970   Ureteral endoscopy through ureterotomy, with or without irrigation, instillation, or ureteropyelography, exclusive of radiologic service;

(For ureterotomy, use 50600)

50972   with ureteral catheterization, with or without dilation of ureter

50974   with biopsy

50976   with fulguration and/or incision, with or without biopsy

(50978 has been deleted)

50980   with removal of foreign body or calculus

Surgery: Urinary System

Bladder

Incision

51000 Aspiration of bladder by needle

51005 Aspiration of bladder; by trocar or intracatheter

51010 with insertion of suprapubic catheter

►(If imaging guidance is performed, see 76942, 77002, 77012)◄

51020 Cystotomy or cystostomy; with fulguration and/or insertion of radioactive material

51030 with cryosurgical destruction of intravesical lesion

51040 Cystostomy, cystotomy with drainage

51045 Cystotomy, with insertion of ureteral catheter or stent (separate procedure)

51050 Cystolithotomy, cystotomy with removal of calculus, without vesical neck resection

51060 Transvesical ureterolithotomy

51065 Cystotomy, with calculus basket extraction and/or ultrasonic or electrohydraulic fragmentation of ureteral calculus

51080 Drainage of perivesical or prevesical space abscess

Excision

51500 Excision of urachal cyst or sinus, with or without umbilical hernia repair

51520 Cystotomy; for simple excision of vesical neck (separate procedure)

51525 for excision of bladder diverticulum, single or multiple (separate procedure)

51530 for excision of bladder tumor

(For transurethral resection, see 52234-52240, 52305)

51535 Cystotomy for excision, incision, or repair of ureterocele

(For bilateral procedure, report 51535 with modifier 50)

(For transurethral excision, use 52300)

51550 Cystectomy, partial; simple

51555 complicated (eg, postradiation, previous surgery, difficult location)

51565 Cystectomy, partial, with reimplantation of ureter(s) into bladder (ureteroneocystostomy)

51570 Cystectomy, complete; (separate procedure)

51575 with bilateral pelvic lymphadenectomy, including external iliac, hypogastric, and obturator nodes

51580 Cystectomy, complete, with ureterosigmoidostomy or ureterocutaneous transplantations;

51585 with bilateral pelvic lymphadenectomy, including external iliac, hypogastric, and obturator nodes

51590 Cystectomy, complete, with ureteroileal conduit or sigmoid bladder, including intestine anastomosis;

51595 with bilateral pelvic lymphadenectomy, including external iliac, hypogastric, and obturator nodes

51596 Cystectomy, complete, with continent diversion, any open technique, using any segment of small and/or large intestine to construct neobladder

51597 Pelvic exenteration, complete, for vesical, prostatic or urethral malignancy, with removal of bladder and ureteral transplantations, with or without hysterectomy and/or abdominoperineal resection of rectum and colon and colostomy, or any combination thereof

(For pelvic exenteration for gynecologic malignancy, use 58240)

Introduction

51600 Injection procedure for cystography or voiding urethrocystography

(For radiological supervision and interpretation, see 74430, 74455)

51605 Injection procedure and placement of chain for contrast and/or chain urethrocystography

(For radiological supervision and interpretation, use 74430)

51610 Injection procedure for retrograde urethrocystography

(For radiological supervision and interpretation, use 74450)

51700 Bladder irrigation, simple, lavage and/or instillation

(Codes 51701-51702 are reported only when performed independently. Do not report 51701-51702 when catheter insertion is an inclusive component of another procedure.)

51701 Insertion of non-indwelling bladder catheter (eg, straight catheterization for residual urine)

51702 Insertion of temporary indwelling bladder catheter; simple (eg, Foley)

51703 complicated (eg, altered anatomy, fractured catheter/balloon)

51705 Change of cystostomy tube; simple

51710 complicated

(If imaging guidance is performed, use 75984)

51715 Endoscopic injection of implant material into the submucosal tissues of the urethra and/or bladder neck

▲ **51720** Bladder instillation of anticarcinogenic agent (including retention time)

Urodynamics

The following section (51725-51797) lists procedures that may be used separately or in many and varied combinations.

When multiple procedures are performed in the same investigative session, modifier 51 should be employed.

All procedures in this section imply that these services are performed by, or are under the direct supervision of, a physician and that all instruments, equipment, fluids, gases, probes, catheters, technician's fees, medications, gloves, trays, tubing and other sterile supplies be provided by the physician. When the physician only interprets the results and/or operates the equipment, a professional component, modifier 26, should be used to identify physicians' services.

51725 Simple cystometrogram (CMG) (eg, spinal manometer)

51726 Complex cystometrogram (eg, calibrated electronic equipment)

51736 Simple uroflowmetry (UFR) (eg, stop-watch flow rate, mechanical uroflowmeter)

51741 Complex uroflowmetry (eg, calibrated electronic equipment)

51772 Urethral pressure profile studies (UPP) (urethral closure pressure profile), any technique

51784 Electromyography studies (EMG) of anal or urethral sphincter, other than needle, any technique

51785 Needle electromyography studies (EMG) of anal or urethral sphincter, any technique

51792 Stimulus evoked response (eg, measurement of bulbocavernosus reflex latency time)

51795 Voiding pressure studies (VP); bladder voiding pressure, any technique

51797 intra-abdominal voiding pressure (AP) (rectal, gastric, intraperitoneal)

51798 Measurement of post-voiding residual urine and/or bladder capacity by ultrasound, non-imaging

Repair

51800 Cystoplasty or cystourethroplasty, plastic operation on bladder and/or vesical neck (anterior Y-plasty, vesical fundus resection), any procedure, with or without wedge resection of posterior vesical neck

51820 Cystourethroplasty with unilateral or bilateral ureteroneocystostomy

51840 Anterior vesicourethropexy, or urethropexy (eg, Marshall-Marchetti-Krantz, Burch); simple

51841 complicated (eg, secondary repair)

(For urethropexy (Pereyra type), use 57289)

51845 Abdomino-vaginal vesical neck suspension, with or without endoscopic control (eg, Stamey, Raz, modified Pereyra)

51860 Cystorrhaphy, suture of bladder wound, injury or rupture; simple

51865 complicated

51880 Closure of cystostomy (separate procedure)

51900 Closure of vesicovaginal fistula, abdominal approach

(For vaginal approach, see 57320-57330)

51920 Closure of vesicouterine fistula;

51925 with hysterectomy

(For closure of vesicoenteric fistula, see 44660, 44661)

(For closure of rectovesical fistula, see 45800-45805)

51940 Closure, exstrophy of bladder

(See also 54390)

51960 Enterocystoplasty, including intestinal anastomosis

51980 Cutaneous vesicostomy

Laparoscopy

Surgical laparoscopy always includes diagnostic laparoscopy. To report a diagnostic laparoscopy (peritoneoscopy) (separate procedure), use 49320.

51990 Laparoscopy, surgical; urethral suspension for stress incontinence

51992 sling operation for stress incontinence (eg, fascia or synthetic)

(For open sling operation for stress incontinence, use 57288)

(For reversal or removal of sling operation for stress incontinence, use 57287)

51999 Unlisted laparoscopy procedure, bladder

Endoscopy—Cystoscopy, Urethroscopy, Cystourethroscopy

Endoscopic descriptions are listed so that the main procedure can be identified without having to list all the minor related functions performed at the same time. For example: meatotomy, urethral calibration and/or dilation, urethro-scopy, and cystoscopy prior to a transurethral resection of prostate; ureteral catheterization following extraction of ureteral calculus; internal urethrotomy and bladder neck fulguration when performing a cystourethroscopy for the female urethral syndrome. When the secondary procedure requires significant additional time and effort, it may be identified by the addition of modifier 22.

For example: urethrotomy performed for a documented pre-existing stricture or bladder neck contracture.

52000	Cystourethroscopy (separate procedure)
52001	Cystourethroscopy with irrigation and evacuation of multiple obstructing clots
	(Do not report 52001 in conjunction with 52000)
52005	Cystourethroscopy, with ureteral catheterization, with or without irrigation, instillation, or ureteropyelography, exclusive of radiologic service;
52007	with brush biopsy of ureter and/or renal pelvis
52010	Cystourethroscopy, with ejaculatory duct catheterization, with or without irrigation, instillation, or duct radiography, exclusive of radiologic service
	(For radiological supervision and interpretation, use 74440)

Transurethral Surgery

Urethra and Bladder

▲ 52204	Cystourethroscopy, with biopsy(s)
52214	Cystourethroscopy, with fulguration (including cryosurgery or laser surgery) of trigone, bladder neck, prostatic fossa, urethra, or periurethral glands
52224	Cystourethroscopy, with fulguration (including cryosurgery or laser surgery) or treatment of MINOR (less than 0.5 cm) lesion(s) with or without biopsy
52234	Cystourethroscopy, with fulguration (including cryosurgery or laser surgery) and/or resection of; SMALL bladder tumor(s) (0.5 up to 2.0 cm)
52235	MEDIUM bladder tumor(s) (2.0 to 5.0 cm)
52240	LARGE bladder tumor(s)
52250	Cystourethroscopy with insertion of radioactive substance, with or without biopsy or fulguration
52260	Cystourethroscopy, with dilation of bladder for interstitial cystitis; general or conduction (spinal) anesthesia
52265	local anesthesia
52270	Cystourethroscopy, with internal urethrotomy; female
52275	male
52276	Cystourethroscopy with direct vision internal urethrotomy
52277	Cystourethroscopy, with resection of external sphincter (sphincterotomy)
52281	Cystourethroscopy, with calibration and/or dilation of urethral stricture or stenosis, with or without meatotomy, with or without injection procedure for cystography, male or female
52282	Cystourethroscopy, with insertion of urethral stent
52283	Cystourethroscopy, with steroid injection into stricture

52285	Cystourethroscopy for treatment of the female urethral syndrome with any or all of the following: urethral meatotomy, urethral dilation, internal urethrotomy, lysis of urethrovaginal septal fibrosis, lateral incisions of the bladder neck, and fulguration of polyp(s) of urethra, bladder neck, and/or trigone
52290	Cystourethroscopy; with ureteral meatotomy, unilateral or bilateral
52300	with resection or fulguration of orthotopic ureterocele(s), unilateral or bilateral
52301	with resection or fulguration of ectopic ureterocele(s), unilateral or bilateral
52305	with incision or resection of orifice of bladder diverticulum, single or multiple
52310	Cystourethroscopy, with removal of foreign body, calculus, or ureteral stent from urethra or bladder (separate procedure); simple
52315	complicated
52317	Litholapaxy: crushing or fragmentation of calculus by any means in bladder and removal of fragments; simple or small (less than 2.5 cm)
52318	complicated or large (over 2.5 cm)

Ureter and Pelvis

▶Therapeutic cystourethroscopy always includes diagnostic cystourethroscopy. To report a diagnostic cystourethroscopy, use 52000. Therapeutic cystourethroscopy with ureteroscopy and/or pyeloscopy always includes diagnostic cystourethroscopy with ureteroscopy and/or pyeloscopy. To report a diagnostic cystourethroscopy with ureteroscopy and/or pyeloscopy, use 52351.

Do not report 52000 in conjunction with 52320-52343.

Do not report 52351 in conjunction with 52344-52346, 52352-52355.

The insertion and removal of a temporary ureteral catheter (52005) during diagnostic or therapeutic cystourethroscopic with ureteroscopy and/or pyeloscopy is included in 52320-52355 and should not be reported separately.

To report insertion of a self-retaining, indwelling stent performed during diagnostic or therapeutic cystourethroscopy with ureteroscopy and/or pyeloscopy, report 52332, in addition to primary procedure(s) performed (52320-52355), and append modifier 51. 52332 is used to report a unilateral procedure unless otherwise specified.◀

For bilateral insertion of self-retaining, indwelling ureteral stents, use code 52332, and append modifier 50.

►To report cystourethroscopic removal of a self-retaining, indwelling ureteral stent, see 52310, 52315, and append modifier 58, if appropriate.◄

52320   Cystourethroscopy (including ureteral catheterization); with removal of ureteral calculus

52325   with fragmentation of ureteral calculus (eg, ultrasonic or electro-hydraulic technique)

52327   with subureteric injection of implant material

52330   with manipulation, without removal of ureteral calculus

52332   Cystourethroscopy, with insertion of indwelling ureteral stent (eg, Gibbons or double-J type)

52334   Cystourethroscopy with insertion of ureteral guide wire through kidney to establish a percutaneous nephrostomy, retrograde

(For percutaneous nephrostolithotomy, see 50080, 50081; for establishment of nephrostomy tract only, use 50395)

(For cystourethroscopy, with ureteroscopy and/or pyeloscopy, see 52351-52355)

(For cystourethroscopy with incision, fulguration, or resection of congenital posterior urethral valves or obstructive hypertrophic mucosal folds, use 52400)

52341   Cystourethroscopy; with treatment of ureteral stricture (eg, balloon dilation, laser, electrocautery, and incision)

52342   with treatment of ureteropelvic junction stricture (eg, balloon dilation, laser, electrocautery, and incision)

52343   with treatment of intra-renal stricture (eg, balloon dilation, laser, electrocautery, and incision)

52344   Cystourethroscopy with ureteroscopy; with treatment of ureteral stricture (eg, balloon dilation, laser, electrocautery, and incision)

52345   with treatment of ureteropelvic junction stricture (eg, balloon dilation, laser, electrocautery, and incision)

52346   with treatment of intra-renal stricture (eg, balloon dilation, laser, electrocautery, and incision)

(52347 has been deleted)

(For transurethral resection or incision of ejaculatory ducts, use 52402)

52351   Cystourethroscopy, with ureteroscopy and/or pyeloscopy; diagnostic

(For radiological supervision and interpretation, use 74485)

(Do not report 52351 in conjunction with 52341-52346, 52352-52355)

52352   with removal or manipulation of calculus (ureteral catheterization is included)

52353   with lithotripsy (ureteral catheterization is included)

52354   with biopsy and/or fulguration of ureteral or renal pelvic lesion

52355   with resection of ureteral or renal pelvic tumor

Vesical Neck and Prostate

52400   Cystourethroscopy with incision, fulguration, or resection of congenital posterior urethral valves, or congenital obstructive hypertrophic mucosal folds

52402   Cystourethroscopy with transurethral resection or incision of ejaculatory ducts

52450   Transurethral incision of prostate

52500   Transurethral resection of bladder neck (separate procedure)

52510   Transurethral balloon dilation of the prostatic urethra

52601   Transurethral electrosurgical resection of prostate, including control of postoperative bleeding, complete (vasectomy, meatotomy, cystourethroscopy, urethral calibration and/or dilation, and internal urethrotomy are included)

(For other approaches, see 55801-55845)

52606   Transurethral fulguration for postoperative bleeding occurring after the usual follow-up time

52612   Transurethral resection of prostate; first stage of two-stage resection (partial resection)

52614   second stage of two-stage resection (resection completed)

52620   Transurethral resection; of residual obstructive tissue after 90 days postoperative

52630   of regrowth of obstructive tissue longer than one year postoperative

52640   of postoperative bladder neck contracture

52647   Laser coagulation of prostate, including control of postoperative bleeding, complete (vasectomy, meatotomy, cystourethroscopy, urethral calibration and/or dilation, and internal urethrotomy are included if performed)

52648   Laser vaporization of prostate, including control of postoperative bleeding, complete (vasectomy, meatotomy, cystourethroscopy, urethral calibration and/or dilation, internal urethrotomy and transurethral resection of prostate are included if performed)

52700   Transurethral drainage of prostatic abscess

(For litholapaxy, use 52317, 52318)

Surgery: Urinary System

Urethra

(For endoscopy, see cystoscopy, urethroscopy, cystourethroscopy, 52000-52700)

(For injection procedure for urethrocystography, see 51600-51610)

Incision

53000 Urethrotomy or urethrostomy, external (separate procedure); pendulous urethra

53010 perineal urethra, external

53020 Meatotomy, cutting of meatus (separate procedure); except infant

53025 infant

(Do not report modifier 63 in conjunction with 53025)

53040 Drainage of deep periurethral abscess

(For subcutaneous abscess, see 10060, 10061)

53060 Drainage of Skene's gland abscess or cyst

53080 Drainage of perineal urinary extravasation; uncomplicated (separate procedure)

53085 complicated

Excision

53200 Biopsy of urethra

53210 Urethrectomy, total, including cystostomy; female

53215 male

53220 Excision or fulguration of carcinoma of urethra

53230 Excision of urethral diverticulum (separate procedure); female

53235 male

53240 Marsupialization of urethral diverticulum, male or female

53250 Excision of bulbourethral gland (Cowper's gland)

53260 Excision or fulguration; urethral polyp(s), distal urethra

(For endoscopic approach, see 52214, 52224)

53265 urethral caruncle

53270 Skene's glands

53275 urethral prolapse

Repair

(For hypospadias, see 54300-54352)

53400 Urethroplasty; first stage, for fistula, diverticulum, or stricture (eg, Johannsen type)

53405 second stage (formation of urethra), including urinary diversion

53410 Urethroplasty, one-stage reconstruction of male anterior urethra

53415 Urethroplasty, transpubic or perineal, one stage, for reconstruction or repair of prostatic or membranous urethra

53420 Urethroplasty, two-stage reconstruction or repair of prostatic or membranous urethra; first stage

53425 second stage

53430 Urethroplasty, reconstruction of female urethra

53431 Urethroplasty with tubularization of posterior urethra and/or lower bladder for incontinence (eg, Tenago, Leadbetter procedure)

53440 Sling operation for correction of male urinary incontinence (eg, fascia or synthetic)

53442 Removal or revision of sling for male urinary incontinence (eg, fascia or synthetic)

53444 Insertion of tandem cuff (dual cuff)

53445 Insertion of inflatable urethral/bladder neck sphincter, including placement of pump, reservoir, and cuff

53446 Removal of inflatable urethral/bladder neck sphincter, including pump, reservoir, and cuff

53447 Removal and replacement of inflatable urethral/bladder neck sphincter including pump, reservoir, and cuff at the same operative session

53448 Removal and replacement of inflatable urethral/bladder neck sphincter including pump, reservoir, and cuff through an infected field at the same operative session including irrigation and debridement of infected tissue

(Do not report 11040-11043 in addition to 53448)

53449 Repair of inflatable urethral/bladder neck sphincter, including pump, reservoir, and cuff

53450 Urethromeatoplasty, with mucosal advancement

(For meatotomy, see 53020, 53025)

53460 Urethromeatoplasty, with partial excision of distal urethral segment (Richardson type procedure)

53500 Urethrolysis, transvaginal, secondary, open, including cystourethroscopy (eg, postsurgical obstruction, scarring)

(For urethrolysis by retropubic approach, use 53899)

(Do not report 53500 in conjunction with 52000)

53502 Urethrorrhaphy, suture of urethral wound or injury, female

53505 Urethrorrhaphy, suture of urethral wound or injury; penile

53510 perineal

53515 prostatomembranous

53520 Closure of urethrostomy or urethrocutaneous fistula, male (separate procedure)

(For closure of urethrovaginal fistula, use 57310)

(For closure of urethrorectal fistula, see 45820, 45825)

Surgery: Urinary System

Manipulation

(For radiological supervision and interpretation, use 74485)

53600   Dilation of urethral stricture by passage of sound or urethral dilator, male; initial

53601   subsequent

53605   Dilation of urethral stricture or vesical neck by passage of sound or urethral dilator, male, general or conduction (spinal) anesthesia

53620   Dilation of urethral stricture by passage of filiform and follower, male; initial

53621   subsequent

53660   Dilation of female urethra including suppository and/or instillation; initial

53661   subsequent

53665   Dilation of female urethra, general or conduction (spinal) anesthesia

(For urethral catheterization, see 51701-51703)

Other Procedures

(For two or three glass urinalysis, use 81020)

53850   Transurethral destruction of prostate tissue; by microwave thermotherapy

53852   by radiofrequency thermotherapy

53853   by water-induced thermotherapy

53899   Unlisted procedure, urinary system

Notes

⊙=Moderate sedation ✚=Add-on code ✗=FDA approval pending

Male Genital System

Penis

Incision

(For abdominal perineal gangrene debridement, see 11004-11006)

54000   Slitting of prepuce, dorsal or lateral (separate procedure); newborn

(Do not report modifier 63 in conjunction with 54000)

54001   except newborn

54015   Incision and drainage of penis, deep

(For skin and subcutaneous abscess, see 10060-10160)

Destruction

54050   Destruction of lesion(s), penis (eg, condyloma, papilloma, molluscum contagiosum, herpetic vesicle), simple; chemical

54055   electrodesiccation

54056   cryosurgery

54057   laser surgery

54060   surgical excision

54065   Destruction of lesion(s), penis (eg, condyloma, papilloma, molluscum contagiosum, herpetic vesicle), extensive (eg, laser surgery, electrosurgery, cryosurgery, chemosurgery)

(For destruction or excision of other lesions, see **Integumentary System**)

Excision

54100   Biopsy of penis; (separate procedure)

54105   deep structures

54110   Excision of penile plaque (Peyronie disease);

54111   with graft to 5 cm in length

54112   with graft greater than 5 cm in length

54115   Removal foreign body from deep penile tissue (eg, plastic implant)

54120   Amputation of penis; partial

54125   complete

54130   Amputation of penis, radical; with bilateral inguinofemoral lymphadenectomy

54135   in continuity with bilateral pelvic lymphadenectomy, including external iliac, hypogastric and obturator nodes

(For lymphadenectomy (separate procedure), see 38760-38770)

▲ **54150**   Circumcision, using clamp or other device with regional dorsal penile or ring block

(Do not report modifier 63 in conjunction with 54150)

►(Report 54150 with modifier 52 when performed without dorsal penile or ring block)◄

►(54152 has been deleted. To report, use 54150)◄

▲ **54160**   Circumcision, surgical excision other than clamp, device, or dorsal slit; neonate (28 days of age or less)

(Do not report modifier 63 in conjunction with 54160)

▲ **54161**   older than 28 days of age

54162   Lysis or excision of penile post-circumcision adhesions

54163   Repair incomplete circumcision

54164   Frenulotomy of penis

(Do not report 54164 with circumcision codes 54150-54161, 54162, 54163)

Introduction

54200   Injection procedure for Peyronie disease;

54205   with surgical exposure of plaque

54220   Irrigation of corpora cavernosa for priapism

54230   Injection procedure for corpora cavernosography

(For radiological supervision and interpretation, use 74445)

54231   Dynamic cavernosometry, including intracavernosal injection of vasoactive drugs (eg, papaverine, phentolamine)

54235   Injection of corpora cavernosa with pharmacologic agent(s) (eg, papaverine, phentolamine)

54240   Penile plethysmography

54250   Nocturnal penile tumescence and/or rigidity test

Repair

(For other urethroplasties, see 53400-53430)

(For penile revascularization, use 37788)

54300   Plastic operation of penis for straightening of chordee (eg, hypospadias), with or without mobilization of urethra

54304   Plastic operation on penis for correction of chordee or for first stage hypospadias repair with or without transplantation of prepuce and/or skin flaps

54308   Urethroplasty for second stage hypospadias repair (including urinary diversion); less than 3 cm

54312   greater than 3 cm

54316   Urethroplasty for second stage hypospadias repair (including urinary diversion) with free skin graft obtained from site other than genitalia

Surgery: Male/Female Genital System

54318 Urethroplasty for third stage hypospadias repair to release penis from scrotum (eg, third stage Cecil repair)

54322 One stage distal hypospadias repair (with or without chordee or circumcision); with simple meatal advancement (eg, Magpi, V-flap)

54324 with urethroplasty by local skin flaps (eg, flip-flap, prepucial flap)

54326 with urethroplasty by local skin flaps and mobilization of urethra

54328 with extensive dissection to correct chordee and urethroplasty with local skin flaps, skin graft patch, and/or island flap

(For urethroplasty and straightening of chordee, use 54308)

54332 One stage proximal penile or penoscrotal hypospadias repair requiring extensive dissection to correct chordee and urethroplasty by use of skin graft tube and/or island flap

54336 One stage perineal hypospadias repair requiring extensive dissection to correct chordee and urethroplasty by use of skin graft tube and/or island flap

54340 Repair of hypospadias complications (ie, fistula, stricture, diverticula); by closure, incision, or excision, simple

54344 requiring mobilization of skin flaps and urethroplasty with flap or patch graft

54348 requiring extensive dissection and urethroplasty with flap, patch or tubed graft (includes urinary diversion)

54352 Repair of hypospadias cripple requiring extensive dissection and excision of previously constructed structures including re-release of chordee and reconstruction of urethra and penis by use of local skin as grafts and island flaps and skin brought in as flaps or grafts

54360 Plastic operation on penis to correct angulation

54380 Plastic operation on penis for epispadias distal to external sphincter;

54385 with incontinence

54390 with exstrophy of bladder

54400 Insertion of penile prosthesis; non-inflatable (semi-rigid)

54401 inflatable (self-contained)

(For removal or replacement of penile prosthesis, see 54415, 54416)

54405 Insertion of multi-component, inflatable penile prosthesis, including placement of pump, cylinders, and reservoir

(For reduced services, report 54405 with modifier 52)

54406 Removal of all components of a multi-component, inflatable penile prosthesis without replacement of prosthesis

(For reduced services, report 54406 with modifier 52)

54408 Repair of component(s) of a multi-component, inflatable penile prosthesis

54410 Removal and replacement of all component(s) of a multi-component, inflatable penile prosthesis at the same operative session

54411 Removal and replacement of all components of a multi-component inflatable penile prosthesis through an infected field at the same operative session, including irrigation and debridement of infected tissue

(For reduced services, report 54411 with modifier 52)

(Do not report 11040-11043 in addition to 54411)

54415 Removal of non-inflatable (semi-rigid) or inflatable (self-contained) penile prosthesis, without replacement of prosthesis

54416 Removal and replacement of non-inflatable (semi-rigid) or inflatable (self-contained) penile prosthesis at the same operative session

54417 Removal and replacement of non-inflatable (semi-rigid) or inflatable (self-contained) penile prosthesis through an infected field at the same operative session, including irrigation and debridement of infected tissue

(Do not report 11040-11043 in addition to 54417)

54420 Corpora cavernosa-saphenous vein shunt (priapism operation), unilateral or bilateral

54430 Corpora cavernosa-corpus spongiosum shunt (priapism operation), unilateral or bilateral

54435 Corpora cavernosa-glans penis fistulization (eg, biopsy needle, Winter procedure, rongeur, or punch) for priapism

54440 Plastic operation of penis for injury

Manipulation

54450 Foreskin manipulation including lysis of preputial adhesions and stretching

Testis

Excision

(For abdominal perineal gangrene debridement, see 11004-11006)

54500 Biopsy of testis, needle (separate procedure)

(For fine needle aspiration, see 10021, 10022)

(For evaluation of fine needle aspirate, see 88172, 88173)

54505 Biopsy of testis, incisional (separate procedure)

(For bilateral procedure, report 54505 with modifier 50)

(When combined with vasogram, seminal vesiculogram, or epididymogram, use 55300)

54512 Excision of extraparenchymal lesion of testis

54520   Orchiectomy, simple (including subcapsular), with or without testicular prosthesis, scrotal or inguinal approach

(For bilateral procedure, report 54520 with modifier 50)

54522   Orchiectomy, partial

54530   Orchiectomy, radical, for tumor; inguinal approach

54535   with abdominal exploration

(For orchiectomy with repair of hernia, see 49505 or 49507 and 54520)

(For radical retroperitoneal lymphadenectomy, use 38780)

►Exploration◄

54550   Exploration for undescended testis (inguinal or scrotal area)

(For bilateral procedure, report 54550 with modifier 50)

54560   Exploration for undescended testis with abdominal exploration

(For bilateral procedure, report 54560 with modifier 50)

Repair

54600   Reduction of torsion of testis, surgical, with or without fixation of contralateral testis

54620   Fixation of contralateral testis (separate procedure)

54640   Orchiopexy, inguinal approach, with or without hernia repair

(For bilateral procedure, report 54640 with modifier 50)

(For inguinal hernia repair performed in conjunction with inguinal orchiopexy, see 49495-49525)

54650   Orchiopexy, abdominal approach, for intra-abdominal testis (eg, Fowler-Stephens)

(For laparoscopic approach, use 54692)

54660   Insertion of testicular prosthesis (separate procedure)

(For bilateral procedure, report 54660 with modifier 50)

54670   Suture or repair of testicular injury

54680   Transplantation of testis(es) to thigh (because of scrotal destruction)

Laparoscopy

Surgical laparoscopy always includes diagnostic laparoscopy. To report a diagnostic laparoscopy (peritoneoscopy) (separate procedure), use 49320.

54690   Laparoscopy, surgical; orchiectomy

54692   orchiopexy for intra-abdominal testis

54699   Unlisted laparoscopy procedure, testis

Epididymis

Incision

54700   Incision and drainage of epididymis, testis and/or scrotal space (eg, abscess or hematoma)

Excision

54800   Biopsy of epididymis, needle

(For fine needle aspiration, see 10021, 10022)

(For evaluation of fine needle aspirate, see 88172, 88173)

►(54820 has been deleted. To report, use 54865)◄

54830   Excision of local lesion of epididymis

54840   Excision of spermatocele, with or without epididymectomy

54860   Epididymectomy; unilateral

54861   bilateral

►Exploration◄

● **54865**   Exploration of epididymis, with or without biopsy

Repair

54900   Epididymovasostomy, anastomosis of epididymis to vas deferens; unilateral

54901   bilateral

(For operating microscope, use 69990)

Tunica Vaginalis

Incision

55000   Puncture aspiration of hydrocele, tunica vaginalis, with or without injection of medication

Excision

55040   Excision of hydrocele; unilateral

55041   bilateral

(With hernia repair, see 49495-49501)

Repair

55060   Repair of tunica vaginalis hydrocele (Bottle type)

Surgery: Male/Female Genital System

Scrotum

Incision

55100   Drainage of scrotal wall abscess

         (See also 54700)

55110   Scrotal exploration

55120   Removal of foreign body in scrotum

Excision

         (For excision of local lesion of skin of scrotum, see **Integumentary System**)

55150   Resection of scrotum

Repair

55175   Scrotoplasty; simple

55180   complicated

Vas Deferens

Incision

55200   Vasotomy, cannulization with or without incision of vas, unilateral or bilateral (separate procedure)

Excision

55250   Vasectomy, unilateral or bilateral (separate procedure), including postoperative semen examination(s)

Introduction

55300   Vasotomy for vasograms, seminal vesiculograms, or epididymograms, unilateral or bilateral

         (For radiological supervision and interpretation, use 74440)

         (When combined with biopsy of testis, see 54505 and use modifier 51)

Repair

55400   Vasovasostomy, vasovasorrhaphy

         (For bilateral procedure, report 55400 with modifier 50)

         (For operating microscope, use 69990)

Suture

55450   Ligation (percutaneous) of vas deferens, unilateral or bilateral (separate procedure)

Spermatic Cord

Excision

55500   Excision of hydrocele of spermatic cord, unilateral (separate procedure)

55520   Excision of lesion of spermatic cord (separate procedure)

55530   Excision of varicocele or ligation of spermatic veins for varicocele; (separate procedure)

55535   abdominal approach

55540   with hernia repair

Laparoscopy

Surgical laparoscopy always includes diagnostic laparoscopy. To report a diagnostic laparoscopy (peritoneoscopy) (separate procedure), use 49320.

55550   Laparoscopy, surgical, with ligation of spermatic veins for varicocele

55559   Unlisted laparoscopy procedure, spermatic cord

Seminal Vesicles

Incision

55600   Vesiculotomy;

         (For bilateral procedure, report 55600 with modifier 50)

55605   complicated

Excision

55650   Vesiculectomy, any approach

         (For bilateral procedure, report 55650 with modifier 50)

55680   Excision of Mullerian duct cyst

         (For injection procedure, see 52010, 55300)

Prostate

Incision

55700   Biopsy, prostate; needle or punch, single or multiple, any approach

         (For prostate needle biopsy saturation sampling for prostate mapping, use Category III code 0137T)

         (If imaging guidance is performed, use 76942)

         (For fine needle aspiration, see 10021, 10022)

         (For evaluation of fine needle aspirate, see 88172, 88173)

55705   incisional, any approach

55720   Prostatotomy, external drainage of prostatic abscess, any approach; simple

55725   complicated

        (For transurethral drainage, use 52700)

Excision

        (For transurethral removal of prostate, see 52601-52640)

        (For transurethral destruction of prostate, see 53850-53852)

        (For limited pelvic lymphadenectomy for staging (separate procedure), use 38562)

        (For independent node dissection, see 38770-38780)

55801   Prostatectomy, perineal, subtotal (including control of postoperative bleeding, vasectomy, meatotomy, urethral calibration and/or dilation, and internal urethrotomy)

55810   Prostatectomy, perineal radical;

55812   with lymph node biopsy(s) (limited pelvic lymphadenectomy)

55815   with bilateral pelvic lymphadenectomy, including external iliac, hypogastric and obturator nodes

        (If 55815 is carried out on separate days, use 38770 with modifier 50 and 55810)

55821   Prostatectomy (including control of postoperative bleeding, vasectomy, meatotomy, urethral calibration and/or dilation, and internal urethrotomy); suprapubic, subtotal, one or two stages

55831   retropubic, subtotal

55840   Prostatectomy, retropubic radical, with or without nerve sparing;

55842   with lymph node biopsy(s) (limited pelvic lymphadenectomy)

55845   with bilateral pelvic lymphadenectomy, including external iliac, hypogastric, and obturator nodes

        (If 55845 is carried out on separate days, use 38770 with modifier 50 and 55840)

        (For laparoscopic retropubic radical prostatectomy, use 55866)

        ►(55859 has been deleted. To report, use 55875)◄

55860   Exposure of prostate, any approach, for insertion of radioactive substance;

        (For application of interstitial radioelement, see 77776-77778)

55862   with lymph node biopsy(s) (limited pelvic lymphadenectomy)

55865   with bilateral pelvic lymphadenectomy, including external iliac, hypogastric and obturator nodes

Laparoscopy

Surgical laparoscopy always includes diagnostic laparoscopy. To report a diagnostic laparoscopy (peritoneoscopy) (separate procedure), use 49320.

55866   Laparoscopy, surgical prostatectomy, retropubic radical, including nerve sparing

        (For open procedure, use 55840)

Other Procedures

        (For artificial insemination, see 58321, 58322)

55870   Electroejaculation

55873   Cryosurgical ablation of the prostate (includes ultrasonic guidance for interstitial cryosurgical probe placement)

● **55875**   Transperineal placement of needles or catheters into prostate for interstitial radioelement application, with or without cystoscopy

        ►(For interstitial radioelement application, see 77776-77784)◄

        ►(For ultrasonic guidance for interstitial radioelement application, use 76965)◄

● **55876**   Placement of interstitial device(s) for radiation therapy guidance (eg, fiducial markers, dosimeter), prostate (via needle, any approach), single or multiple

        ►(Report supply of device separately)◄

        ►(For imaging guidance, see 76942, 77002, 77012, 77021)◄

55899   Unlisted procedure, male genital system

Intersex Surgery

55970   Intersex surgery; male to female

55980   female to male

Notes

⊙=Moderate sedation   ✚=Add-on code   ✗=FDA approval pending

Female Genital System

(For pelvic laparotomy, use 49000)

(For excision or destruction of endometriomas, open method, see 49200, 49201)

(For paracentesis, see 49080, 49081)

(For secondary closure of abdominal wall evisceration or disruption, use 49900)

(For fulguration or excision of lesions, laparoscopic approach, use 58662)

►(For chemotherapy, see 96401-96549)◄

Vulva, Perineum, and Introitus

Definitions

The following definitions apply to the vulvectomy codes (56620-56640).

A *simple* procedure is the removal of skin and superficial subcutaneous tissues.

A *radical* procedure is the removal of skin and deep subcutaneous tissue.

A *partial* procedure is the removal of less than 80% of the vulvar area.

A *complete* procedure is the removal of greater than 80% of the vulvar area.

Incision

(For incision and drainage of sebaceous cyst, furuncle, or abscess, see 10040, 10060, 10061)

56405 Incision and drainage of vulva or perineal abscess

56420 Incision and drainage of Bartholin's gland abscess

(For incision and drainage of Skene's gland abscess or cyst, use 53060)

56440 Marsupialization of Bartholin's gland cyst

56441 Lysis of labial adhesions

● **56442** Hymenotomy, simple incision

Destruction

56501 Destruction of lesion(s), vulva; simple (eg, laser surgery, electrosurgery, cryosurgery, chemosurgery)

56515   extensive (eg, laser surgery, electrosurgery, cryosurgery, chemosurgery)

(For destruction of Skene's gland cyst or abscess, use 53270)

(For cautery destruction of urethral caruncle, use 53265)

Excision

56605 Biopsy of vulva or perineum (separate procedure); one lesion

+ **56606**   each separate additional lesion (List separately in addition to code for primary procedure)

(Use 56606 in conjunction with 56605)

(For excision of local lesion, see 11420-11426, 11620-11626)

56620 Vulvectomy simple; partial

56625   complete

►(For skin graft, see 15002 et seq)◄

56630 Vulvectomy, radical, partial;

►(For skin graft, if used, see 15004-15005, 15120, 15121, 15240, 15241)◄

56631   with unilateral inguinofemoral lymphadenectomy

56632   with bilateral inguinofemoral lymphadenectomy

56633 Vulvectomy, radical, complete;

56634   with unilateral inguinofemoral lymphadenectomy

56637   with bilateral inguinofemoral lymphadenectomy

56640 Vulvectomy, radical, complete, with inguinofemoral, iliac, and pelvic lymphadenectomy

(For bilateral procedure, report 56640 with modifier 50)

(For lymphadenectomy, see 38760-38780)

56700 Partial hymenectomy or revision of hymenal ring

►(56720 has been deleted. To report, use 56442)◄

56740 Excision of Bartholin's gland or cyst

(For excision of Skene's gland, use 53270)

(For excision of urethral caruncle, use 53265)

(For excision or fulguration of urethral carcinoma, use 53220)

(For excision or marsupialization of urethral diverticulum, see 53230, 53240)

Repair

(For repair of urethra for mucosal prolapse, use 53275)

56800 Plastic repair of introitus

56805 Clitoroplasty for intersex state

56810 Perineoplasty, repair of perineum, nonobstetrical (separate procedure)

(See also 56800)

(For repair of wounds to genitalia, see 12001-12007, 12041-12047, 13131-13133)

(For repair of recent injury of vagina and perineum, nonobstetrical, use 57210)

Surgery: Male/Female Genital System

(For anal sphincteroplasty, see 46750, 46751)

(For episiorrhaphy, episioperineorrhaphy for recent injury of vulva and/or perineum, nonobstetrical, use 57210)

Endoscopy

56820   Colposcopy of the vulva;

56821   with biopsy(s)

(For colposcopic examinations/procedures involving the vagina, see 57420, 57421; cervix, see 57452-57461)

Vagina

Incision

57000   Colpotomy; with exploration

57010   with drainage of pelvic abscess

57020   Colpocentesis (separate procedure)

57022   Incision and drainage of vaginal hematoma; obstetrical/postpartum

57023   non-obstetrical (eg, post-trauma, spontaneous bleeding)

Destruction

57061   Destruction of vaginal lesion(s); simple (eg, laser surgery, electrosurgery, cryosurgery, chemosurgery)

57065   extensive (eg, laser surgery, electrosurgery, cryosurgery, chemosurgery)

Excision

57100   Biopsy of vaginal mucosa; simple (separate procedure)

57105   extensive, requiring suture (including cysts)

57106   Vaginectomy, partial removal of vaginal wall;

57107   with removal of paravaginal tissue (radical vaginectomy)

57109   with removal of paravaginal tissue (radical vaginectomy) with bilateral total pelvic lymphadenectomy and para-aortic lymph node sampling (biopsy)

57110   Vaginectomy, complete removal of vaginal wall;

57111   with removal of paravaginal tissue (radical vaginectomy)

57112   with removal of paravaginal tissue (radical vaginectomy) with bilateral total pelvic lymphadenectomy and para-aortic lymph node sampling (biopsy)

57120   Colpocleisis (Le Fort type)

57130   Excision of vaginal septum

57135   Excision of vaginal cyst or tumor

Introduction

57150   Irrigation of vagina and/or application of medicament for treatment of bacterial, parasitic, or fungoid disease

57155   Insertion of uterine tandems and/or vaginal ovoids for clinical brachytherapy

(For insertion of radioelement sources or ribbons, see 77761-77763, 77781-77784)

57160   Fitting and insertion of pessary or other intravaginal support device

57170   Diaphragm or cervical cap fitting with instructions

57180   Introduction of any hemostatic agent or pack for spontaneous or traumatic nonobstetrical vaginal hemorrhage (separate procedure)

Repair

(For urethral suspension, Marshall-Marchetti-Krantz type, abdominal approach, see 51840, 51841)

(For laparoscopic suspension, use 51990)

57200   Colporrhaphy, suture of injury of vagina (nonobstetrical)

57210   Colpoperineorrhaphy, suture of injury of vagina and/or perineum (nonobstetrical)

57220   Plastic operation on urethral sphincter, vaginal approach (eg, Kelly urethral plication)

57230   Plastic repair of urethrocele

57240   Anterior colporrhaphy, repair of cystocele with or without repair of urethrocele

57250   Posterior colporrhaphy, repair of rectocele with or without perineorrhaphy

(For repair of rectocele (separate procedure) without posterior colporrhaphy, use 45560)

57260   Combined anteroposterior colporrhaphy;

57265   with enterocele repair

+ 57267   Insertion of mesh or other prosthesis for repair of pelvic floor defect, each site (anterior, posterior compartment), vaginal approach (List separately in addition to code for primary procedure)

(Use 57267 in addition to 45560, 57240-57265)

57268   Repair of enterocele, vaginal approach (separate procedure)

57270   Repair of enterocele, abdominal approach (separate procedure)

57280   Colpopexy, abdominal approach

57282   Colpopexy, vaginal; extra-peritoneal approach (sacrospinous, iliococcygeus)

57283   intra-peritoneal approach (uterosacral, levator myorrhaphy)

57284 Paravaginal defect repair (including repair of cystocele, stress urinary incontinence, and/or incomplete vaginal prolapse)

57287 Removal or revision of sling for stress incontinence (eg, fascia or synthetic)

57288 Sling operation for stress incontinence (eg, fascia or synthetic)

(For laparoscopic approach, use 51992)

57289 Pereyra procedure, including anterior colporrhaphy

57291 Construction of artificial vagina; without graft

57292   with graft

57295 Revision (including removal) of prosthetic vaginal graft; vaginal approach

● 57296   open abdominal approach

57300 Closure of rectovaginal fistula; vaginal or transanal approach

57305   abdominal approach

57307   abdominal approach, with concomitant colostomy

57308   transperineal approach, with perineal body reconstruction, with or without levator plication

57310 Closure of urethrovaginal fistula;

57311   with bulbocavernosus transplant

57320 Closure of vesicovaginal fistula; vaginal approach

(For concomitant cystostomy, see 51005-51040)

57330   transvesical and vaginal approach

(For abdominal approach, use 51900)

57335 Vaginoplasty for intersex state

Manipulation

57400 Dilation of vagina under anesthesia

57410 Pelvic examination under anesthesia

57415 Removal of impacted vaginal foreign body (separate procedure) under anesthesia

(For removal without anesthesia of an impacted vaginal foreign body, use the appropriate E/M code)

Endoscopy

(For speculoscopy, see Category III codes 0031T, 0032T)

57420 Colposcopy of the entire vagina, with cervix if present;

57421   with biopsy(s) of vagina/cervix

(For colposcopic visualization of cervix and adjacent upper vagina, use 57452)

(When reporting colposcopies of multiple sites, use modifier 51 as appropriate. For colposcopic examinations/procedures involving the vulva, see 56820, 56821; cervix, see 57452-57461)

(For endometrial sampling (biopsy) performed in conjunction with colposcopy, use 58110)

57425 Laparoscopy, surgical, colpopexy (suspension of vaginal apex)

Cervix Uteri

(For cervicography, see Category III code 0003T)

Endoscopy

(For colposcopic examinations/procedures involving the vulva, see 56820, 56821; vagina, see 57420, 57421)

57452 Colposcopy of the cervix including upper/adjacent vagina;

(Do not report 57452 in addition to 57454-57461)

57454   with biopsy(s) of the cervix and endocervical curettage

57455   with biopsy(s) of the cervix

57456   with endocervical curettage

57460   with loop electrode biopsy(s) of the cervix

57461   with loop electrode conization of the cervix

(Do not report 57456 in addition to 57461)

(For endometrial sampling (biopsy) performed in conjunction with colposcopy, use 58110)

Excision

(For radical surgical procedures, see 58200-58240)

57500 Biopsy, single or multiple, or local excision of lesion, with or without fulguration (separate procedure)

57505 Endocervical curettage (not done as part of a dilation and curettage)

57510 Cautery of cervix; electro or thermal

57511   cryocautery, initial or repeat

57513   laser ablation

57520 Conization of cervix, with or without fulguration, with or without dilation and curettage, with or without repair; cold knife or laser

(See also 58120)

57522   loop electrode excision

57530 Trachelectomy (cervicectomy), amputation of cervix (separate procedure)

57531 Radical trachelectomy, with bilateral total pelvic lymphadenectomy and para-aortic lymph node sampling biopsy, with or without removal of tube(s), with or without removal of ovary(s)

(For radical abdominal hysterectomy, use 58210)

57540 Excision of cervical stump, abdominal approach;

57545   with pelvic floor repair

Surgery: Male/Female Genital System

57550   Excision of cervical stump, vaginal approach;

57555   with anterior and/or posterior repair

57556   with repair of enterocele

(For insertion of intrauterine device, use 58300)

(For insertion of any hemostatic agent or pack for control of spontaneous non-obstetrical hemorrhage, see 57180)

● **57558**   Dilation and curettage of cervical stump

Repair

57700   Cerclage of uterine cervix, nonobstetrical

57720   Trachelorrhaphy, plastic repair of uterine cervix, vaginal approach

Manipulation

57800   Dilation of cervical canal, instrumental (separate procedure)

►(57820 has been deleted. To report, use 57558)◄

Corpus Uteri

Excision

58100   Endometrial sampling (biopsy) with or without endocervical sampling (biopsy), without cervical dilation, any method (separate procedure)

(For endocervical curettage only, use 57505)

(For endometrial sampling (biopsy) performed in conjunction with colposcopy (57420, 57421, 57452-57461), use 58110)

+ **58110**   Endometrial sampling (biopsy) performed in conjunction with colposcopy (List separately in addition to code for primary procedure)

(Use 58110 in conjunction with 57420, 57421, 57452-57461)

58120   Dilation and curettage, diagnostic and/or therapeutic (nonobstetrical)

(For postpartum hemorrhage, use 59160)

58140   Myomectomy, excision of fibroid tumor(s) of uterus, 1 to 4 intramural myoma(s) with total weight of 250 g or less and/or removal of surface myomas; abdominal approach

58145   vaginal approach

58146   Myomectomy, excision of fibroid tumor(s) of uterus, 5 or more intramural myomas and/or intramural myomas with total weight greater than 250 g, abdominal approach

(Do not report 58146 in addition to 58140-58145, 58150-58240)

►Hysterectomy Procedures◄

58150   Total abdominal hysterectomy (corpus and cervix), with or without removal of tube(s), with or without removal of ovary(s);

58152   with colpo-urethrocystopexy (eg, Marshall-Marchetti-Krantz, Burch)

(For urethrocystopexy without hysterectomy, see 51840, 51841)

58180   Supracervical abdominal hysterectomy (subtotal hysterectomy), with or without removal of tube(s), with or without removal of ovary(s)

58200   Total abdominal hysterectomy, including partial vaginectomy, with para-aortic and pelvic lymph node sampling, with or without removal of tube(s), with or without removal of ovary(s)

58210   Radical abdominal hysterectomy, with bilateral total pelvic lymphadenectomy and para-aortic lymph node sampling (biopsy), with or without removal of tube(s), with or without removal of ovary(s)

(For radical hysterectomy with ovarian transposition, use also 58825)

58240   Pelvic exenteration for gynecologic malignancy, with total abdominal hysterectomy or cervicectomy, with or without removal of tube(s), with or without removal of ovary(s), with removal of bladder and ureteral transplantations, and/or abdominoperineal resection of rectum and colon and colostomy, or any combination thereof

(For pelvic exenteration for lower urinary tract or male genital malignancy, use 51597)

58260   Vaginal hysterectomy, for uterus 250 g or less;

58262   with removal of tube(s), and/or ovary(s)

58263   with removal of tube(s), and/or ovary(s), with repair of enterocele

(Do not report 58263 in addition to 57283)

58267   with colpo-urethrocystopexy (Marshall-Marchetti-Krantz type, Pereyra type) with or without endoscopic control

58270   with repair of enterocele

(For repair of enterocele with removal of tubes and/or ovaries, use 58263)

58275   Vaginal hysterectomy, with total or partial vaginectomy;

58280   with repair of enterocele

58285   Vaginal hysterectomy, radical (Schauta type operation)

58290   Vaginal hysterectomy, for uterus greater than 250 g;

58291   with removal of tube(s) and/or ovary(s)

58292   with removal of tube(s) and/or ovary(s), with repair of enterocele

58293	with colpo-urethrocystopexy (Marshall-Marchetti-Krantz type, Pereyra type) with or without endoscopic control
58294	with repair of enterocele

Introduction

(For insertion/removal of implantable contraceptive capsules, see 11975, 11976, 11977)

58300	Insertion of intrauterine device (IUD)
58301	Removal of intrauterine device (IUD)
58321	Artificial insemination; intra-cervical
58322	intra-uterine
58323	Sperm washing for artificial insemination
58340	Catheterization and introduction of saline or contrast material for saline infusion sonohysterography (SIS) or hysterosalpingography

(For radiological supervision and interpretation of saline infusion sonohysterography, use 76831)

(For radiological supervision and interpretation of hysterosalpingography, use 74740)

58345	Transcervical introduction of fallopian tube catheter for diagnosis and/or re-establishing patency (any method), with or without hysterosalpingography

(For radiological supervision and interpretation, use 74742)

58346	Insertion of Heyman capsules for clinical brachytherapy

(For insertion of radioelement sources or ribbons, see 77761-77763, 77781-77784)

58350	Chromotubation of oviduct, including materials

(For materials supplied by physician, use 99070)

58353	Endometrial ablation, thermal, without hysteroscopic guidance

(For hysteroscopic procedure, use 58563)

58356	Endometrial cryoablation with ultrasonic guidance, including endometrial curettage, when performed

(Do not report 58356 in conjunction with 58100, 58120, 58340, 76700, 76856)

Repair

58400	Uterine suspension, with or without shortening of round ligaments, with or without shortening of sacrouterine ligaments; (separate procedure)
58410	with presacral sympathectomy

(For anastomosis of tubes to uterus, use 58752)

58520	Hysterorrhaphy, repair of ruptured uterus (nonobstetrical)
58540	Hysteroplasty, repair of uterine anomaly (Strassman type)

(For closure of vesicouterine fistula, use 51920)

Laparoscopy/Hysteroscopy

Surgical laparoscopy always includes diagnostic laparoscopy. To report a diagnostic laparoscopy (peritoneoscopy) (separate procedure), use 49320. To report a diagnostic hysteroscopy (separate procedure), use 58555.

● 58541	Laparoscopy, surgical, supracervical hysterectomy, for uterus 250 g or less;
● 58542	with removal of tube(s) and/or ovary(s)

►(Do not report 58541, 58542 in conjunction with 49320, 57410, 58140, 58150, 58661, 58670, 58671)◄

● 58543	Laparoscopy, surgical, supracervical hysterectomy, for uterus greater than 250 g;
● 58544	with removal of tube(s) and/or ovary(s)

►(Do not report 58543, 58544 in conjunction with 49320, 57410, 58140, 58150, 58661, 58670, 58671)◄

58545	Laparoscopy, surgical, myomectomy, excision; 1 to 4 intramural myomas with total weight of 250 g or less and/or removal of surface myomas
58546	5 or more intramural myomas and/or intramural myomas with total weight greater than 250 g
● 58548	Laparoscopy, surgical, with radical hysterectomy, with bilateral total pelvic lymphadenectomy and para-aortic lymph node sampling (biopsy), with removal of tube(s) and ovary(s), if performed

►(Do not report 58548 in conjunction with 38570-38572, 58210, 58285, 58550-58554)◄

58550	Laparoscopy, surgical, with vaginal hysterectomy, for uterus 250 g or less;
58552	with removal of tube(s) and/or ovary(s)
58553	Laparoscopy, surgical, with vaginal hysterectomy, for uterus greater than 250 g;
58554	with removal of tube(s) and/or ovary(s)
58555	Hysteroscopy, diagnostic (separate procedure)
58558	Hysteroscopy, surgical; with sampling (biopsy) of endometrium and/or polypectomy, with or without D & C
58559	with lysis of intrauterine adhesions (any method)
58560	with division or resection of intrauterine septum (any method)
58561	with removal of leiomyomata
58562	with removal of impacted foreign body
58563	with endometrial ablation (eg, endometrial resection, electrosurgical ablation, thermoablation)
58565	with bilateral fallopian tube cannulation to induce occlusion by placement of permanent implants

(Do not report 58565 in conjunction with 58555 or 57800)

(For unilateral procedure, use modifier 52)

Surgery: Male/Female Genital System

58578 Unlisted laparoscopy procedure, uterus

58579 Unlisted hysteroscopy procedure, uterus

Oviduct/Ovary

Incision

58600 Ligation or transection of fallopian tube(s), abdominal or vaginal approach, unilateral or bilateral

58605 Ligation or transection of fallopian tube(s), abdominal or vaginal approach, postpartum, unilateral or bilateral, during same hospitalization (separate procedure)

(For laparoscopic procedures, use 58670, 58671)

+ 58611 Ligation or transection of fallopian tube(s) when done at the time of cesarean delivery or intra-abdominal surgery (not a separate procedure) (List separately in addition to code for primary procedure)

58615 Occlusion of fallopian tube(s) by device (eg, band, clip, Falope ring) vaginal or suprapubic approach

(For laparoscopic approach, use 58671)

(For lysis of adnexal adhesions, use 58740)

Laparoscopy

Surgical laparoscopy always includes diagnostic laparoscopy. To report a diagnostic laparoscopy (peritoneoscopy) (separate procedure), use 49320.

58660 Laparoscopy, surgical; with lysis of adhesions (salpingolysis, ovariolysis) (separate procedure)

58661 with removal of adnexal structures (partial or total oophorectomy and/or salpingectomy)

58662 with fulguration or excision of lesions of the ovary, pelvic viscera, or peritoneal surface by any method

58670 with fulguration of oviducts (with or without transection)

58671 with occlusion of oviducts by device (eg, band, clip, or Falope ring)

58672 with fimbrioplasty

58673 with salpingostomy (salpingoneostomy)

(Codes 58672 and 58673 are used to report unilateral procedures. For bilateral procedure, use modifier 50)

58679 Unlisted laparoscopy procedure, oviduct, ovary

▶(For laparoscopic aspiration of ovarian cyst, use 49322)◀

▶(For laparoscopic biopsy of the ovary or fallopian tube, use 49321)◀

Excision

58700 Salpingectomy, complete or partial, unilateral or bilateral (separate procedure)

58720 Salpingo-oophorectomy, complete or partial, unilateral or bilateral (separate procedure)

Repair

58740 Lysis of adhesions (salpingolysis, ovariolysis)

(For laparoscopic approach, use 58660)

(For excision or destruction of endometriomas, open method, see 49200, 49201)

(For fulguration or excision of lesions, laparoscopic approach, use 58662)

58750 Tubotubal anastomosis

58752 Tubouterine implantation

58760 Fimbrioplasty

(For laparoscopic approach, use 58672)

58770 Salpingostomy (salpingoneostomy)

(For laparoscopic approach, use 58673)

Ovary

Incision

58800 Drainage of ovarian cyst(s), unilateral or bilateral, (separate procedure); vaginal approach

58805 abdominal approach

58820 Drainage of ovarian abscess; vaginal approach, open

58822 abdominal approach

⊙ 58823 Drainage of pelvic abscess, transvaginal or transrectal approach, percutaneous (eg, ovarian, pericolic)

(For radiological supervision and interpretation, use 75989)

58825 Transposition, ovary(s)

Excision

58900 Biopsy of ovary, unilateral or bilateral (separate procedure)

(For laparoscopic biopsy of the ovary or fallopian tube, use 49321)

58920 Wedge resection or bisection of ovary, unilateral or bilateral

58925 Ovarian cystectomy, unilateral or bilateral

58940 Oophorectomy, partial or total, unilateral or bilateral;

(For oophorectomy with concomitant debulking for ovarian malignancy, use 58952)

58943   for ovarian, tubal or primary peritoneal malignancy, with para-aortic and pelvic lymph node biopsies, peritoneal washings, peritoneal biopsies, diaphragmatic assessments, with or without salpingectomy(s), with or without omentectomy

▲ **58950** Resection (initial) of ovarian, tubal or primary peritoneal malignancy with bilateral salpingo-oophorectomy and omentectomy;

58951   with total abdominal hysterectomy, pelvic and limited para-aortic lymphadenectomy

58952   with radical dissection for debulking (ie, radical excision or destruction, intra-abdominal or retroperitoneal tumors)

▶(For resection of recurrent ovarian, tubal, primary peritoneal, or uterine malignancy, see 58957, 58958)◀

58953   Bilateral salpingo-oophorectomy with omentectomy, total abdominal hysterectomy and radical dissection for debulking;

58954   with pelvic lymphadenectomy and limited para-aortic lymphadenectomy

58956   Bilateral salpingo-oophorectomy with total omentectomy, total abdominal hysterectomy for malignancy

▶(Do not report 58956 in conjunction with 49255, 58150, 58180, 58262, 58263, 58550, 58661, 58700, 58720, 58900, 58925, 58940, 58957, 58958)◀

● **58957** Resection (tumor debulking) of recurrent ovarian, tubal, primary peritoneal, uterine malignancy (intra-abdominal, retroperitoneal tumors), with omentectomy, if performed;

● **58958**   with pelvic lymphadenectomy and limited para-aortic lymphadenectomy

▶(Do not report 58957, 58958 in conjunction with 38770, 38780, 44005, 49000, 49200-49215, 49255, 58900-58960)◀

58960   Laparotomy, for staging or restaging of ovarian, tubal, or primary peritoneal malignancy (second look), with or without omentectomy, peritoneal washing, biopsy of abdominal and pelvic peritoneum, diaphragmatic assessment with pelvic and limited para-aortic lymphadenectomy

▶(Do not report 58960 in conjunction with 58957, 58958)◀

In Vitro Fertilization

58970   Follicle puncture for oocyte retrieval, any method

(For radiological supervision and interpretation, use 76948)

58974   Embryo transfer, intrauterine

58976   Gamete, zygote, or embryo intrafallopian transfer, any method

(For laparoscopic adnexal procedures, see 58660-58673)

Other Procedures

58999   Unlisted procedure, female genital system (nonobstetrical)

Maternity Care and Delivery

The services normally provided in uncomplicated maternity cases include antepartum care, delivery, and postpartum care.

Antepartum care includes the initial and subsequent history, physical examinations, recording of weight, blood pressures, fetal heart tones, routine chemical urinalysis, and monthly visits up to 28 weeks gestation, biweekly visits to 36 weeks gestation, and weekly visits until delivery. Any other visits or services within this time period should be coded separately.

Delivery services include admission to the hospital, the admission history and physical examination, management of uncomplicated labor, vaginal delivery (with or without episiotomy, with or without forceps), or cesarean delivery. Medical problems complicating labor and delivery management may require additional resources and should be identified by utilizing the codes in the **Medicine** and **Evaluation and Management Services** section in addition to codes for maternity care.

Postpartum care includes hospital and office visits following vaginal or cesarean section delivery.

For medical complications of pregnancy (eg, cardiac problems, neurological problems, diabetes, hypertension, toxemia, hyperemesis, pre-term labor, premature rupture of membranes), see services in the **Medicine** and **Evaluation and Management Services** section.

For surgical complications of pregnancy (eg, appendectomy, hernia, ovarian cyst, Bartholin cyst), see services in the **Surgery** section.

If a physician provides all or part of the antepartum and/or postpartum patient care but does not perform delivery due to termination of pregnancy by abortion or referral to another physician for delivery, see the antepartum and postpartum care codes 59425-59426 and 59430.

(For circumcision of newborn, see 54150, 54160)

Antepartum Services

(For insertion of transcervical or transvaginal fetal oximetry sensor, use Category III code 0021T)

59000   Amniocentesis; diagnostic

(For radiological supervision and interpretation, use 76946)

59001   therapeutic amniotic fluid reduction (includes ultrasound guidance)

59012 Cordocentesis (intrauterine), any method

(For radiological supervision and interpretation, use 76941)

59015 Chorionic villus sampling, any method

(For radiological supervision and interpretation, use 76945)

59020 Fetal contraction stress test

59025 Fetal non-stress test

59030 Fetal scalp blood sampling

(For repeat fetal scalp blood sampling, use 59030 and see modifiers 76 and 77)

59050 Fetal monitoring during labor by consulting physician (ie, non-attending physician) with written report; supervision and interpretation

59051 interpretation only

59070 Transabdominal amnioinfusion, including ultrasound guidance

59072 Fetal umbilical cord occlusion, including ultrasound guidance

59074 Fetal fluid drainage (eg, vesicocentesis, thoracocentesis, paracentesis), including ultrasound guidance

59076 Fetal shunt placement, including ultrasound guidance

(For unlisted fetal invasive procedure, use 59897)

Excision

59100 Hysterotomy, abdominal (eg, for hydatidiform mole, abortion)

(When tubal ligation is performed at the same time as hysterotomy, use 58611 in addition to 59100)

59120 Surgical treatment of ectopic pregnancy; tubal or ovarian, requiring salpingectomy and/or oophorectomy, abdominal or vaginal approach

59121 tubal or ovarian, without salpingectomy and/or oophorectomy

59130 abdominal pregnancy

59135 interstitial, uterine pregnancy requiring total hysterectomy

59136 interstitial, uterine pregnancy with partial resection of uterus

59140 cervical, with evacuation

59150 Laparoscopic treatment of ectopic pregnancy; without salpingectomy and/or oophorectomy

59151 with salpingectomy and/or oophorectomy

59160 Curettage, postpartum

Introduction

(For intrauterine fetal transfusion, use 36460)

(For introduction of hypertonic solution and/or prostaglandins to initiate labor, see 59850-59857)

59200 Insertion of cervical dilator (eg, laminaria, prostaglandin) (separate procedure)

Repair

(For tracheloplasty, use 57700)

59300 Episiotomy or vaginal repair, by other than attending physician

59320 Cerclage of cervix, during pregnancy; vaginal

59325 abdominal

59350 Hysterorrhaphy of ruptured uterus

Vaginal Delivery, Antepartum and Postpartum Care

(For insertion of transcervical or transvaginal fetal oximetry sensor, use Category III code 0021T)

59400 Routine obstetric care including antepartum care, vaginal delivery (with or without episiotomy, and/or forceps) and postpartum care

59409 Vaginal delivery only (with or without episiotomy and/or forceps);

59410 including postpartum care

59412 External cephalic version, with or without tocolysis

(Use 59412 in addition to code(s) for delivery)

59414 Delivery of placenta (separate procedure)

(For antepartum care only, see 59425, 59426 or appropriate E/M code(s))

(For 1-3 antepartum care visits, see appropriate E/M code(s))

59425 Antepartum care only; 4-6 visits

59426 7 or more visits

59430 Postpartum care only (separate procedure)

Cesarean Delivery

(For insertion of transcervical or transvaginal fetal oximetry sensor, use Category III code 0021T)

(For standby attendance for infant, use 99360)

(For low cervical cesarean section, see 59510, 59515, 59525)

59510 Routine obstetric care including antepartum care, cesarean delivery, and postpartum care

59514 Cesarean delivery only;

59515   including postpartum care

(For classic cesarean section, see 59510, 59515, 59525)

+ 59525 Subtotal or total hysterectomy after cesarean delivery (List separately in addition to code for primary procedure)

(Use 59525 in conjunction with 59510, 59514, 59515, 59618, 59620, 59622)

(For extraperitoneal cesarean section, or cesarean section with subtotal or total hysterectomy, see 59510, 59515, 59525)

Delivery After Previous Cesarean Delivery

Patients who have had a previous cesarean delivery and now present with the expectation of a vaginal delivery are coded using codes 59610-59622. If the patient has a successful vaginal delivery after a previous cesarean delivery (VBAC), use codes 59610-59614. If the attempt is unsuccessful and another cesarean delivery is carried out, use codes 59618-59622. To report elective cesarean deliveries use code 59510, 59514 or 59515.

(For insertion of transcervical or transvaginal fetal oximetry sensor, use Category III code 0021T)

59610 Routine obstetric care including antepartum care, vaginal delivery (with or without episiotomy, and/or forceps) and postpartum care, after previous cesarean delivery

59612 Vaginal delivery only, after previous cesarean delivery (with or without episiotomy and/or forceps);

59614   including postpartum care

59618 Routine obstetric care including antepartum care, cesarean delivery, and postpartum care, following attempted vaginal delivery after previous cesarean delivery

59620 Cesarean delivery only, following attempted vaginal delivery after previous cesarean delivery;

59622   including postpartum care

Abortion

(For medical treatment of spontaneous complete abortion, any trimester, use E/M codes 99201-99233)

(For surgical treatment of spontaneous abortion, use 59812)

59812 Treatment of incomplete abortion, any trimester, completed surgically

59820 Treatment of missed abortion, completed surgically; first trimester

59821   second trimester

59830 Treatment of septic abortion, completed surgically

59840 Induced abortion, by dilation and curettage

59841 Induced abortion, by dilation and evacuation

59850 Induced abortion, by one or more intra-amniotic injections (amniocentesis-injections), including hospital admission and visits, delivery of fetus and secundines;

59851   with dilation and curettage and/or evacuation

59852   with hysterotomy (failed intra-amniotic injection)

(For insertion of cervical dilator, use 59200)

59855 Induced abortion, by one or more vaginal suppositories (eg, prostaglandin) with or without cervical dilation (eg, laminaria), including hospital admission and visits, delivery of fetus and secundines;

59856   with dilation and curettage and/or evacuation

59857   with hysterotomy (failed medical evacuation)

Other Procedures

59866 Multifetal pregnancy reduction(s) (MPR)

59870 Uterine evacuation and curettage for hydatidiform mole

59871 Removal of cerclage suture under anesthesia (other than local)

59897 Unlisted fetal invasive procedure, including ultrasound guidance

59898 Unlisted laparoscopy procedure, maternity care and delivery

59899 Unlisted procedure, maternity care and delivery

Surgery: Male/Female Genital System

Notes

⊙=Moderate sedation　✚=Add-on code　✔=FDA approval pending

Endocrine System

(For pituitary and pineal surgery, see **Nervous System**)

Thyroid Gland

Incision

60000   Incision and drainage of thyroglossal duct cyst, infected

Excision

60001   Aspiration and/or injection, thyroid cyst

(For fine needle aspiration, see 10021, 10022)

▶(If imaging guidance is performed, see 76942, 77012)◀

60100   Biopsy thyroid, percutaneous core needle

▶(If imaging guidance is performed, see 76942, 77002, 77012, 77021)◀

(For fine needle aspiration, use 10021 or 10022)

(For evaluation of fine needle aspirate, see 88172, 88173)

60200   Excision of cyst or adenoma of thyroid, or transection of isthmus

60210   Partial thyroid lobectomy, unilateral; with or without isthmusectomy

60212   with contralateral subtotal lobectomy, including isthmusectomy

60220   Total thyroid lobectomy, unilateral; with or without isthmusectomy

60225   with contralateral subtotal lobectomy, including isthmusectomy

60240   Thyroidectomy, total or complete

(For thyroidectomy, subtotal or partial, use 60271)

60252   Thyroidectomy, total or subtotal for malignancy; with limited neck dissection

60254   with radical neck dissection

60260   Thyroidectomy, removal of all remaining thyroid tissue following previous removal of a portion of thyroid

(For bilateral procedure, report 60260 with modifier 50)

60270   Thyroidectomy, including substernal thyroid; sternal split or transthoracic approach

60271   cervical approach

60280   Excision of thyroglossal duct cyst or sinus;

60281   recurrent

(For thyroid ultrasonography, use 76536)

Parathyroid, Thymus, Adrenal Glands, Pancreas, and Carotid Body

Excision

(For pituitary and pineal surgery, see **Nervous System**)

60500   Parathyroidectomy or exploration of parathyroid(s);

60502   re-exploration

60505   with mediastinal exploration, sternal split or transthoracic approach

+ 60512   Parathyroid autotransplantation (List separately in addition to code for primary procedure)

(Use 60512 in conjunction with 60500, 60502, 60505, 60212, 60225, 60240, 60252, 60254, 60260, 60270, 60271)

60520   Thymectomy, partial or total; transcervical approach (separate procedure)

60521   sternal split or transthoracic approach, without radical mediastinal dissection (separate procedure)

60522   sternal split or transthoracic approach, with radical mediastinal dissection (separate procedure)

60540   Adrenalectomy, partial or complete, or exploration of adrenal gland with or without biopsy, transabdominal, lumbar or dorsal (separate procedure);

60545   with excision of adjacent retroperitoneal tumor

(Do not report 60540, 60545 in conjunction with 50323)

(For bilateral procedure, report 60540 with modifier 50)

(For excision of remote or disseminated pheochromocytoma, see 49200, 49201)

(For laparoscopic approach, use 60650)

60600   Excision of carotid body tumor; without excision of carotid artery

60605   with excision of carotid artery

Laparoscopy

Surgical laparoscopy always includes diagnostic laparoscopy. To report a diagnostic laparoscopy (peritoneoscopy) (separate procedure), use 49320.

60650   Laparoscopy, surgical, with adrenalectomy, partial or complete, or exploration of adrenal gland with or without biopsy, transabdominal, lumbar or dorsal

60659   Unlisted laparoscopy procedure, endocrine system

Other Procedures

60699   Unlisted procedure, endocrine system

Surgery: Nervous System

Notes

⊙=Moderate sedation ✚=Add-on code ✔=FDA approval pending

Nervous System

Skull, Meninges, and Brain

(For injection procedure for cerebral angiography, see 36100-36218)

(For injection procedure for ventriculography, see 61026, 61120)

(For injection procedure for pneumoencephalography, use 61055)

Injection, Drainage, or Aspiration

61000 Subdural tap through fontanelle, or suture, infant, unilateral or bilateral; initial

61001   subsequent taps

61020 Ventricular puncture through previous burr hole, fontanelle, suture, or implanted ventricular catheter/reservoir; without injection

61026   with injection of medication or other substance for diagnosis or treatment

61050 Cisternal or lateral cervical (C1-C2) puncture; without injection (separate procedure)

61055   with injection of medication or other substance for diagnosis or treatment (eg, C1-C2)

(For radiological supervision and interpretation, see **Radiology**)

61070 Puncture of shunt tubing or reservoir for aspiration or injection procedure

(For radiological supervision and interpretation, use 75809)

Twist Drill, Burr Hole(s), or Trephine

61105 Twist drill hole for subdural or ventricular puncture

⊘▲ **61107** Twist drill hole(s) for subdural, intracerebral, or ventricular puncture; for implanting ventricular catheter, pressure recording device, or other intracerebral monitoring device

(For intracranial neuroendoscopic ventricular catheter placement, use 62160)

(For twist drill or burr hole performed to place thermal perfusion probe, use Category III code 0077T)

61108   for evacuation and/or drainage of subdural hematoma

61120 Burr hole(s) for ventricular puncture (including injection of gas, contrast media, dye, or radioactive material)

61140 Burr hole(s) or trephine; with biopsy of brain or intracranial lesion

61150   with drainage of brain abscess or cyst

61151   with subsequent tapping (aspiration) of intracranial abscess or cyst

61154 Burr hole(s) with evacuation and/or drainage of hematoma, extradural or subdural

(For bilateral procedure, report 61154 with modifier 50)

61156 Burr hole(s); with aspiration of hematoma or cyst, intracerebral

⊘▲ **61210**   for implanting ventricular catheter, reservoir, EEG electrode(s), pressure recording device, or other cerebral monitoring device (separate procedure)

(For intracranial neuroendoscopic ventricular catheter placement, use 62160)

61215 Insertion of subcutaneous reservoir, pump or continuous infusion system for connection to ventricular catheter

(For refilling and maintenance of an implantable infusion pump for spinal or brain drug therapy, use 95990)

(For chemotherapy, use 96450)

61250 Burr hole(s) or trephine, supratentorial, exploratory, not followed by other surgery

(For bilateral procedure, report 61250 with modifier 50)

61253 Burr hole(s) or trephine, infratentorial, unilateral or bilateral

(If burr hole(s) or trephine are followed by craniotomy at same operative session, use 61304-61321; do not use 61250 or 61253)

Craniectomy or Craniotomy

61304 Craniectomy or craniotomy, exploratory; supratentorial

61305   infratentorial (posterior fossa)

61312 Craniectomy or craniotomy for evacuation of hematoma, supratentorial; extradural or subdural

61313   intracerebral

61314 Craniectomy or craniotomy for evacuation of hematoma, infratentorial; extradural or subdural

61315   intracerebellar

+ **61316** Incision and subcutaneous placement of cranial bone graft (List separately in addition to code for primary procedure)

(Use 61316 in conjunction with 61304, 61312, 61313, 61322, 61323, 61340, 61570, 61571, 61680-61705)

61320 Craniectomy or craniotomy, drainage of intracranial abscess; supratentorial

61321   infratentorial

Surgery: Nervous System

61322 Craniectomy or craniotomy, decompressive, with or without duraplasty, for treatment of intracranial hypertension, without evacuation of associated intraparenchymal hematoma; without lobectomy

(Do not report 61313 in addition to 61322)

(For subtemporal decompression, use 61340)

61323 　　with lobectomy

(Do not report 61313 in addition to 61323)

(For subtemporal decompression, use 61340)

61330 Decompression of orbit only, transcranial approach

(For bilateral procedure, report 61330 with modifier 50)

61332 Exploration of orbit (transcranial approach); with biopsy

61333 　　with removal of lesion

61334 　　with removal of foreign body

61340 Subtemporal cranial decompression (pseudotumor cerebri, slit ventricle syndrome)

(For bilateral procedure, report 61340 with modifier 50)

(For decompressive craniotomy or craniectomy for intracranial hypertension, without hematoma evacuation, see 61322, 61323)

61343 Craniectomy, suboccipital with cervical laminectomy for decompression of medulla and spinal cord, with or without dural graft (eg, Arnold-Chiari malformation)

61345 Other cranial decompression, posterior fossa

(For orbital decompression by lateral wall approach, Kroenlein type, use 67445)

61440 Craniotomy for section of tentorium cerebelli (separate procedure)

61450 Craniectomy, subtemporal, for section, compression, or decompression of sensory root of gasserian ganglion

61458 Craniectomy, suboccipital; for exploration or decompression of cranial nerves

61460 　　for section of one or more cranial nerves

61470 　　for medullary tractotomy

61480 　　for mesencephalic tractotomy or pedunculotomy

61490 Craniotomy for lobotomy, including cingulotomy

(For bilateral procedure, report 61490 with modifier 50)

61500 Craniectomy; with excision of tumor or other bone lesion of skull

61501 　　for osteomyelitis

61510 Craniectomy, trephination, bone flap craniotomy; for excision of brain tumor, supratentorial, except meningioma

61512 　　for excision of meningioma, supratentorial

⊙ **61514** 　　for excision of brain abscess, supratentorial

61516 　　for excision or fenestration of cyst, supratentorial

(For excision of pituitary tumor or craniopharyngioma, see 61545, 61546, 61548)

+ 61517 Implantation of brain intracavitary chemotherapy agent (List separately in addition to code for primary procedure)

(Use 61517 only in conjunction with 61510 or 61518)

(Do not report 61517 for brachytherapy insertion. For intracavitary insertion of radioelement sources or ribbons, see 77781-77784)

61518 Craniectomy for excision of brain tumor, infratentorial or posterior fossa; except meningioma, cerebellopontine angle tumor, or midline tumor at base of skull

61519 　　meningioma

61520 　　cerebellopontine angle tumor

61521 　　midline tumor at base of skull

61522 Craniectomy, infratentorial or posterior fossa; for excision of brain abscess

61524 　　for excision or fenestration of cyst

61526 Craniectomy, bone flap craniotomy, transtemporal (mastoid) for excision of cerebellopontine angle tumor;

61530 　　combined with middle/posterior fossa craniotomy/craniectomy

61531 Subdural implantation of strip electrodes through one or more burr or trephine hole(s) for long term seizure monitoring

(For stereotactic implantation of electrodes, use 61760)

(For craniotomy for excision of intracranial arteriovenous malformation, see 61680-61692)

61533 Craniotomy with elevation of bone flap; for subdural implantation of an electrode array, for long term seizure monitoring

(For continuous EEG monitoring, see 95950-95954)

61534 　　for excision of epileptogenic focus without electrocorticography during surgery

61535 　　for removal of epidural or subdural electrode array, without excision of cerebral tissue (separate procedure)

61536 　　for excision of cerebral epileptogenic focus, with electrocorticography during surgery (includes removal of electrode array)

61537 　　for lobectomy, temporal lobe, without electrocorticography during surgery

61538 　　for lobectomy, temporal lobe, with electrocorticography during surgery

61539   for lobectomy, other than temporal lobe, partial or total, with electrocorticography during surgery

61540   for lobectomy, other than temporal lobe, partial or total, without electrocorticography during surgery

61541   for transection of corpus callosum

61542   for total hemispherectomy

61543   for partial or subtotal (functional) hemispherectomy

61544   for excision or coagulation of choroid plexus

61545   for excision of craniopharyngioma

(For craniotomy for selective amygdalohippocampectomy, use 61566)

(For craniotomy for multiple subpial transections during surgery, use 61567)

61546   Craniotomy for hypophysectomy or excision of pituitary tumor, intracranial approach

61548   Hypophysectomy or excision of pituitary tumor, transnasal or transseptal approach, nonstereotactic

(Do not report code 69990 in addition to code 61548)

61550   Craniectomy for craniosynostosis; single cranial suture

61552   multiple cranial sutures

(For cranial reconstruction for orbital hypertelorism, see 21260-21263)

(For reconstruction, see 21172-21180)

61556   Craniotomy for craniosynostosis; frontal or parietal bone flap

61557   bifrontal bone flap

61558   Extensive craniectomy for multiple cranial suture craniosynostosis (eg, cloverleaf skull); not requiring bone grafts

61559   recontouring with multiple osteotomies and bone autografts (eg, barrel-stave procedure) (includes obtaining grafts)

(For reconstruction, see 21172-21180)

61563   Excision, intra and extracranial, benign tumor of cranial bone (eg, fibrous dysplasia); without optic nerve decompression

61564   with optic nerve decompression

(For reconstruction, see 21181-21183)

61566   Craniotomy with elevation of bone flap; for selective amygdalohippocampectomy

61567   for multiple subpial transections, with electrocorticography during surgery

61570   Craniectomy or craniotomy; with excision of foreign body from brain

61571   with treatment of penetrating wound of brain

(For sequestrectomy for osteomyelitis, use 61501)

61575   Transoral approach to skull base, brain stem or upper spinal cord for biopsy, decompression or excision of lesion;

61576   requiring splitting of tongue and/or mandible (including tracheostomy)

(For arthrodesis, use 22548)

Surgery of Skull Base

The surgical management of lesions involving the skull base (base of anterior, middle, and posterior cranial fossae) often requires the skills of several surgeons of different surgical specialties working together or in tandem during the operative session. These operations are usually not staged because of the need for definitive closure of dura, subcutaneous tissues, and skin to avoid serious infections such as osteomyelitis and/or meningitis.

The procedures are categorized according to: 1) *approach procedure* necessary to obtain adequate exposure to the lesion (pathologic entity), 2) *definitive procedure(s)* necessary to biopsy, excise or otherwise treat the lesion, and 3) *repair/reconstruction* of the defect present following the definitive procedure(s).

The *approach procedure* is described according to anatomical area involved, ie, anterior cranial fossa, middle cranial fossa, posterior cranial fossa, and brain stem or upper spinal cord.

The *definitive procedure(s)* describes the repair, biopsy, resection, or excision of various lesions of the skull base and, when appropriate, primary closure of the dura, mucous membranes, and skin.

The *repair/reconstruction procedure(s)* is reported separately if extensive dural grafting, cranioplasty, local or regional myocutaneous pedicle flaps, or extensive skin grafts are required.

For primary closure, see the appropriate codes, ie, 15732, 15756-15758.

When one surgeon performs the approach procedure, another surgeon performs the definitive procedure, and another surgeon performs the repair/reconstruction procedure, each surgeon reports only the code for the specific procedure performed.

If one surgeon performs more than one procedure (ie, approach procedure and definitive procedure), then both codes are reported, adding modifier 51 to the secondary, additional procedure(s).

Surgery: Nervous System

Approach Procedures

Anterior Cranial Fossa

61580 Craniofacial approach to anterior cranial fossa; extradural, including lateral rhinotomy, ethmoidectomy, sphenoidectomy, without maxillectomy or orbital exenteration

61581 extradural, including lateral rhinotomy, orbital exenteration, ethmoidectomy, sphenoidectomy and/or maxillectomy

61582 extradural, including unilateral or bifrontal craniotomy, elevation of frontal lobe(s), osteotomy of base of anterior cranial fossa

61583 intradural, including unilateral or bifrontal craniotomy, elevation or resection of frontal lobe, osteotomy of base of anterior cranial fossa

61584 Orbitocranial approach to anterior cranial fossa, extradural, including supraorbital ridge osteotomy and elevation of frontal and/or temporal lobe(s); without orbital exenteration

61585 with orbital exenteration

61586 Bicoronal, transzygomatic and/or LeFort I osteotomy approach to anterior cranial fossa with or without internal fixation, without bone graft

Middle Cranial Fossa

61590 Infratemporal pre-auricular approach to middle cranial fossa (parapharyngeal space, infratemporal and midline skull base, nasopharynx), with or without disarticulation of the mandible, including parotidectomy, craniotomy, decompression and/or mobilization of the facial nerve and/or petrous carotid artery

61591 Infratemporal post-auricular approach to middle cranial fossa (internal auditory meatus, petrous apex, tentorium, cavernous sinus, parasellar area, infratemporal fossa) including mastoidectomy, resection of sigmoid sinus, with or without decompression and/or mobilization of contents of auditory canal or petrous carotid artery

61592 Orbitocranial zygomatic approach to middle cranial fossa (cavernous sinus and carotid artery, clivus, basilar artery or petrous apex) including osteotomy of zygoma, craniotomy, extra- or intradural elevation of temporal lobe

Posterior Cranial Fossa

61595 Transtemporal approach to posterior cranial fossa, jugular foramen or midline skull base, including mastoidectomy, decompression of sigmoid sinus and/or facial nerve, with or without mobilization

61596 Transcochlear approach to posterior cranial fossa, jugular foramen or midline skull base, including labyrinthectomy, decompression, with or without mobilization of facial nerve and/or petrous carotid artery

61597 Transcondylar (far lateral) approach to posterior cranial fossa, jugular foramen or midline skull base, including occipital condylectomy, mastoidectomy, resection of C1-C3 vertebral body(s), decompression of vertebral artery, with or without mobilization

61598 Transpetrosal approach to posterior cranial fossa, clivus or foramen magnum, including ligation of superior petrosal sinus and/or sigmoid sinus

Definitive Procedures

Base of Anterior Cranial Fossa

61600 Resection or excision of neoplastic, vascular or infectious lesion of base of anterior cranial fossa; extradural

61601 intradural, including dural repair, with or without graft

Base of Middle Cranial Fossa

61605 Resection or excision of neoplastic, vascular or infectious lesion of infratemporal fossa, parapharyngeal space, petrous apex; extradural

61606 intradural, including dural repair, with or without graft

61607 Resection or excision of neoplastic, vascular or infectious lesion of parasellar area, cavernous sinus, clivus or midline skull base; extradural

61608 intradural, including dural repair, with or without graft

Codes 61609-61612 are reported in addition to code(s) for primary procedure(s) 61605-61608. Report only one transection or ligation of carotid artery code per operative session.

+ 61609 Transection or ligation, carotid artery in cavernous sinus; without repair (List separately in addition to code for primary procedure)

+ 61610 with repair by anastomosis or graft (List separately in addition to code for primary procedure)

+ 61611 Transection or ligation, carotid artery in petrous canal; without repair (List separately in addition to code for primary procedure)

+ 61612 with repair by anastomosis or graft (List separately in addition to code for primary procedure)

61613 Obliteration of carotid aneurysm, arteriovenous malformation, or carotid-cavernous fistula by dissection within cavernous sinus

Surgery: Nervous System

Base of Posterior Cranial Fossa

61615   Resection or excision of neoplastic, vascular or infectious lesion of base of posterior cranial fossa, jugular foramen, foramen magnum, or C1-C3 vertebral bodies; extradural

61616   intradural, including dural repair, with or without graft

Repair and/or Reconstruction of Surgical Defects of Skull Base

61618   Secondary repair of dura for cerebrospinal fluid leak, anterior, middle or posterior cranial fossa following surgery of the skull base; by free tissue graft (eg, pericranium, fascia, tensor fascia lata, adipose tissue, homologous or synthetic grafts)

61619   by local or regionalized vascularized pedicle flap or myocutaneous flap (including galea, temporalis, frontalis or occipitalis muscle)

Endovascular Therapy

61623   Endovascular temporary balloon arterial occlusion, head or neck (extracranial/intracranial) including selective catheterization of vessel to be occluded, positioning and inflation of occlusion balloon, concomitant neurological monitoring, and radiologic supervision and interpretation of all angiography required for balloon occlusion and to exclude vascular injury post occlusion

(If selective catheterization and angiography of arteries other than artery to be occluded is performed, use appropriate catheterization and radiologic supervision and interpretation codes)

(If complete diagnostic angiography of the artery to be occluded is performed immediately prior to temporary occlusion, use appropriate radiologic supervision and interpretation codes only)

61624   Transcatheter permanent occlusion or embolization (eg, for tumor destruction, to achieve hemostasis, to occlude a vascular malformation), percutaneous, any method; central nervous system (intracranial, spinal cord)

(See also 37204)

(For radiological supervision and interpretation, use 75894)

61626   non-central nervous system, head or neck (extracranial, brachiocephalic branch)

(See also 37204)

(For radiological supervision and interpretation, use 75894)

61630   Balloon angioplasty, intracranial (eg, atherosclerotic stenosis), percutaneous

61635   Transcatheter placement of intravascular stent(s), intracranial (eg, atherosclerotic stenosis), including balloon angioplasty, if performed

(61630 and 61635 include all selective vascular catheterization of the target vascular family, all diagnostic imaging for arteriography of the target vascular family, and all related radiological supervision and interpretation. When diagnostic arteriogram (including imaging and selective catheterization) confirms the need for angioplasty or stent placement, 61630 and 61635 are inclusive of these services. If angioplasty or stenting are not indicated, then the appropriate codes for selective catheterization and imaging should be reported in lieu of 61630 and 61635)

61640   Balloon dilatation of intracranial vasospasm, percutaneous; initial vessel

+ 61641   each additional vessel in same vascular family (List separately in addition to code for primary procedure)

+ 61642   each additional vessel in different vascular family (List separately in addition to code for primary procedure)

(Use 61641 and 61642 in conjunction with 61640)

(61640, 61641, 61642 include all selective vascular catheterization of the target vessel, contrast injection(s), vessel measurement, roadmapping, postdilatation angiography, and fluoroscopic guidance for the balloon dilatation)

Surgery for Aneurysm, Arteriovenous Malformation or Vascular Disease

Includes craniotomy when appropriate for procedure.

61680   Surgery of intracranial arteriovenous malformation; supratentorial, simple

61682   supratentorial, complex

61684   infratentorial, simple

61686   infratentorial, complex

61690   dural, simple

61692   dural, complex

61697   Surgery of complex intracranial aneurysm, intracranial approach; carotid circulation

61698   vertebrobasilar circulation

(61697, 61698 involve aneurysms that are larger than 15 mm or with calcification of the aneurysm neck, or with incorporation of normal vessels into the aneurysm neck, or a procedure requiring temporary vessel occlusion, trapping or cardiopulmonary bypass to successfully treat the aneurysm)

61700   Surgery of simple intracranial aneurysm, intracranial approach; carotid circulation

61702   vertebrobasilar circulation

Surgery: Nervous System

61703   Surgery of intracranial aneurysm, cervical approach by application of occluding clamp to cervical carotid artery (Selverstone-Crutchfield type)

(For cervical approach for direct ligation of carotid artery, see 37600-37606)

61705   Surgery of aneurysm, vascular malformation or carotid-cavernous fistula; by intracranial and cervical occlusion of carotid artery

61708   by intracranial electrothrombosis

(For ligation or gradual occlusion of internal/common carotid artery, see 37605, 37606)

61710   by intra-arterial embolization, injection procedure, or balloon catheter

61711   Anastomosis, arterial, extracranial-intracranial (eg, middle cerebral/cortical) arteries

(For carotid or vertebral thromboendarterectomy, use 35301)

(Use 69990 when the surgical microscope is employed for the microsurgical procedure. Do not use 69990 for visualization with magnifying loupes or corrected vision)

Stereotaxis

61720   Creation of lesion by stereotactic method, including burr hole(s) and localizing and recording techniques, single or multiple stages; globus pallidus or thalamus

61735   subcortical structure(s) other than globus pallidus or thalamus

61750   Stereotactic biopsy, aspiration, or excision, including burr hole(s), for intracranial lesion;

61751   with computed tomography and/or magnetic resonance guidance

(For radiological supervision and interpretation of computerized tomography, see 70450, 70460, or 70470 as appropriate)

(For radiological supervision and interpretation of magnetic resonance imaging, see 70551, 70552, or 70553 as appropriate)

61760   Stereotactic implantation of depth electrodes into the cerebrum for long term seizure monitoring

61770   Stereotactic localization, including burr hole(s), with insertion of catheter(s) or probe(s) for placement of radiation source

61790   Creation of lesion by stereotactic method, percutaneous, by neurolytic agent (eg, alcohol, thermal, electrical, radiofrequency); gasserian ganglion

61791   trigeminal medullary tract

61793   Stereotactic radiosurgery (particle beam, gamma ray or linear accelerator), one or more sessions

(For intensity modulated beam delivery plan and treatment, see 77301, 77418)

+ 61795   Stereotactic computer-assisted volumetric (navigational) procedure, intracranial, extracranial, or spinal (List separately in addition to code for primary procedure)

Neurostimulators (Intracranial)

Codes 61850-61888 apply to both simple and complex neurostimulators. For initial or subsequent electronic analysis and programming of neurostimulator pulse generators, see codes 95970-95975.

Microelectrode recording, when performed by the operating surgeon in association with implantation of neurostimulator electrode arrays, is an inclusive service and should not be reported separately. If another physician participates in neurophysiological mapping during a deep brain stimulator implantation procedure, this service may be reported by the other physician with codes 95961-95962.

61850   Twist drill or burr hole(s) for implantation of neurostimulator electrodes, cortical

61860   Craniectomy or craniotomy for implantation of neurostimulator electrodes, cerebral, cortical

61863   Twist drill, burr hole, craniotomy, or craniectomy with stereotactic implantation of neurostimulator electrode array in subcortical site (eg, thalamus, globus pallidus, subthalamic nucleus, periventricular, periaqueductal gray), without use of intraoperative microelectrode recording; first array

+ 61864   each additional array (List separately in addition to primary procedure)

(Use 61864 in conjunction with 61863)

61867   Twist drill, burr hole, craniotomy, or craniectomy with stereotactic implantation of neurostimulator electrode array in subcortical site (eg, thalamus, globus pallidus, subthalamic nucleus, periventricular, periaqueductal gray), with use of intraoperative microelectrode recording; first array

+ 61868   each additional array (List separately in addition to primary procedure)

(Use 61868 in conjunction with 61867)

61870   Craniectomy for implantation of neurostimulator electrodes, cerebellar; cortical

61875   subcortical

61880   Revision or removal of intracranial neurostimulator electrodes

61885   Insertion or replacement of cranial neurostimulator pulse generator or receiver, direct or inductive coupling; with connection to a single electrode array

61886   with connection to two or more electrode arrays

(For open placement of cranial nerve (eg, vagal, trigeminal) neurostimulator electrode(s), use 64573)

(For percutaneous placement of cranial nerve (eg, vagal, trigeminal) neurostimulator electrode(s), use 64553)

(For revision or removal of cranial nerve (eg, vagal, trigeminal) neurostimulator electrode(s), use 64585)

61888   Revision or removal of cranial neurostimulator pulse generator or receiver

(Do not report 61888 in conjunction with 61885 or 61886 for the same pulse generator)

Repair

62000   Elevation of depressed skull fracture; simple, extradural

62005   compound or comminuted, extradural

62010   with repair of dura and/or debridement of brain

62100   Craniotomy for repair of dural/cerebrospinal fluid leak, including surgery for rhinorrhea/otorrhea

(For repair of spinal dural/CSF leak, see 63707, 63709)

62115   Reduction of craniomegalic skull (eg, treated hydrocephalus); not requiring bone grafts or cranioplasty

62116   with simple cranioplasty

62117   requiring craniotomy and reconstruction with or without bone graft (includes obtaining grafts)

62120   Repair of encephalocele, skull vault, including cranioplasty

62121   Craniotomy for repair of encephalocele, skull base

62140   Cranioplasty for skull defect; up to 5 cm diameter

62141   larger than 5 cm diameter

62142   Removal of bone flap or prosthetic plate of skull

62143   Replacement of bone flap or prosthetic plate of skull

62145   Cranioplasty for skull defect with reparative brain surgery

62146   Cranioplasty with autograft (includes obtaining bone grafts); up to 5 cm diameter

62147   larger than 5 cm diameter

+ 62148   Incision and retrieval of subcutaneous cranial bone graft for cranioplasty (List separately in addition to code for primary procedure)

(Use 62148 in conjunction with 62140-62147)

Neuroendoscopy

Surgical endoscopy always includes diagnostic endoscopy.

+ 62160   Neuroendoscopy, intracranial, for placement or replacement of ventricular catheter and attachment to shunt system or external drainage (List separately in addition to code for primary procedure)

▶(Use 62160 only in conjunction with 61107, 61210, 62220-62230, 62258)◀

62161   Neuroendoscopy, intracranial; with dissection of adhesions, fenestration of septum pellucidum or intraventricular cysts (including placement, replacement, or removal of ventricular catheter)

62162   with fenestration or excision of colloid cyst, including placement of external ventricular catheter for drainage

62163   with retrieval of foreign body

62164   with excision of brain tumor, including placement of external ventricular catheter for drainage

62165   with excision of pituitary tumor, transnasal or trans-sphenoidal approach

Cerebrospinal Fluid (CSF) Shunt

62180   Ventriculocisternostomy (Torkildsen type operation)

62190   Creation of shunt; subarachnoid/subdural-atrial, -jugular, -auricular

62192   subarachnoid/subdural-peritoneal, -pleural, other terminus

62194   Replacement or irrigation, subarachnoid/subdural catheter

62200   Ventriculocisternostomy, third ventricle;

62201   stereotactic, neuroendoscopic method

(For intracranial neuroendoscopic procedures, see 62161-62165)

62220   Creation of shunt; ventriculo-atrial, -jugular, -auricular

(For intracranial neuroendoscopic ventricular catheter placement, use 62160)

62223   ventriculo-peritoneal, -pleural, other terminus

(For intracranial neuroendoscopic ventricular catheter placement, use 62160)

62225   Replacement or irrigation, ventricular catheter

(For intracranial neuroendoscopic ventricular catheter placement, use 62160)

62230   Replacement or revision of cerebrospinal fluid shunt, obstructed valve, or distal catheter in shunt system

(For intracranial neuroendoscopic ventricular catheter placement, use 62160)

62252   Reprogramming of programmable cerebrospinal shunt

62256   Removal of complete cerebrospinal fluid shunt system; without replacement

62258   with replacement by similar or other shunt at same operation

(For percutaneous irrigation or aspiration of shunt reservoir, use 61070)

(For reprogramming of programmable CSF shunt, use 62252)

▶(For intracranial neuroendoscopic ventricular catheter placement, use 62160)◀

Surgery: Nervous System

Spine and Spinal Cord

(For application of caliper or tongs, use 20660)

(For treatment of fracture or dislocation of spine, see 22305-22327)

Injection, Drainage, or Aspiration

►Injection of contrast during fluoroscopic guidance and localization is an inclusive component of codes 62263-62264, 62270-62273, 62280-62282, 62310-62319, 0027T. Fluoroscopic guidance and localization is reported by code 77003, unless a formal contrast study (myelography, epidurography, or arthrography) is performed, in which case the use of fluoroscopy is included in the supervision and interpretation codes.◄

For radiologic supervision and interpretation of epidurography, use 72275. Code 72275 is only to be used when an epidurogram is performed, images documented, and a formal radiologic report is issued.

Code 62263 describes a catheter-based treatment involving targeted injection of various substances (eg, hypertonic saline, steroid, anesthetic) via an indwelling epidural catheter. Code 62263 includes percutaneous insertion and removal of an epidural catheter (remaining in place over a several-day period), for the administration of multiple injections of a neurolytic agent(s) performed during serial treatment sessions (ie, spanning two or more treatment days). If required, adhesions or scarring may also be lysed by mechanical means. Code 62263 is NOT reported for each adhesiolysis treatment, but should be reported ONCE to describe the entire series of injections/infusions spanning two or more treatment days. For endoscopic lysis of adhesions, use 0027T.

Code 62264 describes multiple adhesiolysis treatment sessions performed on the same day. Adhesions or scarring may be lysed by injections of neurolytic agent(s). If required, adhesions or scarring may also be lysed mechanically using a percutaneously-deployed catheter.

►Codes 62263 and 62264 include the procedure of injections of contrast for epidurography (72275) and fluoroscopic guidance and localization (77003) during initial or subsequent sessions.◄

(Report 01996 for daily hospital management of continuous epidural or subarachnoid drug administration performed in conjunction with 62318-62319)

(For endoscopic lysis of epidural adhesions, use Category III code 0027T)

62263   Percutaneous lysis of epidural adhesions using solution injection (eg, hypertonic saline, enzyme) or mechanical means (eg, catheter) including radiologic localization (includes contrast when administered), multiple adhesiolysis sessions; 2 or more days

►(62263 includes codes 72275 and 77003)◄

62264   1 day

(Do not report 62264 with 62263)

►(62264 includes codes 72275 and 77003)◄

62268   Percutaneous aspiration, spinal cord cyst or syrinx

►(For radiological supervision and interpretation, see 76942, 77002, 77012)◄

62269   Biopsy of spinal cord, percutaneous needle

►(For radiological supervision and interpretation, see 76942, 77002, 77012)◄

(For fine needle aspiration, see 10021, 10022)

(For evaluation of fine needle aspirate, see 88172, 88173)

62270   Spinal puncture, lumbar, diagnostic

62272   Spinal puncture, therapeutic, for drainage of cerebrospinal fluid (by needle or catheter)

62273   Injection, epidural, of blood or clot patch

(For injection of diagnostic or therapeutic substance(s), see 62310, 62311, 62318, 62319)

62280   Injection/infusion of neurolytic substance (eg, alcohol, phenol, iced saline solutions), with or without other therapeutic substance; subarachnoid

62281   epidural, cervical or thoracic

62282   epidural, lumbar, sacral (caudal)

⊘ **62284**   Injection procedure for myelography and/or computed tomography, spinal (other than C1-C2 and posterior fossa)

(For injection procedure at C1-C2, use 61055)

(For radiological supervision and interpretation, see **Radiology**)

62287   Aspiration or decompression procedure, percutaneous, of nucleus pulposus of intervertebral disc, any method, single or multiple levels, lumbar (eg, manual or automated percutaneous discectomy, percutaneous laser discectomy)

►(For fluoroscopic guidance, use 77002)◄

(For injection of non-neurolytic diagnostic or therapeutic substance(s), see 62310, 62311)

62290   Injection procedure for discography, each level; lumbar

62291   cervical or thoracic

(For radiological supervision and interpretation, see 72285, 72295)

62292   Injection procedure for chemonucleolysis, including discography, intervertebral disc, single or multiple levels, lumbar

62294   Injection procedure, arterial, for occlusion of arteriovenous malformation, spinal

62310   Injection, single (not via indwelling catheter), not including neurolytic substances, with or without contrast (for either localization or epidurography), of diagnostic or therapeutic substance(s) (including anesthetic, antispasmodic, opioid, steroid, other solution), epidural or subarachnoid; cervical or thoracic

62311   lumbar, sacral (caudal)

62318   Injection, including catheter placement, continuous infusion or intermittent bolus, not including neurolytic substances, with or without contrast (for either localization or epidurography), of diagnostic or therapeutic substance(s) (including anesthetic, antispasmodic, opioid, steroid, other solution), epidural or subarachnoid; cervical or thoracic

62319   lumbar, sacral (caudal)

(For transforaminal epidural injection, see 64479-64484)

(Report 01996 for daily hospital management of continuous epidural or subarachnoid drug administration performed in conjunction with 62318-62319)

Catheter Implantation

(For percutaneous placement of intrathecal or epidural catheter, see codes 62270-62273, 62280-62284, 62310-62319)

62350   Implantation, revision or repositioning of tunneled intrathecal or epidural catheter, for long-term medication administration via an external pump or implantable reservoir/infusion pump; without laminectomy

62351   with laminectomy

(For refilling and maintenance of an implantable infusion pump for spinal or brain drug therapy, see 95990, 95991)

62355   Removal of previously implanted intrathecal or epidural catheter

Reservoir/Pump Implantation

62360   Implantation or replacement of device for intrathecal or epidural drug infusion; subcutaneous reservoir

62361   non-programmable pump

62362   programmable pump, including preparation of pump, with or without programming

62365   Removal of subcutaneous reservoir or pump, previously implanted for intrathecal or epidural infusion

62367   Electronic analysis of programmable, implanted pump for intrathecal or epidural drug infusion (includes evaluation of reservoir status, alarm status, drug prescription status); without reprogramming

62368   with reprogramming

(For refilling and maintenance of an implantable infusion pump for spinal or brain drug therapy, use 95990-95991)

Posterior Extradural Laminotomy or Laminectomy for Exploration/ Decompression of Neural Elements or Excision of Herniated Intervertebral Discs

(When 63001-63048 are followed by arthrodesis, see 22590-22614)

63001   Laminectomy with exploration and/or decompression of spinal cord and/or cauda equina, without facetectomy, foraminotomy or discectomy, (eg, spinal stenosis), one or two vertebral segments; cervical

63003   thoracic

63005   lumbar, except for spondylolisthesis

63011   sacral

63012   Laminectomy with removal of abnormal facets and/or pars inter-articularis with decompression of cauda equina and nerve roots for spondylolisthesis, lumbar (Gill type procedure)

63015   Laminectomy with exploration and/or decompression of spinal cord and/or cauda equina, without facetectomy, foraminotomy or discectomy, (eg, spinal stenosis), more than 2 vertebral segments; cervical

63016   thoracic

63017   lumbar

63020   Laminotomy (hemilaminectomy), with decompression of nerve root(s), including partial facetectomy, foraminotomy and/or excision of herniated intervertebral disc; one interspace, cervical

(For bilateral procedure, report 63020 with modifier 50)

63030   one interspace, lumbar (including open or endoscopically-assisted approach)

(For bilateral procedure, report 63030 with modifier 50)

+ 63035   each additional interspace, cervical or lumbar (List separately in addition to code for primary procedure)

(Use 63035 in conjunction with 63020-63030)

(For bilateral procedure, report 63035 with modifier 50)

Surgery: Nervous System

63040 Laminotomy (hemilaminectomy), with decompression of nerve root(s), including partial facetectomy, foraminotomy and/or excision of herniated intervertebral disc, reexploration, single interspace; cervical

(For bilateral procedure, report 63040 with modifier 50)

63042 lumbar

(For bilateral procedure, report 63042 with modifier 50)

+ 63043 each additional cervical interspace (List separately in addition to code for primary procedure)

(Use 63043 in conjunction with 63040)

(For bilateral procedure, report 63043 with modifier 50)

+ 63044 each additional lumbar interspace (List separately in addition to code for primary procedure)

(Use 63044 in conjunction with 63042)

(For bilateral procedure, report 63044 with modifier 50)

63045 Laminectomy, facetectomy and foraminotomy (unilateral or bilateral with decompression of spinal cord, cauda equina and/or nerve root(s), (eg, spinal or lateral recess stenosis)), single vertebral segment; cervical

63046 thoracic

63047 lumbar

+ 63048 each additional segment, cervical, thoracic, or lumbar (List separately in addition to code for primary procedure)

(Use 63048 in conjunction with 63045-63047)

63050 Laminoplasty, cervical, with decompression of the spinal cord, two or more vertebral segments;

63051 with reconstruction of the posterior bony elements (including the application of bridging bone graft and non-segmental fixation devices (eg, wire, suture, mini-plates), when performed)

(Do not report 63050 or 63051 in conjunction with 22600, 22614, 22840-22842, 63001, 63015, 63045, 63048, 63295 for the same vertebral segment(s))

Transpedicular or Costovertebral Approach for Posterolateral Extradural Exploration/Decompression

63055 Transpedicular approach with decompression of spinal cord, equina and/or nerve root(s) (eg, herniated intervertebral disc), single segment; thoracic

63056 lumbar (including transfacet, or lateral extraforaminal approach) (eg, far lateral herniated intervertebral disc)

+ 63057 each additional segment, thoracic or lumbar (List separately in addition to code for primary procedure)

(Use 63057 in conjunction with 63055, 63056)

63064 Costovertebral approach with decompression of spinal cord or nerve root(s), (eg, herniated intervertebral disc), thoracic; single segment

+ 63066 each additional segment (List separately in addition to code for primary procedure)

(Use 63066 in conjunction with 63064)

(For excision of thoracic intraspinal lesions by laminectomy, see 63266, 63271, 63276, 63281, 63286)

Anterior or Anterolateral Approach for Extradural Exploration/Decompression

For the following codes, when two surgeons work together as primary surgeons performing distinct part(s) of spinal cord exploration/decompression operation, each surgeon should report his/her distinct operative work by appending modifier 62 to the procedure code (and any associated add-on codes for that procedure code as long as both surgeons continue to work together as primary surgeons). In this situation, modifier 62 may be appended to the definitive procedure code(s) 63075, 63077, 63081, 63085, 63087, 63090 and, as appropriate, to associated additional interspace add-on code(s) 63076, 63078 or additional segment add-on code(s) 63082, 63086, 63088, 63091 as long as both surgeons continue to work together as primary surgeons.

63075 Discectomy, anterior, with decompression of spinal cord and/or nerve root(s), including osteophytectomy; cervical, single interspace

+ 63076 cervical, each additional interspace (List separately in addition to code for primary procedure)

(Use 63076 in conjunction with 63075)

63077 thoracic, single interspace

+ 63078 thoracic, each additional interspace (List separately in addition to code for primary procedure)

(Use 63078 in conjunction with 63077)

(Do not report code 69990 in addition to codes 63075-63078)

63081 Vertebral corpectomy (vertebral body resection), partial or complete, anterior approach with decompression of spinal cord and/or nerve root(s); cervical, single segment

+ 63082 cervical, each additional segment (List separately in addition to code for primary procedure)

(Use 63082 in conjunction with 63081)

(For transoral approach, see 61575, 61576)

63085 Vertebral corpectomy (vertebral body resection), partial or complete, transthoracic approach with decompression of spinal cord and/or nerve root(s); thoracic, single segment

+ 63086 thoracic, each additional segment (List separately in addition to code for primary procedure)

(Use 63086 in conjunction with 63085)

Surgery: Nervous System

63087 Vertebral corpectomy (vertebral body resection), partial or complete, combined thoracolumbar approach with decompression of spinal cord, cauda equina or nerve root(s), lower thoracic or lumbar; single segment

+ 63088   each additional segment (List separately in addition to code for primary procedure)

(Use 63088 in conjunction with 63087)

63090 Vertebral corpectomy (vertebral body resection), partial or complete, transperitoneal or retroperitoneal approach with decompression of spinal cord, cauda equina or nerve root(s), lower thoracic, lumbar, or sacral; single segment

+ 63091   each additional segment (List separately in addition to code for primary procedure)

(Use 63091 in conjunction with 63090)

(Procedures 63081-63091 include discectomy above and/or below vertebral segment)

(If followed by arthrodesis, see 22548-22812)

(For reconstruction of spine, use appropriate vertebral corpectomy codes 63081-63091, bone graft codes 20930-20938, arthrodesis codes 22548-22812, and spinal instrumentation codes 22840-22855)

Lateral Extracavitary Approach for Extradural Exploration/Decompression

63101 Vertebral corpectomy (vertebral body resection), partial or complete, lateral extracavitary approach with decompression of spinal cord and/or nerve root(s) (eg, for tumor or retropulsed bone fragments); thoracic, single segment

63102   lumbar, single segment

+ 63103   thoracic or lumbar, each additional segment (List separately in addition to code for primary procedure)

(Use 63103 in conjunction with 63101 and 63102)

Incision

63170 Laminectomy with myelotomy (eg, Bischof or DREZ type), cervical, thoracic, or thoracolumbar

63172 Laminectomy with drainage of intramedullary cyst/syrinx; to subarachnoid space

63173   to peritoneal or pleural space

63180 Laminectomy and section of dentate ligaments, with or without dural graft, cervical; one or two segments

63182   more than two segments

63185 Laminectomy with rhizotomy; one or two segments

63190   more than two segments

63191 Laminectomy with section of spinal accessory nerve

(For bilateral procedure, report 63191 with modifier 50)

(For resection of sternocleidomastoid muscle, use 21720)

63194 Laminectomy with cordotomy, with section of one spinothalamic tract, one stage; cervical

63195   thoracic

63196 Laminectomy with cordotomy, with section of both spinothalamic tracts, one stage; cervical

63197   thoracic

63198 Laminectomy with cordotomy with section of both spinothalamic tracts, two stages within 14 days; cervical

63199   thoracic

63200 Laminectomy, with release of tethered spinal cord, lumbar

Excision by Laminectomy of Lesion Other Than Herniated Disc

63250 Laminectomy for excision or occlusion of arteriovenous malformation of spinal cord; cervical

63251   thoracic

63252   thoracolumbar

63265 Laminectomy for excision or evacuation of intraspinal lesion other than neoplasm, extradural; cervical

63266   thoracic

63267   lumbar

63268   sacral

63270 Laminectomy for excision of intraspinal lesion other than neoplasm, intradural; cervical

63271   thoracic

63272   lumbar

63273   sacral

63275 Laminectomy for biopsy/excision of intraspinal neoplasm; extradural, cervical

63276   extradural, thoracic

63277   extradural, lumbar

63278   extradural, sacral

63280   intradural, extramedullary, cervical

63281   intradural, extramedullary, thoracic

63282   intradural, extramedullary, lumbar

63283   intradural, sacral

63285   intradural, intramedullary, cervical

63286   intradural, intramedullary, thoracic

63287   intradural, intramedullary, thoracolumbar

63290   combined extradural-intradural lesion, any level

(For drainage of intramedullary cyst/syrinx, use 63172, 63173)

Surgery: Nervous System

Surgery: Nervous System

+ 63295   Osteoplastic reconstruction of dorsal spinal elements, following primary intraspinal procedure (List separately in addition to code for primary procedure)

(Use 63295 in conjunction with 63172, 63173, 63185, 63190, 63200-63290)

(Do not report 63295 in conjunction with 22590-22614, 22840-22844, 63050, 63051 for the same vertebral segment(s))

Excision, Anterior or Anterolateral Approach, Intraspinal Lesion

For the following codes, when two surgeons work together as primary surgeons performing distinct part(s) of an anterior approach for an intraspinal excision, each surgeon should report his/her distinct operative work by appending modifier 62 to the single definitive procedure code. In this situation, modifier 62 may be appended to the definitive procedure code(s) 63300-63307 and, as appropriate, to the associated additional segment add-on code 63308 as long as both surgeons continue to work together as primary surgeons.

(For arthrodesis, see 22548-22585)

(For reconstruction of spine, see 20930-20938)

63300   Vertebral corpectomy (vertebral body resection), partial or complete, for excision of intraspinal lesion, single segment; extradural, cervical

63301   extradural, thoracic by transthoracic approach

63302   extradural, thoracic by thoracolumbar approach

63303   extradural, lumbar or sacral by transperitoneal or retroperitoneal approach

63304   intradural, cervical

63305   intradural, thoracic by transthoracic approach

63306   intradural, thoracic by thoracolumbar approach

63307   intradural, lumbar or sacral by transperitoneal or retroperitoneal approach

+ 63308   each additional segment (List separately in addition to codes for single segment)

(Use 63308 in conjunction with 63300-63307)

Stereotaxis

63600   Creation of lesion of spinal cord by stereotactic method, percutaneous, any modality (including stimulation and/or recording)

63610   Stereotactic stimulation of spinal cord, percutaneous, separate procedure not followed by other surgery

63615   Stereotactic biopsy, aspiration, or excision of lesion, spinal cord

Neurostimulators (Spinal)

Codes 63650-63688 apply to both simple and complex neurostimulators. For initial or subsequent electronic analysis and programming of neurostimulator pulse generators, see codes 95970-95975.

Codes 63650, 63655, and 63660 describe the operative placement, revision, or removal of the spinal neurostimulator system components to provide spinal electrical stimulation. A neurostimulator system includes an implanted neurostimulator, external controller, extension, and collection of contacts. Multiple contacts or electrodes (4 or more) provide the actual electrical stimulation in the epidural space.

For percutaneously placed neurostimulator systems (63650, 63660), the contacts are on a catheter-like lead. An array defines the collection of contacts that are on one catheter.

For systems placed via an open surgical exposure (63655, 63660), the contacts are on a plate or paddle-shaped surface.

63650   Percutaneous implantation of neurostimulator electrode array, epidural

63655   Laminectomy for implantation of neurostimulator electrodes, plate/paddle, epidural

63660   Revision or removal of spinal neurostimulator electrode percutaneous array(s) or plate/paddle(s)

63685   Insertion or replacement of spinal neurostimulator pulse generator or receiver, direct or inductive coupling

(Do not report 63685 in conjunction with 63688 for the same pulse generator or receiver)

63688   Revision or removal of implanted spinal neurostimulator pulse generator or receiver

(For electronic analysis of implanted neurostimulator pulse generator system, see 95970-95975)

Repair

63700   Repair of meningocele; less than 5 cm diameter

63702   larger than 5 cm diameter

(Do not use modifier 63 in conjunction with 63700, 63702)

63704   Repair of myelomeningocele; less than 5 cm diameter

63706   larger than 5 cm diameter

(Do not use modifier 63 in conjunction with 63704, 63706)

(For complex skin closure, see **Integumentary System**)

63707   Repair of dural/cerebrospinal fluid leak, not requiring laminectomy

63709	Repair of dural/cerebrospinal fluid leak or pseudomeningocele, with laminectomy
63710	Dural graft, spinal

(For laminectomy and section of dentate ligaments, with or without dural graft, cervical, see 63180, 63182)

Shunt, Spinal CSF

63740	Creation of shunt, lumbar, subarachnoid-peritoneal, -pleural, or other; including laminectomy
63741	percutaneous, not requiring laminectomy
63744	Replacement, irrigation or revision of lumbosubarachnoid shunt
63746	Removal of entire lumbosubarachnoid shunt system without replacement

(For insertion of subarachnoid catheter with reservoir and/or pump for intermittent or continuous infusion of drug including laminectomy, see 62351 and 62360, 62361 or 62362)

(For insertion or replacement of subarachnoid or epidural catheter, with reservoir and/or pump for drug infusion without laminectomy, see 62350 and 62360, 62361 or 62362)

Extracranial Nerves, Peripheral Nerves, and Autonomic Nervous System

(For intracranial surgery on cranial nerves, see 61450, 61460, 61790)

Introduction/Injection of Anesthetic Agent (Nerve Block), Diagnostic or Therapeutic

Somatic Nerves

64400	Injection, anesthetic agent; trigeminal nerve, any division or branch
64402	facial nerve
64405	greater occipital nerve
64408	vagus nerve
64410	phrenic nerve
64412	spinal accessory nerve
64413	cervical plexus
64415	brachial plexus, single
64416	brachial plexus, continuous infusion by catheter (including catheter placement) including daily management for anesthetic agent administration

(Do not report 64416 in conjunction with 01996)

64417	axillary nerve
64418	suprascapular nerve
64420	intercostal nerve, single
64421	intercostal nerves, multiple, regional block
64425	ilioinguinal, iliohypogastric nerves
64430	pudendal nerve
64435	paracervical (uterine) nerve
64445	sciatic nerve, single
64446	sciatic nerve, continuous infusion by catheter, (including catheter placement) including daily management for anesthetic agent administration

(Do not report 64446 in conjunction with 01996)

64447	femoral nerve, single

(Do not report 64447 in conjunction with 01996)

64448	femoral nerve, continuous infusion by catheter (including catheter placement) including daily management for anesthetic agent administration

(Do not report 64448 in conjunction with 01996)

64449	lumbar plexus, posterior approach, continuous infusion by catheter (including catheter placement) including daily management for anesthetic agent administration

(Do not report 64449 in conjunction with 01996)

64450	other peripheral nerve or branch

(For phenol destruction, see 64622-64627)

(For subarachnoid or subdural injection, see 62280, 62310-62319)

(For epidural or caudal injection, see 62273, 62281-62282, 62310-62319)

(Codes 64470-64484 are unilateral procedures. For bilateral procedures, use modifier 50)

►(For fluoroscopic guidance and localization for needle placement and injection in conjunction with 64470-64484, use 77003)◄

64470	Injection, anesthetic agent and/or steroid, paravertebral facet joint or facet joint nerve; cervical or thoracic, single level
+ 64472	cervical or thoracic, each additional level (List separately in addition to code for primary procedure)

(Use 64472 in conjunction with 64470)

64475	lumbar or sacral, single level
+ 64476	lumbar or sacral, each additional level (List separately in addition to code for primary procedure)

(Use 64476 in conjunction with 64475)

Surgery: Nervous System

64479 Injection, anesthetic agent and/or steroid, transforaminal epidural; cervical or thoracic, single level

+ 64480 cervical or thoracic, each additional level (List separately in addition to code for primary procedure)

(Use 64480 in conjunction with 64479)

64483 lumbar or sacral, single level

+ 64484 lumbar or sacral, each additional level (List separately in addition to code for primary procedure)

(Use 64484 in conjunction with 64483)

Sympathetic Nerves

64505 Injection, anesthetic agent; sphenopalatine ganglion

64508 carotid sinus (separate procedure)

64510 stellate ganglion (cervical sympathetic)

64517 superior hypogastric plexus

64520 lumbar or thoracic (paravertebral sympathetic)

64530 celiac plexus, with or without radiologic monitoring

Neurostimulators (Peripheral Nerve)

Codes 64553-64595 apply to both simple and complex neurostimulators. For initial or subsequent electronic analysis and programming of neurostimulator pulse generators, see codes 95970-95975.

64550 Application of surface (transcutaneous) neurostimulator

64553 Percutaneous implantation of neurostimulator electrodes; cranial nerve

(For open placement of cranial nerve (eg, vagal, trigeminal) neurostimulator pulse generator or receiver, see 61885, 61886, as appropriate)

64555 peripheral nerve (excludes sacral nerve)

64560 autonomic nerve

64561 sacral nerve (transforaminal placement)

64565 neuromuscular

64573 Incision for implantation of neurostimulator electrodes; cranial nerve

(For open placement of cranial nerve (eg, vagal, trigeminal) neurostimulator pulse generator or receiver, see 61885, 61886, as appropriate)

(For revision or removal of cranial nerve (eg, vagal, trigeminal) neurostimulator pulse generator or receiver, use 61888)

64575 peripheral nerve (excludes sacral nerve)

64577 autonomic nerve

64580 neuromuscular

64581 sacral nerve (transforaminal placement)

64585 Revision or removal of peripheral neurostimulator electrodes

▲ 64590 Insertion or replacement of peripheral or gastric neurostimulator pulse generator or receiver, direct or inductive coupling

(Do not report 64590 in conjunction with 64595)

▲ 64595 Revision or removal of peripheral or gastric neurostimulator pulse generator or receiver

Destruction by Neurolytic Agent (eg, Chemical, Thermal, Electrical or Radiofrequency)

Codes 64600-64681 include the injection of other therapeutic agents (eg, corticosteroids).

Somatic Nerves

64600 Destruction by neurolytic agent, trigeminal nerve; supraorbital, infraorbital, mental, or inferior alveolar branch

64605 second and third division branches at foramen ovale

64610 second and third division branches at foramen ovale under radiologic monitoring

64612 Chemodenervation of muscle(s); muscle(s) innervated by facial nerve (eg, for blepharospasm, hemifacial spasm)

64613 neck muscle(s) (eg, for spasmodic torticollis, spasmodic dysphonia)

64614 extremity(s) and/or trunk muscle(s) (eg, for dystonia, cerebral palsy, multiple sclerosis)

(For chemodenervation guided by needle electromyography or muscle electrical stimulation, see 95873, 95874)

(For chemodenervation for strabismus involving the extraocular muscles, use 67345)

(For chemodenervation of internal anal sphincter, use 46505)

64620 Destruction by neurolytic agent, intercostal nerve

▶(For fluoroscopic guidance and localization for needle placement and neurolysis in conjunction with 64622-64627, use 77003)◀

64622 Destruction by neurolytic agent, paravertebral facet joint nerve; lumbar or sacral, single level

(For bilateral procedure, report 64622 with modifier 50)

+ 64623 lumbar or sacral, each additional level (List separately in addition to code for primary procedure)

(Use 64623 in conjunction with 64622)

(For bilateral procedure, report 64623 with modifier 50)

64626 cervical or thoracic, single level

(For bilateral procedure, report 64626 with modifier 50)

+ **64627**   cervical or thoracic, each additional level (List separately in addition to code for primary procedure)

(Use 64627 in conjunction with 64626)

(For bilateral procedure, report 64627 with modifier 50)

64630   Destruction by neurolytic agent; pudendal nerve

64640   other peripheral nerve or branch

Sympathetic Nerves

64650   Chemodenervation of eccrine glands; both axillae

64653   other area(s) (eg, scalp, face, neck), per day

(Report the specific service in conjunction with code(s) for the specific substance(s) or drug(s) provided)

(For chemodenervation of extremities (eg, hands or feet), use 64999)

64680   Destruction by neurolytic agent, with or without radiologic monitoring; celiac plexus

64681   superior hypogastric plexus

Neuroplasty (Exploration, Neurolysis or Nerve Decompression)

Neuroplasty is the decompression or freeing of intact nerve from scar tissue, including external neurolysis and/or transposition.

(For internal neurolysis requiring use of operating microscope, use 64727)

(For facial nerve decompression, use 69720)

64702   Neuroplasty; digital, one or both, same digit

64704   nerve of hand or foot

64708   Neuroplasty, major peripheral nerve, arm or leg; other than specified

64712   sciatic nerve

64713   brachial plexus

64714   lumbar plexus

64716   Neuroplasty and/or transposition; cranial nerve (specify)

64718   ulnar nerve at elbow

64719   ulnar nerve at wrist

64721   median nerve at carpal tunnel

(For arthroscopic procedure, use 29848)

64722   Decompression; unspecified nerve(s) (specify)

64726   plantar digital nerve

+ **64727**   Internal neurolysis, requiring use of operating microscope (List separately in addition to code for neuroplasty) (Neuroplasty includes external neurolysis)

(Do not report code 69990 in addition to code 64727)

Transection or Avulsion

(For stereotactic lesion of gasserian ganglion, use 61790)

64732   Transection or avulsion of; supraorbital nerve

64734   infraorbital nerve

64736   mental nerve

64738   inferior alveolar nerve by osteotomy

64740   lingual nerve

64742   facial nerve, differential or complete

64744   greater occipital nerve

64746   phrenic nerve

(For section of recurrent laryngeal nerve, use 31595)

64752   vagus nerve (vagotomy), transthoracic

64755   vagus nerves limited to proximal stomach (selective proximal vagotomy, proximal gastric vagotomy, parietal cell vagotomy, supra- or highly selective vagotomy)

(For laparoscopic approach, use 43652)

64760   vagus nerve (vagotomy), abdominal

(For laparoscopic approach, use 43651)

64761   pudendal nerve

(For bilateral procedure, report 64761 with modifier 50)

64763   Transection or avulsion of obturator nerve, extrapelvic, with or without adductor tenotomy

(For bilateral procedure, report 64763 with modifier 50)

64766   Transection or avulsion of obturator nerve, intrapelvic, with or without adductor tenotomy

(For bilateral procedure, report 64766 with modifier 50)

64771   Transection or avulsion of other cranial nerve, extradural

64772   Transection or avulsion of other spinal nerve, extradural

(For excision of tender scar, skin and subcutaneous tissue, with or without tiny neuroma, see 11400-11446, 13100-13153)

Excision

Somatic Nerves

(For Morton neurectomy, use 28080)

64774   Excision of neuroma; cutaneous nerve, surgically identifiable

64776   digital nerve, one or both, same digit

+ **64778**   digital nerve, each additional digit (List separately in addition to code for primary procedure)

(Use 64778 in conjunction with 64776)

Surgery: Nervous System

64782   hand or foot, except digital nerve

+ 64783   hand or foot, each additional nerve, except same digit (List separately in addition to code for primary procedure)

(Use 64783 in conjunction with 64782)

64784   major peripheral nerve, except sciatic

64786   sciatic nerve

+ 64787   Implantation of nerve end into bone or muscle (List separately in addition to neuroma excision)

(Use 64787 in conjunction with 64774-64786)

64788   Excision of neurofibroma or neurolemmoma; cutaneous nerve

64790   major peripheral nerve

64792   extensive (including malignant type)

64795   Biopsy of nerve

Sympathetic Nerves

64802   Sympathectomy, cervical

(For bilateral procedure, report 64802 with modifier 50)

64804   Sympathectomy, cervicothoracic

(For bilateral procedure, report 64804 with modifier 50)

64809   Sympathectomy, thoracolumbar

(For bilateral procedure, report 64809 with modifier 50)

64818   Sympathectomy, lumbar

(For bilateral procedure, report 64818 with modifier 50)

64820   Sympathectomy; digital arteries, each digit

(Do not report 69990 in addition to code 64820)

64821   radial artery

(Do not report 69990 in addition to code 64821)

64822   ulnar artery

(Do not report 69990 in addition to code 64822)

64823   superficial palmar arch

(Do not report 69990 in addition to code 64823)

Neurorrhaphy

64831   Suture of digital nerve, hand or foot; one nerve

+ 64832   each additional digital nerve (List separately in addition to code for primary procedure)

(Use 64832 in conjunction with 64831)

64834   Suture of one nerve, hand or foot; common sensory nerve

64835   median motor thenar

64836   ulnar motor

+ 64837   Suture of each additional nerve, hand or foot (List separately in addition to code for primary procedure)

(Use 64837 in conjunction with 64834-64836)

64840   Suture of posterior tibial nerve

64856   Suture of major peripheral nerve, arm or leg, except sciatic; including transposition

64857   without transposition

64858   Suture of sciatic nerve

+ 64859   Suture of each additional major peripheral nerve (List separately in addition to code for primary procedure)

(Use 64859 in conjunction with 64856, 64857)

64861   Suture of; brachial plexus

64862   lumbar plexus

64864   Suture of facial nerve; extracranial

64865   infratemporal, with or without grafting

64866   Anastomosis; facial-spinal accessory

64868   facial-hypoglossal

64870   facial-phrenic

+ 64872   Suture of nerve; requiring secondary or delayed suture (List separately in addition to code for primary neurorrhaphy)

(Use 64872 in conjunction with 64831-64865)

+ 64874   requiring extensive mobilization, or transposition of nerve (List separately in addition to code for nerve suture)

(Use 64874 in conjunction with 64831-64865)

+ 64876   requiring shortening of bone of extremity (List separately in addition to code for nerve suture)

(Use 64876 in conjunction with 64831-64865)

▶Neurorrhaphy With Nerve Graft, Vein Graft, or Conduit◀

64885   Nerve graft (includes obtaining graft), head or neck; up to 4 cm in length

64886   more than 4 cm length

64890   Nerve graft (includes obtaining graft), single strand, hand or foot; up to 4 cm length

64891   more than 4 cm length

64892   Nerve graft (includes obtaining graft), single strand, arm or leg; up to 4 cm length

64893   more than 4 cm length

64895   Nerve graft (includes obtaining graft), multiple strands (cable), hand or foot; up to 4 cm length

64896   more than 4 cm length

64897   Nerve graft (includes obtaining graft), multiple strands (cable), arm or leg; up to 4 cm length

64898   more than 4 cm length

+ 64901   Nerve graft, each additional nerve; single strand (List separately in addition to code for primary procedure)

        (Use 64901 in conjunction with 64885-64893)

+ 64902   multiple strands (cable) (List separately in addition to code for primary procedure)

        (Use 64902 in conjunction with 64885, 64886, 64895-64898)

64905   Nerve pedicle transfer; first stage

64907   second stage

● **64910**   Nerve repair; with synthetic conduit or vein allograft (eg, nerve tube), each nerve

● **64911**   with autogenous vein graft (includes harvest of vein graft), each nerve

        ▶(Do not report 69990 in addition to 64910, 64911)◀

Other Procedures

64999   Unlisted procedure, nervous system

Notes

⊙=Moderate sedation　✚=Add-on code　✗=FDA approval pending

Eye and Ocular Adnexa

(For diagnostic and treatment ophthalmological services, see **Medicine, Ophthalmology,** and 92002 et seq)

(Do not report code 69990 in addition to codes 65091-68850)

Eyeball

Removal of Eye

65091 Evisceration of ocular contents; without implant

65093   with implant

65101 Enucleation of eye; without implant

65103   with implant, muscles not attached to implant

65105   with implant, muscles attached to implant

(For conjunctivoplasty after enucleation, see 68320 et seq)

65110 Exenteration of orbit (does not include skin graft), removal of orbital contents; only

65112   with therapeutic removal of bone

65114   with muscle or myocutaneous flap

(For skin graft to orbit (split skin), see 15120, 15121; free, full thickness, see 15260, 15261)

(For eyelid repair involving more than skin, see 67930 et seq)

Secondary Implant(s) Procedures

An ocular implant is an implant inside muscular cone; an orbital implant is an implant outside muscular cone.

65125 Modification of ocular implant with placement or replacement of pegs (eg, drilling receptacle for prosthesis appendage) (separate procedure)

65130 Insertion of ocular implant secondary; after evisceration, in scleral shell

65135   after enucleation, muscles not attached to implant

65140   after enucleation, muscles attached to implant

65150 Reinsertion of ocular implant; with or without conjunctival graft

65155   with use of foreign material for reinforcement and/or attachment of muscles to implant

65175 Removal of ocular implant

(For orbital implant (implant outside muscle cone) insertion, use 67550; removal, use 67560)

Removal of Foreign Body

(For removal of implanted material: ocular implant, use 65175; anterior segment implant, use 65920; posterior segment implant, use 67120; orbital implant, use 67560)

(For diagnostic x-ray for foreign body, use 70030)

(For diagnostic echography for foreign body, use 76529)

(For removal of foreign body from orbit: frontal approach, use 67413; lateral approach, use 67430; transcranial approach, use 61334)

(For removal of foreign body from eyelid, embedded, use 67938)

(For removal of foreign body from lacrimal system, use 68530)

65205 Removal of foreign body, external eye; conjunctival superficial

65210   conjunctival embedded (includes concretions), subconjunctival, or scleral nonperforating

65220   corneal, without slit lamp

65222   corneal, with slit lamp

(For repair of corneal laceration with foreign body, use 65275)

65235 Removal of foreign body, intraocular; from anterior chamber of eye or lens

(For removal of implanted material from anterior segment, use 65920)

65260   from posterior segment, magnetic extraction, anterior or posterior route

65265   from posterior segment, nonmagnetic extraction

(For removal of implanted material from posterior segment, use 67120)

Repair of Laceration

(For fracture of orbit, see 21385 et seq)

(For repair of wound of eyelid, skin, linear, simple, see 12011-12018; intermediate, layered closure, see 12051-12057; linear, complex, see 13150-13160; other, see 67930, 67935)

(For repair of wound of lacrimal system, use 68700)

(For repair of operative wound, use 66250)

65270 Repair of laceration; conjunctiva, with or without nonperforating laceration sclera, direct closure

65272   conjunctiva, by mobilization and rearrangement, without hospitalization

65273   conjunctiva, by mobilization and rearrangement, with hospitalization

65275   cornea, nonperforating, with or without removal foreign body

Surgery: Eye and Ocular Adnexa

65280   cornea and/or sclera, perforating, not involving uveal tissue

65285   cornea and/or sclera, perforating, with reposition or resection of uveal tissue

65286   application of tissue glue, wounds of cornea and/or sclera

(Repair of laceration includes use of conjunctival flap and restoration of anterior chamber, by air or saline injection when indicated)

(For repair of iris or ciliary body, use 66680)

65290   Repair of wound, extraocular muscle, tendon and/or Tenon's capsule

Anterior Segment

Cornea

Excision

65400   Excision of lesion, cornea (keratectomy, lamellar, partial), except pterygium

65410   Biopsy of cornea

65420   Excision or transposition of pterygium; without graft

65426   with graft

Removal or Destruction

65430   Scraping of cornea, diagnostic, for smear and/or culture

65435   Removal of corneal epithelium; with or without chemocauterization (abrasion, curettage)

65436   with application of chelating agent (eg, EDTA)

65450   Destruction of lesion of cornea by cryotherapy, photocoagulation or thermocauterization

65600   Multiple punctures of anterior cornea (eg, for corneal erosion, tattoo)

Keratoplasty

Corneal transplant includes use of fresh or preserved grafts, and preparation of donor material.

(Keratoplasty excludes refractive keratoplasty procedures, 65760, 65765, and 65767)

65710   Keratoplasty (corneal transplant); lamellar

65730   penetrating (except in aphakia)

65750   penetrating (in aphakia)

65755   penetrating (in pseudophakia)

Other Procedures

65760   Keratomileusis

65765   Keratophakia

65767   Epikeratoplasty

65770   Keratoprosthesis

65771   Radial keratotomy

65772   Corneal relaxing incision for correction of surgically induced astigmatism

65775   Corneal wedge resection for correction of surgically induced astigmatism

(For fitting of contact lens for treatment of disease, use 92070)

(For unlisted procedures on cornea, use 66999)

65780   Ocular surface reconstruction; amniotic membrane transplantation

65781   limbal stem cell allograft (eg, cadaveric or living donor)

65782   limbal conjunctival autograft (includes obtaining graft)

(For harvesting conjunctival allograft, living donor, use 68371)

Anterior Chamber

Incision

65800   Paracentesis of anterior chamber of eye (separate procedure); with diagnostic aspiration of aqueous

65805   with therapeutic release of aqueous

65810   with removal of vitreous and/or discission of anterior hyaloid membrane, with or without air injection

65815   with removal of blood, with or without irrigation and/or air injection

(For injection, see 66020-66030)

(For removal of blood clot, use 65930)

65820   Goniotomy

(Do not report modifier 63 in conjunction with 65820)

►(For use of ophthalmic endoscope with 65820, use 66990)◄

65850   Trabeculotomy ab externo

65855   Trabeculoplasty by laser surgery, one or more sessions (defined treatment series)

(If re-treatment is necessary after several months because of disease progression, a new treatment or treatment series should be reported with a modifier, if necessary, to indicate lesser or greater complexity)

(For trabeculectomy, use 66170)

65860   Severing adhesions of anterior segment, laser technique (separate procedure)

Other Procedures

65865   Severing adhesions of anterior segment of eye, incisional technique (with or without injection of air or liquid) (separate procedure); goniosynechiae

(For trabeculoplasty by laser surgery, use 65855)

65870   anterior synechiae, except goniosynechiae

65875   posterior synechiae

►(For use of ophthalmic endoscope with 65875, use 66990)◄

65880   corneovitreal adhesions

(For laser surgery, use 66821)

65900   Removal of epithelial downgrowth, anterior chamber of eye

65920   Removal of implanted material, anterior segment of eye

►(For use of ophthalmic endoscope with 65920, use 66990)◄

65930   Removal of blood clot, anterior segment of eye

66020   Injection, anterior chamber of eye (separate procedure); air or liquid

66030   medication

(For unlisted procedures on anterior segment, use 66999)

Anterior Sclera

Excision

(For removal of intraocular foreign body, use 65235)

(For operations on posterior sclera, use 67250, 67255)

66130   Excision of lesion, sclera

66150   Fistulization of sclera for glaucoma; trephination with iridectomy

66155   thermocauterization with iridectomy

66160   sclerectomy with punch or scissors, with iridectomy

66165   iridencleisis or iridotasis

66170   trabeculectomy ab externo in absence of previous surgery

(For trabeculotomy ab externo, use 65850)

(For repair of operative wound, use 66250)

66172   trabeculectomy ab externo with scarring from previous ocular surgery or trauma (includes injection of antifibrotic agents)

(For transciliary body sclera fistulization, use Category III code 0123T)

►Aqueous Shunt◄

66180   Aqueous shunt to extraocular reservoir (eg, Molteno, Schocket, Denver-Krupin)

66185   Revision of aqueous shunt to extraocular reservoir

(For removal of implanted shunt, use 67120)

Repair or Revision

(For scleral procedures in retinal surgery, see 67101 et seq)

66220   Repair of scleral staphyloma; without graft

66225   with graft

(For scleral reinforcement, see 67250, 67255)

66250   Revision or repair of operative wound of anterior segment, any type, early or late, major or minor procedure

(For unlisted procedures on anterior sclera, use 66999)

Iris, Ciliary Body

Incision

66500   Iridotomy by stab incision (separate procedure); except transfixion

66505   with transfixion as for iris bombe

(For iridotomy by photocoagulation, use 66761)

Excision

66600   Iridectomy, with corneoscleral or corneal section; for removal of lesion

66605   with cyclectomy

66625   peripheral for glaucoma (separate procedure)

66630   sector for glaucoma (separate procedure)

66635   optical (separate procedure)

(For coreoplasty by photocoagulation, use 66762)

Repair

66680   Repair of iris, ciliary body (as for iridodialysis)

(For reposition or resection of uveal tissue with perforating wound of cornea or sclera, use 65285)

66682   Suture of iris, ciliary body (separate procedure) with retrieval of suture through small incision (eg, McCannel suture)

Destruction

66700 Ciliary body destruction; diathermy

66710 cyclophotocoagulation, transscleral

66711 cyclophotocoagulation, endoscopic

(Do not report 66711 in conjunction with 66990)

⊙ **66720** cryotherapy

66740 cyclodialysis

66761 Iridotomy/iridectomy by laser surgery (eg, for glaucoma) (one or more sessions)

66762 Iridoplasty by photocoagulation (one or more sessions) (eg, for improvement of vision, for widening of anterior chamber angle)

66770 Destruction of cyst or lesion iris or ciliary body (nonexcisional procedure)

(For excision lesion iris, ciliary body, see 66600, 66605; for removal of epithelial downgrowth, use 65900)

(For unlisted procedures on iris, ciliary body, use 66999)

Lens

Incision

66820 Discission of secondary membranous cataract (opacified posterior lens capsule and/or anterior hyaloid); stab incision technique (Ziegler or Wheeler knife)

66821 laser surgery (eg, YAG laser) (one or more stages)

66825 Repositioning of intraocular lens prosthesis, requiring an incision (separate procedure)

Removal Cataract

Lateral canthotomy, iridectomy, iridotomy, anterior capsulotomy, posterior capsulotomy, the use of viscoelastic agents, enzymatic zonulysis, use of other pharmacologic agents, and subconjunctival or sub-tenon injections are included as part of the code for the extraction of lens.

66830 Removal of secondary membranous cataract (opacified posterior lens capsule and/or anterior hyaloid) with corneo-scleral section, with or without iridectomy (iridocapsulotomy, iridocapsulectomy)

66840 Removal of lens material; aspiration technique, one or more stages

66850 phacofragmentation technique (mechanical or ultrasonic) (eg, phacoemulsification), with aspiration

66852 pars plana approach, with or without vitrectomy

66920 intracapsular

66930 intracapsular, for dislocated lens

66940 extracapsular (other than 66840, 66850, 66852)

(For removal of intralenticular foreign body without lens extraction, use 65235)

(For repair of operative wound, use 66250)

66982 Extracapsular cataract removal with insertion of intraocular lens prosthesis (one stage procedure), manual or mechanical technique (eg, irrigation and aspiration or phacoemulsification), complex, requiring devices or techniques not generally used in routine cataract surgery (eg, iris expansion device, suture support for intraocular lens, or primary posterior capsulorrhexis) or performed on patients in the amblyogenic developmental stage

66983 Intracapsular cataract extraction with insertion of intraocular lens prosthesis (one stage procedure)

66984 Extracapsular cataract removal with insertion of intraocular lens prosthesis (one stage procedure), manual or mechanical technique (eg, irrigation and aspiration or phacoemulsification)

(For complex extracapsular cataract removal, use 66982)

66985 Insertion of intraocular lens prosthesis (secondary implant), not associated with concurrent cataract removal

(To code implant at time of concurrent cataract surgery, see 66982, 66983, 66984)

(For intraocular lens prosthesis supplied by physician, use 99070)

(For ultrasonic determination of intraocular lens power, use 76519)

(For removal of implanted material from anterior segment, use 65920)

(For secondary fixation (separate procedure), use 66682)

▶(For use of ophthalmic endoscope with 66985, use 66990)◀

66986 Exchange of intraocular lens

▶(For use of ophthalmic endoscope with 66986, use 66990)◀

✛ **66990** Use of ophthalmic endoscope (List separately in addition to code for primary procedure)

▶(66990 may be used only with codes 65820, 65875, 65920, 66985, 66986, 67036, 67038, 67039, 67040, 67112)◀

Other Procedures

66999 Unlisted procedure, anterior segment of eye

Posterior Segment

Vitreous

67005   Removal of vitreous, anterior approach (open sky technique or limbal incision); partial removal

67010   subtotal removal with mechanical vitrectomy

(For removal of vitreous by paracentesis of anterior chamber, use 65810)

(For removal of corneovitreal adhesions, use 65880)

67015   Aspiration or release of vitreous, subretinal or choroidal fluid, pars plana approach (posterior sclerotomy)

67025   Injection of vitreous substitute, pars plana or limbal approach, (fluid-gas exchange), with or without aspiration (separate procedure)

67027   Implantation of intravitreal drug delivery system (eg, ganciclovir implant), includes concomitant removal of vitreous

(For removal, use 67121)

67028   Intravitreal injection of a pharmacologic agent (separate procedure)

67030   Discission of vitreous strands (without removal), pars plana approach

67031   Severing of vitreous strands, vitreous face adhesions, sheets, membranes or opacities, laser surgery (one or more stages)

67036   Vitrectomy, mechanical, pars plana approach;

67038   with epiretinal membrane stripping

67039   with focal endolaser photocoagulation

67040   with endolaser panretinal photocoagulation

▶(For use of ophthalmic endoscope with 67036, 67038, 67039, 67040, use 66990)◀

(For associated lensectomy, use 66850)

(For use of vitrectomy in retinal detachment surgery, use 67108)

(For associated removal of foreign body, see 65260, 65265)

(For unlisted procedures on vitreous, use 67299)

Retina or Choroid

Repair

(If diathermy, cryotherapy and/or photocoagulation are combined, report under principal modality used)

67101   Repair of retinal detachment, one or more sessions; cryotherapy or diathermy, with or without drainage of subretinal fluid

67105   photocoagulation, with or without drainage of subretinal fluid

67107   Repair of retinal detachment; scleral buckling (such as lamellar scleral dissection, imbrication or encircling procedure), with or without implant, with or without cryotherapy, photocoagulation, and drainage of subretinal fluid

67108   with vitrectomy, any method, with or without air or gas tamponade, focal endolaser photocoagulation, cryotherapy, drainage of subretinal fluid, scleral buckling, and/or removal of lens by same technique

67110   by injection of air or other gas (eg, pneumatic retinopexy)

67112   by scleral buckling or vitrectomy, on patient having previous ipsilateral retinal detachment repair(s) using scleral buckling or vitrectomy techniques

(For aspiration or drainage of subretinal or subchoroidal fluid, use 67015)

▶(For use of ophthalmic endoscope with 67112, use 66990)◀

67115   Release of encircling material (posterior segment)

67120   Removal of implanted material, posterior segment; extraocular

67121   intraocular

(For removal from anterior segment, use 65920)

(For removal of foreign body, see 65260, 65265)

Prophylaxis

Repetitive services. The services listed below are often performed in multiple sessions or groups of sessions. The methods of reporting vary.

The following descriptors are intended to include all sessions in a defined treatment period.

67141   Prophylaxis of retinal detachment (eg, retinal break, lattice degeneration) without drainage, one or more sessions; cryotherapy, diathermy

67145   photocoagulation (laser or xenon arc)

Destruction

67208   Destruction of localized lesion of retina (eg, macular edema, tumors), one or more sessions; cryotherapy, diathermy

67210   photocoagulation

67218   radiation by implantation of source (includes removal of source)

67220   Destruction of localized lesion of choroid (eg, choroidal neovascularization); photocoagulation (eg, laser), one or more sessions

(For destruction of macular drusen, photocoagulation, use Category III code 0017T)

(For destruction of localized lesion of choroid by transpupillary thermotherapy, use Category III code 0016T)

67221   photodynamic therapy (includes intravenous infusion)

+ 67225   photodynamic therapy, second eye, at single session (List separately in addition to code for primary eye treatment)

(Use 67225 in conjunction with 67221)

67227   Destruction of extensive or progressive retinopathy (eg, diabetic retinopathy), one or more sessions; cryotherapy, diathermy

67228   photocoagulation (laser or xenon arc)

(For unlisted procedures on retina, use 67299)

►Posterior Sclera◄

Repair

(For excision lesion sclera, use 66130)

67250   Scleral reinforcement (separate procedure); without graft

67255   with graft

(For repair scleral staphyloma, see 66220, 66225)

Other Procedures

67299   Unlisted procedure, posterior segment

Ocular Adnexa

Extraocular Muscles

67311   Strabismus surgery, recession or resection procedure; one horizontal muscle

67312   two horizontal muscles

67314   one vertical muscle (excluding superior oblique)

67316   two or more vertical muscles (excluding superior oblique)

(For adjustable sutures, use 67335 in addition to codes 67311-67334 for primary procedure reflecting number of muscles operated on)

67318   Strabismus surgery, any procedure, superior oblique muscle

+ 67320   Transposition procedure (eg, for paretic extraocular muscle), any extraocular muscle (specify) (List separately in addition to code for primary procedure)

(Use 67320 in conjunction with 67311-67318)

+ 67331   Strabismus surgery on patient with previous eye surgery or injury that did not involve the extraocular muscles (List separately in addition to code for primary procedure)

(Use 67331 in conjunction with 67311-67318)

+ 67332   Strabismus surgery on patient with scarring of extraocular muscles (eg, prior ocular injury, strabismus or retinal detachment surgery) or restrictive myopathy (eg, dysthyroid ophthalmopathy) (List separately in addition to code for primary procedure)

(Use 67332 in conjunction with 67311-67318)

+ 67334   Strabismus surgery by posterior fixation suture technique, with or without muscle recession (List separately in addition to code for primary procedure)

(Use 67334 in conjunction with 67311-67318)

+ 67335   Placement of adjustable suture(s) during strabismus surgery, including postoperative adjustment(s) of suture(s) (List separately in addition to code for specific strabismus surgery)

(Use 67335 in conjunction with 67311-67334)

+ 67340   Strabismus surgery involving exploration and/or repair of detached extraocular muscle(s) (List separately in addition to code for primary procedure)

(Use 67340 in conjunction with 67311-67334)

67343   Release of extensive scar tissue without detaching extraocular muscle (separate procedure)

(Use 67343 in conjunction with 67311-67340, when such procedures are performed other than on the affected muscle)

67345   Chemodenervation of extraocular muscle

(For chemodenervation for blepharospasm and other neurological disorders, see 64612 and 64613)

● 67346   Biopsy of extraocular muscle

►(For repair of wound, extraocular muscle, tendon or Tenon's capsule, use 65290)◄

Other Procedures

►(67350 has been deleted. To report, use 67346)◄

67399   Unlisted procedure, ocular muscle

Orbit

Exploration, Excision, Decompression

67400   Orbitotomy without bone flap (frontal or transconjunctival approach); for exploration, with or without biopsy

67405   with drainage only

67412   with removal of lesion

67413   with removal of foreign body

67414   with removal of bone for decompression

67415   Fine needle aspiration of orbital contents

(For exenteration, enucleation, and repair, see 65101 et seq; for optic nerve decompression, use 67570)

67420   Orbitotomy with bone flap or window, lateral approach (eg, Kroenlein); with removal of lesion

67430   with removal of foreign body

67440   with drainage

67445   with removal of bone for decompression

         (For optic nerve sheath decompression, use 67570)

67450   for exploration, with or without biopsy

         (For orbitotomy, transcranial approach, see 61330-61334)

         (For orbital implant, see 67550, 67560)

         (For removal of eyeball or for repair after removal, see 65091-65175)

Other Procedures

67500   Retrobulbar injection; medication (separate procedure, does not include supply of medication)

67505   alcohol

67515   Injection of medication or other substance into Tenon's capsule

         (For subconjunctival injection, use 68200)

67550   Orbital implant (implant outside muscle cone); insertion

67560   removal or revision

         (For ocular implant (implant inside muscle cone), see 65093-65105, 65130-65175)

         (For treatment of fractures of malar area, orbit, see 21355 et seq)

67570   Optic nerve decompression (eg, incision or fenestration of optic nerve sheath)

67599   Unlisted procedure, orbit

Eyelids

Incision

67700   Blepharotomy, drainage of abscess, eyelid

67710   Severing of tarsorrhaphy

67715   Canthotomy (separate procedure)

         (For canthoplasty, use 67950)

         (For division of symblepharon, use 68340)

►Excision, Destruction◄

Codes for removal of lesion include more than skin (ie, involving lid margin, tarsus, and/or palpebral conjunctiva).

         (For removal of lesion, involving mainly skin of eyelid, see 11310-11313; 11440-11446, 11640-11646; 17000-17004)

         (For repair of wounds, blepharoplasty, grafts, reconstructive surgery, see 67930-67975)

67800   Excision of chalazion; single

67801   multiple, same lid

67805   multiple, different lids

67808   under general anesthesia and/or requiring hospitalization, single or multiple

67810   Biopsy of eyelid

67820   Correction of trichiasis; epilation, by forceps only

67825   epilation by other than forceps (eg, by electrosurgery, cryotherapy, laser surgery)

67830   incision of lid margin

67835   incision of lid margin, with free mucous membrane graft

67840   Excision of lesion of eyelid (except chalazion) without closure or with simple direct closure

         (For excision and repair of eyelid by reconstructive surgery, see 67961, 67966)

67850   Destruction of lesion of lid margin (up to 1 cm)

         ►(For Mohs micrographic surgery, see 17311-17315)◄

         (For initiation or follow-up care of topical chemotherapy (eg, 5-FU or similar agents), see appropriate office visits)

Tarsorrhaphy

67875   Temporary closure of eyelids by suture (eg, Frost suture)

67880   Construction of intermarginal adhesions, median tarsorrhaphy, or canthorrhaphy;

67882   with transposition of tarsal plate

         (For severing of tarsorrhaphy, use 67710)

         (For canthoplasty, reconstruction canthus, use 67950)

         (For canthotomy, use 67715)

Repair (Brow Ptosis, Blepharoptosis, Lid Retraction, Ectropion, Entropion)

67900   Repair of brow ptosis (supraciliary, mid-forehead or coronal approach)

         (For forehead rhytidectomy, use 15824)

67901   Repair of blepharoptosis; frontalis muscle technique with suture or other material (eg, banked fascia)

67902   frontalis muscle technique with autologous fascial sling (includes obtaining fascia)

67903   (tarso) levator resection or advancement, internal approach

67904   (tarso) levator resection or advancement, external approach

67906   superior rectus technique with fascial sling (includes obtaining fascia)

67908   conjunctivo-tarso-Muller's muscle-levator resection (eg, Fasanella-Servat type)

▲=Revised code   ●=New code   ►◄=Contains new or revised text   ⊘=Modifier 51 exempt   American Medical Association   **225**

67909   Reduction of overcorrection of ptosis

67911   Correction of lid retraction

(For obtaining autogenous graft materials, see 20920, 20922 or 20926)

(For correction of trichiasis by mucous membrane graft, use 67835)

67912   Correction of lagophthalmos, with implantation of upper eyelid lid load (eg, gold weight)

67914   Repair of ectropion; suture

67915   thermocauterization

67916   excision tarsal wedge

67917   extensive (eg, tarsal strip operations)

(For correction of everted punctum, use 68705)

67921   Repair of entropion; suture

67922   thermocauterization

67923   excision tarsal wedge

67924   extensive (eg, tarsal strip or capsulopalpebral fascia repairs operation)

(For repair of cicatricial ectropion or entropion requiring scar excision or skin graft, see also 67961 et seq)

Reconstruction

Codes for blepharoplasty involve more than skin (ie, involving lid margin, tarsus, and/or palpebral conjunctiva).

67930   Suture of recent wound, eyelid, involving lid margin, tarsus, and/or palpebral conjunctiva direct closure; partial thickness

67935   full thickness

67938   Removal of embedded foreign body, eyelid

(For repair of skin of eyelid, see 12011-12018; 12051-12057; 13150-13153)

(For tarsorrhaphy, canthorrhaphy, see 67880, 67882)

(For repair of blepharoptosis and lid retraction, see 67901-67911)

(For blepharoplasty for entropion, ectropion, see 67916, 67917, 67923, 67924)

(For correction of blepharochalasis (blepharorhytidectomy), see 15820-15823)

▶(For repair of skin of eyelid, adjacent tissue transfer, see 14060, 14061; preparation for graft, use 15004; free graft, see 15120, 15121, 15260, 15261)◀

(For excision of lesion of eyelid, use 67800 et seq)

(For repair of lacrimal canaliculi, use 68700)

67950   Canthoplasty (reconstruction of canthus)

67961   Excision and repair of eyelid, involving lid margin, tarsus, conjunctiva, canthus, or full thickness, may include preparation for skin graft or pedicle flap with adjacent tissue transfer or rearrangement; up to one-fourth of lid margin

67966   over one-fourth of lid margin

(For canthoplasty, use 67950)

(For free skin grafts, see 15120, 15121, 15260, 15261)

(For tubed pedicle flap preparation, use 15576; for delay, use 15630; for attachment, use 15650)

67971   Reconstruction of eyelid, full thickness by transfer of tarsoconjunctival flap from opposing eyelid; up to two-thirds of eyelid, one stage or first stage

67973   total eyelid, lower, one stage or first stage

67974   total eyelid, upper, one stage or first stage

67975   second stage

Other Procedures

67999   Unlisted procedure, eyelids

Conjunctiva

(For removal of foreign body, see 65205 et seq)

Incision and Drainage

68020   Incision of conjunctiva, drainage of cyst

68040   Expression of conjunctival follicles (eg, for trachoma)

Excision and/or Destruction

68100   Biopsy of conjunctiva

68110   Excision of lesion, conjunctiva; up to 1 cm

68115   over 1 cm

68130   with adjacent sclera

68135   Destruction of lesion, conjunctiva

Injection

(For injection into Tenon's capsule or retrobulbar injection, see 67500-67515)

68200   Subconjunctival injection

Conjunctivoplasty

(For wound repair, see 65270-65273)

68320   Conjunctivoplasty; with conjunctival graft or extensive rearrangement

68325   with buccal mucous membrane graft (includes obtaining graft)

68326 Conjunctivoplasty, reconstruction cul-de-sac; with conjunctival graft or extensive rearrangement

68328   with buccal mucous membrane graft (includes obtaining graft)

68330 Repair of symblepharon; conjunctivoplasty, without graft

68335   with free graft conjunctiva or buccal mucous membrane (includes obtaining graft)

68340   division of symblepharon, with or without insertion of conformer or contact lens

Other Procedures

68360 Conjunctival flap; bridge or partial (separate procedure)

68362   total (such as Gunderson thin flap or purse string flap)

(For conjunctival flap for perforating injury, see 65280, 65285)

(For repair of operative wound, use 66250)

(For removal of conjunctival foreign body, see 65205, 65210)

68371 Harvesting conjunctival allograft, living donor

68399 Unlisted procedure, conjunctiva

Lacrimal System

Incision

68400 Incision, drainage of lacrimal gland

68420 Incision, drainage of lacrimal sac (dacryocystotomy or dacryocystostomy)

68440 Snip incision of lacrimal punctum

Excision

68500 Excision of lacrimal gland (dacryoadenectomy), except for tumor; total

68505   partial

68510 Biopsy of lacrimal gland

68520 Excision of lacrimal sac (dacryocystectomy)

68525 Biopsy of lacrimal sac

68530 Removal of foreign body or dacryolith, lacrimal passages

68540 Excision of lacrimal gland tumor; frontal approach

68550   involving osteotomy

Repair

68700 Plastic repair of canaliculi

68705 Correction of everted punctum, cautery

68720 Dacryocystorhinostomy (fistulization of lacrimal sac to nasal cavity)

68745 Conjunctivorhinostomy (fistulization of conjunctiva to nasal cavity); without tube

68750   with insertion of tube or stent

68760 Closure of the lacrimal punctum; by thermocauterization, ligation, or laser surgery

68761   by plug, each

68770 Closure of lacrimal fistula (separate procedure)

Probing and/or Related Procedures

68801 Dilation of lacrimal punctum, with or without irrigation

(To report a bilateral procedure, use 68801 with modifier 50)

68810 Probing of nasolacrimal duct, with or without irrigation;

(For bilateral procedure, report 68810 with modifier 50)

68811   requiring general anesthesia

(For bilateral procedure, report 68811 with modifier 50)

68815   with insertion of tube or stent

(See also 92018)

(For bilateral procedure, report 68815 with modifier 50)

68840 Probing of lacrimal canaliculi, with or without irrigation

68850 Injection of contrast medium for dacryocystography

(For radiological supervision and interpretation, see 70170, 78660)

Other Procedures

68899 Unlisted procedure, lacrimal system

Surgery: Eye and Ocular Adnexa

Notes

Auditory System

(For diagnostic services (eg, audiometry, vestibular tests), see 92502 et seq)

External Ear

Incision

69000   Drainage external ear, abscess or hematoma; simple

69005   complicated

69020   Drainage external auditory canal, abscess

69090   Ear piercing

Excision

69100   Biopsy external ear

69105   Biopsy external auditory canal

69110   Excision external ear; partial, simple repair

69120   complete amputation

(For reconstruction of ear, see 15120 et seq)

69140   Excision exostosis(es), external auditory canal

69145   Excision soft tissue lesion, external auditory canal

69150   Radical excision external auditory canal lesion; without neck dissection

69155   with neck dissection

(For resection of temporal bone, use 69535)

►(For skin grafting, see 15004-15261)◄

►Removal◄

69200   Removal foreign body from external auditory canal; without general anesthesia

69205   with general anesthesia

69210   Removal impacted cerumen (separate procedure), one or both ears

69220   Debridement, mastoidectomy cavity, simple (eg, routine cleaning)

(For bilateral procedure, report 69220 with modifier 50)

69222   Debridement, mastoidectomy cavity, complex (eg, with anesthesia or more than routine cleaning)

(For bilateral procedure, report 69222 with modifier 50)

Repair

(For suture of wound or injury of external ear, see 12011-14300)

⊙ **69300**   Otoplasty, protruding ear, with or without size reduction

(For bilateral procedure, report 69300 with modifier 50)

69310   Reconstruction of external auditory canal (meatoplasty) (eg, for stenosis due to injury, infection) (separate procedure)

69320   Reconstruction external auditory canal for congenital atresia, single stage

(For combination with middle ear reconstruction, see 69631, 69641)

(For other reconstructive procedures with grafts (eg, skin, cartilage, bone), see 13150-15760, 21230-21235)

Other Procedures

(For otoscopy under general anesthesia, use 92502)

69399   Unlisted procedure, external ear

Middle Ear

Introduction

69400   Eustachian tube inflation, transnasal; with catheterization

69401   without catheterization

69405   Eustachian tube catheterization, transtympanic

(69410 has been deleted)

Incision

69420   Myringotomy including aspiration and/or eustachian tube inflation

69421   Myringotomy including aspiration and/or eustachian tube inflation requiring general anesthesia

69424   Ventilating tube removal requiring general anesthesia

(For bilateral procedure, report 69424 with modifier 50)

(Do not report code 69424 in conjunction with 69205, 69210, 69420, 69421, 69433-69676, 69710-69745, 69801-69930)

69433   Tympanostomy (requiring insertion of ventilating tube), local or topical anesthesia

(For bilateral procedure, report 69433 with modifier 50)

69436   Tympanostomy (requiring insertion of ventilating tube), general anesthesia

(For bilateral procedure, report 69436 with modifier 50)

69440   Middle ear exploration through postauricular or ear canal incision

(For atticotomy, see 69601 et seq)

69450   Tympanolysis, transcanal

Surgery: Auditory System

Excision

69501   Transmastoid antrotomy (simple mastoidectomy)

69502   Mastoidectomy; complete

69505   modified radical

69511   radical

▶(For skin graft, see 15004 et seq)◀

(For mastoidectomy cavity debridement, see 69220, 69222)

69530   Petrous apicectomy including radical mastoidectomy

69535   Resection temporal bone, external approach

(For middle fossa approach, see 69950-69970)

69540   Excision aural polyp

69550   Excision aural glomus tumor; transcanal

69552   transmastoid

69554   extended (extratemporal)

Repair

69601   Revision mastoidectomy; resulting in complete mastoidectomy

69602   resulting in modified radical mastoidectomy

69603   resulting in radical mastoidectomy

69604   resulting in tympanoplasty

(For planned secondary tympanoplasty after mastoidectomy, see 69631, 69632)

69605   with apicectomy

(For skin graft, see 15120, 15121, 15260, 15261)

69610   Tympanic membrane repair, with or without site preparation of perforation for closure, with or without patch

69620   Myringoplasty (surgery confined to drumhead and donor area)

69631   Tympanoplasty without mastoidectomy (including canalplasty, atticotomy and/or middle ear surgery), initial or revision; without ossicular chain reconstruction

69632   with ossicular chain reconstruction (eg, postfenestration)

69633   with ossicular chain reconstruction and synthetic prosthesis (eg, partial ossicular replacement prosthesis (PORP), total ossicular replacement prosthesis (TORP))

69635   Tympanoplasty with antrotomy or mastoidotomy (including canalplasty, atticotomy, middle ear surgery, and/or tympanic membrane repair); without ossicular chain reconstruction

69636   with ossicular chain reconstruction

69637   with ossicular chain reconstruction and synthetic prosthesis (eg, partial ossicular replacement prosthesis (PORP), total ossicular replacement prosthesis (TORP))

69641   Tympanoplasty with mastoidectomy (including canalplasty, middle ear surgery, tympanic membrane repair); without ossicular chain reconstruction

69642   with ossicular chain reconstruction

69643   with intact or reconstructed wall, without ossicular chain reconstruction

69644   with intact or reconstructed canal wall, with ossicular chain reconstruction

69645   radical or complete, without ossicular chain reconstruction

69646   radical or complete, with ossicular chain reconstruction

69650   Stapes mobilization

69660   Stapedectomy or stapedotomy with reestablishment of ossicular continuity, with or without use of foreign material;

69661   with footplate drill out

69662   Revision of stapedectomy or stapedotomy

69666   Repair oval window fistula

69667   Repair round window fistula

69670   Mastoid obliteration (separate procedure)

69676   Tympanic neurectomy

(For bilateral procedure, report 69676 with modifier 50)

Other Procedures

69700   Closure postauricular fistula, mastoid (separate procedure)

69710   Implantation or replacement of electromagnetic bone conduction hearing device in temporal bone

(Replacement procedure includes removal of old device)

69711   Removal or repair of electromagnetic bone conduction hearing device in temporal bone

69714   Implantation, osseointegrated implant, temporal bone, with percutaneous attachment to external speech processor/cochlear stimulator; without mastoidectomy

69715   with mastoidectomy

69717   Replacement (including removal of existing device), osseointegrated implant, temporal bone, with percutaneous attachment to external speech processor/cochlear stimulator; without mastoidectomy

69718   with mastoidectomy

Surgery: Auditory System

69720   Decompression facial nerve, intratemporal; lateral to geniculate ganglion

69725   including medial to geniculate ganglion

69740   Suture facial nerve, intratemporal, with or without graft or decompression; lateral to geniculate ganglion

69745   including medial to geniculate ganglion

      (For extracranial suture of facial nerve, use 64864)

69799   Unlisted procedure, middle ear

Inner Ear

Incision and/or Destruction

69801   Labyrinthotomy, with or without cryosurgery including other nonexcisional destructive procedures or perfusion of vestibuloactive drugs (single or multiple perfusions); transcanal

      (69801 includes all required infusions performed on initial and subsequent days of treatment)

69802   with mastoidectomy

69805   Endolymphatic sac operation; without shunt

69806   with shunt

69820   Fenestration semicircular canal

69840   Revision fenestration operation

Excision

69905   Labyrinthectomy; transcanal

69910   with mastoidectomy

69915   Vestibular nerve section, translabyrinthine approach

      (For transcranial approach, use 69950)

Introduction

69930   Cochlear device implantation, with or without mastoidectomy

Other Procedures

69949   Unlisted procedure, inner ear

Temporal Bone, Middle Fossa Approach

      (For external approach, use 69535)

69950   Vestibular nerve section, transcranial approach

69955   Total facial nerve decompression and/or repair (may include graft)

69960   Decompression internal auditory canal

69970   Removal of tumor, temporal bone

Other Procedures

69979   Unlisted procedure, temporal bone, middle fossa approach

Operating Microscope

The surgical microscope is employed when the surgical services are performed using the techniques of microsurgery. Code 69990 should be reported (without modifier 51 appended) in addition to the code for the primary procedure performed. Do not use 69990 for visualization with magnifying loupes or corrected vision. Do not report code 69990 in addition to procedures where use of the operating microscope is an inclusive component (15756-15758, 15842, 19364, 19368, 20955-20962, 20969-20973, 26551-26554, 26556, 31526, 31531, 31536, 31541, 31545, 31546, 31561, 31571, 43116, 43496, 49906, 61548, 63075-63078, 64727, 64820-64823, 65091-68850).

+ 69990   Microsurgical techniques, requiring use of operating microscope (List separately in addition to code for primary procedure)

Surgery: Auditory System

Notes

⊙=Moderate sedation   ✚=Add-on code   ✗=FDA approval pending

Radiology Guidelines (Including Nuclear Medicine and Diagnostic Ultrasound)

Items used by all physicians in reporting their services are presented in the **Introduction.** Some of the commonalities are repeated here for the convenience of those physicians referring to this section on **Radiology (Including Nuclear Medicine and Diagnostic Ultrasound).** Other definitions and items unique to Radiology are also listed.

Subject Listings

Subject listings apply when radiological services are performed by or under the responsible supervision of a physician.

Separate Procedures

Some of the procedures or services listed in the CPT codebook that are commonly carried out as an integral component of a total service or procedure have been identified by the inclusion of the term "separate procedure." The codes designated as "separate procedure" should not be reported in addition to the code for the total procedure or service of which it is considered an integral component.

However, when a procedure or service that is designated as a "separate procedure" is carried out independently or considered to be unrelated or distinct from other procedures/services provided at that time, it may be reported by itself, or in addition to other procedures/services by appending modifier 59 to the specific "separate procedure" code to indicate that the procedure is not considered to be a component of another procedure, but is a distinct, independent procedure. This may represent a different session or patient encounter, different procedure or surgery, different site or organ system, separate incision/excision, separate lesion, or separate injury (or area of injury in extensive injuries).

Subsection Information

Several of the subheadings or subsections have special needs or instructions unique to that section. Where these are indicated (eg, "Radiation Oncology") special **"Notes"** will be presented preceding those procedural terminology listings, referring to that subsection specifically. If there is an "Unlisted Procedure" code number (see section below) for the individual subsection, it will be shown. Those subsections with **"Notes"** are as follows:

▶**Functional MRI** . . . . 70554-70555◀
Aorta and Arteries 75600-75790
Veins and Lymphatics 75801-75893
Transcatheter Procedures. 75894-75989
Diagnostic Ultrasound 76506-76999
Abdomen and Retroperitoneum 76700-76776
Obstetrical 76801-76828
Non-Obstetrical 76830-76857
Radiation Oncology 77261-77799
Clinical Treatment Planning 77261-77299
Radiation Treatment Management 77427-77499
Proton Beam Treatment Delivery 77520-77525
Hyperthermia 77600-77620
Clinical Brachytherapy 77750-77799
Nuclear Medicine. 78000-78299
Musculoskeletal System 78300-78399
Cardiovascular System 78414-78499
Therapeutic 79005-79999

Unlisted Service or Procedure

A service or procedure may be provided that is not listed in this edition of the CPT codebook. When reporting such a service, the appropriate "Unlisted Procedure" code may be used to indicate the service, identifying it by "Special Report" as discussed below. The "Unlisted Procedures" and accompanying codes for **Radiology (Including Nuclear Medicine and Diagnostic Ultrasound)** are as follows:

76496   Unlisted fluoroscopic procedure (eg, diagnostic, interventional)

76497   Unlisted computed tomography procedure (eg, diagnostic, interventional)

76498   Unlisted magnetic resonance procedure (eg, diagnostic, interventional)

Radiology Guidelines

76499   Unlisted diagnostic radiographic procedure

76999   Unlisted ultrasound procedure (eg, diagnostic, interventional)

77299   Unlisted procedure, therapeutic radiology clinical treatment planning

77399   Unlisted procedure, medical radiation physics, dosimetry and treatment devices, and special services

77499   Unlisted procedure, therapeutic radiology treatment management

77799   Unlisted procedure, clinical brachytherapy

78099   Unlisted endocrine procedure, diagnostic nuclear medicine

78199   Unlisted hematopoietic, reticuloendothelial and lymphatic procedure, diagnostic nuclear medicine

78299   Unlisted gastrointestinal procedure, diagnostic nuclear medicine

78399   Unlisted musculoskeletal procedure, diagnostic nuclear medicine

78499   Unlisted cardiovascular procedure, diagnostic nuclear medicine

78599   Unlisted respiratory procedure, diagnostic nuclear medicine

78699   Unlisted nervous system procedure, diagnostic nuclear medicine

78799   Unlisted genitourinary procedure, diagnostic nuclear medicine

78999   Unlisted miscellaneous procedure, diagnostic nuclear medicine

79999   Radiopharmaceutical therapy, unlisted procedure

►Results/Testing/Reports◄

►Results are the technical component of a service. Testing leads to results; results lead to interpretation. Reports are the work product of the interpretation of numerous test results.◄

Special Report

A service that is rarely provided, unusual, variable, or new may require a special report in determining medical appropriateness of the service. Pertinent information should include an adequate definition or description of the nature, extent, and need for the procedure; and the time, effort, and equipment necessary to provide the service. Additional items that may be included are:

- Complexity of symptoms
- Final diagnosis
- Pertinent physical findings
- Diagnostic and therapeutic procedures
- Concurrent problems
- Follow-up care

Supervision and Interpretation

When a procedure is performed by two physicians, the radiologic portion of the procedure is designated as "radiological supervision and interpretation." When a physician performs both the procedure and provides imaging supervision and interpretation, a combination of procedure codes outside the 70000 series and imaging supervision and interpretation codes are to be used.

(The Radiological Supervision and Interpretation codes are not applicable to the Radiation Oncology subsection.)

Administration of Contrast Material(s)

The phrase "with contrast" used in the codes for procedures performed using contrast for imaging enhancement represents contrast material administered intravascularly, intra-articularly or intrathecally.

For intra-articular injection, use the appropriate joint injection code. If radiographic arthrography is performed, also use the arthrography supervision and interpretation code for the appropriate joint (which includes fluoroscopy). If computed tomography (CT) or magnetic resonance (MR) arthrography are performed without radiographic arthrography, use the appropriate joint injection code, the appropriate CT or MR code ("with contrast" or "without followed by contrast"), and the appropriate imaging guidance code for needle placement for contrast injection.

For spine examinations using computed tomography, magnetic resonance imaging, magnetic resonance angiography, "with contrast" includes intrathecal or intravascular injection. For intrathecal injection, use also 61055 or 62284.

Injection of intravascular contrast material is part of the "with contrast" CT, computed tomographic angiography (CTA), magnetic resonance imaging (MRI), and magnetic resonance angiography (MRA) procedures.

Oral and/or rectal contrast administration alone does not qualify as a study "with contrast."

Written Report(s)

A written report, signed by the interpreting physician, should be considered an integral part of a radiologic procedure or interpretation.

Radiology

Diagnostic Radiology (Diagnostic Imaging)

Head and Neck

70010 Myelography, posterior fossa, radiological supervision and interpretation

70015 Cisternography, positive contrast, radiological supervision and interpretation

70030 Radiologic examination, eye, for detection of foreign body

70100 Radiologic examination, mandible; partial, less than four views

70110 complete, minimum of four views

70120 Radiologic examination, mastoids; less than three views per side

70130 complete, minimum of three views per side

70134 Radiologic examination, internal auditory meati, complete

70140 Radiologic examination, facial bones; less than three views

70150 complete, minimum of three views

70160 Radiologic examination, nasal bones, complete, minimum of three views

70170 Dacryocystography, nasolacrimal duct, radiological supervision and interpretation

70190 Radiologic examination; optic foramina

70200 orbits, complete, minimum of four views

70210 Radiologic examination, sinuses, paranasal, less than three views

70220 Radiologic examination, sinuses, paranasal, complete, minimum of three views

70240 Radiologic examination, sella turcica

70250 Radiologic examination, skull; less than four views

70260 complete, minimum of four views

70300 Radiologic examination, teeth; single view

70310 partial examination, less than full mouth

70320 complete, full mouth

70328 Radiologic examination, temporomandibular joint, open and closed mouth; unilateral

70330 bilateral

70332 Temporomandibular joint arthrography, radiological supervision and interpretation

▶(Do not report 70332 in conjunction with 77002)◀

70336 Magnetic resonance (eg, proton) imaging, temporomandibular joint(s)

70350 Cephalogram, orthodontic

70355 Orthopantogram

70360 Radiologic examination; neck, soft tissue

70370 pharynx or larynx, including fluoroscopy and/or magnification technique

70371 Complex dynamic pharyngeal and speech evaluation by cine or video recording

70373 Laryngography, contrast, radiological supervision and interpretation

70380 Radiologic examination, salivary gland for calculus

70390 Sialography, radiological supervision and interpretation

70450 Computed tomography, head or brain; without contrast material

70460 with contrast material(s)

70470 without contrast material, followed by contrast material(s) and further sections

(To report 3D rendering, see 76376, 76377)

70480 Computed tomography, orbit, sella, or posterior fossa or outer, middle, or inner ear; without contrast material

70481 with contrast material(s)

70482 without contrast material, followed by contrast material(s) and further sections

(To report 3D rendering, see 76376, 76377)

70486 Computed tomography, maxillofacial area; without contrast material

70487 with contrast material(s)

70488 without contrast material, followed by contrast material(s) and further sections

(To report 3D rendering, see 76376, 76377)

70490 Computed tomography, soft tissue neck; without contrast material

70491 with contrast material(s)

70492 without contrast material followed by contrast material(s) and further sections

(To report 3D rendering, see 76376, 76377)

(For cervical spine, see 72125, 72126)

Radiology

70496   Computed tomographic angiography, head, without contrast material(s), followed by contrast material(s) and further sections, including image post-processing

70498   Computed tomographic angiography, neck, without contrast material(s), followed by contrast material(s) and further sections, including image post-processing

▲ **70540**   Magnetic resonance (eg, proton) imaging, orbit, face, and/or neck; without contrast material(s)

(For head or neck magnetic resonance angiography studies, see 70544-70546, 70547-70549)

70542   with contrast material(s)

70543   without contrast material(s), followed by contrast material(s) and further sequences

►(Report 70540-70543 once per imaging session)◄

70544   Magnetic resonance angiography, head; without contrast material(s)

70545   with contrast material(s)

70546   without contrast material(s), followed by contrast material(s) and further sequences

70547   Magnetic resonance angiography, neck; without contrast material(s)

70548   with contrast material(s)

70549   without contrast material(s), followed by contrast material(s) and further sequences

70551   Magnetic resonance (eg, proton) imaging, brain (including brain stem); without contrast material

70552   with contrast material(s)

70553   without contrast material, followed by contrast material(s) and further sequences

(For magnetic spectroscopy, use 76390)

►Functional MRI involves identification and mapping of stimulation of brain function. When neurofunctional tests are administered by a technologist or other non-physician or non-psychologist, use 70554. When neurofunctional tests are entirely administered by a physician or psychologist, use 70555.◄

● **70554**   Magnetic resonance imaging, brain, functional MRI; including test selection and administration of repetitive body part movement and/or visual stimulation, not requiring physician or psychologist administration

►(Do not report 70554 in conjunction with 96020)◄

● **70555**   requiring physician or psychologist administration of entire neurofunctional testing

►(Do not report 70555 unless 96020 is performed)◄

►(Do not report 70554, 70555 in conjunction with 70551-70553 unless a separate diagnostic MRI is performed)◄

70557   Magnetic resonance (eg, proton) imaging, brain (including brain stem and skull base), during open intracranial procedure (eg, to assess for residual tumor or residual vascular malformation); without contrast material

70558   with contrast material(s)

70559   without contrast material(s), followed by contrast material(s) and further sequences

►(For stereotactic biopsy of intracranial lesion with magnetic resonance guidance, use 61751. 70557, 70558 or 70559 may be reported only if a separate report is generated. Report only one of the above codes once per operative session. Do not use these codes in conjunction with 61751, 77021, 77022)◄

Chest

►(For fluoroscopic or ultrasonic guidance for needle placement procedures (eg, biopsy, aspiration, injection, localization device) of the thorax, see 76942, 77002)◄

71010   Radiologic examination, chest; single view, frontal

71015   stereo, frontal

71020   Radiologic examination, chest, two views, frontal and lateral;

71021   with apical lordotic procedure

71022   with oblique projections

71023   with fluoroscopy

71030   Radiologic examination, chest, complete, minimum of four views;

71034   with fluoroscopy

(For separate chest fluoroscopy, use 76000)

71035   Radiologic examination, chest, special views (eg, lateral decubitus, Bucky studies)

71040   Bronchography, unilateral, radiological supervision and interpretation

71060   Bronchography, bilateral, radiological supervision and interpretation

71090   Insertion pacemaker, fluoroscopy and radiography, radiological supervision and interpretation

(For procedure, see appropriate organ or site)

71100   Radiologic examination, ribs, unilateral; two views

71101   including posteroanterior chest, minimum of three views

71110   Radiologic examination, ribs, bilateral; three views

71111   including posteroanterior chest, minimum of four views

71120   Radiologic examination; sternum, minimum of two views

71130   sternoclavicular joint or joints, minimum of three views

Radiology

71250   Computed tomography, thorax; without contrast material

71260   with contrast material(s)

71270   without contrast material, followed by contrast material(s) and further sections

▶(For cardiac computed tomography of the heart, see Category III codes 0144T-0151T)◀

(To report 3D rendering, see 76376, 76377)

▲ **71275**   Computed tomographic angiography, chest (noncoronary), without contrast material(s), followed by contrast material(s) and further sections, including image postprocessing

▶(For coronary artery computed tomographic angiography including calcification score and/or cardiac morphology, see Category III codes 0146T-0149T)◀

71550   Magnetic resonance (eg, proton) imaging, chest (eg, for evaluation of hilar and mediastinal lymphadenopathy); without contrast material(s)

71551   with contrast material(s)

71552   without contrast material(s), followed by contrast material(s) and further sequences

▶(For breast MRI, see 77058, 77059)◀

71555   Magnetic resonance angiography, chest (excluding myocardium), with or without contrast material(s)

Spine and Pelvis

72010   Radiologic examination, spine, entire, survey study, anteroposterior and lateral

72020   Radiologic examination, spine, single view, specify level

72040   Radiologic examination, spine, cervical; two or three views

72050   minimum of four views

72052   complete, including oblique and flexion and/or extension studies

72069   Radiologic examination, spine, thoracolumbar, standing (scoliosis)

72070   Radiologic examination, spine; thoracic, two views

72072   thoracic, three views

72074   thoracic, minimum of four views

72080   thoracolumbar, two views

72090   scoliosis study, including supine and erect studies

72100   Radiologic examination, spine, lumbosacral; two or three views

72110   minimum of four views

72114   complete, including bending views

72120   Radiologic examination, spine, lumbosacral, bending views only, minimum of four views

(Contrast material in CT of spine is either by intrathecal or intravenous injection. For intrathecal injection, use also 61055 or 62284. IV injection of contrast material is part of the CT procedure)

72125   Computed tomography, cervical spine; without contrast material

72126   with contrast material

72127   without contrast material, followed by contrast material(s) and further sections

(For intrathecal injection procedure, see 61055, 62284)

72128   Computed tomography, thoracic spine; without contrast material

72129   with contrast material

(For intrathecal injection procedure, see 61055, 62284)

72130   without contrast material, followed by contrast material(s) and further sections

(For intrathecal injection procedure, see 61055, 62284)

72131   Computed tomography, lumbar spine; without contrast material

72132   with contrast material

72133   without contrast material, followed by contrast material(s) and further sections

(For intrathecal injection procedure, see 61055, 62284)

(To report 3D rendering, see 76376, 76377)

72141   Magnetic resonance (eg, proton) imaging, spinal canal and contents, cervical; without contrast material

72142   with contrast material(s)

(For cervical spinal canal imaging without contrast material followed by contrast material, use 72156)

72146   Magnetic resonance (eg, proton) imaging, spinal canal and contents, thoracic; without contrast material

72147   with contrast material(s)

(For thoracic spinal canal imaging without contrast material followed by contrast material, use 72157)

72148   Magnetic resonance (eg, proton) imaging, spinal canal and contents, lumbar; without contrast material

72149   with contrast material(s)

(For lumbar spinal canal imaging without contrast material followed by contrast material, use 72158)

72156   Magnetic resonance (eg, proton) imaging, spinal canal and contents, without contrast material, followed by contrast material(s) and further sequences; cervical

72157   thoracic

72158   lumbar

Radiology

72159 Magnetic resonance angiography, spinal canal and contents, with or without contrast material(s)

72170 Radiologic examination, pelvis; one or two views

72190 complete, minimum of three views

(For pelvimetry, use 74710)

72191 Computed tomographic angiography, pelvis, without contrast material(s), followed by contrast material(s) and further sections, including image post-processing

(For CTA aorto-iliofemoral runoff, use 75635)

72192 Computed tomography, pelvis; without contrast material

72193 with contrast material(s)

72194 without contrast material, followed by contrast material(s) and further sections

(To report 3D rendering, see 76376, 76377)

(For computed tomographic colonography, see Category III codes 0066T, 0067T. Do not report 72192-72194 in conjunction with 0066T, 0067T)

72195 Magnetic resonance (eg, proton) imaging, pelvis; without contrast material(s)

72196 with contrast material(s)

72197 without contrast material(s), followed by contrast material(s) and further sequences

72198 Magnetic resonance angiography, pelvis, with or without contrast material(s)

72200 Radiologic examination, sacroiliac joints; less than three views

72202 three or more views

72220 Radiologic examination, sacrum and coccyx, minimum of two views

72240 Myelography, cervical, radiological supervision and interpretation

(For complete cervical myelography, see 61055, 62284, 72240)

72255 Myelography, thoracic, radiological supervision and interpretation

(For complete thoracic myelography, see 61055, 62284, 72255)

72265 Myelography, lumbosacral, radiological supervision and interpretation

(For complete lumbosacral myelography, see 61055, 62284, 72265)

72270 Myelography, two or more regions (eg, lumbar/thoracic, cervical/thoracic, lumbar/cervical, lumbar/thoracic/cervical), radiological supervision and interpretation

(For complete myelography of entire spinal canal, see 61055, 62284, 72270)

72275 Epidurography, radiological supervision and interpretation

►(72275 includes 77003)◄

(For injection procedure, see 62280-62282, 62310-62319, 64479-64484, 0027T)

(Use 72275 only when an epidurogram is performed, images documented, and a formal radiologic report is issued)

72285 Discography, cervical or thoracic, radiological supervision and interpretation

● **72291** Radiological supervision and interpretation, percutaneous vertebroplasty or vertebral augmentation including cavity creation, per vertebral body; under fluoroscopic guidance

● **72292** under CT guidance

►(For procedure, see 22520-22525)◄

72295 Discography, lumbar, radiological supervision and interpretation

Upper Extremities

►(For stress views, any joint, use 77071)◄

73000 Radiologic examination; clavicle, complete

73010 scapula, complete

73020 Radiologic examination, shoulder; one view

73030 complete, minimum of two views

73040 Radiologic examination, shoulder, arthrography, radiological supervision and interpretation

►(Do not report 77002 in conjunction with 73040)◄

73050 Radiologic examination; acromioclavicular joints, bilateral, with or without weighted distraction

73060 humerus, minimum of two views

73070 Radiologic examination, elbow; two views

73080 complete, minimum of three views

73085 Radiologic examination, elbow, arthrography, radiological supervision and interpretation

►(Do not report 77002 in conjunction with 73085)◄

73090 Radiologic examination; forearm, two views

73092 upper extremity, infant, minimum of two views

73100 Radiologic examination, wrist; two views

73110 complete, minimum of three views

73115 Radiologic examination, wrist, arthrography, radiological supervision and interpretation

►(Do not report 77002 in conjunction with 73115)◄

73120 Radiologic examination, hand; two views

73130 minimum of three views

73140 Radiologic examination, finger(s), minimum of two views

Radiology

73200   Computed tomography, upper extremity; without contrast material

73201   with contrast material(s)

73202   without contrast material, followed by contrast material(s) and further sections

      (To report 3D rendering, see 76376, 76377)

73206   Computed tomographic angiography, upper extremity, without contrast material(s), followed by contrast material(s) and further sections, including image post-processing

73218   Magnetic resonance (eg, proton) imaging, upper extremity, other than joint; without contrast material(s)

73219   with contrast material(s)

73220   without contrast material(s), followed by contrast material(s) and further sequences

73221   Magnetic resonance (eg, proton) imaging, any joint of upper extremity; without contrast material(s)

73222   with contrast material(s)

73223   without contrast material(s), followed by contrast material(s) and further sequences

73225   Magnetic resonance angiography, upper extremity, with or without contrast material(s)

Lower Extremities

      ►(For stress views, any joint, use 77071)◄

73500   Radiologic examination, hip, unilateral; one view

73510   complete, minimum of two views

73520   Radiologic examination, hips, bilateral, minimum of two views of each hip, including anteroposterior view of pelvis

73525   Radiologic examination, hip, arthrography, radiological supervision and interpretation

      ►(Do not report 73525 in conjunction with 77002)◄

73530   Radiologic examination, hip, during operative procedure

73540   Radiologic examination, pelvis and hips, infant or child, minimum of two views

73542   Radiological examination, sacroiliac joint arthrography, radiological supervision and interpretation

      ►(Do not report 73542 in conjunction with 77002)◄

      ►(For procedure, use 27096. If formal arthrography is not performed, recorded, and a formal radiologic report is not issued, use 77003 for fluoroscopic guidance for sacroiliac joint injections)◄

73550   Radiologic examination, femur, two views

73560   Radiologic examination, knee; one or two views

73562   three views

73564   complete, four or more views

73565   both knees, standing, anteroposterior

73580   Radiologic examination, knee, arthrography, radiological supervision and interpretation

      ►(Do not report 73580 in conjunction with 77002)◄

73590   Radiologic examination; tibia and fibula, two views

73592   lower extremity, infant, minimum of two views

73600   Radiologic examination, ankle; two views

73610   complete, minimum of three views

73615   Radiologic examination, ankle, arthrography, radiological supervision and interpretation

      ►(Do not report 73615 in conjunction with 77002)◄

73620   Radiologic examination, foot; two views

73630   complete, minimum of three views

73650   Radiologic examination; calcaneus, minimum of two views

73660   toe(s), minimum of two views

73700   Computed tomography, lower extremity; without contrast material

73701   with contrast material(s)

73702   without contrast material, followed by contrast material(s) and further sections

      (To report 3D rendering, see 76376, 76377)

73706   Computed tomographic angiography, lower extremity, without contrast material(s), followed by contrast material(s) and further sections, including image post-processing

      (For CTA aorto-iliofemoral runoff, use 75635)

73718   Magnetic resonance (eg, proton) imaging, lower extremity other than joint; without contrast material(s)

73719   with contrast material(s)

73720   without contrast material(s), followed by contrast material(s) and further sequences

73721   Magnetic resonance (eg, proton) imaging, any joint of lower extremity; without contrast material

73722   with contrast material(s)

73723   without contrast material(s), followed by contrast material(s) and further sequences

73725   Magnetic resonance angiography, lower extremity, with or without contrast material(s)

Abdomen

74000   Radiologic examination, abdomen; single anteroposterior view

74010   anteroposterior and additional oblique and cone views

74020   complete, including decubitus and/or erect views

74022   complete acute abdomen series, including supine, erect, and/or decubitus views, single view chest

Radiology

74150 Computed tomography, abdomen; without contrast material

74160 with contrast material(s)

74170 without contrast material, followed by contrast material(s) and further sections

(To report 3D rendering, see 76376, 76377)

(For computed tomographic colonography, see Category III codes 0066T, 0067T. Do not report 74150-74170 in conjunction with 0066T, 0067T)

74175 Computed tomographic angiography, abdomen, without contrast material(s), followed by contrast material(s) and further sections, including image post-processing

(For CTA aorto-iliofemoral runoff, use 75635)

74181 Magnetic resonance (eg, proton) imaging, abdomen; without contrast material(s)

74182 with contrast material(s)

74183 without contrast material(s), followed by with contrast material(s) and further sequences

74185 Magnetic resonance angiography, abdomen, with or without contrast material(s)

74190 Peritoneogram (eg, after injection of air or contrast), radiological supervision and interpretation

(For procedure, use 49400)

(For computed tomography, see 72192 or 74150)

Gastrointestinal Tract

(For percutaneous placement of gastrostomy tube, use 43750)

74210 Radiologic examination; pharynx and/or cervical esophagus

74220 esophagus

74230 Swallowing function, with cineradiography/videoradiography

74235 Removal of foreign body(s), esophageal, with use of balloon catheter, radiological supervision and interpretation

(For procedure, see 43215, 43247)

74240 Radiologic examination, gastrointestinal tract, upper; with or without delayed films, without KUB

74241 with or without delayed films, with KUB

74245 with small intestine, includes multiple serial films

74246 Radiological examination, gastrointestinal tract, upper, air contrast, with specific high density barium, effervescent agent, with or without glucagon; with or without delayed films, without KUB

74247 with or without delayed films, with KUB

74249 with small intestine follow-through

74250 Radiologic examination, small intestine, includes multiple serial films;

74251 via enteroclysis tube

74260 Duodenography, hypotonic

74270 Radiologic examination, colon; barium enema, with or without KUB

74280 air contrast with specific high density barium, with or without glucagon

74283 Therapeutic enema, contrast or air, for reduction of intussusception or other intraluminal obstruction (eg, meconium ileus)

74290 Cholecystography, oral contrast;

74291 additional or repeat examination or multiple day examination

74300 Cholangiography and/or pancreatography; intraoperative, radiological supervision and interpretation

+ 74301 additional set intraoperative, radiological supervision and interpretation (List separately in addition to code for primary procedure)

(Use 74301 in conjunction with 74300)

74305 through existing catheter, radiological supervision and interpretation

(For procedure, see 47505, 48400, 47560-47561, 47563)

(For biliary duct stone extraction, percutaneous, see 47630, 74327)

74320 Cholangiography, percutaneous, transhepatic, radiological supervision and interpretation

74327 Postoperative biliary duct calculus removal, percutaneous via T-tube tract, basket, or snare (eg, Burhenne technique), radiological supervision and interpretation

(For procedure, use 47630)

74328 Endoscopic catheterization of the biliary ductal system, radiological supervision and interpretation

(For procedure, see 43260-43272 as appropriate)

74329 Endoscopic catheterization of the pancreatic ductal system, radiological supervision and interpretation

(For procedure, see 43260-43272 as appropriate)

74330 Combined endoscopic catheterization of the biliary and pancreatic ductal systems, radiological supervision and interpretation

(For procedure, see 43260-43272 as appropriate)

74340 Introduction of long gastrointestinal tube (eg, Miller-Abbott), including multiple fluoroscopies and films, radiological supervision and interpretation

(For tube placement, use 44500)

74350 Percutaneous placement of gastrostomy tube, radiological supervision and interpretation

Radiology

74355   Percutaneous placement of enteroclysis tube, radiological supervision and interpretation

74360   Intraluminal dilation of strictures and/or obstructions (eg, esophagus), radiological supervision and interpretation

74363   Percutaneous transhepatic dilation of biliary duct stricture with or without placement of stent, radiological supervision and interpretation

      (For procedure, see 47510, 47511, 47555, 47556)

Urinary Tract

74400   Urography (pyelography), intravenous, with or without KUB, with or without tomography

74410   Urography, infusion, drip technique and/or bolus technique;

74415   with nephrotomography

74420   Urography, retrograde, with or without KUB

74425   Urography, antegrade, (pyelostogram, nephrostogram, loopogram), radiological supervision and interpretation

74430   Cystography, minimum of three views, radiological supervision and interpretation

74440   Vasography, vesiculography, or epididymography, radiological supervision and interpretation

74445   Corpora cavernosography, radiological supervision and interpretation

74450   Urethrocystography, retrograde, radiological supervision and interpretation

74455   Urethrocystography, voiding, radiological supervision and interpretation

74470   Radiologic examination, renal cyst study, translumbar, contrast visualization, radiological supervision and interpretation

74475   Introduction of intracatheter or catheter into renal pelvis for drainage and/or injection, percutaneous, radiological supervision and interpretation

74480   Introduction of ureteral catheter or stent into ureter through renal pelvis for drainage and/or injection, percutaneous, radiological supervision and interpretation

      (For transurethral surgery (ureter and pelvis), see 52320-52355)

74485   Dilation of nephrostomy, ureters, or urethra, radiological supervision and interpretation

      (For dilation of ureter without radiologic guidance, use 52341, 52344)

      (For change of nephrostomy or pyelostomy tube, use 50398)

Gynecological and Obstetrical

      (For abdomen and pelvis, see 72170-72190, 74000-74170)

74710   Pelvimetry, with or without placental localization

74740   Hysterosalpingography, radiological supervision and interpretation

      (For introduction of saline or contrast for hysterosalpingography, see 58340)

74742   Transcervical catheterization of fallopian tube, radiological supervision and interpretation

      (For procedure, use 58345)

74775   Perineogram (eg, vaginogram, for sex determination or extent of anomalies)

Heart

      (For separate injection procedures for vascular radiology, see **Surgery** section, 36000-36299)

      (For cardiac catheterization procedures, see 93501-93556)

75552   Cardiac magnetic resonance imaging for morphology; without contrast material

75553   with contrast material

75554   Cardiac magnetic resonance imaging for function, with or without morphology; complete study

75555   limited study

75556   Cardiac magnetic resonance imaging for velocity flow mapping

Vascular Procedures

Aorta and Arteries

Selective vascular catheterizations should be coded to include introduction and all lesser order selective catheterizations used in the approach (eg, the description for a selective right middle cerebral artery catheterization includes the introduction and placement catheterization of the right common and internal carotid arteries).

Additional second and/or third order arterial catheterizations within the same family of arteries supplied by a single first order artery should be expressed by 36218 or 36248. Additional first order or higher catheterizations in vascular families supplied by a first order vessel different from a previously selected and coded family should be separately coded using the conventions described above.

For angiography performed in conjunction with therapeutic transcatheter radiological supervision and interpretation services, see the Radiology Transcatheter Procedures guidelines.

Radiology

Diagnostic angiography (radiological supervision and interpretation) codes should NOT be used with interventional procedures for:

1. Contrast injections, angiography, roadmapping, and/or fluoroscopic guidance for the intervention,

2. Vessel measurement, and

3. Post-angioplasty/stent angiography,

as this work is captured in the radiological supervision and interpretation code(s).

Diagnostic angiography performed at the time of an interventional procedure is separately reportable if:

1. No prior catheter-based angiographic study is available and a full diagnostic study is performed, and the decision to intervene is based on the diagnostic study, OR

2. A prior study is available, but as documented in the medical record:

  a. The patient's condition with respect to the clinical indication has changed since the prior study, OR

  b. There is inadequate visualization of the anatomy and/or pathology, OR

  c. There is a clinical change during the procedure that requires new evaluation outside the target area of intervention.

Diagnostic angiography performed at a separate setting from an interventional procedure is separately reported.

Diagnostic angiography performed at the time of an interventional procedure is NOT separately reportable if it is specifically included in the interventional code descriptor.

> (For intravenous procedure, see 36000-36013, 36400-36425 and 36100-36248 for intra-arterial procedure)
>
> (For radiological supervision and interpretation, see 75600-75978)

75600 Aortography, thoracic, without serialography, radiological supervision and interpretation

> (For injection procedure, use 93544)

75605 Aortography, thoracic, by serialography, radiological supervision and interpretation

> (For injection procedure, use 93544)

75625 Aortography, abdominal, by serialography, radiological supervision and interpretation

> (For injection procedure, use 93544)

75630 Aortography, abdominal plus bilateral iliofemoral lower extremity, catheter, by serialography, radiological supervision and interpretation

75635 Computed tomographic angiography, abdominal aorta and bilateral iliofemoral lower extremity runoff, radiological supervision and interpretation, without contrast material(s), followed by contrast material(s) and further sections, including image post-processing

75650 Angiography, cervicocerebral, catheter, including vessel origin, radiological supervision and interpretation

75658 Angiography, brachial, retrograde, radiological supervision and interpretation

75660 Angiography, external carotid, unilateral, selective, radiological supervision and interpretation

75662 Angiography, external carotid, bilateral, selective, radiological supervision and interpretation

75665 Angiography, carotid, cerebral, unilateral, radiological supervision and interpretation

75671 Angiography, carotid, cerebral, bilateral, radiological supervision and interpretation

75676 Angiography, carotid, cervical, unilateral, radiological supervision and interpretation

75680 Angiography, carotid, cervical, bilateral, radiological supervision and interpretation

75685 Angiography, vertebral, cervical, and/or intracranial, radiological supervision and interpretation

75705 Angiography, spinal, selective, radiological supervision and interpretation

75710 Angiography, extremity, unilateral, radiological supervision and interpretation

75716 Angiography, extremity, bilateral, radiological supervision and interpretation

75722 Angiography, renal, unilateral, selective (including flush aortogram), radiological supervision and interpretation

75724 Angiography, renal, bilateral, selective (including flush aortogram), radiological supervision and interpretation

75726 Angiography, visceral, selective or supraselective, (with or without flush aortogram), radiological supervision and interpretation

> (For selective angiography, each additional visceral vessel studied after basic examination, use 75774)

75731 Angiography, adrenal, unilateral, selective, radiological supervision and interpretation

75733 Angiography, adrenal, bilateral, selective, radiological supervision and interpretation

75736 Angiography, pelvic, selective or supraselective, radiological supervision and interpretation

75741 Angiography, pulmonary, unilateral, selective, radiological supervision and interpretation

> (For injection procedure, use 93541)

75743 Angiography, pulmonary, bilateral, selective, radiological supervision and interpretation

> (For injection procedure, use 93541)

Radiology

75746   Angiography, pulmonary, by nonselective catheter or venous injection, radiological supervision and interpretation

(For injection procedure, use 93541)

(For introduction of catheter, injection procedure, see 93501-93533, 93539, 93540, 93545, 93556)

(For introduction of catheter, injection procedure, see 93501-93533, 93545, 93556)

(For introduction of catheter, injection procedure, see 93501-93533, 93539, 93540, 93545, 93556)

75756   Angiography, internal mammary, radiological supervision and interpretation

(For introduction of catheter, injection procedure, see 93501-93533, 93545, 93556)

+ 75774   Angiography, selective, each additional vessel studied after basic examination, radiological supervision and interpretation (List separately in addition to code for primary procedure)

(Use 75774 in addition to code for specific initial vessel studied)

(For angiography, see codes 75600-75790)

(For catheterizations, see codes 36215-36248)

(For introduction of catheter, injection procedure, see 93501-93533, 93545, 93555, 93556)

75790   Angiography, arteriovenous shunt (eg, dialysis patient), radiological supervision and interpretation

(For introduction of catheter, use 36140, 36145, 36215-36217, 36245-36247)

Veins and Lymphatics

For venography performed in conjunction with therapeutic transcatheter radiological supervision and interpretation services, see the Radiology Transcatheter Procedures guidelines.

Diagnostic venography (radiological supervision and interpretation) codes should NOT be used with interventional procedures for:

1. Contrast injections, venography, roadmapping, and/or fluoroscopic guidance for the intervention,

2. Vessel measurement, and

3. Post-angioplasty/stent venography,

as this work is captured in the radiological supervision and interpretation code(s).

Diagnostic venography performed at the time of an interventional procedure is separately reportable if:

1. No prior catheter-based venographic study is available and a full diagnostic study is performed, and decision to intervene is based on the diagnostic study, OR

2. A prior study is available, but as documented in the medical record:

a. The patient's condition with respect to the clinical indication has changed since the prior study, OR

b. There is inadequate visualization of the anatomy and/or pathology, OR

c. There is a clinical change during the procedure that requires new evaluation outside the target area of intervention.

Diagnostic venography performed at a separate setting from an interventional procedure is separately reported.

Diagnostic venography performed at the time of an interventional procedure is NOT separately reportable if it is specifically included in the interventional code descriptor.

(For injection procedure for venous system, see 36000-36015, 36400-36510)

(For injection procedure for lymphatic system, use 38790)

75801   Lymphangiography, extremity only, unilateral, radiological supervision and interpretation

75803   Lymphangiography, extremity only, bilateral, radiological supervision and interpretation

75805   Lymphangiography, pelvic/abdominal, unilateral, radiological supervision and interpretation

75807   Lymphangiography, pelvic/abdominal, bilateral, radiological supervision and interpretation

75809   Shuntogram for investigation of previously placed indwelling nonvascular shunt (eg, LeVeen shunt, ventriculoperitoneal shunt, indwelling infusion pump), radiological supervision and interpretation

(For procedure, see 49427 or 61070)

75810   Splenoportography, radiological supervision and interpretation

75820   Venography, extremity, unilateral, radiological supervision and interpretation

75822   Venography, extremity, bilateral, radiological supervision and interpretation

75825   Venography, caval, inferior, with serialography, radiological supervision and interpretation

75827   Venography, caval, superior, with serialography, radiological supervision and interpretation

75831   Venography, renal, unilateral, selective, radiological supervision and interpretation

75833   Venography, renal, bilateral, selective, radiological supervision and interpretation

75840   Venography, adrenal, unilateral, selective, radiological supervision and interpretation

75842   Venography, adrenal, bilateral, selective, radiological supervision and interpretation

Radiology

75860 Venography, venous sinus (eg, petrosal and inferior sagittal) or jugular, catheter, radiological supervision and interpretation

75870 Venography, superior sagittal sinus, radiological supervision and interpretation

75872 Venography, epidural, radiological supervision and interpretation

75880 Venography, orbital, radiological supervision and interpretation

75885 Percutaneous transhepatic portography with hemodynamic evaluation, radiological supervision and interpretation

75887 Percutaneous transhepatic portography without hemodynamic evaluation, radiological supervision and interpretation

75889 Hepatic venography, wedged or free, with hemodynamic evaluation, radiological supervision and interpretation

75891 Hepatic venography, wedged or free, without hemodynamic evaluation, radiological supervision and interpretation

75893 Venous sampling through catheter, with or without angiography (eg, for parathyroid hormone, renin), radiological supervision and interpretation

(For procedure, use 36500)

Transcatheter Procedures

Therapeutic transcatheter radiological supervision and interpretation code(s) include the following services associated with that intervention:

1. Contrast injections, angiography/venography, roadmapping, and fluoroscopic guidance for the intervention,

2. Vessel measurement, and

3. Completion angiography/venography (except for those uses permitted by 75898).

Unless specifically included in the code descriptor, diagnostic angiography/venography performed at the time of transcatheter therapeutic radiological and interpretation service(s) is separately reportable (eg, no prior catheter-based diagnostic angiography/venography study of the target vessel is available, prior diagnostic study is inadequate, patient's condition with respect to the clinical indication has changed since the prior study or during the intervention). See 75600-75893.

Codes 75956 and 75957 include all angiography of the thoracic aorta and its branches for diagnostic imaging prior to deployment of the primary endovascular devices (including all routine components of modular devices), fluoroscopic guidance in the delivery of the endovascular components, and intraprocedural arterial angiography (eg, confirm position, detect endoleak, evaluate runoff).

Code 75958 includes the analogous services for placement of each proximal thoracic endovascular extension. Code 75959 includes the analogous services for placement of a distal thoracic endovascular extension(s) placed during a procedure after the primary repair.

75894 Transcatheter therapy, embolization, any method, radiological supervision and interpretation

▶(For uterine fibroid embolization [uterine artery embolization performed to treat uterine fibroids], use 37210)◀

▶(For obstetrical and gynecologic embolization procedures other than uterine fibroid embolization [eg, embolization to treat obstetrical or postpartum hemorrhage], use 37204)◀

75896 Transcatheter therapy, infusion, any method (eg, thrombolysis other than coronary), radiological supervision and interpretation

(For infusion for coronary disease, see 92975, 92977)

75898 Angiography through existing catheter for follow-up study for transcatheter therapy, embolization or infusion

75900 Exchange of a previously placed intravascular catheter during thrombolytic therapy with contrast monitoring, radiological supervision and interpretation

(For procedure, use 37209)

75901 Mechanical removal of pericatheter obstructive material (eg, fibrin sheath) from central venous device via separate venous access, radiologic supervision and interpretation

(For procedure, use 36595)

(For venous catheterization, see 36010-36012)

75902 Mechanical removal of intraluminal (intracatheter) obstructive material from central venous device through device lumen, radiologic supervision and interpretation

(For procedure, use 36596)

(For venous catheterization, see 36010-36012)

75940 Percutaneous placement of IVC filter, radiological supervision and interpretation

75945 Intravascular ultrasound (non-coronary vessel), radiological supervision and interpretation; initial vessel

+ 75946 each additional non-coronary vessel (List separately in addition to code for primary procedure)

(Use 75946 in conjunction with 75945)

(For catheterizations, see codes 36215-36248)

(For transcatheter therapies, see codes 37200-37208, 61624, 61626)

(For procedure, see 37250, 37251)

Radiology

75952   Endovascular repair of infrarenal abdominal aortic aneurysm or dissection, radiological supervision and interpretation

(For implantation of endovascular grafts, see 34800-34808)

(For radiologic supervision and interpretation of endovascular repair of abdominal aortic aneurysm involving visceral vessels, see Category III codes 0078T-0081T)

75953   Placement of proximal or distal extension prosthesis for endovascular repair of infrarenal aortic or iliac artery aneurysm, pseudoaneurysm, or dissection, radiological supervision and interpretation

(For implantation of endovascular extension prostheses, see 34825, 34826)

75954   Endovascular repair of iliac artery aneurysm, pseudoaneurysm, arteriovenous malformation, or trauma, radiological supervision and interpretation

(For implantation of endovascular graft, see 34900)

75956   Endovascular repair of descending thoracic aorta (eg, aneurysm, pseudoaneurysm, dissection, penetrating ulcer, intramural hematoma, or traumatic disruption); involving coverage of left subclavian artery origin, initial endoprosthesis plus descending thoracic aortic extension(s), if required, to level of celiac artery origin, radiological supervision and interpretation

(For implantation of endovascular graft, use 33880)

75957   not involving coverage of left subclavian artery origin, initial endoprosthesis plus descending thoracic aortic extension(s), if required, to level of celiac artery origin, radiological supervision and interpretation

(For implantation of endovascular graft, use 33881)

75958   Placement of proximal extension prosthesis for endovascular repair of descending thoracic aorta (eg, aneurysm, pseudoaneurysm, dissection, penetrating ulcer, intramural hematoma, or traumatic disruption), radiological supervision and interpretation

(Report 75958 for each proximal extension)

(For implantation of proximal endovascular extension, see 33883, 33884)

75959   Placement of distal extension prosthesis(s) (delayed) after endovascular repair of descending thoracic aorta, as needed, to level of celiac origin, radiological supervision and interpretation

(Do not report 75959 in conjunction with 75956, 75957)

(Report 75959 once, regardless of number of modules deployed)

(For implantation of distal endovascular extension, use 33886)

75960   Transcatheter introduction of intravascular stent(s), (except coronary, carotid, and vertebral vessel), percutaneous and/or open, radiological supervision and interpretation, each vessel

(For procedure, see 37205-37208)

(For radiologic supervision and interpretation for transcatheter placement of extracranial vertebral or intrathoracic carotid artery stent(s), see Category III codes 0075T, 0076T)

75961   Transcatheter retrieval, percutaneous, of intravascular foreign body (eg, fractured venous or arterial catheter), radiological supervision and interpretation

(For procedure, use 37203)

75962   Transluminal balloon angioplasty, peripheral artery, radiological supervision and interpretation

+ 75964   Transluminal balloon angioplasty, each additional peripheral artery, radiological supervision and interpretation (List separately in addition to code for primary procedure)

(Use 75964 in conjunction with 75962)

75966   Transluminal balloon angioplasty, renal or other visceral artery, radiological supervision and interpretation

+ 75968   Transluminal balloon angioplasty, each additional visceral artery, radiological supervision and interpretation (List separately in addition to code for primary procedure)

(Use 75968 in conjunction with 75966)

(For percutaneous transluminal coronary angioplasty, see 92982-92984)

75970   Transcatheter biopsy, radiological supervision and interpretation

(For injection procedure only for transcatheter therapy or biopsy, see 36100-36299)

(For transcatheter renal and ureteral biopsy, use 52007)

(For percutaneous needle biopsy of pancreas, use 48102; of retroperitoneal lymph node or mass, use 49180)

75978   Transluminal balloon angioplasty, venous (eg, subclavian stenosis), radiological supervision and interpretation

75980   Percutaneous transhepatic biliary drainage with contrast monitoring, radiological supervision and interpretation

75982   Percutaneous placement of drainage catheter for combined internal and external biliary drainage or of a drainage stent for internal biliary drainage in patients with an inoperable mechanical biliary obstruction, radiological supervision and interpretation

75984   Change of percutaneous tube or drainage catheter with contrast monitoring (eg, gastrointestinal system, genitourinary system, abscess), radiological supervision and interpretation

(For change of nephrostomy or pyelostomy tube only, use 50398)

Radiology

(For introduction procedure only for percutaneous biliary drainage, see 47510, 47511)

(For percutaneous cholecystostomy, use 47490)

(For change of percutaneous biliary drainage catheter only, use 47525)

(For percutaneous nephrostolithotomy or pyelostolithotomy, see 50080, 50081)

75989 Radiological guidance (ie, fluoroscopy, ultrasound, or computed tomography), for percutaneous drainage (eg, abscess, specimen collection), with placement of catheter, radiological supervision and interpretation

Transluminal Atherectomy

75992 Transluminal atherectomy, peripheral artery, radiological supervision and interpretation

(For procedure, see 35481-35485, 35491-35495)

+ 75993 Transluminal atherectomy, each additional peripheral artery, radiological supervision and interpretation (List separately in addition to code for primary procedure)

(Use 75993 in conjunction with 75992)

(For procedure, see 35481-35485, 35491-35495)

75994 Transluminal atherectomy, renal, radiological supervision and interpretation

(For procedure, see 35480, 35490)

75995 Transluminal atherectomy, visceral, radiological supervision and interpretation

(For procedure, see 35480, 35490)

+ 75996 Transluminal atherectomy, each additional visceral artery, radiological supervision and interpretation (List separately in addition to code for primary procedure)

(Use 75996 in conjunction with 75995)

(For procedure, see 35480, 35490)

Other Procedures

(For computed tomography cerebral perfusion analysis, see Category III code 0042T)

(For arthrography of shoulder, use 73040; elbow, use 73085; wrist, use 73115; hip, use 73525; knee, use 73580; ankle, use 73615)

▶(75998 has been deleted. To report, use 77001)◀

76000 Fluoroscopy (separate procedure), up to 1 hour physician time, other than 71023 or 71034 (eg, cardiac fluoroscopy)

76001 Fluoroscopy, physician time more than 1 hour, assisting a nonradiologic physician (eg, nephrostolithotomy, ERCP, bronchoscopy, transbronchial biopsy)

▶(76003 has been deleted. To report, use 77002)◀

▶(76005 has been deleted. To report, use 77003)◀

▶(76006 has been deleted. To report, use 77071)◀

76010 Radiologic examination from nose to rectum for foreign body, single view, child

▶(76012, 76013 have been deleted. To report, see 72291, 72292)◀

▶(76020 has been deleted. To report, use 77072)◀

▶(76040 has been deleted. To report, use 77073)◀

▶(76061, 76062 have been deleted. To report, see 77074, 77075)◀

▶(76065 has been deleted. To report, use 77076)◀

▶(76066 has been deleted. To report, use 77077)◀

▶(76070, 76071 have been deleted. To report, see 77078, 77079)◀

▶(76075-76077 have been deleted. To report, see 77080-77082)◀

▶(76078 has been deleted. To report, use 77083)◀

76080 Radiologic examination, abscess, fistula or sinus tract study, radiological supervision and interpretation

▶(76082, 76083 have been deleted. To report, see 77051, 77052)◀

(76085 has been deleted. To report, see 77051, 77052)

▶(76086 has been deleted. To report, use 77053)◀

▶(76088 has been deleted. To report, use 77054)◀

▶(76090, 76091 have been deleted. To report, see 77055, 77056)◀

▶(76092 has been deleted. To report, use 77057)◀

▶(76093, 76094 have been deleted. To report, see 77058, 77059)◀

▶(76095 has been deleted. To report, use 77031)◀

▶(76096 has been deleted. To report, use 77032)◀

76098 Radiological examination, surgical specimen

76100 Radiologic examination, single plane body section (eg, tomography), other than with urography

76101 Radiologic examination, complex motion (ie, hypercycloidal) body section (eg, mastoid polytomography), other than with urography; unilateral

76102   bilateral

(For nephrotomography, use 74415)

76120 Cineradiography/videoradiography, except where specifically included

+ 76125 Cineradiography/videoradiography to complement routine examination (List separately in addition to code for primary procedure)

76140 Consultation on X-ray examination made elsewhere, written report

76150 Xeroradiography

(76150 is to be used for non-mammographic studies only)

Radiology

76350   Subtraction in conjunction with contrast studies

▶(76355 has been deleted. To report, use 77011)◀

▶(76360 has been deleted. To report, use 77012)◀

▶(76362 has been deleted. To report, use 77013)◀

▶(76370 has been deleted. To report, use 77014)◀

(76375 has been deleted)

(2D reformatting is no longer separately reported. To report 3D rendering, see 76376, 76377)

(76376, 76377 require concurrent physician supervision of image postprocessing 3D manipulation of volumetric data set and image rendering)

76376   3D rendering with interpretation and reporting of computed tomography, magnetic resonance imaging, ultrasound, or other tomographic modality; not requiring image postprocessing on an independent workstation

(Use 76376 in conjunction with code[s] for base imaging procedure[s])

▶(Do not report 76376 in conjunction with 70496, 70498, 70544-70549, 71275, 71555, 72159, 72191, 72198, 73206, 73225, 73706, 73725, 74175, 74185, 75635, 76377, 78000-78999, 0066T, 0067T, 0144T-0151T)◀

76377   requiring image postprocessing on an independent workstation

(Use 76377 in conjunction with code[s] for base imaging procedure[s])

▶(Do not report 76377 in conjunction with 70496, 70498, 70544-70549, 71275, 71555, 72159, 72191, 72198, 73206, 73225, 73706, 73725, 74175, 74185, 75635, 76376, 78000-78999, 0066T, 0067T, 0144T-0151T)◀

76380   Computed tomography, limited or localized follow-up study

76390   Magnetic resonance spectroscopy

(For magnetic resonance imaging, use appropriate MRI body site code)

▶(76393 has been deleted. To report, use 77021)◀

▶(76394 has been deleted. To report, use 77022)◀

▶(76400 has been deleted. To report, use 77084)◀

76496   Unlisted fluoroscopic procedure (eg, diagnostic, interventional)

76497   Unlisted computed tomography procedure (eg, diagnostic, interventional)

76498   Unlisted magnetic resonance procedure (eg, diagnostic, interventional)

76499   Unlisted diagnostic radiographic procedure

Diagnostic Ultrasound

All diagnostic ultrasound examinations require permanently recorded images with measurements, when such measurements are clinically indicated. For those codes whose sole diagnostic goal is a biometric measure (ie, 76514, 76516, and 76519), permanently recorded images are not required. A final, written report should be issued for inclusion in the patient's medical record. The prescription form for the intraocular lens satisfies the written report requirement for 76519. For those anatomic regions that have "complete" and "limited" ultrasound codes, note the elements that comprise a "complete" exam. The report should contain a description of these elements or the reason that an element could not be visualized (eg, obscured by bowel gas, surgically absent).

If less than the required elements for a "complete" exam are reported (eg, limited number of organs or limited portion of region evaluated), the "limited" code for that anatomic region should be used once per patient exam session. A "limited" exam of an anatomic region should not be reported for the same exam session as a "complete" exam of that same region.

Doppler evaluation of vascular structures (other than color flow used only for anatomic structure identification) is separately reportable. To report, see Non-Invasive Vascular Diagnostic Studies (93875-93990).

Ultrasound guidance procedures also require permanently recorded images of the site to be localized, as well as a documented description of the localization process, either separately or within the report of the procedure for which the guidance is utilized.

Use of ultrasound, without thorough evaluation of organ(s) or anatomic region, image documentation, and final, written report, is not separately reportable.

Definitions

A-mode implies a one-dimensional ultrasonic measurement procedure.

M-mode implies a one-dimensional ultrasonic measurement procedure with movement of the trace to record amplitude and velocity of moving echo-producing structures.

B-scan implies a two-dimensional ultrasonic scanning procedure with a two-dimensional display.

Real-time scan implies a two-dimensional ultrasonic scanning procedure with display of both two-dimensional structure and motion with time.

(To report diagnostic vascular ultrasound studies, see 93875-93990)

(For focused ultrasound ablation treatment of uterine leiomyomata, see Category III codes 0071T, 0072T)

Radiology

Head and Neck

▲ **76506**   Echoencephalography, real time with image documentation (gray scale) (for determination of ventricular size, delineation of cerebral contents, and detection of fluid masses or other intracranial abnormalities), including A-mode encephalography as secondary component where indicated

76510   Ophthalmic ultrasound, diagnostic; B-scan and quantitative A-scan performed during the same patient encounter

76511   quantitative A-scan only

76512   B-scan (with or without superimposed non-quantitative A-scan)

76513   anterior segment ultrasound, immersion (water bath) B-scan or high resolution biomicroscopy

76514   corneal pachymetry, unilateral or bilateral (determination of corneal thickness)

76516   Ophthalmic biometry by ultrasound echography, A-scan;

76519   with intraocular lens power calculation

(For partial coherence interferometry, use 92136)

76529   Ophthalmic ultrasonic foreign body localization

▲ **76536**   Ultrasound, soft tissues of head and neck (eg, thyroid, parathyroid, parotid), real time with image documentation

Chest

▲ **76604**   Ultrasound, chest (includes mediastinum), real time with image documentation

▲ **76645**   Ultrasound, breast(s) (unilateral or bilateral), real time with image documentation

Abdomen and Retroperitoneum

►A complete ultrasound examination of the abdomen (76700) consists of real time scans of the liver, gall bladder, common bile duct, pancreas, spleen, kidneys, and the upper abdominal aorta and inferior vena cava including any demonstrated abdominal abnormality.

A complete ultrasound examination of the retroperitoneum (76770) consists of real time scans of the kidneys, abdominal aorta, common iliac artery origins, and inferior vena cava, including any demonstrated retroperitoneal abnormality. Alternatively, if clinical history suggests urinary tract pathology, complete evaluation of the kidneys and urinary bladder also comprises a complete retroperitoneal ultrasound.◄

Use of ultrasound, without thorough evaluation of organ(s) or anatomic region, image documentation and final, written report, is not separately reportable.

▲ **76700**   Ultrasound, abdominal, real time with image documentation; complete

76705   limited (eg, single organ, quadrant, follow-up)

▲ **76770**   Ultrasound, retroperitoneal (eg, renal, aorta, nodes), real time with image documentation; complete

76775   limited

● **76776**   Ultrasound, transplanted kidney, real time and duplex Doppler with image documentation

►(For ultrasound of transplanted kidney without duplex Doppler, use 76775)◄

►(Do not report 76776 in conjunction with 93975, 93976)◄

►(76778 has been deleted. To report, see 76775, 76776)◄

Spinal Canal

76800   Ultrasound, spinal canal and contents

Pelvis

Obstetrical

Codes 76801 and 76802 include determination of the number of gestational sacs and fetuses, gestational sac/fetal measurements appropriate for gestation (younger than 14 weeks 0 days), survey of visible fetal and placental anatomic structure, qualitative assessment of amniotic fluid volume/gestational sac shape and examination of the maternal uterus and adnexa.

Codes 76805 and 76810 include determination of number of fetuses and amniotic/chorionic sacs, measurements appropriate for gestational age (older than or equal to 14 weeks 0 days), survey of intracranial/spinal/abdominal anatomy, 4 chambered heart, umbilical cord insertion site, placenta location and amniotic fluid assessment and, when visible, examination of maternal adnexa.

Codes 76811 and 76812 include all elements of codes 76805 and 76810 plus detailed anatomic evaluation of the fetal brain/ventricles, face, heart/outflow tracts and chest anatomy, abdominal organ specific anatomy, number/length/architecture of limbs and detailed evaluation of the umbilical cord and placenta and other fetal anatomy as clinically indicated.

Report should document the results of the evaluation of each element described above or the reason for non-visualization.

Code 76815 represents a focused "quick look" exam limited to the assessment of one or more of the elements listed in code 76815.

Code 76816 describes an examination designed to reassess fetal size and interval growth or reevaluate one or more anatomic abnormalities of a fetus previously demonstrated on ultrasound, and should be coded once for each fetus requiring reevaluation using modifier 59 for each fetus after the first.

Radiology

Code 76817 describes a transvaginal obstetric ultrasound performed separately or in addition to one of the transabdominal examinations described above. For transvaginal examinations performed for non-obstetrical purposes, use code 76830.

76801   Ultrasound, pregnant uterus, real time with image documentation, fetal and maternal evaluation, first trimester (< 14 weeks 0 days), transabdominal approach; single or first gestation

►(To report first trimester fetal nuchal translucency measurement, use 76813)◄

+ 76802   each additional gestation (List separately in addition to code for primary procedure)

(Use 76802 in conjunction with 76801)

►(To report first trimester fetal nuchal translucency measurement, use 76814)◄

76805   Ultrasound, pregnant uterus, real time with image documentation, fetal and maternal evaluation, after first trimester (> or = 14 weeks 0 days), transabdominal approach; single or first gestation

+ 76810   each additional gestation (List separately in addition to code for primary procedure)

(Use 76810 in conjunction with 76805)

76811   Ultrasound, pregnant uterus, real time with image documentation, fetal and maternal evaluation plus detailed fetal anatomic examination, transabdominal approach; single or first gestation

+ 76812   each additional gestation (List separately in addition to code for primary procedure)

(Use 76812 in conjunction with 76811)

● 76813   Ultrasound, pregnant uterus, real time with image documentation, first trimester fetal nuchal translucency measurement, transabdominal or transvaginal approach; single or first gestation

+● 76814   each additional gestation (List separately in addition to code for primary procedure)

►(Use 76814 in conjunction with 76813)◄

76815   Ultrasound, pregnant uterus, real time with image documentation, limited (eg, fetal heart beat, placental location, fetal position and/or qualitative amniotic fluid volume), one or more fetuses

(Use 76815 only once per exam and not per element)

►(To report first trimester fetal nuchal translucency measurement, see 76813, 76814)◄

76816   Ultrasound, pregnant uterus, real time with image documentation, follow-up (eg, re-evaluation of fetal size by measuring standard growth parameters and amniotic fluid volume, re-evaluation of organ system(s) suspected or confirmed to be abnormal on a previous scan), transabdominal approach, per fetus

(Report 76816 with modifier 59 for each additional fetus examined in a multiple pregnancy)

76817   Ultrasound, pregnant uterus, real time with image documentation, transvaginal

(For non-obstetrical transvaginal ultrasound, use 76830)

(If transvaginal examination is done in addition to transabdominal obstetrical ultrasound exam, use 76817 in addition to appropriate transabdominal exam code)

76818   Fetal biophysical profile; with non-stress testing

76819   without non-stress testing

(Fetal biophysical profile assessments for the second and any additional fetuses, should be reported separately by code 76818 or 76819 with the modifier 59 appended)

(For amniotic fluid index without non-stress test, use 76815)

76820   Doppler velocimetry, fetal; umbilical artery

76821   middle cerebral artery

76825   Echocardiography, fetal, cardiovascular system, real time with image documentation (2D), with or without M-mode recording;

76826   follow-up or repeat study

76827   Doppler echocardiography, fetal, pulsed wave and/or continuous wave with spectral display; complete

76828   follow-up or repeat study

(To report the use of color mapping, use 93325)

Nonobstetrical

Code 76856 includes the complete evaluation of the female pelvic anatomy. Elements of this examination include a description and measurements of the uterus and adnexal structures, measurement of the endometrium, measurement of the bladder (when applicable), and a description of any pelvic pathology (eg, ovarian cysts, uterine leiomyomata, free pelvic fluid).

Code 76856 is also applicable to a complete evaluation of the male pelvis. Elements of the examination include evaluation and measurement (when applicable) of the urinary bladder, evaluation of the prostate and seminal vesicles to the extent that they are visualized transabdominally, and any pelvic pathology (eg, bladder tumor, enlarged prostate, free pelvic fluid, pelvic abscess).

Code 76857 represents a focused examination limited to the assessment of one or more elements listed in code 76856 and/or the reevaluation of one or more pelvic abnormalities previously demonstrated on ultrasound. Code 76857, rather than 76770, should be utilized if the urinary bladder alone (ie, not including the kidneys) is imaged, whereas code 51798 should be utilized if a bladder volume or post-void residual measurement is obtained without imaging the bladder.

Radiology

Use of ultrasound, without thorough evaluation of organ(s) or anatomic region, image documentation, and final, written report, is not separately reportable.

76830 Ultrasound, transvaginal

(For obstetrical transvaginal ultrasound, use 76817)

(If transvaginal examination is done in addition to transabdominal non-obstetrical ultrasound exam, use 76830 in addition to appropriate transabdominal exam code)

76831 Saline infusion sonohysterography (SIS), including color flow Doppler, when performed

(For introduction of saline for saline infusion sonohysterography, use 58340)

▲ **76856** Ultrasound, pelvic (nonobstetric), real time with image documentation; complete

76857 limited or follow-up (eg, for follicles)

Genitalia

76870 Ultrasound, scrotum and contents

76872 Ultrasound, transrectal;

76873 prostate volume study for brachytherapy treatment planning (separate procedure)

Extremities

▲ **76880** Ultrasound, extremity, nonvascular, real time with image documentation

76885 Ultrasound, infant hips, real time with imaging documentation; dynamic (requiring physician manipulation)

76886 limited, static (not requiring physician manipulation)

Ultrasonic Guidance Procedures

76930 Ultrasonic guidance for pericardiocentesis, imaging supervision and interpretation

76932 Ultrasonic guidance for endomyocardial biopsy, imaging supervision and interpretation

76936 Ultrasound guided compression repair of arterial pseudoaneurysm or arteriovenous fistulae (includes diagnostic ultrasound evaluation, compression of lesion and imaging)

+ **76937** Ultrasound guidance for vascular access requiring ultrasound evaluation of potential access sites, documentation of selected vessel patency, concurrent realtime ultrasound visualization of vascular needle entry, with permanent recording and reporting (List separately in addition to code for primary procedure)

(Do not use 76937 in conjunction with 76942)

(If extremity venous non-invasive vascular diagnostic study is performed separate from venous access guidance, use 93965, 93970 or 93971)

▲ **76940** Ultrasound guidance for, and monitoring of, parenchymal tissue ablation

►(Do not report 76940 in conjunction with 76998)◄

►(For ablation, see 32998, 47370-47382, 50592)◄

(For percutaneous cryotherapy ablation of renal tumors, use 0135T)

76941 Ultrasonic guidance for intrauterine fetal transfusion or cordocentesis, imaging supervision and interpretation

(For procedure, see 36460, 59012)

76942 Ultrasonic guidance for needle placement (eg, biopsy, aspiration, injection, localization device), imaging supervision and interpretation

(Do not report 76942 in conjunction with 43232, 43237, 43242, 45341, 45342, or 76975)

(For microwave thermotherapy of the breast, use Category III code 0061T)

76945 Ultrasonic guidance for chorionic villus sampling, imaging supervision and interpretation

(For procedure, use 59015)

76946 Ultrasonic guidance for amniocentesis, imaging supervision and interpretation

76948 Ultrasonic guidance for aspiration of ova, imaging supervision and interpretation

76950 Ultrasonic guidance for placement of radiation therapy fields

76965 Ultrasonic guidance for interstitial radioelement application

Other Procedures

76970 Ultrasound study follow-up (specify)

76975 Gastrointestinal endoscopic ultrasound, supervision and interpretation

(Do not report 76975 in conjunction with 43231, 43232, 43237, 43238, 43242, 43259, 45341, 45342, or 76942)

76977 Ultrasound bone density measurement and interpretation, peripheral site(s), any method

►(76986 has been deleted. To report, use 76998)◄

● **76998** Ultrasonic guidance, intraoperative

►(Do not report 76998 in conjunction with 47370-47382)◄

►(For ultrasound guidance for open and laparoscopic radiofrequency tissue ablation, use 76940)◄

76999 Unlisted ultrasound procedure (eg, diagnostic, interventional)

Radiology

►Radiologic Guidance◄

►Fluoroscopic Guidance◄

+● 77001 Fluoroscopic guidance for central venous access device placement, replacement (catheter only or complete), or removal (includes fluoroscopic guidance for vascular access and catheter manipulation, any necessary contrast injections through access site or catheter with related venography radiologic supervision and interpretation, and radiographic documentation of final catheter position) (List separately in addition to code for primary procedure

►(Do not use 77001 in conjunction with 77002)◄

►(If formal extremity venography is performed from separate venous access and separately interpreted, use 36005 and 75820, 75822, 75825, or 75827)◄

● 77002 Fluoroscopic guidance for needle placement (eg, biopsy, aspiration, injection, localization device)

►(See appropriate surgical code for procedure and anatomic location)◄

►(77002 includes all radiographic arthrography with the exception of supervision and interpretation for CT and MR arthrography)◄

►(Do not report 77002 in addition to 70332, 73040, 73085, 73115, 73525, 73580, 73615)◄

►(77002 is included in the organ/anatomic specific radiological supervision and interpretation procedures 74320, 74350, 74355, 74445, 74470, 74475, 75809, 75810, 75885, 75887, 75980, 75982, 75989)◄

● 77003 Fluoroscopic guidance and localization of needle or catheter tip for spine or paraspinous diagnostic or therapeutic injection procedures (epidural, transforaminal epidural, subarachnoid, paravertebral facet joint, paravertebral facet joint nerve, or sacroiliac joint), including neurolytic agent destruction

►(Injection of contrast during fluoroscopic guidance and localization [77003] is included in 22526, 22527, 62263, 62264, 62270-62282, 62310-62319, 0027T)◄

►(Fluoroscopic guidance for subarachnoid puncture for diagnostic radiographic myelography is included in supervision and interpretation codes 72240-72270)◄

►(For epidural or subarachnoid needle or catheter placement and injection, see 62270-62282, 62310-62319)◄

►(For sacroiliac joint arthrography, see 27096, 73542. If formal arthrography is not performed and recorded, and a formal radiographic report is not issued, use 77003 for fluoroscopic guidance for sacroiliac joint injections)◄

►(For paravertebral facet joint injection, see 64470-64476. For transforaminal epidural needle placement and injection, see 64479-64484)◄

►(For destruction by neurolytic agent, see 64600-64680)◄

►(For percutaneous or endoscopic lysis of epidural adhesions, 62263, 62264, 0027T include fluoroscopic guidance and localization)◄

►Computed Tomography Guidance◄

● 77011 Computed tomography guidance for stereotactic localization

● 77012 Computed tomography guidance for needle placement (eg, biopsy, aspiration, injection, localization device), radiological supervision and interpretation

● 77013 Computerized tomography guidance for, and monitoring of, parenchymal tissue ablation

►(Do not report 77013 in conjunction with 20982)◄

►(For percutaneous cryotherapy ablation of renal tumors, use 0135T)◄

►(For percutaneous radiofrequency ablation, see 32998, 47382, 50592)◄

● 77014 Computed tomography guidance for placement of radiation therapy fields

►Magnetic Resonance Guidance◄

● 77021 Magnetic resonance guidance for needle placement (eg, for biopsy, needle aspiration, injection, or placement of localization device) radiological supervision and interpretation

►(For procedure, see appropriate organ or site)◄

● 77022 Magnetic resonance guidance for, and monitoring of, parenchymal tissue ablation

►(For percutaneous radiofrequency ablation, see 32998, 47382, 50592)◄

►(For focused ultrasound ablation treatment of uterine leiomyomata, see Category III codes 0071T, 0072T)◄

►(For percutaneous cryotherapy ablation of renal tumors, use 0135T)◄

►Other Radiologic Guidance◄

● 77031 Stereotactic localization guidance for breast biopsy or needle placement (eg, for wire localization or for injection), each lesion, radiological supervision and interpretation

►(For procedure, see 10022, 19000-19103, 19290, 19291)◄

►(For injection for sentinel node localization without lymphoscintigraphy, use 38792)◄

● 77032 Mammographic guidance for needle placement, breast (eg, for wire localization or for injection), each lesion, radiological supervision and interpretation

►(For procedure, see 10022, 19000, 19102, 19103, 19290, 19291)◄

►(For injection for sentinel node localization without lymphoscintigraphy, use 38792)◄

Radiology

►Breast, Mammography◄

►(For mammographic guidance for needle placement of breast lesion, use 77032)◄

+● 77051   Computer-aided detection (computer algorithm analysis of digital image data for lesion detection) with further physician review for interpretation, with or without digitization of film radiographic images; diagnostic mammography (List separately in addition to code for primary procedure)

►(Use 77051 in conjunction with 77055, 77056)◄

+● 77052   screening mammography (List separately in addition to code for primary procedure)

►(Use 77052 in conjunction with 77057)◄

● 77053   Mammary ductogram or galactogram, single duct, radiological supervision and interpretation

►(For mammary ductogram or galactogram injection, use 19030)◄

● 77054   Mammary ductogram or galactogram, multiple ducts, radiological supervision and interpretation

● 77055   Mammography; unilateral

● 77056   bilateral

►(Use 77055, 77056 in conjunction with 77051 for computer-aided detection applied to a diagnostic mammogram)◄

● 77057   Screening mammography, bilateral (2-view film study of each breast)

►(Use 77057 in conjunction with 77052 for computer-aided detection applied to a screening mammogram)◄

►(To report electrical impedance scan of the breast, bilateral, use Category III code 0060T)◄

● 77058   Magnetic resonance imaging, breast, without and/or with contrast material(s); unilateral

● 77059   bilateral

►Bone/Joint Studies◄

● 77071   Manual application of stress performed by physician for joint radiography, including contralateral joint if indicated

►(For radiographic interpretation of stressed images, see appropriate anatomic site and number of views)◄

● 77072   Bone age studies

● 77073   Bone length studies (orthoroentgenogram, scanogram)

● 77074   Radiologic examination, osseous survey; limited (eg, for metastases)

● 77075   complete (axial and appendicular skeleton)

● 77076   Radiologic examination, osseous survey, infant

● 77077   Joint survey, single view, 2 or more joints (specify)

● 77078   Computed tomography, bone mineral density study, 1 or more sites; axial skeleton (eg, hips, pelvis, spine)

● 77079   appendicular skeleton (peripheral) (eg, radius, wrist, heel)

● 77080   Dual-energy X-ray absorptiometry (DXA), bone density study, 1 or more sites; axial skeleton (eg, hips, pelvis, spine)

● 77081   appendicular skeleton (peripheral) (eg, radius, wrist, heel)

● 77082   vertebral fracture assessment

►(To report dual-energy X-ray absorptiometry [DXA] body composition study, 1 or more sites, use Category III code 0028T)◄

● 77083   Radiographic absorptiometry (eg, photodensitometry, radiogrammetry), 1 or more sites

● 77084   Magnetic resonance (eg, proton) imaging, bone marrow blood supply

Radiation Oncology

Listings for Radiation Oncology provide for teletherapy and brachytherapy to include initial consultation, clinical treatment planning, simulation, medical radiation physics, dosimetry, treatment devices, special services, and clinical treatment management procedures. They include normal follow-up care during course of treatment and for three months following its completion.

When a service or procedure is provided that is not listed in this edition of the CPT codebook it should be identified by a Special Report (see page 234) and one of the following unlisted procedure codes:

77299 Unlisted procedure, therapeutic radiology clinical treatment planning

77399 Unlisted procedure, medical radiation physics, dosimetry and treatment devices, and special services

77499 Unlisted procedure, therapeutic radiology treatment management

77799 Unlisted procedure, clinical brachytherapy

For treatment by injectable or ingestible isotopes, see subsection **Nuclear Medicine.**

Consultation: Clinical Management

Preliminary consultation, evaluation of patient prior to decision to treat, or full medical care (in addition to treatment management) when provided by the therapeutic radiologist may be identified by the appropriate procedure codes from **Evaluation and Management, Medicine,** or **Surgery** sections.

Clinical Treatment Planning (External and Internal Sources)

The clinical treatment planning process is a complex service including interpretation of special testing, tumor localization, treatment volume determination, treatment time/dosage determination, choice of treatment modality, determination of number and size of treatment ports, selection of appropriate treatment devices, and other procedures.

Definitions

Simple planning requires a single treatment area of interest encompassed in a single port or simple parallel opposed ports with simple or no blocking.

Intermediate planning requires three or more converging ports, two separate treatment areas, multiple blocks, or special time dose constraints.

Complex planning requires highly complex blocking, custom shielding blocks, tangential ports, special wedges or compensators, three or more separate treatment areas, rotational or special beam considerations, combination of therapeutic modalities.

77261   Therapeutic radiology treatment planning; simple

77262   intermediate

77263   complex

Definitions

Simple simulation of a single treatment area with either a single port or parallel opposed ports. Simple or no blocking.

Intermediate simulation of three or more converging ports, two separate treatment areas, multiple blocks.

Complex simulation of tangential portals, three or more treatment areas, rotation or arc therapy, complex blocking, custom shielding blocks, brachytherapy source verification, hyperthermia probe verification, any use of contrast materials.

Three-dimensional (3D) computer-generated 3D reconstruction of tumor volume and surrounding critical normal tissue structures from direct CT scans and/or MRI data in preparation for non-coplanar or coplanar therapy. The simulation uses documented 3D beam's eye view volume-dose displays of multiple or moving beams. Documentation with 3D volume reconstruction and dose distribution is required.

Simulation may be carried out on a dedicated simulator, a radiation therapy treatment unit, or diagnostic X-ray machine.

77280   Therapeutic radiology simulation-aided field setting; simple

77285   intermediate

77290   complex

77295   3-dimensional

77299   Unlisted procedure, therapeutic radiology clinical treatment planning

Medical Radiation Physics, Dosimetry, Treatment Devices, and Special Services

77300   Basic radiation dosimetry calculation, central axis depth dose calculation, TDF, NSD, gap calculation, off axis factor, tissue inhomogeneity factors, calculation of non-ionizing radiation surface and depth dose, as required during course of treatment, only when prescribed by the treating physician

77301   Intensity modulated radiotherapy plan, including dose-volume histograms for target and critical structure partial tolerance specifications

(Dose plan is optimized using inverse or forward planning technique for modulated beam delivery (eg, binary, dynamic MLC) to create highly conformal dose distribution. Computer plan distribution must be verified for positional accuracy based on dosimetric verification of the intensity map with verification of treatment set-up and interpretation of verification methodology)

77305   Teletherapy, isodose plan (whether hand or computer calculated); simple (one or two parallel opposed unmodified ports directed to a single area of interest)

77310   intermediate (three or more treatment ports directed to a single area of interest)

77315   complex (mantle or inverted Y, tangential ports, the use of wedges, compensators, complex blocking, rotational beam, or special beam considerations)

(Only one teletherapy isodose plan may be reported for a given course of therapy to a specific treatment area)

77321   Special teletherapy port plan, particles, hemibody, total body

77326   Brachytherapy isodose plan; simple (calculation made from single plane, one to four sources/ribbon application, remote afterloading brachytherapy, 1 to 8 sources)

(For definition of source/ribbon, see page 255)

77327   intermediate (multiplane dosage calculations, application involving 5 to 10 sources/ribbons, remote afterloading brachytherapy, 9 to 12 sources)

77328   complex (multiplane isodose plan, volume implant calculations, over 10 sources/ribbons used, special spatial reconstruction, remote afterloading brachytherapy, over 12 sources)

77331   Special dosimetry (eg, TLD, microdosimetry) (specify), only when prescribed by the treating physician

77332   Treatment devices, design and construction; simple (simple block, simple bolus)

77333   intermediate (multiple blocks, stents, bite blocks, special bolus)

77334   complex (irregular blocks, special shields, compensators, wedges, molds or casts)

Radiology

77336 Continuing medical physics consultation, including assessment of treatment parameters, quality assurance of dose delivery, and review of patient treatment documentation in support of the radiation oncologist, reported per week of therapy

77370 Special medical radiation physics consultation

►Stereotactic Radiation Treatment Delivery◄

● **77371** Radiation treatment delivery, stereotactic radiosurgery (SRS), complete course of treatment of cerebral lesion(s) consisting of 1 session; multi-source Cobalt 60 based

● **77372**   linear accelerator based

    ►(For radiation treatment management, use 77432)◄

● **77373** Stereotactic body radiation therapy, treatment delivery, per fraction to 1 or more lesions, including image guidance, entire course not to exceed 5 fractions

    ►(Do not report 77373 in conjunction with 77401-77416, 77418)◄

    ►(For single fraction cranial lesion[s], see 77371, 77372)◄

►Other Procedures◄

77399 Unlisted procedure, medical radiation physics, dosimetry and treatment devices, and special services

Radiation Treatment Delivery

(Radiation treatment delivery [77401-77416] recognizes the technical component and the various energy levels)

77401 Radiation treatment delivery, superficial and/or ortho voltage

77402 Radiation treatment delivery, single treatment area, single port or parallel opposed ports, simple blocks or no blocks; up to 5 MeV

77403   6-10 MeV

77404   11-19 MeV

77406   20 MeV or greater

77407 Radiation treatment delivery, two separate treatment areas, three or more ports on a single treatment area, use of multiple blocks; up to 5 MeV

77408   6-10 MeV

77409   11-19 MeV

77411   20 MeV or greater

77412 Radiation treatment delivery, three or more separate treatment areas, custom blocking, tangential ports, wedges, rotational beam, compensators, electron beam; up to 5 MeV

77413   6-10 MeV

77414   11-19 MeV

77416   20 MeV or greater

77417 Therapeutic radiology port film(s)

77418 Intensity modulated treatment delivery, single or multiple fields/arcs, via narrow spatially and temporally modulated beams, binary, dynamic MLC, per treatment session

(For intensity modulated treatment planning, use 77301)

(For compensator-based beam modulation treatment delivery, use Category III code 0073T)

77421 Stereoscopic X-ray guidance for localization of target volume for the delivery of radiation therapy

    ►(Do not report 77421 in conjunction with 77432, 77435)◄

    ►(For placement of interstitial device[s] for radiation therapy guidance, prostate, use 55876)◄

Neutron Beam Treatment Delivery

77422 High energy neutron radiation treatment delivery; single treatment area using a single port or parallel-opposed ports with no blocks or simple blocking

77423   1 or more isocenter(s) with coplanar or non-coplanar geometry with blocking and/or wedge, and/or compensator(s)

Radiation Treatment Management

Radiation treatment management is reported in units of five fractions or treatment sessions, regardless of the actual time period in which the services are furnished. The services need not be furnished on consecutive days. Multiple fractions representing two or more treatment sessions furnished on the same day may be counted separately as long as there has been a distinct break in therapy sessions, and the fractions are of the character usually furnished on different days. Code 77427 is also reported if there are three or four fractions beyond a multiple of five at the end of a course of treatment; one or two fractions beyond a multiple of five at the end of a course of treatment are not reported separately. The professional services furnished during treatment management typically consist of:

■ Review of port films;

■ Review of dosimetry, dose delivery, and treatment parameters;

■ Review of patient treatment set-up;

■ Examination of patient for medical evaluation and management (eg, assessment of the patient's response to treatment, coordination of care and treatment, review of imaging and/or lab test results).

77427 Radiation treatment management, five treatments

77431 Radiation therapy management with complete course of therapy consisting of one or two fractions only

(77431 is not to be used to fill in the last week of a long course of therapy)

Radiology

77432   Stereotactic radiation treatment management of cerebral lesion(s) (complete course of treatment consisting of one session)

● 77435   Stereotactic body radiation therapy, treatment management, per treatment course, to one or more lesions, including image guidance, entire course not to exceed 5 fractions

►(Do not report 77435 in conjunction with 77427-77432)◄

►(When stereotactic radiation therapy is performed jointly by a surgeon and a radiation oncologist [eg, spinal or cranial], the surgeon reports radiosurgery with 61793)◄

77470   Special treatment procedure (eg, total body irradiation, hemibody radiation, per oral, endocavitary or intraoperative cone irradiation)

(77470 assumes that the procedure is performed one or more times during the course of therapy, in addition to daily or weekly patient management)

77499   Unlisted procedure, therapeutic radiology treatment management

Proton Beam Treatment Delivery

Definitions

Simple proton treatment delivery to a single treatment area utilizing a single non-tangential/oblique port, custom block with compensation (77522) and without compensation (77520).

Intermediate proton treatment delivery to one or more treatment areas utilizing two or more ports or one or more tangential/oblique ports, with custom blocks and compensators.

Complex proton treatment delivery to one or more treatment areas utilizing two or more ports per treatment area with matching or patching fields and/or multiple isocenters, with custom blocks and compensators.

77520   Proton treatment delivery; simple, without compensation

77522   simple, with compensation

77523   intermediate

77525   complex

Hyperthermia

Hyperthermia treatments as listed in this section include external (superficial and deep), interstitial, and intracavitary.

Radiation therapy when given concurrently is listed separately.

Hyperthermia is used only as an adjunct to radiation therapy or chemotherapy. It may be induced by a variety of sources (eg, microwave, ultrasound, low energy radio-frequency conduction, or by probes).

The listed treatments include management during the course of therapy and follow-up care for three months after completion.

Preliminary consultation is not included (see **Evaluation and Management** 99241-99255).

Physics planning and interstitial insertion of temperature sensors, and use of external or interstitial heat generating sources are included.

The following descriptors are included in the treatment schedule:

⊙ 77600   Hyperthermia, externally generated; superficial (ie, heating to a depth of 4 cm or less)

⊙ 77605   deep (ie, heating to depths greater than 4 cm)

⊙ 77610   Hyperthermia generated by interstitial probe(s); 5 or fewer interstitial applicators

⊙ 77615   more than 5 interstitial applicators

Clinical Intracavitary Hyperthermia

77620   Hyperthermia generated by intracavitary probe(s)

Clinical Brachytherapy

Clinical brachytherapy requires the use of either natural or man-made radioelements applied into or around a treatment field of interest. The supervision of radioelements and dose interpretation are performed solely by the therapeutic radiologist.

Services 77750-77799 include admission to the hospital and daily visits.

For insertion of ovoids and tandems, use 57155.

For insertion of Heyman capsules, use 58346.

Definitions

(Sources refer to intracavitary placement or permanent interstitial placement; ribbons refer to temporary interstitial placement)

A simple application has one to four sources/ribbons.

An intermediate application has five to 10 sources/ribbons.

A complex application has greater than 10 sources/ribbons.

77750   Infusion or instillation of radioelement solution (includes 3 months follow-up care)

(For administration of radiolabeled monoclonal antibodies, use 79403)

(For non-antibody radiopharmaceutical therapy by intravenous administration only, not including 3-month follow-up care, use 79101)

77761   Intracavitary radiation source application; simple

77762   intermediate

77763   complex

Radiology

77776	Interstitial radiation source application; simple
77777	intermediate
77778	complex
77781	Remote afterloading high intensity brachytherapy; 1-4 source positions or catheters
77782	5-8 source positions or catheters
77783	9-12 source positions or catheters
77784	over 12 source positions or catheters
77789	Surface application of radiation source
77790	Supervision, handling, loading of radiation source
77799	Unlisted procedure, clinical brachytherapy

Nuclear Medicine

Listed procedures may be performed independently or in the course of overall medical care. If the physician providing these services is also responsible for diagnostic work-up and/or follow-up care of patient, see appropriate sections also.

Radioimmunoassay tests are found in the **Clinical Pathology** section (codes 82000-84999). These codes can be appropriately used by any specialist performing such tests in a laboratory licensed and/or certified for radioimmunoassays. The reporting of these tests is not confined to clinical pathology laboratories alone.

The services listed do not include the radiopharmaceutical or drug. Diagnostic and therapeutic radiopharmaceuticals and drugs supplied by the physician should be reported separately using the appropriate supply code(s), in addition to the procedure code.

Diagnostic

Endocrine System

78000	Thyroid uptake; single determination
78001	multiple determinations
78003	stimulation, suppression or discharge (not including initial uptake studies)
78006	Thyroid imaging, with uptake; single determination
78007	multiple determinations
78010	Thyroid imaging; only
78011	with vascular flow
78015	Thyroid carcinoma metastases imaging; limited area (eg, neck and chest only)
78016	with additional studies (eg, urinary recovery)
78018	whole body

+ 78020	Thyroid carcinoma metastases uptake (List separately in addition to code for primary procedure)
	(Use 78020 in conjunction with 78018 only)
78070	Parathyroid imaging
78075	Adrenal imaging, cortex and/or medulla
78099	Unlisted endocrine procedure, diagnostic nuclear medicine
	(For chemical analysis, see **Chemistry** section)

Hematopoietic, Reticuloendothelial and Lymphatic System

78102	Bone marrow imaging; limited area
78103	multiple areas
78104	whole body
78110	Plasma volume, radiopharmaceutical volume-dilution technique (separate procedure); single sampling
78111	multiple samplings
78120	Red cell volume determination (separate procedure); single sampling
78121	multiple samplings
78122	Whole blood volume determination, including separate measurement of plasma volume and red cell volume (radiopharmaceutical volume-dilution technique)
78130	Red cell survival study;
78135	differential organ/tissue kinetics, (eg, splenic and/or hepatic sequestration)
78140	Labeled red cell sequestration, differential organ/tissue, (eg, splenic and/or hepatic)
	(78160, 78162, 78170, 78172 have been deleted)
78185	Spleen imaging only, with or without vascular flow
	(If combined with liver study, use procedures 78215 and 78216)
78190	Kinetics, study of platelet survival, with or without differential organ/tissue localization
78191	Platelet survival study
78195	Lymphatics and lymph nodes imaging
	(For sentinel node identification without scintigraphy imaging, use 38792)
	(For sentinal node excision, see 38500-38542)
78199	Unlisted hematopoietic, reticuloendothelial and lymphatic procedure, diagnostic nuclear medicine
	(For chemical analysis, see **Chemistry** section)

Gastrointestinal System

78201   Liver imaging; static only

78202   with vascular flow

       (For spleen imaging only, use 78185)

78205   Liver imaging (SPECT);

78206   with vascular flow

78215   Liver and spleen imaging; static only

78216   with vascular flow

78220   Liver function study with hepatobiliary agents, with serial images

78223   Hepatobiliary ductal system imaging, including gallbladder, with or without pharmacologic intervention, with or without quantitative measurement of gallbladder function

78230   Salivary gland imaging;

78231   with serial images

78232   Salivary gland function study

78258   Esophageal motility

78261   Gastric mucosa imaging

78262   Gastroesophageal reflux study

78264   Gastric emptying study

78267   Urea breath test, C-14 (isotopic); acquisition for analysis

78268   analysis

78270   Vitamin B-12 absorption study (eg, Schilling test); without intrinsic factor

78271   with intrinsic factor

78272   Vitamin B-12 absorption studies combined, with and without intrinsic factor

78278   Acute gastrointestinal blood loss imaging

78282   Gastrointestinal protein loss

78290   Intestine imaging (eg, ectopic gastric mucosa, Meckel's localization, volvulus)

78291   Peritoneal-venous shunt patency test (eg, for LeVeen, Denver shunt)

       (For injection procedure, use 49427)

78299   Unlisted gastrointestinal procedure, diagnostic nuclear medicine

Musculoskeletal System

Bone and joint imaging can be used in the diagnosis of a variety of inflammatory processes (eg, osteomyelitis), as well as for localization of primary and/or metastatic neoplasms.

78300   Bone and/or joint imaging; limited area

78305   multiple areas

78306   whole body

78315   three phase study

78320   tomographic (SPECT)

78350   Bone density (bone mineral content) study, one or more sites; single photon absorptiometry

78351   dual photon absorptiometry, one or more sites

       ►(For radiographic bone density [photodensitometry], use 77083)◄

78399   Unlisted musculoskeletal procedure, diagnostic nuclear medicine

Cardiovascular System

Myocardial perfusion and cardiac blood pool imaging studies may be performed at rest and/or during stress. When performed during exercise and/or pharmacologic stress, the appropriate stress testing code from the 93015-93018 series should be reported in addition to 78460-78465, 78472-78492.

78414   Determination of central c-v hemodynamics (non-imaging) (eg, ejection fraction with probe technique) with or without pharmacologic intervention or exercise, single or multiple determinations

78428   Cardiac shunt detection

78445   Non-cardiac vascular flow imaging (ie, angiography, venography)

       (78455 has been deleted)

78456   Acute venous thrombosis imaging, peptide

78457   Venous thrombosis imaging, venogram; unilateral

78458   bilateral

78459   Myocardial imaging, positron emission tomography (PET), metabolic evaluation

       (For myocardial perfusion study, see 78491-78492)

78460   Myocardial perfusion imaging; (planar) single study, at rest or stress (exercise and/or pharmacologic), with or without quantification

78461   multiple studies, (planar) at rest and/or stress (exercise and/or pharmacologic), and redistribution and/or rest injection, with or without quantification

Radiology

78464   tomographic (SPECT), single study (including attenuation correction when performed), at rest or stress (exercise and/or pharmacologic), with or without quantification

78465   tomographic (SPECT), multiple studies (including attenuation correction when performed), at rest and/or stress (exercise and/or pharmacologic) and redistribution and/or rest injection, with or without quantification

78466   Myocardial imaging, infarct avid, planar; qualitative or quantitative

78468   with ejection fraction by first pass technique

78469   tomographic SPECT with or without quantification

78472   Cardiac blood pool imaging, gated equilibrium; planar, single study at rest or stress (exercise and/or pharmacologic), wall motion study plus ejection fraction, with or without additional quantitative processing

(For assessment of right ventricular ejection fraction by first pass technique, use 78496)

78473   multiple studies, wall motion study plus ejection fraction, at rest and stress (exercise and/or pharmacologic), with or without additional quantification

+ 78478   Myocardial perfusion study with wall motion, qualitative or quantitative study (List separately in addition to code for primary procedure)

(Use 78478 in conjunction with 78460, 78461, 78464, 78465)

+ 78480   Myocardial perfusion study with ejection fraction (List separately in addition to code for primary procedure)

(Use 78480 in conjunction with 78460, 78461, 78464, 78465)

78481   Cardiac blood pool imaging, (planar), first pass technique; single study, at rest or with stress (exercise and/or pharmacologic), wall motion study plus ejection fraction, with or without quantification

78483   multiple studies, at rest and with stress (exercise and/ or pharmacologic), wall motion study plus ejection fraction, with or without quantification

(For cerebral blood flow study, use 78615)

78491   Myocardial imaging, positron emission tomography (PET), perfusion; single study at rest or stress

78492   multiple studies at rest and/or stress

78494   Cardiac blood pool imaging, gated equilibrium, SPECT, at rest, wall motion study plus ejection fraction, with or without quantitative processing

+ 78496   Cardiac blood pool imaging, gated equilibrium, single study, at rest, with right ventricular ejection fraction by first pass technique (List separately in addition to code for primary procedure)

(Use 78496 in conjunction with 78472)

78499   Unlisted cardiovascular procedure, diagnostic nuclear medicine

Respiratory System

78580   Pulmonary perfusion imaging, particulate

78584   Pulmonary perfusion imaging, particulate, with ventilation; single breath

78585   rebreathing and washout, with or without single breath

78586   Pulmonary ventilation imaging, aerosol; single projection

78587   multiple projections (eg, anterior, posterior, lateral views)

78588   Pulmonary perfusion imaging, particulate, with ventilation imaging, aerosol, one or multiple projections

78591   Pulmonary ventilation imaging, gaseous, single breath, single projection

78593   Pulmonary ventilation imaging, gaseous, with rebreathing and washout with or without single breath; single projection

78594   multiple projections (eg, anterior, posterior, lateral views)

78596   Pulmonary quantitative differential function (ventilation/perfusion) study

78599   Unlisted respiratory procedure, diagnostic nuclear medicine

Nervous System

78600   Brain imaging, limited procedure; static

78601   with vascular flow

78605   Brain imaging, complete study; static

78606   with vascular flow

78607   tomographic (SPECT)

78608   Brain imaging, positron emission tomography (PET); metabolic evaluation

78609   perfusion evaluation

78610   Brain imaging, vascular flow only

78615   Cerebral vascular flow

78630   Cerebrospinal fluid flow, imaging (not including introduction of material); cisternography

(For injection procedure, see 61000-61070, 62270-62319)

78635   ventriculography

(For injection procedure, see 61000-61070, 62270-62294)

78645   shunt evaluation

(For injection procedure, see 61000-61070, 62270-62294)

78647   tomographic (SPECT)

Radiology

78650   Cerebrospinal fluid leakage detection and localization

(For injection procedure, see 61000-61070, 62270-62294)

78660   Radiopharmaceutical dacryocystography

78699   Unlisted nervous system procedure, diagnostic nuclear medicine

Genitourinary System

▲ **78700**   Kidney imaging morphology;

78701   with vascular flow

►(78704 has been deleted. To report, see 78707-78709)◄

▲ **78707**   with vascular flow and function, single study without pharmacological intervention

▲ **78708**   with vascular flow and function, single study, with pharmacological intervention (eg, angiotensin converting enzyme inhibitor and/or diuretic)

▲ **78709**   with vascular flow and function, multiple studies, with and without pharmacological intervention (eg, angiotensin converting enzyme inhibitor and/or diuretic)

►(For introduction of radioactive substance in association with renal endoscopy, see 77776-77778)◄

▲ **78710**   tomographic (SPECT)

►(78715 has been deleted. To report, see 78701-78709)◄

78725   Kidney function study, non-imaging radioisotopic study

+▲ **78730**   Urinary bladder residual study (List separately in addition to code for primary procedure)

►(Use 78730 in conjunction with 78740)◄

►(For measurement of postvoid residual urine and/or bladder capacity by ultrasound, nonimaging, use 51798)◄

►(For ultrasound imaging of the bladder only, with measurement of postvoid residual urine when performed, use 76857)◄

78740   Ureteral reflux study (radiopharmaceutical voiding cystogram)

►(Use 78740 in conjunction with 78730 for urinary bladder residual study)◄

(For catheterization, see 51701, 51702, 51703)

►(78760 has been deleted. To report, use 78761)◄

▲ **78761**   Testicular imaging with vascular flow

78799   Unlisted genitourinary procedure, diagnostic nuclear medicine

(For chemical analysis, see **Chemistry** section)

Other Procedures

(For specific organ, see appropriate heading)

(For radiophosphorus tumor identification, ocular, see 78800)

78800   Radiopharmaceutical localization of tumor or distribution of radiopharmaceutical agent(s); limited area

(For specific organ, see appropriate heading)

78801   multiple areas

78802   whole body, single day imaging

78803   tomographic (SPECT)

78804   whole body, requiring two or more days imaging

78805   Radiopharmaceutical localization of inflammatory process; limited area

78806   whole body

78807   tomographic (SPECT)

(For imaging bone infectious or inflammatory disease with a bone imaging radiopharmaceutical, see 78300, 78305, 78306)

(78810 has been deleted. To report, see 78811-78813)

(For PET of brain, see 78608, 78609)

(For PET myocardial imaging, see 78459, 78491, 78492)

78811   Tumor imaging, positron emission tomography (PET); limited area (eg, chest, head/neck)

78812   skull base to mid-thigh

78813   whole body

78814   Tumor imaging, positron emission tomography (PET) with concurrently acquired computed tomography (CT) for attenuation correction and anatomical localization; limited area (eg, chest, head/neck)

78815   skull base to mid-thigh

78816   whole body

(Report 78811-78816 only once per imaging session)

(Computed tomography (CT) performed for other than attenuation correction and anatomical localization is reported using the appropriate site specific CT code with modifier 59)

78890   Generation of automated data: interactive process involving nuclear physician and/or allied health professional personnel; simple manipulations and interpretation, not to exceed 30 minutes

78891   complex manipulations and interpretation, exceeding 30 minutes

(Use 78890 or 78891 in addition to primary procedure)

(78990 has been deleted)

78999   Unlisted miscellaneous procedure, diagnostic nuclear medicine

Radiology

Therapeutic

The oral and intravenous administration codes in this section are inclusive of the mode of administration. For intra-arterial, intra-cavitary, and intra-articular administration, also use the appropriate injection and/or procedure codes, as well as imaging guidance and radiological supervision and interpretation codes, when appropriate.

(79000, 79001 have been deleted. To report, use 79005)

79005   Radiopharmaceutical therapy, by oral administration

(79020, 79030, 79035 have been deleted. To report, use 79005)

(79100 has been deleted. To report, use 79101)

(For monoclonal antibody therapy, use 79403)

79101   Radiopharmaceutical therapy, by intravenous administration

(Do not report 79101 in conjunction with 36400, 36410, 79403, 90760, 90774 or 90775, 96409)

(For radiolabeled monoclonal antibody by intravenous infusion, use 79403)

(For infusion or instillation of non-antibody radioelement solution that includes 3 months follow-up care, use 77750)

79200   Radiopharmaceutical therapy, by intracavitary administration

79300   Radiopharmaceutical therapy, by interstitial radioactive colloid administration

(79400 has been deleted. To report, use 79101)

79403   Radiopharmaceutical therapy, radiolabeled monoclonal antibody by intravenous infusion

(For pre-treatment imaging, see 78802, 78804)

(Do not report 79403 in conjunction with 79101)

(79420 has been deleted. To report use 79445)

79440   Radiopharmaceutical therapy, by intra-articular administration

79445   Radiopharmaceutical therapy, by intra-arterial particulate administration

(Do not report 79445 in conjunction with 90773, 96420)

(Use appropriate procedural and radiological supervision and interpretation codes for the angiographic and interventional procedures provided prerequisite to intra-arterial radiopharmaceutical therapy)

(79900 has been deleted)

79999   Radiopharmaceutical therapy, unlisted procedure

Radiology

Pathology and Laboratory Guidelines

Items used by all physicians in reporting their services are presented in the **Introduction.** Some of the commonalities are repeated here for the convenience of those physicians referring to this section on **Pathology and Laboratory.** Other definitions and items unique to Pathology and Laboratory are also listed.

Services in Pathology and Laboratory

Services in Pathology and Laboratory are provided by a physician or by technologists under responsible supervision of a physician.

Separate or Multiple Procedures

It is appropriate to designate multiple procedures that are rendered on the same date by separate entries.

Subsection Information

Several of the subheadings or subsections have special needs or instructions unique to that section. Where these are indicated (eg, "Panel Tests"), special **"Notes"** will be presented preceding those procedural terminology listings referring to that subsection specifically. If there is an "Unlisted Procedure" code number (see the following section) for the individual subsection, it will be shown. Those subsections with **"Notes"** are as follows:

Organ or Disease Panels	80048-80076
Drug Testing	80100-80103
Therapeutic Drug Assays	80150-80299
Evocative/Suppression Testing	80400-80440
Consultations	
(Clinical Pathology)	80500-80502
Urinalysis	81000-81099
Chemistry	82000-84999
Molecular Diagnostics	83890-83912
Infectious Agent: Detection	
of Antibodies	86602-86804
Microbiology	87001-87255
Infectious Agent Detection	87260-87999
Anatomic Pathology	88000-88099
Cytopathology	88104-88199
Cytogenetic Studies	88230-88299
Surgical Pathology	88300-88399

Unlisted Service or Procedure

A service or procedure may be provided that is not listed in this edition of the CPT codebook. When reporting such a service, the appropriate "Unlisted Procedure" code may be used to indicate the service, identifying it by "Special Report" as discussed below. The "Unlisted Procedures" and accompanying codes for **Pathology and Laboratory** are as follows:

81099	Unlisted urinalysis procedure
84999	Unlisted chemistry procedure
85999	Unlisted hematology and coagulation procedure
86586	Unlisted antigen, each
86849	Unlisted immunology procedure
86999	Unlisted transfusion medicine procedure
87999	Unlisted microbiology procedure
88099	Unlisted necropsy (autopsy) procedure
88199	Unlisted cytopathology procedure
88299	Unlisted cytogenetic study
88399	Unlisted surgical pathology procedure
89240	Unlisted miscellaneous pathology test

►Results/Testing/Reports◄

►Results are the technical component of a service. Testing leads to results; results lead to interpretation. Reports are the work product of the interpretation of numerous test results.◄

Special Report

A service that is rarely provided, unusual, variable, or new may require a special report in determining medical appropriateness of the service. Pertinent information should include an adequate definition or description of the nature, extent, and need for the procedure; and the time, effort, and equipment necessary to provide the service. Additional items that may be included are:

- Complexity of symptoms
- Final diagnosis
- Pertinent physical findings
- Diagnostic and therapeutic procedures
- Concurrent problems
- Follow-up care

Notes

⊙=Moderate sedation　✚=Add-on code　✔=FDA approval pending

Pathology and Laboratory

Organ or Disease-Oriented Panels

These panels were developed for coding purposes only and should not be interpreted as clinical parameters. The tests listed with each panel identify the defined components of that panel.

These panel components are not intended to limit the performance of other tests. If one performs tests in addition to those specifically indicated for a particular panel, those tests should be reported separately in addition to the panel code.

80048   Basic metabolic panel

This panel must include the following:

Calcium (82310)

Carbon dioxide (82374)

Chloride (82435)

Creatinine (82565)

Glucose (82947)

Potassium (84132)

Sodium (84295)

Urea nitrogen (BUN) (84520)

(Do not use 80048 in addition to 80053)

80050   General health panel

This panel must include the following:

Comprehensive metabolic panel (80053)

Blood count, complete (CBC), automated and automated differential WBC count (85025 or 85027 and 85004)

OR

Blood count, complete (CBC), automated (85027) and appropriate manual differential WBC count (85007 or 85009)

Thyroid stimulating hormone (TSH) (84443)

80051   Electrolyte panel

This panel must include the following:

Carbon dioxide (82374)

Chloride (82435)

Potassium (84132)

Sodium (84295)

80053   Comprehensive metabolic panel

This panel must include the following:

Albumin (82040)

Bilirubin, total (82247)

Calcium (82310)

Carbon dioxide (bicarbonate) (82374)

Chloride (82435)

Creatinine (82565)

Glucose (82947)

Phosphatase, alkaline (84075)

Potassium (84132)

Protein, total (84155)

Sodium (84295)

Transferase, alanine amino (ALT) (SGPT) (84460)

Transferase, aspartate amino (AST) (SGOT) (84450)

Urea nitrogen (BUN) (84520)

(Do not use 80053 in addition to 80048, 80076)

80055   Obstetric panel

This panel must include the following:

Blood count, complete (CBC), automated and automated differential WBC count (85025 or 85027 and 85004)

OR

Blood count, complete (CBC), automated (85027) and appropriate manual differential WBC count (85007 or 85009)

Hepatitis B surface antigen (HBsAg) (87340)

Antibody, rubella (86762)

Syphilis test, qualitative (eg, VDRL, RPR, ART) (86592)

Antibody screen, RBC, each serum technique (86850)

Blood typing, ABO (86900) AND

Blood typing, Rh (D) (86901)

80061   Lipid panel

This panel must include the following:

Cholesterol, serum, total (82465)

Lipoprotein, direct measurement, high density cholesterol (HDL cholesterol) (83718)

Triglycerides (84478)

80069   Renal function panel

This panel must include the following:

Albumin (82040)

Calcium (82310)

Carbon dioxide (bicarbonate) (82374)

Chloride (82435)

Pathology and Laboratory

Creatinine (82565)

Glucose (82947)

Phosphorus inorganic (phosphate) (84100)

Potassium (84132)

Sodium (84295)

Urea nitrogen (BUN) (84520)

80074 Acute hepatitis panel

This panel must include the following:

Hepatitis A antibody (HAAb), IgM antibody (86709)

Hepatitis B core antibody (HBcAb), IgM antibody (86705)

Hepatitis B surface antigen (HBsAg) (87340)

Hepatitis C antibody (86803)

80076 Hepatic function panel

This panel must include the following:

Albumin (82040)

Bilirubin, total (82247)

Bilirubin, direct (82248)

Phosphatase, alkaline (84075)

Protein, total (84155)

Transferase, alanine amino (ALT) (SGPT) (84460)

Transferase, aspartate amino (AST) (SGOT) (84450)

(Do not use 80076 in addition to 80053)

Drug Testing

The following list contains examples of drugs or classes of drugs that are commonly assayed by qualitative screen, followed by confirmation with a second method:

- Alcohols
- Amphetamines
- Barbiturates
- Benzodiazepines
- Cocaine and metabolites
- Methadones
- Methaqualones
- Opiates
- Phencyclidines
- Phenothiazines
- Propoxyphenes
- Tetrahydrocannabinoids
- Tricyclic antidepressants

Confirmed drugs may also be quantitated.

Use 80100 for each multiple drug class chromatographic procedure. Use 80102 for each procedure necessary for confirmation. For chromatography, each combination of stationary and mobile phase is to be counted as one procedure. For example, if detection of three drugs by chromatography requires one stationary phase with three mobile phases, use 80100 three (3) times. However, if multiple drugs can be detected using a single analysis (eg, one stationary phase with one mobile phase), use 80100 only once.

For quantitation of drugs screened, use appropriate code in **Chemistry** section (82000-84999) or **Therapeutic Drug Assay** section (80150-80299).

80100 Drug screen, qualitative; multiple drug classes chromatographic method, each procedure

80101 single drug class method (eg, immunoassay, enzyme assay), each drug class

80102 Drug confirmation, each procedure

80103 Tissue preparation for drug analysis

Therapeutic Drug Assays

The material for examination may be from any source. Examination is quantitative. For nonquantitative testing, see Drug Testing (80100-80103).

80150 Amikacin

80152 Amitriptyline

80154 Benzodiazepines

80156 Carbamazepine; total

80157   free

80158 Cyclosporine

80160 Desipramine

80162 Digoxin

80164 Dipropylacetic acid (valproic acid)

80166 Doxepin

80168 Ethosuximide

80170 Gentamicin

80172 Gold

80173 Haloperidol

80174 Imipramine

80176 Lidocaine

80178 Lithium

80182 Nortriptyline

80184 Phenobarbital

80185 Phenytoin; total

80186   free

80188   Primidone

80190   Procainamide;

80192   with metabolites (eg, n-acetyl procainamide)

80194   Quinidine

80195   Sirolimus

80196   Salicylate

80197   Tacrolimus

80198   Theophylline

80200   Tobramycin

80201   Topiramate

80202   Vancomycin

80299   Quantitation of drug, not elsewhere specified

Evocative/Suppression Testing

The following test panels involve the administration of evocative or suppressive agents, and the baseline and subsequent measurement of their effects on chemical constituents. These codes are to be used for the reporting of the laboratory component of the overall testing protocol. For the physician's administration of the evocative or suppressive agents, see 90760, 90761, 90772-90774, 90775; for the supplies and drugs, see 99070. To report physician attendance and monitoring during the testing, use the appropriate evaluation and management code, including the prolonged physician care codes if required. Prolonged physician care codes are not separately reported when evocative/suppression testing involves prolonged infusions reported with 90760-90761. In the code descriptors where reference is made to a particular analyte (eg, Cortisol (82533 x 2)) the "x 2" refers to the number of times the test for that particular analyte is performed.

80400   ACTH stimulation panel; for adrenal insufficiency

     This panel must include the following:

     Cortisol (82533 x 2)

80402   for 21 hydroxylase deficiency

     This panel must include the following:

     Cortisol (82533 x 2)

     17 hydroxyprogesterone (83498 x 2)

80406   for 3 beta-hydroxydehydrogenase deficiency

     This panel must include the following:

     Cortisol (82533 x 2)

     17 hydroxypregnenolone (84143 x 2)

80408   Aldosterone suppression evaluation panel (eg, saline infusion)

     This panel must include the following:

     Aldosterone (82088 x 2)

     Renin (84244 x 2)

80410   Calcitonin stimulation panel (eg, calcium, pentagastrin)

     This panel must include the following:

     Calcitonin (82308 x 3)

80412   Corticotropic releasing hormone (CRH) stimulation panel

     This panel must include the following:

     Cortisol (82533 x 6)

     Adrenocorticotropic hormone (ACTH) (82024 x 6)

80414   Chorionic gonadotropin stimulation panel; testosterone response

     This panel must include the following:

     Testosterone (84403 x 2 on three pooled blood samples)

80415   estradiol response

     This panel must include the following:

     Estradiol (82670 x 2 on three pooled blood samples)

80416   Renal vein renin stimulation panel (eg, captopril)

     This panel must include the following:

     Renin (84244 x 6)

80417   Peripheral vein renin stimulation panel (eg, captopril)

     This panel must include the following:

     Renin (84244 x 2)

80418   Combined rapid anterior pituitary evaluation panel

     This panel must include the following:

     Adrenocorticotropic hormone (ACTH) (82024 x 4)

     Luteinizing hormone (LH) (83002 x 4)

     Follicle stimulating hormone (FSH) (83001 x 4)

     Prolactin (84146 x 4)

     Human growth hormone (HGH) (83003 x 4)

     Cortisol (82533 x 4)

     Thyroid stimulating hormone (TSH) (84443 x 4)

80420   Dexamethasone suppression panel, 48 hour

     This panel must include the following:

     Free cortisol, urine (82530 x 2)

     Cortisol (82533 x 2)

     Volume measurement for timed collection (81050 x 2)

     (For single dose dexamethasone, use 82533)

Pathology and Laboratory

Pathology and Laboratory

80422 Glucagon tolerance panel; for insulinoma

This panel must include the following:

Glucose (82947 x 3)

Insulin (83525 x 3)

80424 　for pheochromocytoma

This panel must include the following:

Catecholamines, fractionated (82384 x 2)

80426 Gonadotropin releasing hormone stimulation panel

This panel must include the following:

Follicle stimulating hormone (FSH) (83001 x 4)

Luteinizing hormone (LH) (83002 x 4)

80428 Growth hormone stimulation panel (eg, arginine infusion, l-dopa administration)

This panel must include the following:

Human growth hormone (HGH) (83003 x 4)

80430 Growth hormone suppression panel (glucose administration)

This panel must include the following:

Glucose (82947 x 3)

Human growth hormone (HGH) (83003 x 4)

80432 Insulin-induced C-peptide suppression panel

This panel must include the following:

Insulin (83525)

C-peptide (84681 x 5)

Glucose (82947 x 5)

80434 Insulin tolerance panel; for ACTH insufficiency

This panel must include the following:

Cortisol (82533 x 5)

Glucose (82947 x 5)

80435 　for growth hormone deficiency

This panel must include the following:

Glucose (82947 x 5)

Human growth hormone (HGH) (83003 x 5)

80436 Metyrapone panel

This panel must include the following:

Cortisol (82533 x 2)

11 deoxycortisol (82634 x 2)

80438 Thyrotropin releasing hormone (TRH) stimulation panel; one hour

This panel must include the following:

Thyroid stimulating hormone (TSH) (84443 x 3)

80439 　two hour

This panel must include the following:

Thyroid stimulating hormone (TSH) (84443 x 4)

80440 　for hyperprolactinemia

This panel must include the following:

Prolactin (84146 x 3)

Consultations (Clinical Pathology)

A clinical pathology consultation is a service, including a written report, rendered by the pathologist in response to a request from an attending physician in relation to a test result(s) requiring additional medical interpretive judgment.

Reporting of a test result(s) without medical interpretive judgment is not considered a clinical pathology consultation.

80500 Clinical pathology consultation; limited, without review of patient's history and medical records

80502 　comprehensive, for a complex diagnostic problem, with review of patient's history and medical records

(These codes may also be used for pharmacokinetic consultations)

(For consultations involving the examination and evaluation of the patient, see 99241-99255)

Urinalysis

For specific analyses, see appropriate section.

(For urinalysis, infectious agent detection, semi-quantitative analysis of volatile compounds, use Category III code 0041T)

81000 Urinalysis, by dip stick or tablet reagent for bilirubin, glucose, hemoglobin, ketones, leukocytes, nitrite, pH, protein, specific gravity, urobilinogen, any number of these constituents; non-automated, with microscopy

81001 　automated, with microscopy

81002 　non-automated, without microscopy

81003 　automated, without microscopy

81005 Urinalysis; qualitative or semiquantitative, except immunoassays

(For non-immunoassay reagent strip urinalysis, see 81000, 81002)

(For immunoassay, qualitative or semiquantitative, use 83518)

(For microalbumin, see 82043, 82044)

81007	bacteriuria screen, except by culture or dipstick
	(For culture, see 87086-87088)
	(For dipstick, use 81000 or 81002)
81015	microscopic only
81020	two or three glass test
81025	Urine pregnancy test, by visual color comparison methods
81050	Volume measurement for timed collection, each
81099	Unlisted urinalysis procedure

Chemistry

The material for examination may be from any source unless otherwise specified in the code descriptor. When an analyte is measured in multiple specimens from different sources, or in specimens that are obtained at different times, the analyte is reported separately for each source and for each specimen. The examination is quantitative unless specified. To report an organ or disease oriented panel, see codes 80048-80076.

When a code describes a method where measurement of multiple analytes may require one or several procedures, each procedure is coded separately (eg, 82491-82492, 82541-82544). For example, if two (2) analytes are measured using column chromatography using a single stationary or mobile phase, use 82492. If the same two analytes are measured using different stationary or mobile phase conditions, 82491 would be used twice. If a total of four (4) analytes are measured where two (2) analytes are measured with a single stationary and mobile phase, and the other two (2) analytes are measured using a different stationary and mobile phase, use 82492 twice. If a total of three (3) analytes are measured where two (2) analytes are measured using a single stationary or mobile phase condition, and the third analyte is measured separately using a different stationary or mobile phase procedure, use 82492 once for the two (2) analytes measured under the same condition, and use 82491 once for the third analyte measured separately.

Clinical information derived from the results of laboratory data that is mathematically calculated (eg, free thyroxine index (T7)) is considered part of the test procedure and therefore is not a separately reportable service.

82000	Acetaldehyde, blood
82003	Acetaminophen
82009	Acetone or other ketone bodies, serum; qualitative
82010	quantitative
82013	Acetylcholinesterase
	(Acid, gastric, see gastric acid, 82926, 82928)
	(Acid phosphatase, see 84060-84066)

82016	Acylcarnitines; qualitative, each specimen
82017	quantitative, each specimen
	(For carnitine, use 82379)
82024	Adrenocorticotropic hormone (ACTH)
82030	Adenosine, 5-monophosphate, cyclic (cyclic AMP)
82040	Albumin; serum
82042	urine or other source, quantitative, each specimen
82043	urine, microalbumin, quantitative
82044	urine, microalbumin, semiquantitative (eg, reagent strip assay)
	(For prealbumin, use 84134)
82045	ischemia modified
82055	Alcohol (ethanol); any specimen except breath
	(For other volatiles, alcohol, use 84600)
82075	breath
82085	Aldolase
82088	Aldosterone
	(Alkaline phosphatase, see 84075, 84080)
82101	Alkaloids, urine, quantitative
	(Alphaketoglutarate, see 82009, 82010)
	(Alpha tocopherol (Vitamin E), use 84446)
82103	Alpha-1-antitrypsin; total
82104	phenotype
82105	Alpha-fetoprotein (AFP); serum
82106	amniotic fluid
● **82107**	AFP-L3 fraction isoform and total AFP (including ratio)
82108	Aluminum
82120	Amines, vaginal fluid, qualitative
	(For combined pH and amines test for vaginitis, use 82120 and 83986)
82127	Amino acids; single, qualitative, each specimen
82128	multiple, qualitative, each specimen
82131	single, quantitative, each specimen
82135	Aminolevulinic acid, delta (ALA)
82136	Amino acids, 2 to 5 amino acids, quantitative, each specimen
82139	Amino acids, 6 or more amino acids, quantitative, each specimen
82140	Ammonia
82143	Amniotic fluid scan (spectrophotometric)
	(For L/S ratio, use 83661)
	(Amobarbital, see 80100-80103 for qualitative analysis, 82205 for quantitative analysis)

Pathology and Laboratory

Pathology and Laboratory

82145   Amphetamine or methamphetamine

    (For qualitative analysis, see 80100-80103)

82150   Amylase

82154   Androstanediol glucuronide

82157   Androstenedione

82160   Androsterone

82163   Angiotensin II

82164   Angiotensin I - converting enzyme (ACE)

    (Antidiuretic hormone (ADH), use 84588)

    (Antimony, use 83015)

    (Antitrypsin, alpha-1-, see 82103, 82104)

82172   Apolipoprotein, each

82175   Arsenic

    (For heavy metal screening, use 83015)

82180   Ascorbic acid (Vitamin C), blood

    (Aspirin, see acetylsalicylic acid, 80196)

    (Atherogenic index, blood, ultracentrifugation, quantitative, use 83701)

82190   Atomic absorption spectroscopy, each analyte

82205   Barbiturates, not elsewhere specified

    (For qualitative analysis, see 80100-80103)

    (For B-Natriuretic peptide, use 83880)

82232   Beta-2 microglobulin

    (Bicarbonate, use 82374)

82239   Bile acids; total

82240   cholylglycine

    (For bile pigments, urine, see 81000-81005)

82247   Bilirubin; total

82248   direct

82252   feces, qualitative

82261   Biotinidase, each specimen

82270   Blood, occult, by peroxidase activity (eg, guaiac), qualitative; feces, consecutive collected specimens with single determination, for colorectal neoplasm screening (ie, patient was provided three cards or single triple card for consecutive collection)

82271   other sources

82272   Blood, occult, by peroxidase activity (eg, guaiac), qualitative, feces, single specimen (eg, from digital rectal exam)

    (82273 has been deleted. To report, use 82271)

    (Blood urea nitrogen (BUN), see 84520, 84525)

82274   Blood, occult, by fecal hemoglobin determination by immunoassay, qualitative, feces, 1-3 simultaneous determinations

82286   Bradykinin

82300   Cadmium

82306   Calcifediol (25-OH Vitamin D-3)

82307   Calciferol (Vitamin D)

    (For 1,25-Dihydroxyvitamin D, use 82652)

82308   Calcitonin

82310   Calcium; total

82330   ionized

82331   after calcium infusion test

82340   urine quantitative, timed specimen

82355   Calculus; qualitative analysis

82360   quantitative analysis, chemical

82365   infrared spectroscopy

82370   x-ray diffraction

    (Carbamates, see individual listings)

82373   Carbohydrate deficient transferrin

82374   Carbon dioxide (bicarbonate)

    (See also 82803)

82375   Carbon monoxide, (carboxyhemoglobin); quantitative

82376   qualitative

    (To report end-tidal carbon monoxide, use Category III code 0043T)

82378   Carcinoembryonic antigen (CEA)

82379   Carnitine (total and free), quantitative, each specimen

    (For acylcarnitine, see 82016, 82017)

82380   Carotene

82382   Catecholamines; total urine

82383   blood

82384   fractionated

    (For urine metabolites, see 83835, 84585)

82387   Cathepsin-D

82390   Ceruloplasmin

82397   Chemiluminescent assay

82415   Chloramphenicol

82435   Chloride; blood

82436   urine

82438   other source

    (For sweat collection by iontophoresis, use 89230)

82441   Chlorinated hydrocarbons, screen

      (Chlorpromazine, use 84022)

      (Cholecalciferol (Vitamin D), use 82307)

82465   Cholesterol, serum or whole blood, total

      (For high density lipoprotein (HDL), use 83718)

82480   Cholinesterase; serum

82482   RBC

82485   Chondroitin B sulfate, quantitative

      (Chorionic gonadotropin, see gonadotropin, 84702, 84703)

82486   Chromatography, qualitative; column (eg, gas liquid or HPLC), analyte not elsewhere specified

82487   paper, 1-dimensional, analyte not elsewhere specified

82488   paper, 2-dimensional, analyte not elsewhere specified

82489   thin layer, analyte not elsewhere specified

82491   Chromatography, quantitative, column (eg, gas liquid or HPLC); single analyte not elsewhere specified, single stationary and mobile phase

82492   multiple analytes, single stationary and mobile phase

82495   Chromium

82507   Citrate

82520   Cocaine or metabolite

      (Cocaine, qualitative analysis, see 80100-80103)

      (Codeine, qualitative analysis, see 80100-80103)

      (Codeine, quantitative analysis, see 82101)

      (Complement, see 86160-86162)

82523   Collagen cross links, any method

82525   Copper

      (Coproporphyrin, see 84119, 84120)

      (Corticosteroids, use 83491)

82528   Corticosterone

82530   Cortisol; free

82533   total

      (C-peptide, use 84681)

82540   Creatine

82541   Column chromatography/mass spectrometry (eg, GC/MS, or HPLC/MS), analyte not elsewhere specified; qualitative, single stationary and mobile phase

82542   quantitative, single stationary and mobile phase

82543   stable isotope dilution, single analyte, quantitative, single stationary and mobile phase

82544   stable isotope dilution, multiple analytes, quantitative, single stationary and mobile phase

82550   Creatine kinase (CK), (CPK); total

82552   isoenzymes

82553   MB fraction only

82554   isoforms

82565   Creatinine; blood

82570   other source

82575   clearance

82585   Cryofibrinogen

82595   Cryoglobulin, qualitative or semi-quantitative (eg, cryocrit)

      (For quantitative, cryoglobulin, see 82784, 82785)

      (Crystals, pyrophosphate vs. urate, use 89060)

82600   Cyanide

82607   Cyanocobalamin (Vitamin B-12);

82608   unsaturated binding capacity

      (Cyclic AMP, use 82030)

      (Cyclic GMP, use 83008)

      (Cyclosporine, use 80158)

82615   Cystine and homocystine, urine, qualitative

82626   Dehydroepiandrosterone (DHEA)

82627   Dehydroepiandrosterone-sulfate (DHEA-S)

      (Delta-aminolevulinic acid (ALA), use 82135)

82633   Desoxycorticosterone, 11-

82634   Deoxycortisol, 11-

      (Dexamethasone suppression test, use 80420)

      (Diastase, urine, use 82150)

82638   Dibucaine number

      (Dichloroethane, use 84600)

      (Dichloromethane, use 84600)

      (Diethylether, use 84600)

82646   Dihydrocodeinone

      (For qualitative analysis, see 80100-80103)

82649   Dihydromorphinone

      (For qualitative analysis, see 80100-80103)

82651   Dihydrotestosterone (DHT)

82652   Dihydroxyvitamin D, 1,25-

82654   Dimethadione

      (For qualitative analysis, see 80100-80103)

      (Diphenylhydantoin, use 80185)

      (Dipropylacetic acid, use 80164)

Pathology and Laboratory

(Dopamine, see 82382-82384)

(Duodenal contents, see individual enzymes; for intubation and collection, use 89100)

82656 Elastase, pancreatic (EL-1), fecal, qualitative or semi-quantitative

82657 Enzyme activity in blood cells, cultured cells, or tissue, not elsewhere specified; nonradioactive substrate, each specimen

82658   radioactive substrate, each specimen

82664 Electrophoretic technique, not elsewhere specified

(Endocrine receptor assays, see 84233-84235)

82666 Epiandrosterone

(Epinephrine, see 82382-82384)

82668 Erythropoietin

82670 Estradiol

82671 Estrogens; fractionated

82672   total

(Estrogen receptor assay, use 84233)

82677 Estriol

82679 Estrone

(Ethanol, see 82055 and 82075)

82690 Ethchlorvynol

(Ethyl alcohol, see 82055 and 82075)

82693 Ethylene glycol

82696 Etiocholanolone

(For fractionation of ketosteroids, use 83593)

82705 Fat or lipids, feces; qualitative

82710   quantitative

82715 Fat differential, feces, quantitative

82725 Fatty acids, nonesterified

82726 Very long chain fatty acids

(For long-chain (C20-22) omega-3 fatty acids in red blood cell (RBC) membranes, use Category III code 0111T)

82728 Ferritin

(Fetal hemoglobin, see hemoglobin 83030, 83033, and 85460)

(Fetoprotein, alpha-1, see 82105, 82106)

82731 Fetal fibronectin, cervicovaginal secretions, semi-quantitative

82735 Fluoride

82742 Flurazepam

(For qualitative analysis, see 80100-80103)

(Foam stability test, use 83662)

82746 Folic acid; serum

82747   RBC

(Follicle stimulating hormone (FSH), use 83001)

82757 Fructose, semen

(Fructosamine, use 82985)

(Fructose, TLC screen, use 84375)

82759 Galactokinase, RBC

82760 Galactose

82775 Galactose-1-phosphate uridyl transferase; quantitative

82776   screen

82784 Gammaglobulin; IgA, IgD, IgG, IgM, each

82785   IgE

(For allergen specific IgE, see 86003, 86005)

82787   immunoglobulin subclasses, (IgG1, 2, 3, or 4), each

(Gamma-glutamyltransferase (GGT), use 82977)

82800 Gases, blood, pH only

82803 Gases, blood, any combination of pH, pCO_2, pO_2, CO_2, HCO_3 (including calculated O_2 saturation);

(Use 82803 for two or more of the above listed analytes)

82805   with O_2 saturation, by direct measurement, except pulse oximetry

82810 Gases, blood, O_2 saturation only, by direct measurement, except pulse oximetry

(For pulse oximetry, use 94760)

82820 Hemoglobin-oxygen affinity (pO_2 for 50% hemoglobin saturation with oxygen)

82926 Gastric acid, free and total, each specimen

82928 Gastric acid, free or total, each specimen

82938 Gastrin after secretin stimulation

82941 Gastrin

(Gentamicin, use 80170)

(GGT, use 82977)

(GLC, gas liquid chromatography, use 82486)

82943 Glucagon

82945 Glucose, body fluid, other than blood

82946 Glucagon tolerance test

82947 Glucose; quantitative, blood (except reagent strip)

82948   blood, reagent strip

82950   post glucose dose (includes glucose)

82951   tolerance test (GTT), three specimens (includes glucose)

Pathology and Laboratory

82952	tolerance test, each additional beyond three specimens	**83015**	Heavy metal (eg, arsenic, barium, beryllium, bismuth, antimony, mercury); screen
82953	tolbutamide tolerance test	**83018**	quantitative, each

82952   tolerance test, each additional beyond three specimens

82953   tolbutamide tolerance test

(For insulin tolerance test, see 80434, 80435)

(For leucine tolerance test, use 80428)

(For semiquantitative urine glucose, see 81000, 81002, 81005, 81099)

82955   Glucose-6-phosphate dehydrogenase (G6PD); quantitative

82960   screen

►(For glucose tolerance test with medication, use 90774 in addition)◄

82962   Glucose, blood by glucose monitoring device(s) cleared by the FDA specifically for home use

82963   Glucosidase, beta

82965   Glutamate dehydrogenase

82975   Glutamine (glutamic acid amide)

82977   Glutamyltransferase, gamma (GGT)

82978   Glutathione

82979   Glutathione reductase, RBC

82980   Glutethimide

(Glycohemoglobin, use 83036)

82985   Glycated protein

(Gonadotropin, chorionic, see 84702, 84703)

83001   Gonadotropin; follicle stimulating hormone (FSH)

83002   luteinizing hormone (LH)

(For luteinizing releasing factor (LRH), use 83727)

83003   Growth hormone, human (HGH) (somatotropin)

(For antibody to human growth hormone, use 86277)

83008   Guanosine monophosphate (GMP), cyclic

83009   Helicobacter pylori, blood test analysis for urease activity, non-radioactive isotope (eg, C-13)

(For H. pylori, breath test analysis for urease activity, see 83013, 83014)

83010   Haptoglobin; quantitative

83012   phenotypes

83013   Helicobacter pylori; breath test analysis for urease activity, non-radioactive isotope (eg, C-13)

83014   drug administration

(For H. pylori, stool, use 87338. For H. pylori, liquid scintillation counter, see 78267, 78268. For H. pylori, enzyme immunoassay, use 87339)

(For H. pylori, blood test analysis for urease activity, use 83009)

83015   Heavy metal (eg, arsenic, barium, beryllium, bismuth, antimony, mercury); screen

83018   quantitative, each

83020   Hemoglobin fractionation and quantitation; electrophoresis (eg, A2, S, C, and/or F)

83021   chromatography (eg, A2, S, C, and/or F)

83026   Hemoglobin; by copper sulfate method, non-automated

83030   F (fetal), chemical

83033   F (fetal), qualitative

83036   glycosylated (A1C)

(For fecal hemoglobin detection by immunoassay, use 82274)

83037   glycosylated (A1C) by device cleared by FDA for home use

83045   methemoglobin, qualitative

83050   methemoglobin, quantitative

83051   plasma

83055   sulfhemoglobin, qualitative

83060   sulfhemoglobin, quantitative

83065   thermolabile

83068   unstable, screen

83069   urine

83070   Hemosiderin; qualitative

83071   quantitative

(Heroin, see 80100-80103)

(HIAA, use 83497)

(High performance liquid chromatography (HPLC), use 82486)

83080   b-Hexosaminidase, each assay

83088   Histamine

(Hollander test, use 91052)

83090   Homocysteine

83150   Homovanillic acid (HVA)

(Hormones, see individual alphabetic listings in **Chemistry** section)

(Hydrogen breath test, use 91065)

83491   Hydroxycorticosteroids, 17- (17-OHCS)

(For cortisol, see 82530, 82533. For deoxycortisol, use 82634)

83497   Hydroxyindolacetic acid, 5-(HIAA)

(For urine qualitative test, use 81005)

(5-Hydroxytryptamine, use 84260)

83498   Hydroxyprogesterone, 17-d

Pathology and Laboratory

Pathology and Laboratory

83499	Hydroxyprogesterone, 20-
83500	Hydroxyproline; free
83505	total
83516	Immunoassay for analyte other than infectious agent antibody or infectious agent antigen, qualitative or semiquantitative; multiple step method
83518	single step method (eg, reagent strip)
83519	Immunoassay, analyte, quantitative; by radiopharmaceutical technique (eg, RIA)
83520	not otherwise specified

(For immunoassays for antibodies to infectious agent antigens, see analyte and method specific codes in the **Immunology** section)

(For immunoassay of tumor antigen not elsewhere specified, use 86316)

(Immunoglobulins, see 82784, 82785)

83525	Insulin; total

(For proinsulin, use 84206)

83527	free
83528	Intrinsic factor

(For intrinsic factor antibodies, use 86340)

83540	Iron
83550	Iron binding capacity
83570	Isocitric dehydrogenase (IDH)

(Isonicotinic acid hydrazide, INH, see code for specific method)

(Isopropyl alcohol, use 84600)

83582	Ketogenic steroids, fractionation

(Ketone bodies, for serum, see 82009, 82010; for urine, see 81000-81003)

83586	Ketosteroids, 17- (17-KS); total
83593	fractionation
83605	Lactate (lactic acid)
83615	Lactate dehydrogenase (LD), (LDH);
83625	isoenzymes, separation and quantitation
83630	Lactoferrin, fecal; qualitative
83631	quantitative
83632	Lactogen, human placental (HPL) human chorionic somatomammotropin
83633	Lactose, urine; qualitative
83634	quantitative

(For tolerance, see 82951, 82952)

(For breath hydrogen test for lactase deficiency, use 91065)

83655	Lead
83661	Fetal lung maturity assessment; lecithin sphingomyelin (L/S) ratio
83662	foam stability test
83663	fluorescence polarization
83664	lamellar body density

(For phosphatidylglycerol, use 84081)

83670	Leucine aminopeptidase (LAP)
83690	Lipase
83695	Lipoprotein (a)
● 83698	Lipoprotein-associated phospholipase A_2, (Lp-PLA$_2$)
83700	Lipoprotein, blood; electrophoretic separation and quantitation
83701	high resolution fractionation and quantitation of lipoproteins including lipoprotein subclasses when performed (eg, electrophoresis, ultracentrifugation)
83704	quantitation of lipoprotein particle numbers and lipoprotein particle subclasses (eg, by nuclear magnetic resonance spectroscopy)

(83715, 83716 have been deleted. To report, use 83700, 83701)

83718	Lipoprotein, direct measurement; high density cholesterol (HDL cholesterol)
83719	VLDL cholesterol
83721	LDL cholesterol

(For fractionation by high resolution electrophoresis or ultracentrifugation, use 83701)

(For lipoprotein particle numbers and subclasses analysis by nuclear magnetic resonance spectroscopy, use 83704)

(To report direct measurement, intermediate density lipoproteins (remnant lipoproteins), use Category III code 0026T)

83727	Luteinizing releasing factor (LRH)

(Luteinizing hormone (LH), use 83002)

(For qualitative analysis, see 80100-80103)

(Macroglobulins, alpha-2, use 86329)

83735	Magnesium
83775	Malate dehydrogenase

(Maltose tolerance, see 82951, 82952)

(Mammotropin, use 84146)

83785	Manganese

(Marijuana, see 80100-80103)

83788	Mass spectrometry and tandem mass spectrometry (MS, MS/MS), analyte not elsewhere specified; qualitative, each specimen
83789	quantitative, each specimen

83805	Meprobamate
	(For qualitative analysis, see 80100-80103)
83825	Mercury, quantitative
	(Mercury screen, use 83015)
83835	Metanephrines
	(For catecholamines, see 82382-82384)
83840	Methadone
	(For methadone qualitative analysis, see 80100-80103)
	(Methamphetamine, see 80100-80103, 82145)
	(Methanol, use 84600)
83857	Methemalbumin
	(Methemoglobin, see hemoglobin 83045, 83050)
83858	Methsuximide
	(Methyl alcohol, use 84600)
	(Microalbumin, see 82043 for quantitative, see 82044 for semiquantitative)
	(Microglobulin, beta-2, use 82232)
83864	Mucopolysaccharides, acid; quantitative
83866	screen
83872	Mucin, synovial fluid (Ropes test)
83873	Myelin basic protein, cerebrospinal fluid
	(For oligoclonal bands, use 83916)
83874	Myoglobin
	(Nalorphine, use 83925)
83880	Natriuretic peptide
83883	Nephelometry, each analyte not elsewhere specified
83885	Nickel
83887	Nicotine

Codes 83890-83914 are intended for use with molecular diagnostic techniques for analysis of nucleic acids.

Codes 83890-83914 are coded by procedure rather than analyte.

Code separately for each procedure used in an analysis. For example, a procedure requiring isolation of DNA, restriction endonuclease digestion, electrophoresis, and nucleic acid probe amplification would be coded 83890, 83892, 83894, and 83898.

When molecular diagnostic procedures are performed to test for oncology, hematology, neurology or inherited disorder, use the appropriate modifier to specify probe type or condition tested. (See **Appendix I** for a listing of appropriate modifiers to report with molecular diagnostic and cytogenetic procedures.)

	▶(For microbial identification, see 87470-87801)◀
	(For array technology using more than 10 probes, see 88384-88386)
83890	Molecular diagnostics; molecular isolation or extraction
83891	isolation or extraction of highly purified nucleic acid
83892	enzymatic digestion
83893	dot/slot blot production
83894	separation by gel electrophoresis (eg, agarose, polyacrylamide)
83896	nucleic acid probe, each
83897	nucleic acid transfer (eg, Southern, Northern)
83898	amplification of patient nucleic acid, each nucleic acid sequence
83900	amplification of patient nucleic acid, multiplex, first two nucleic acid sequences
+ 83901	amplification of patient nucleic acid, multiplex, each additional nucleic acid sequence (List separately in addition to code for primary procedure)
	(Use 83901 in conjunction with 83900)
83902	reverse transcription
83903	mutation scanning, by physical properties (eg, single strand conformational polymorphisms (SSCP), heteroduplex, denaturing gradient gel electrophoresis (DGGE), RNA'ase A), single segment, each
83904	mutation identification by sequencing, single segment, each segment
83905	mutation identification by allele specific transcription, single segment, each segment
83906	mutation identification by allele specific translation, single segment, each segment
83907	lysis of cells prior to nucleic acid extraction (eg, stool specimens, paraffin embedded tissue)
83908	signal amplification of patient nucleic acid, each nucleic acid sequence
	(For multiplex amplification, see 83900, 83901)
83909	separation and identification by high resolution technique (eg, capillary electrophoresis)
83912	interpretation and report
● **83913**	RNA stabilization
83914	Mutation identification by enzymatic ligation or primer extension, single segment, each segment (eg, oligonucleotide ligation assay (OLA), single base chain extension (SBCE), or allele-specific primer extension (ASPE))
83915	Nucleotidase 5'-
83916	Oligoclonal immune (oligoclonal bands)

▲=Revised code   ●=New code   ▶ ◀=Contains new or revised text   ⊘=Modifier 51 exempt

Pathology and Laboratory

83918	Organic acids; total, quantitative, each specimen
83919	qualitative, each specimen
83921	Organic acid, single, quantitative
83925	Opiates, (eg, morphine, meperidine)
83930	Osmolality; blood
83935	urine
83937	Osteocalcin (bone g1a protein)
83945	Oxalate
83950	Oncoprotein, HER-2/neu

(For tissue, see 88342, 88365)

83970	Parathormone (parathyroid hormone)

(Pesticide, quantitative, see code for specific method. For screen for chlorinated hydrocarbons, use 82441)

83986	pH, body fluid, except blood

(For blood pH, see 82800, 82803)

83992	Phencyclidine (PCP)

(For qualitative analysis, see 80100-80103)

(Phenobarbital, use 80184)

84022	Phenothiazine

(For qualitative analysis, see 80100, 80101)

84030	Phenylalanine (PKU), blood

(Phenylalanine-tyrosine ratio, see 84030, 84510)

84035	Phenylketones, qualitative
84060	Phosphatase, acid; total
84061	forensic examination
84066	prostatic
84075	Phosphatase, alkaline;
84078	heat stable (total not included)
84080	isoenzymes
84081	Phosphatidylglycerol

(Phosphates inorganic, use 84100)

(Phosphates, organic, see code for specific method. For cholinesterase, see 82480, 82482)

84085	Phosphogluconate, 6-, dehydrogenase, RBC
84087	Phosphohexose isomerase
84100	Phosphorus inorganic (phosphate);
84105	urine

(Pituitary gonadotropins, see 83001-83002)

(PKU, see 84030, 84035)

84106	Porphobilinogen, urine; qualitative
84110	quantitative
84119	Porphyrins, urine; qualitative
84120	quantitation and fractionation
84126	Porphyrins, feces; quantitative
84127	qualitative

(Porphyrin precursors, see 82135, 84106, 84110)

(For protoporphyrin, RBC, see 84202, 84203)

84132	Potassium; serum
84133	urine
84134	Prealbumin

(For microalbumin, see 82043, 82044)

84135	Pregnanediol
84138	Pregnanetriol
84140	Pregnenolone
84143	17-hydroxypregnenolone
84144	Progesterone

(Progesterone receptor assay, use 84234)

(For proinsulin, use 84206)

84146	Prolactin
84150	Prostaglandin, each
84152	Prostate specific antigen (PSA); complexed (direct measurement)
84153	total
84154	free
84155	Protein, total, except by refractometry; serum
84156	urine
84157	other source (eg, synovial fluid, cerebrospinal fluid)
84160	Protein, total, by refractometry, any source

(For urine total protein by dipstick method, use 81000-81003)

84163	Pregnancy-associated plasma protein-A (PAPP-A)
84165	Protein; electrophoretic fractionation and quantitation, serum
84166	electrophoretic fractionation and quantitation, other fluids with concentration (eg, urine, CSF)
84181	Western Blot, with interpretation and report, blood or other body fluid
84182	Western Blot, with interpretation and report, blood or other body fluid, immunological probe for band identification, each

(For Western Blot tissue analysis, use 88371)

84202	Protoporphyrin, RBC; quantitative
84203	screen
84206	Proinsulin

(Pseudocholinesterase, use 82480)

84207	Pyridoxal phosphate (Vitamin B-6)
84210	Pyruvate
84220	Pyruvate kinase
84228	Quinine
84233	Receptor assay; estrogen
84234	progesterone
84235	endocrine, other than estrogen or progesterone (specify hormone)
84238	non-endocrine (specify receptor)
84244	Renin
84252	Riboflavin (Vitamin B-2)

(Salicylates, use 80196)

(Secretin test, see 99070, 89100 and appropriate analyses)

84255	Selenium
84260	Serotonin

(For urine metabolites (HIAA), use 83497)

84270	Sex hormone binding globulin (SHBG)
84275	Sialic acid

(Sickle hemoglobin, use 85660)

84285	Silica
84295	Sodium; serum
84300	urine
84302	other source

(Somatomammotropin, use 83632)

(Somatotropin, use 83003)

84305	Somatomedin
84307	Somatostatin
84311	Spectrophotometry, analyte not elsewhere specified
84315	Specific gravity (except urine)

(For specific gravity, urine, see 81000-81003)

(Stone analysis, see 82355-82370)

84375	Sugars, chromatographic, TLC or paper chromatography
84376	Sugars (mono-, di-, and oligosaccharides); single qualitative, each specimen
84377	multiple qualitative, each specimen
84378	single quantitative, each specimen
84379	multiple quantitative, each specimen
84392	Sulfate, urine

(Sulfhemoglobin, see hemoglobin, 83055, 83060)

(T-3, see 84479-84481)

(T-4, see 84436-84439)

84402	Testosterone; free
84403	total
84425	Thiamine (Vitamin B-1)
84430	Thiocyanate
84432	Thyroglobulin

(Thyroglobulin, antibody, use 86800)

(Thyrotropin releasing hormone (TRH) test, see 80438, 80439)

84436	Thyroxine; total
84437	requiring elution (eg, neonatal)
84439	free
84442	Thyroxine binding globulin (TBG)
84443	Thyroid stimulating hormone (TSH)
84445	Thyroid stimulating immune globulins (TSI)

(Tobramycin, use 80200)

84446	Tocopherol alpha (Vitamin E)

(Tolbutamide tolerance, use 82953)

84449	Transcortin (cortisol binding globulin)
84450	Transferase; aspartate amino (AST) (SGOT)
84460	alanine amino (ALT) (SGPT)
84466	Transferrin

(Iron binding capacity, use 83550)

84478	Triglycerides
84479	Thyroid hormone (T3 or T4) uptake or thyroid hormone binding ratio (THBR)
84480	Triiodothyronine T3; total (TT-3)
84481	free
84482	reverse
84484	Troponin, quantitative

(For troponin, qualitative assay, use 84512)

84485	Trypsin; duodenal fluid
84488	feces, qualitative
84490	feces, quantitative, 24-hour collection
84510	Tyrosine

(Urate crystal identification, use 89060)

84512	Troponin, qualitative

(For troponin, quantitative assay, use 84484)

84520	Urea nitrogen; quantitative
84525	semiquantitative (eg, reagent strip test)
84540	Urea nitrogen, urine
84545	Urea nitrogen, clearance

Pathology and Laboratory

84550   Uric acid; blood

84560   other source

84577   Urobilinogen, feces, quantitative

84578   Urobilinogen, urine; qualitative

84580   quantitative, timed specimen

84583   semiquantitative

(Uroporphyrins, use 84120)

(Valproic acid (dipropylacetic acid), use 80164)

84585   Vanillylmandelic acid (VMA), urine

84586   Vasoactive intestinal peptide (VIP)

84588   Vasopressin (antidiuretic hormone, ADH)

84590   Vitamin A

(Vitamin B-1, use 84425)

(Vitamin B-2, use 84252)

(Vitamin B-6, use 84207)

(Vitamin B-12, use 82607)

(Vitamin B-12, absorption (Schilling), see 78270, 78271)

(Vitamin C, use 82180)

(Vitamin D, see 82306, 82307, 82652)

(Vitamin E, use 84446)

84591   Vitamin, not otherwise specified

84597   Vitamin K

(VMA, use 84585)

84600   Volatiles (eg, acetic anhydride, carbon tetrachloride, dichloroethane, dichloromethane, diethylether, isopropyl alcohol, methanol)

(For acetaldehyde, use 82000)

(Volume, blood, RISA or Cr-51, see 78110, 78111)

84620   Xylose absorption test, blood and/or urine

(For administration, use 99070)

84630   Zinc

84681   C-peptide

84702   Gonadotropin, chorionic (hCG); quantitative

84703   qualitative

(For urine pregnancy test by visual color comparison, use 81025)

84830   Ovulation tests, by visual color comparison methods for human luteinizing hormone

84999   Unlisted chemistry procedure

Hematology and Coagulation

(For blood banking procedures, see **Transfusion Medicine**)

(Agglutinins, see **Immunology**)

(Antiplasmin, use 85410)

(Antithrombin III, see 85300, 85301)

85002   Bleeding time

85004   Blood count; automated differential WBC count

85007   blood smear, microscopic examination with manual differential WBC count

85008   blood smear, microscopic examination without manual differential WBC count

(For other fluids (eg, CSF), see 89050, 89051)

85009   manual differential WBC count, buffy coat

(Eosinophils, nasal smear, use 89190)

85013   spun microhematocrit

85014   hematocrit (Hct)

85018   hemoglobin (Hgb)

(For other hemoglobin determination, see 83020-83069)

(For immunoassay, hemoglobin, fecal, use 82274)

85025   complete (CBC), automated (Hgb, Hct, RBC, WBC and platelet count) and automated differential WBC count

85027   complete (CBC), automated (Hgb, Hct, RBC, WBC and platelet count)

85032   manual cell count (erythrocyte, leukocyte, or platelet) each

85041   red blood cell (RBC), automated

(Do not report code 85041 in conjunction with 85025 or 85027)

85044   reticulocyte, manual

85045   reticulocyte, automated

85046   reticulocytes, automated, including one or more cellular parameters (eg, reticulocyte hemoglobin content (CHr), immature reticulocyte fraction (IRF), reticulocyte volume (MRV), RNA content), direct measurement

85048   leukocyte (WBC), automated

85049   platelet, automated

85055   Reticulated platelet assay

85060   Blood smear, peripheral, interpretation by physician with written report

85097   Bone marrow, smear interpretation

(For special stains, see 88312, 88313)

(For bone biopsy, see 20220, 20225, 20240, 20245, 20250, 20251)

Pathology and Laboratory

85130   Chromogenic substrate assay

(Circulating anti-coagulant screen (mixing studies), see 85611, 85732)

85170   Clot retraction

85175   Clot lysis time, whole blood dilution

(Clotting factor I (fibrinogen), see 85384, 85385)

85210   Clotting; factor II, prothrombin, specific

(See also 85610-85613)

85220   factor V (AcG or proaccelerin), labile factor

85230   factor VII (proconvertin, stable factor)

85240   factor VIII (AHG), one stage

85244   factor VIII related antigen

85245   factor VIII, VW factor, ristocetin cofactor

85246   factor VIII, VW factor antigen

85247   factor VIII, von Willebrand factor, multimetric analysis

85250   factor IX (PTC or Christmas)

85260   factor X (Stuart-Prower)

85270   factor XI (PTA)

85280   factor XII (Hageman)

85290   factor XIII (fibrin stabilizing)

85291   factor XIII (fibrin stabilizing), screen solubility

85292   prekallikrein assay (Fletcher factor assay)

85293   high molecular weight kininogen assay (Fitzgerald factor assay)

85300   Clotting inhibitors or anticoagulants; antithrombin III, activity

85301   antithrombin III, antigen assay

85302   protein C, antigen

85303   protein C, activity

85305   protein S, total

85306   protein S, free

85307   Activated Protein C (APC) resistance assay

85335   Factor inhibitor test

85337   Thrombomodulin

(For mixing studies for inhibitors, use 85732)

85345   Coagulation time; Lee and White

85347   activated

85348   other methods

(Differential count, see 85007 et seq)

(Duke bleeding time, use 85002)

(Eosinophils, nasal smear, use 89190)

85360   Euglobulin lysis

(Fetal hemoglobin, see 83030, 83033, 85460)

85362   Fibrin(ogen) degradation (split) products (FDP)(FSP); agglutination slide, semiquantitative

(Immunoelectrophoresis, use 86320)

85366   paracoagulation

85370   quantitative

85378   Fibrin degradation products, D-dimer; qualitative or semiquantitative

85379   quantitative

(For ultrasensitive and standard sensitivity quantitative D-dimer, use 85379)

85380   ultrasensitive (eg, for evaluation for venous thromboembolism), qualitative or semiquantitative

85384   Fibrinogen; activity

85385   antigen

85390   Fibrinolysins or coagulopathy screen, interpretation and report

85396   Coagulation/fibrinolysis assay, whole blood (eg, viscoelastic clot assessment), including use of any pharmacologic additive(s), as indicated, including interpretation and written report, per day

85400   Fibrinolytic factors and inhibitors; plasmin

85410   alpha-2 antiplasmin

85415   plasminogen activator

85420   plasminogen, except antigenic assay

85421   plasminogen, antigenic assay

(Fragility, red blood cell, see 85547, 85555-85557)

85441   Heinz bodies; direct

85445   induced, acetyl phenylhydrazine

(Hematocrit (PCV), see 85014, 85025, 85027)

(Hemoglobin, see 83020-83068, 85018, 85025, 85027)

85460   Hemoglobin or RBCs, fetal, for fetomaternal hemorrhage; differential lysis (Kleihauer-Betke)

(See also 83030, 83033)

(Hemolysins, see 86940, 86941)

85461   rosette

85475   Hemolysin, acid

(See also 86940, 86941)

85520   Heparin assay

85525   Heparin neutralization

85530   Heparin-protamine tolerance test

85536   Iron stain, peripheral blood

(For iron stains on bone marrow or other tissues with physician evaluation, use 88313)

Pathology and Laboratory

▲=Revised code   ●=New code   ►◄=Contains new or revised text   ⊘=Modifier 51 exempt

85540   Leukocyte alkaline phosphatase with count

85547   Mechanical fragility, RBC

85549   Muramidase

(Nitroblue tetrazolium dye test, use 86384)

85555   Osmotic fragility, RBC; unincubated

85557   incubated

(Packed cell volume, use 85013)

(Partial thromboplastin time, see 85730, 85732)

(Parasites, blood (eg, malaria smears), use 87207)

(Plasmin, use 85400)

(Plasminogen, use 85420)

(Plasminogen activator, use 85415)

85576   Platelet, aggregation (in vitro), each agent

85597   Platelet neutralization

85610   Prothrombin time;

85611   substitution, plasma fractions, each

85612   Russell viper venom time (includes venom); undiluted

85613   diluted

(Red blood cell count, see 85025, 85027, 85041)

85635   Reptilase test

(Reticulocyte count, see 85044, 85045)

85651   Sedimentation rate, erythrocyte; non-automated

85652   automated

85660   Sickling of RBC, reduction

(Hemoglobin electrophoresis, use 83020)

(Smears (eg, for parasites, malaria), use 87207)

85670   Thrombin time; plasma

85675   titer

85705   Thromboplastin inhibition, tissue

(For individual clotting factors, see 85245-85247)

85730   Thromboplastin time, partial (PTT); plasma or whole blood

85732   substitution, plasma fractions, each

85810   Viscosity

(von Willebrand factor assay, see 85245-85247)

(WBC count, see 85025, 85027, 85048, 89050)

85999   Unlisted hematology and coagulation procedure

Immunology

(Acetylcholine receptor antibody, see 83519, 86255, 86256)

(Actinomyces, antibodies to, use 86602)

(Adrenal cortex antibodies, see 86255, 86256)

86000   Agglutinins, febrile (eg, Brucella, Francisella, Murine typhus, Q fever, Rocky Mountain spotted fever, scrub typhus), each antigen

(For antibodies to infectious agents, see 86602-86804)

86001   Allergen specific IgG quantitative or semiquantitative, each allergen

(Agglutinins and autohemolysins, see 86940, 86941)

86003   Allergen specific IgE; quantitative or semiquantitative, each allergen

(For total quantitative IgE, use 82785)

86005   qualitative, multiallergen screen (dipstick, paddle or disk)

(For total qualitative IgE, use 83518)

(Alpha-1 antitrypsin, see 82103, 82104)

(Alpha-1 feto-protein, see 82105, 82106)

(Anti-AChR (acetylcholine receptor) antibody titer, see 86255, 86256)

(Anticardiolipin antibody, use 86147)

(Anti-DNA, use 86225)

(Anti-deoxyribonuclease titer, use 86215)

86021   Antibody identification; leukocyte antibodies

86022   platelet antibodies

86023   platelet associated immunoglobulin assay

86038   Antinuclear antibodies (ANA);

86039   titer

(Antistreptococcal antibody, ie, anti-DNAse, use 86215)

(Antistreptokinase titer, use 86590)

86060   Antistreptolysin O; titer

(For antibodies to infectious agents, see 86602-86804)

86063   screen

(For antibodies to infectious agents, see 86602-86804)

(Blastomyces, antibodies to, use 86612)

(86064 has been deleted. For B cells, total count, use 86355)

Pathology and Laboratory

86077   Blood bank physician services; difficult cross match and/or evaluation of irregular antibody(s), interpretation and written report

86078   investigation of transfusion reaction including suspicion of transmissible disease, interpretation and written report

86079   authorization for deviation from standard blood banking procedures (eg, use of outdated blood, transfusion of Rh incompatible units), with written report

(Brucella, antibodies to, use 86622)

(Candida, antibodies to, use 86628. For skin testing, use 86485)

86140   C-reactive protein;

(Candidiasis, use 86628)

86141   high sensitivity (hsCRP)

86146   Beta 2 Glycoprotein I antibody, each

86147   Cardiolipin (phospholipid) antibody, each Ig class

86148   Anti-phosphatidylserine (phospholipid) antibody

(To report antiprothrombin (phospholipid cofactor) antibody, use Category III code 0030T)

86155   Chemotaxis assay, specify method

(Clostridium difficile toxin, use 87230)

(Coccidioides, antibodies to, see 86635. For skin testing, use 86490)

86156   Cold agglutinin; screen

86157   titer

86160   Complement; antigen, each component

86161   functional activity, each component

86162   total hemolytic (CH50)

86171   Complement fixation tests, each antigen

(Coombs test, see 86880-86886)

86185   Counterimmunoelectrophoresis, each antigen

(Cryptococcus, antibodies to, use 86641)

86200   Cyclic citrullinated peptide (CCP), antibody

86215   Deoxyribonuclease, antibody

86225   Deoxyribonucleic acid (DNA) antibody; native or double stranded

(Echinococcus, antibodies to, see code for specific method)

(For HIV antibody tests, see 86701-86703)

86226   single stranded

(Anti D.S., DNA, IFA, eg, using C.Lucilae, see 86255 and 86256)

86235   Extractable nuclear antigen, antibody to, any method (eg, nRNP, SS-A, SS-B, Sm, RNP, Sc170, J01), each antibody

86243   Fc receptor

(Filaria, antibodies to, see code for specific method)

86255   Fluorescent noninfectious agent antibody; screen, each antibody

86256   titer, each antibody

(Fluorescent technique for antigen identification in tissue, use 88346; for indirect fluorescence, use 88347)

(FTA, see 86781)

(Gel (agar) diffusion tests, use 86331)

86277   Growth hormone, human (HGH), antibody

86280   Hemagglutination inhibition test (HAI)

(For rubella, use 86762)

(For antibodies to infectious agents, see 86602-86804)

86294   Immunoassay for tumor antigen, qualitative or semiquantitative (eg, bladder tumor antigen)

86300   Immunoassay for tumor antigen, quantitative; CA 15-3 (27.29)

86301   CA 19-9

86304   CA 125

(For measurement of serum HER-2/neu oncoprotein, see 83950)

(For hepatitis delta agent, antibody, use 86692)

86308   Heterophile antibodies; screening

(For antibodies to infectious agents, see 86602-86804)

86309   titer

(For antibodies to infectious agents, see 86602-86804)

86310   titers after absorption with beef cells and guinea pig kidney

(Histoplasma, antibodies to, use 86698. For skin testing, use 86510)

(For antibodies to infectious agents, see 86602-86804)

(Human growth hormone antibody, use 86277)

86316   Immunoassay for tumor antigen, other antigen, quantitative (eg, CA 50, 72-4, 549), each

86317   Immunoassay for infectious agent antibody, quantitative, not otherwise specified

(For immunoassay techniques for antigens, see 83516, 83518, 83519, 83520, 87301-87450, 87810-87899)

(For particle agglutination procedures, use 86403)

86318   Immunoassay for infectious agent antibody, qualitative or semiquantitative, single step method (eg, reagent strip)

86320 Immunoelectrophoresis; serum

86325 other fluids (eg, urine, cerebrospinal fluid) with concentration

86327 crossed (2-dimensional assay)

86329 Immunodiffusion; not elsewhere specified

86331 gel diffusion, qualitative (Ouchterlony), each antigen or antibody

86332 Immune complex assay

86334 Immunofixation electrophoresis; serum

86335 other fluids with concentration (eg, urine, CSF)

86336 Inhibin A

86337 Insulin antibodies

86340 Intrinsic factor antibodies

(Leptospira, antibodies to, use 86720)

(Leukoagglutinins, use 86021)

86341 Islet cell antibody

86343 Leukocyte histamine release test (LHR)

86344 Leukocyte phagocytosis

86353 Lymphocyte transformation, mitogen (phytomitogen) or antigen induced blastogenesis

(Malaria antibodies, use 86750)

86355 B cells, total count

86357 Natural killer (NK) cells, total count

86359 T cells; total count

86360 absolute CD4 and CD8 count, including ratio

86361 absolute CD4 count

86367 Stem cells (ie, CD34), total count

(For flow cytometric immunophenotyping for the assessment of potential hematolymphoid neoplasia, see 88184-88189)

86376 Microsomal antibodies (eg, thyroid or liver-kidney), each

86378 Migration inhibitory factor test (MIF)

(Mitochondrial antibody, liver, see 86255, 86256)

(Mononucleosis, see 86308-86310)

(86379 has been deleted. For natural killer cells, total count, use 86357)

86382 Neutralization test, viral

86384 Nitroblue tetrazolium dye test (NTD)

(Ouchterlony diffusion, use 86331)

(Platelet antibodies, see 86022, 86023)

86403 Particle agglutination; screen, each antibody

86406 titer, each antibody

(Pregnancy test, see 84702, 84703)

(Rapid plasma reagin test (RPR), see 86592, 86593)

86430 Rheumatoid factor; qualitative

86431 quantitative

(Serologic test for syphilis, see 86592, 86593)

86480 Tuberculosis test, cell mediated immunity measurement of gamma interferon antigen response

86485 Skin test; candida

(For antibody, candida, use 86628)

86490 coccidioidomycosis

86510 histoplasmosis

(For histoplasma, antibody, use 86698)

86580 tuberculosis, intradermal

(For tuberculosis test, cell mediated immunity measurement of gamma interferon antigen response, use 86480)

(86585 has been deleted. To report tuberculosis testing by intradermal (Mantoux) test, use 86580)

(For skin tests for allergy, see 95010-95199)

(Smooth muscle antibody, see 86255, 86256)

(Sporothrix, antibodies to, see code for specific method)

86586 Unlisted antigen, each

(86587 has been deleted. For stem cells, total count, use 86367)

86590 Streptokinase, antibody

(For antibodies to infectious agents, see 86602-86804)

(Streptolysin O antibody, see antistreptolysin O, 86060, 86063)

86592 Syphilis test; qualitative (eg, VDRL, RPR, ART)

(For antibodies to infectious agents, see 86602-86804)

86593 quantitative

(For antibodies to infectious agents, see 86602-86804)

(Tetanus antibody, use 86774)

(Thyroglobulin antibody, use 86800)

(Thyroglobulin, use 84432)

(Thyroid microsomal antibody, use 86376)

(For toxoplasma antibody, see 86777-86778)

▶The following codes (86602-86804) are qualitative or semiquantitative immunoassays performed by multiple-step methods for the detection of antibodies to infectious agents. For immunoassays by single-step method (eg, reagent strips), use code 86318. Procedures for the identification of antibodies should be coded as precisely as possible. For example, an antibody to a virus could be coded with increasing specificity for virus, family, genus, species, or type. In some cases, further precision may be added to codes by specifying the class of immunoglobulin being detected. When multiple tests are done to detect antibodies to organisms classified more precisely than the specificity allowed by available codes, it is appropriate to code each as a separate service. For example, a test for antibody to an enterovirus is coded as 86658. Coxsackie viruses are enteroviruses, but there are no codes for the individual species of enterovirus. If assays are performed for antibodies to coxsackie A and B species, each assay should be separately coded. Similarly, if multiple assays are performed for antibodies of different immunoglobulin classes, each assay should be coded separately. When a coding option exists for reporting IgM specific antibodies (eg, 86632), the corresponding nonspecific code (eg, 86631) may be reported for performance of either an antibody analysis not specific for a particular immunoglobulin class or for an IgG analysis.◄

(For the detection of antibodies other than those to infectious agents, see specific antibody [eg, 86021-86023, 86376, 86800, 86850-86870] or specific method [eg, 83516, 86255, 86256]).

(For infectious agent/antigen detection, see 87260-87899)

86602	Antibody; actinomyces
86603	adenovirus
86606	Aspergillus
86609	bacterium, not elsewhere specified
86611	Bartonella
86612	Blastomyces
86615	Bordetella
86617	Borrelia burgdorferi (Lyme disease) confirmatory test (eg, Western Blot or immunoblot)
86618	Borrelia burgdorferi (Lyme disease)
86619	Borrelia (relapsing fever)
86622	Brucella
86625	Campylobacter
86628	Candida

(For skin test, candida, use 86485)

86631	Chlamydia
86632	Chlamydia, IgM

(For chlamydia antigen, see 87270, 87320. For fluorescent antibody technique, see 86255, 86256)

86635	Coccidioides
86638	Coxiella burnetii (Q fever)
86641	Cryptococcus
86644	cytomegalovirus (CMV)
86645	cytomegalovirus (CMV), IgM
86648	Diphtheria
86651	encephalitis, California (La Crosse)

86652	encephalitis, Eastern equine
86653	encephalitis, St. Louis
86654	encephalitis, Western equine
86658	enterovirus (eg, coxsackie, echo, polio)

(Trichinella, antibodies to, use 86784)

(Trypanosoma, antibodies to, see code for specific method)

(Tuberculosis, use 86580 for skin testing)

(Viral antibodies, see code for specific method)

86663	Epstein-Barr (EB) virus, early antigen (EA)
86664	Epstein-Barr (EB) virus, nuclear antigen (EBNA)
86665	Epstein-Barr (EB) virus, viral capsid (VCA)
86666	Ehrlichia
86668	Francisella tularensis
86671	fungus, not elsewhere specified
86674	Giardia lamblia
86677	Helicobacter pylori
86682	helminth, not elsewhere specified
86684	Haemophilus influenza
86687	HTLV-I
86688	HTLV-II
86689	HTLV or HIV antibody, confirmatory test (eg, Western Blot)
86692	hepatitis, delta agent

(For hepatitis delta agent, antigen, use 87380)

86694	herpes simplex, non-specific type test
86695	herpes simplex, type 1
86696	herpes simplex, type 2
86698	histoplasma
86701	HIV-1
86702	HIV-2
86703	HIV-1 and HIV-2, single assay

(For HIV-1 antigen, use 87390)

(For HIV-2 antigen, use 87391)

(For confirmatory test for HIV antibody (eg, Western Blot), use 86689)

86704	Hepatitis B core antibody (HBcAb); total
86705	IgM antibody
86706	Hepatitis B surface antibody (HBsAb)
86707	Hepatitis Be antibody (HBeAb)
86708	Hepatitis A antibody (HAAb); total
86709	IgM antibody

Pathology and Laboratory

86710	Antibody; influenza virus
86713	Legionella
86717	Leishmania
86720	Leptospira
86723	Listeria monocytogenes
86727	lymphocytic choriomeningitis
86729	lymphogranuloma venereum
86732	mucormycosis
86735	mumps
86738	mycoplasma
86741	Neisseria meningitidis
86744	Nocardia
86747	parvovirus
86750	Plasmodium (malaria)
86753	protozoa, not elsewhere specified
86756	respiratory syncytial virus
86757	Rickettsia
86759	rotavirus
86762	rubella
86765	rubeola
86768	Salmonella
86771	Shigella
86774	tetanus
86777	Toxoplasma
86778	Toxoplasma, IgM
86781	Treponema pallidum, confirmatory test (eg, FTA-abs)
86784	Trichinella
86787	varicella-zoster
● 86788	West Nile virus, IgM
● 86789	West Nile virus
86790	virus, not elsewhere specified
86793	Yersinia
86800	Thyroglobulin antibody

(For thyroglobulin, use 84432)

86803	Hepatitis C antibody;
86804	confirmatory test (eg, immunoblot)

Tissue Typing

(For pretransplant cross-match, see appropriate code or codes)

86805	Lymphocytotoxicity assay, visual crossmatch; with titration
86806	without titration

86807	Serum screening for cytotoxic percent reactive antibody (PRA); standard method
86808	quick method
86812	HLA typing; A, B, or C (eg, A10, B7, B27), single antigen
86813	A, B, or C, multiple antigens
86816	DR/DQ, single antigen
86817	DR/DQ, multiple antigens
86821	lymphocyte culture, mixed (MLC)
86822	lymphocyte culture, primed (PLC)
86849	Unlisted immunology procedure

Transfusion Medicine

(For apheresis, use 36511, 36512)

(For therapeutic phlebotomy, use 99195)

86850	Antibody screen, RBC, each serum technique
86860	Antibody elution (RBC), each elution
86870	Antibody identification, RBC antibodies, each panel for each serum technique
86880	Antihuman globulin test (Coombs test); direct, each antiserum
86885	indirect, qualitative, each antiserum
86886	indirect, titer, each antiserum
86890	Autologous blood or component, collection processing and storage; predeposited
86891	intra- or postoperative salvage

(For physician services to autologous donors, see 99201-99204)

86900	Blood typing; ABO
86901	Rh (D)
86903	antigen screening for compatible blood unit using reagent serum, per unit screened
86904	antigen screening for compatible unit using patient serum, per unit screened
86905	RBC antigens, other than ABO or Rh (D), each
86906	Rh phenotyping, complete
86910	Blood typing, for paternity testing, per individual; ABO, Rh and MN
86911	each additional antigen system
86920	Compatibility test each unit; immediate spin technique
86921	incubation technique
86922	antiglobulin technique
86923	electronic

(Do not use 86923 in conjunction with 86920-86922 for same unit crossmatch)

Pathology and Laboratory

86927   Fresh frozen plasma, thawing, each unit

86930   Frozen blood, each unit; freezing (includes preparation)

86931   thawing

86932   freezing (includes preparation) and thawing

86940   Hemolysins and agglutinins; auto, screen, each

86941   incubated

86945   Irradiation of blood product, each unit

86950   Leukocyte transfusion

       (For leukapheresis, use 36511)

86960   Volume reduction of blood or blood product (eg, red blood cells or platelets), each unit

86965   Pooling of platelets or other blood products

86970   Pretreatment of RBCs for use in RBC antibody detection, identification, and/or compatibility testing; incubation with chemical agents or drugs, each

86971   incubation with enzymes, each

86972   by density gradient separation

86975   Pretreatment of serum for use in RBC antibody identification; incubation with drugs, each

86976   by dilution

86977   incubation with inhibitors, each

86978   by differential red cell absorption using patient RBCs or RBCs of known phenotype, each absorption

86985   Splitting of blood or blood products, each unit

86999   Unlisted transfusion medicine procedure

Microbiology

Includes bacteriology, mycology, parasitology, and virology.

Presumptive identification of microorganisms is defined as identification by colony morphology, growth on selective media, Gram stains, or up to three tests (eg, catalase, oxidase, indole, urease). Definitive identification of microorganisms is defined as an identification to the genus or species level that requires additional tests (eg, biochemical panels, slide cultures). If additional studies involve molecular probes, chromatography, or immunologic techniques, these should be separately coded in addition to definitive identification codes (87140-87158). For multiple specimens/sites use modifier 59. For repeat laboratory tests performed on the same day, use modifier 91.

87001   Animal inoculation, small animal; with observation

87003   with observation and dissection

87015   Concentration (any type), for infectious agents

       (Do not report 87015 in conjunction with 87177)

87040   Culture, bacterial; blood, aerobic, with isolation and presumptive identification of isolates (includes anaerobic culture, if appropriate)

87045   stool, aerobic, with isolation and preliminary examination (eg, KIA, LIA), Salmonella and Shigella species

87046   stool, aerobic, additional pathogens, isolation and presumptive identification of isolates, each plate

87070   any other source except urine, blood or stool, aerobic, with isolation and presumptive identification of isolates

       (For urine, use 87088)

87071   quantitative, aerobic with isolation and presumptive identification of isolates, any source except urine, blood or stool

       (For urine, use 87088)

87073   quantitative, anaerobic with isolation and presumptive identification of isolates, any source except urine, blood or stool

       (For definitive identification of isolates, use 87076 or 87077. For typing of isolates see 87140-87158)

87075   any source, except blood, anaerobic with isolation and presumptive identification of isolates

87076   anaerobic isolate, additional methods required for definitive identification, each isolate

       (For gas liquid chromatography (GLC) or high pressure liquid chromatography (HPLC), use 87143)

87077   aerobic isolate, additional methods required for definitive identification, each isolate

       (For gas liquid chromatography (GLC) or high pressure liquid chromatography (HPLC), use 87143)

87081   Culture, presumptive, pathogenic organisms, screening only;

87084   with colony estimation from density chart

87086   Culture, bacterial; quantitative colony count, urine

▲ **87088**   with isolation and presumptive identification of each isolate, urine

87101   Culture, fungi (mold or yeast) isolation, with presumptive identification of isolates; skin, hair, or nail

87102   other source (except blood)

87103   blood

87106   Culture, fungi, definitive identification, each organism; yeast

       (Use 87106 in addition to codes 87101, 87102, or 87103 when appropriate)

87107   mold

87109   Culture, mycoplasma, any source

Pathology and Laboratory

87110   Culture, chlamydia, any source

(For immunofluorescence staining of shell vials, use 87140)

87116   Culture, tubercle or other acid-fast bacilli (eg, TB, AFB, mycobacteria) any source, with isolation and presumptive identification of isolates

(For concentration, use 87015)

87118   Culture, mycobacterial, definitive identification, each isolate

(For nucleic acid probe identification, use 87149)

(For GLC or HPLC identification, use 87143)

87140   Culture, typing; immunofluorescent method, each antiserum

87143   gas liquid chromatography (GLC) or high pressure liquid chromatography (HPLC) method

87147   immunologic method, other than immunofluoresence (eg, agglutination grouping), per antiserum

87149   identification by nucleic acid probe

87152   identification by pulse field gel typing

87158   other methods

87164   Dark field examination, any source (eg, penile, vaginal, oral, skin); includes specimen collection

87166   without collection

87168   Macroscopic examination; arthropod

87169   parasite

87172   Pinworm exam (eg, cellophane tape prep)

87176   Homogenization, tissue, for culture

87177   Ova and parasites, direct smears, concentration and identification

(Do not report 87177 in conjunction with 87015)

(For direct smears from a primary source, use 87207)

(For coccidia or microsporidia exam, use 87207)

(For complex special stain (trichrome, iron hematoxylin), use 87209)

(For nucleic acid probes in cytologic material, use 88365)

(For molecular diagnostics, see 83890-83898, 87470-87799)

87181   Susceptibility studies, antimicrobial agent; agar dilution method, per agent (eg, antibiotic gradient strip)

87184   disk method, per plate (12 or fewer agents)

87185   enzyme detection (eg, beta lactamase), per enzyme

87186   microdilution or agar dilution (minimum inhibitory concentration (MIC) or breakpoint), each multi-antimicrobial, per plate

+ 87187   microdilution or agar dilution, minimum lethal concentration (MLC), each plate (List separately in addition to code for primary procedure)

(Use 87187 in conjunction with 87186 or 87188)

87188   macrobroth dilution method, each agent

87190   mycobacteria, proportion method, each agent

(For other mycobacterial susceptibility studies, see 87181, 87184, 87186, or 87188)

87197   Serum bactericidal titer (Schlicter test)

87205   Smear, primary source with interpretation; Gram or Giemsa stain for bacteria, fungi, or cell types

87206   fluorescent and/or acid fast stain for bacteria, fungi, parasites, viruses or cell types

87207   special stain for inclusion bodies or parasites (eg, malaria, coccidia, microsporidia, trypanosomes, herpes viruses)

(For direct smears with concentration and identification, use 87177)

(For thick smear preparation, use 87015)

(For fat, meat, fibers, nasal eosinophils, and starch, see miscellaneous section)

87209   complex special stain (eg, trichrome, iron hemotoxylin) for ova and parasites

87210   wet mount for infectious agents (eg, saline, India ink, KOH preps)

(For KOH examination of skin, hair or nails, see 87220)

87220   Tissue examination by KOH slide of samples from skin, hair, or nails for fungi or ectoparasite ova or mites (eg, scabies)

87230   Toxin or antitoxin assay, tissue culture (eg, Clostridium difficile toxin)

87250   Virus isolation; inoculation of embryonated eggs, or small animal, includes observation and dissection

87252   tissue culture inoculation, observation, and presumptive identification by cytopathic effect

87253   tissue culture, additional studies or definitive identification (eg, hemabsorption, neutralization, immunofluoresence stain), each isolate

(Electron microscopy, use 88348)

(Inclusion bodies in tissue sections, see 88304-88309; in smears, see 87207-87210; in fluids, use 88106)

87254   centrifuge enhanced (shell vial) technique, includes identification with immunofluorescence stain, each virus

(Report 87254 in addition to 87252 as appropriate)

87255   including identification by non-immunologic method, other than by cytopathic effect (eg, virus specific enzymatic activity)

These codes are intended for primary source only. For similar studies on culture material, refer to codes 87140-87158. Infectious agents by antigen detection, immunofluorescence microscopy, or nucleic acid probe techniques should be reported as precisely as possible. The most specific code possible should be reported. If there is no specific agent code, the general methodology code (eg, 87299, 87449, 87450, 87797, 87798, 87799, 87899) should be used. For identification of antibodies to many of the listed infectious agents, see 86602-86804. When separate assays are performed for different species or strain(s) of organisms, each assay should be reported separately.

87260   Infectious agent antigen detection by immunofluorescent technique; adenovirus

87265   Bordetella pertussis/parapertussis

87267   Enterovirus, direct fluorescent antibody (DFA)

87269   giardia

87270   Chlamydia trachomatis

87271   Cytomegalovirus, direct fluorescent antibody (DFA)

87272   cryptosporidium

87273   Herpes simplex virus type 2

87274   Herpes simplex virus type 1

87275   influenza B virus

87276   influenza A virus

87277   Legionella micdadei

87278   Legionella pneumophila

87279   Parainfluenza virus, each type

87280   respiratory syncytial virus

87281   Pneumocystis carinii

87283   Rubeola

87285   Treponema pallidum

87290   Varicella zoster virus

87299   not otherwise specified, each organism

87300   Infectious agent antigen detection by immunofluorescent technique, polyvalent for multiple organisms, each polyvalent antiserum

(For physician evaluation of infectious disease agents by immunofluorescence, use 88346)

87301   Infectious agent antigen detection by enzyme immunoassay technique, qualitative or semiquantitative, multiple-step method; adenovirus enteric types 40/41

● 87305   Aspergillus

87320   Chlamydia trachomatis

87324   Clostridium difficile toxin(s)

87327   Cryptococcus neoformans

(For Cryptococcus latex agglutination, use 86403)

87328   cryptosporidium

87329   giardia

87332   cytomegalovirus

87335   Escherichia coli 0157

(For giardia antigen, use 87329)

87336   Entamoeba histolytica dispar group

87337   Entamoeba histolytica group

87338   Helicobacter pylori, stool

87339   Helicobacter pylori

(For H. pylori, stool, use 87338. For H. pylori, breath and blood by mass spectrometry, see 83013, 83014. For H. pylori, liquid scintillation counter, see 78267, 78268)

87340   hepatitis B surface antigen (HBsAg)

87341   hepatitis B surface antigen (HBsAg) neutralization

87350   hepatitis Be antigen (HBeAg)

87380   hepatitis, delta agent

87385   Histoplasma capsulatum

87390   HIV-1

87391   HIV-2

87400   Influenza, A or B, each

87420   respiratory syncytial virus

87425   rotavirus

87427   Shiga-like toxin

87430   Streptococcus, group A

87449   Infectious agent antigen detection by enzyme immunoassay technique qualitative or semiquantitative; multiple step method, not otherwise specified, each organism

87450   single step method, not otherwise specified, each organism

87451   multiple step method, polyvalent for multiple organisms, each polyvalent antiserum

87470   Infectious agent detection by nucleic acid (DNA or RNA); Bartonella henselae and Bartonella quintana, direct probe technique

87471   Bartonella henselae and Bartonella quintana, amplified probe technique

87472   Bartonella henselae and Bartonella quintana, quantification

87475   Borrelia burgdorferi, direct probe technique

87476   Borrelia burgdorferi, amplified probe technique

87477   Borrelia burgdorferi, quantification

87480   Candida species, direct probe technique

87481   Candida species, amplified probe technique

87482   Candida species, quantification

Pathology and Laboratory

87485	Chlamydia pneumoniae, direct probe technique
87486	Chlamydia pneumoniae, amplified probe technique
87487	Chlamydia pneumoniae, quantification
87490	Chlamydia trachomatis, direct probe technique
87491	Chlamydia trachomatis, amplified probe technique
87492	Chlamydia trachomatis, quantification
87495	cytomegalovirus, direct probe technique
87496	cytomegalovirus, amplified probe technique
87497	cytomegalovirus, quantification
● 87498	enterovirus, amplified probe technique
87510	Gardnerella vaginalis, direct probe technique
87511	Gardnerella vaginalis, amplified probe technique
87512	Gardnerella vaginalis, quantification
87515	hepatitis B virus, direct probe technique
87516	hepatitis B virus, amplified probe technique
87517	hepatitis B virus, quantification
87520	hepatitis C, direct probe technique
87521	hepatitis C, amplified probe technique
87522	hepatitis C, quantification
87525	hepatitis G, direct probe technique
87526	hepatitis G, amplified probe technique
87527	hepatitis G, quantification
87528	Herpes simplex virus, direct probe technique
87529	Herpes simplex virus, amplified probe technique
87530	Herpes simplex virus, quantification
87531	Herpes virus-6, direct probe technique
87532	Herpes virus-6, amplified probe technique
87533	Herpes virus-6, quantification
87534	HIV-1, direct probe technique
87535	HIV-1, amplified probe technique
87536	HIV-1, quantification
87537	HIV-2, direct probe technique
87538	HIV-2, amplified probe technique
87539	HIV-2, quantification
87540	Legionella pneumophila, direct probe technique
87541	Legionella pneumophila, amplified probe technique
87542	Legionella pneumophila, quantification
87550	Mycobacteria species, direct probe technique
87551	Mycobacteria species, amplified probe technique
87552	Mycobacteria species, quantification
87555	Mycobacteria tuberculosis, direct probe technique

87556	Mycobacteria tuberculosis, amplified probe technique
87557	Mycobacteria tuberculosis, quantification
87560	Mycobacteria avium-intracellulare, direct probe technique
87561	Mycobacteria avium-intracellulare, amplified probe technique
87562	Mycobacteria avium-intracellulare, quantification
87580	Mycoplasma pneumoniae, direct probe technique
87581	Mycoplasma pneumoniae, amplified probe technique
87582	Mycoplasma pneumoniae, quantification
87590	Neisseria gonorrhoeae, direct probe technique
87591	Neisseria gonorrhoeae, amplified probe technique
87592	Neisseria gonorrhoeae, quantification
87620	papillomavirus, human, direct probe technique
87621	papillomavirus, human, amplified probe technique
87622	papillomavirus, human, quantification
● 87640	Staphylococcus aureus, amplified probe technique
● 87641	Staphylococcus aureus, methicillin resistant, amplified probe technique

►(For assays that detect methicillin resistance and identify Staphylococcus aureus using a single nucleic acid sequence, use 87641)◄

87650	Streptococcus, group A, direct probe technique
87651	Streptococcus, group A, amplified probe technique
87652	Streptococcus, group A, quantification
● 87653	Streptococcus, group B, amplified probe technique
87660	Trichomonas vaginalis, direct probe technique
87797	Infectious agent detection by nucleic acid (DNA or RNA), not otherwise specified; direct probe technique, each organism
87798	amplified probe technique, each organism
87799	quantification, each organism
87800	Infectious agent detection by nucleic acid (DNA or RNA), multiple organisms; direct probe(s) technique
87801	amplified probe(s) technique

►(For each specific organism nucleic acid detection from a primary source, see 87470-87660. For detection of specific infectious agents not otherwise specified, see 87797, 87798, or 87799 one time for each agent)◄

87802	Infectious agent antigen detection by immunoassay with direct optical observation; Streptococcus, group B
87803	Clostridium difficile toxin A
87804	Influenza
87807	respiratory syncytial virus
● 87808	Trichomonas vaginalis

Pathology and Laboratory

87810	Infectious agent detection by immunoassay with direct optical observation; Chlamydia trachomatis
87850	Neisseria gonorrhoeae
87880	Streptococcus, group A
87899	not otherwise specified
87900	Infectious agent drug susceptibility phenotype prediction using regularly updated genotypic bioinformatics
87901	Infectious agent genotype analysis by nucleic acid (DNA or RNA); HIV 1, reverse transcriptase and protease

(For infectious agent drug susceptibility phenotype prediction for HIV-1, use 87900)

87902	Hepatitis C virus
87903	Infectious agent phenotype analysis by nucleic acid (DNA or RNA) with drug resistance tissue culture analysis, HIV 1; first through 10 drugs tested
+ 87904	each additional drug tested (List separately in addition to code for primary procedure)

(Use 87904 in conjunction with 87903)

87999	Unlisted microbiology procedure

Anatomic Pathology

Postmortem Examination

Procedures 88000 through 88099 represent physician services only. Use modifier 90 for outside laboratory services.

88000	Necropsy (autopsy), gross examination only; without CNS
88005	with brain
88007	with brain and spinal cord
88012	infant with brain
88014	stillborn or newborn with brain
88016	macerated stillborn
88020	Necropsy (autopsy), gross and microscopic; without CNS
88025	with brain
88027	with brain and spinal cord
88028	infant with brain
88029	stillborn or newborn with brain
88036	Necropsy (autopsy), limited, gross and/or microscopic; regional
88037	single organ
88040	Necropsy (autopsy); forensic examination
88045	coroner's call
88099	Unlisted necropsy (autopsy) procedure

Cytopathology

(For cervicography, see Category III code 0003T)

(For collection of cytology specimens via mammary duct catheter lavage, report 0046T-0047T)

88104	Cytopathology, fluids, washings or brushings, except cervical or vaginal; smears with interpretation
▲ 88106	simple filter method with interpretation
▲ 88107	smears and simple filter preparation with interpretation

►(For nongynecological selective cellular enhancement including filter transfer techniques, use 88112)◄

88108	Cytopathology, concentration technique, smears and interpretation (eg, Saccomanno technique)

(For cervical or vaginal smears, see 88150-88155)

(For gastric intubation with lavage, see 89130-89141, 91055)

(For x-ray localization, use 74340)

88112	Cytopathology, selective cellular enhancement technique with interpretation (eg, liquid based slide preparation method), except cervical or vaginal

(Do not report 88112 with 88108)

88125	Cytopathology, forensic (eg, sperm)
88130	Sex chromatin identification; Barr bodies
88140	peripheral blood smear, polymorphonuclear drumsticks

(For Guard stain, use 88313)

Codes 88141-88155, 88164-88167, 88174-88175 are used to report cervical or vaginal screening by various methods and to report physician interpretation services. Use codes 88150-88154 to report conventional Pap smears that are examined using non-Bethesda reporting. Use codes 88164-88167 to report conventional Pap smears that are examined using the Bethesda System of reporting. Use codes 88142-88143 to report liquid-based specimens processed as thin-layer preparations that are examined using any system of reporting (Bethesda or non-Bethesda). Use codes 88174-88175 to report automated screening of liquid-based specimens that are examined using any system of reporting (Bethesda or non-Bethesda). Within each of these three code families choose the one code that describes the screening method(s) used. Codes 88141 and 88155 should be reported in addition to the screening code chosen when the additional services are provided. Manual rescreening requires a complete visual reassessment of the entire slide initially screened by either an automated or manual process. Manual review represents an assessment of selected cells or regions of a slide identified by initial automated review.

88141 Cytopathology, cervical or vaginal (any reporting system), requiring interpretation by physician

(Use 88141 in conjunction with 88142-88154, 88164-88167, 88174-88175)

88142 Cytopathology, cervical or vaginal (any reporting system), collected in preservative fluid, automated thin layer preparation; manual screening under physician supervision

88143 with manual screening and rescreening under physician supervision

(For automated screening of automated thin layer preparation, see 88174, 88175)

88147 Cytopathology smears, cervical or vaginal; screening by automated system under physician supervision

88148 screening by automated system with manual rescreening under physician supervision

88150 Cytopathology, slides, cervical or vaginal; manual screening under physician supervision

88152 with manual screening and computer-assisted rescreening under physician supervision

88153 with manual screening and rescreening under physician supervision

88154 with manual screening and computer-assisted rescreening using cell selection and review under physician supervision

+ 88155 Cytopathology, slides, cervical or vaginal, definitive hormonal evaluation (eg, maturation index, karyopyknotic index, estrogenic index) (List separately in addition to code(s) for other technical and interpretation services)

(Use 88155 in conjunction with 88142-88154, 88164-88167, 88174-88175)

88160 Cytopathology, smears, any other source; screening and interpretation

88161 preparation, screening and interpretation

88162 extended study involving over 5 slides and/or multiple stains

(For aerosol collection of sputum, use 89220)

(For special stains, see 88312-88314)

88164 Cytopathology, slides, cervical or vaginal (the Bethesda System); manual screening under physician supervision

88165 with manual screening and rescreening under physician supervision

88166 with manual screening and computer-assisted rescreening under physician supervision

88167 with manual screening and computer-assisted rescreening using cell selection and review under physician supervision

(88170, 88171 have been deleted)

(To report collection of specimen via fine needle aspiration, see 10021, 10022)

88172 Cytopathology, evaluation of fine needle aspirate; immediate cytohistologic study to determine adequacy of specimen(s)

88173 interpretation and report

(For fine needle aspirate, see 10021, 10022)

(Do not report 88172, 88173 in conjunction with 88333 and 88334 for the same specimen)

88174 Cytopathology, cervical or vaginal (any reporting system), collected in preservative fluid, automated thin layer preparation; screening by automated system, under physician supervision

88175 with screening by automated system and manual rescreening or review, under physician supervision

(For manual screening, see 88142, 88143)

(88180 has been deleted. To report, see 88184-88189)

88182 Flow cytometry, cell cycle or DNA analysis

(For DNA ploidy analysis by morphometric technique, use 88358)

88184 Flow cytometry, cell surface, cytoplasmic, or nuclear marker, technical component only; first marker

+ 88185 each additional marker (List separately in addition to code for first marker)

(Report 88185 in conjunction with 88184)

88187 Flow cytometry, interpretation; 2 to 8 markers

88188 9 to 15 markers

88189 16 or more markers

88199 Unlisted cytopathology procedure

(For electron microscopy, see 88348, 88349)

Cytogenetic Studies

When molecular diagnostic procedures are performed to test for oncologic or inherited disorder, use the appropriate modifier to specify probe type or condition tested. (See **Appendix I** for a listing of appropriate modifiers to report with molecular diagnostic and cytogenetic procedures.)

(For acetylcholinesterase, use 82013)

(For alpha-fetoprotein, serum or amniotic fluid, see 82105, 82106)

(For laser microdissection of cells from tissue sample, see 88380)

88230 Tissue culture for non-neoplastic disorders; lymphocyte

88233 skin or other solid tissue biopsy

88235 amniotic fluid or chorionic villus cells

88237 Tissue culture for neoplastic disorders; bone marrow, blood cells

88239 solid tumor

88240   Cryopreservation, freezing and storage of cells, each cell line

(For therapeutic cryopreservation and storage, use 38207)

88241   Thawing and expansion of frozen cells, each aliquot

(For therapeutic thawing of previous harvest, use 38208)

88245   Chromosome analysis for breakage syndromes; baseline Sister Chromatid Exchange (SCE), 20-25 cells

88248   baseline breakage, score 50-100 cells, count 20 cells, 2 karyotypes (eg, for ataxia telangiectasia, Fanconi anemia, fragile X)

88249   score 100 cells, clastogen stress (eg, diepoxybutane, mitomycin C, ionizing radiation, UV radiation)

88261   Chromosome analysis; count 5 cells, 1 karyotype, with banding

88262   count 15-20 cells, 2 karyotypes, with banding

88263   count 45 cells for mosaicism, 2 karyotypes, with banding

88264   analyze 20-25 cells

88267   Chromosome analysis, amniotic fluid or chorionic villus, count 15 cells, 1 karyotype, with banding

88269   Chromosome analysis, in situ for amniotic fluid cells, count cells from 6-12 colonies, 1 karyotype, with banding

88271   Molecular cytogenetics; DNA probe, each (eg, FISH)

88272   chromosomal in situ hybridization, analyze 3-5 cells (eg, for derivatives and markers)

88273   chromosomal in situ hybridization, analyze 10-30 cells (eg, for microdeletions)

88274   interphase in situ hybridization, analyze 25-99 cells

88275   interphase in situ hybridization, analyze 100-300 cells

88280   Chromosome analysis; additional karyotypes, each study

88283   additional specialized banding technique (eg, NOR, C-banding)

88285   additional cells counted, each study

88289   additional high resolution study

88291   Cytogenetics and molecular cytogenetics, interpretation and report

88299   Unlisted cytogenetic study

Surgical Pathology

Services 88300 through 88309 include accession, examination, and reporting. They do not include the services designated in codes 88311 through 88365 and 88399, which are coded in addition when provided.

The unit of service for codes 88300 through 88309 is the specimen.

A specimen is defined as tissue or tissues that is (are) submitted for individual and separate attention, requiring individual examination and pathologic diagnosis. Two or more such specimens from the same patient (eg, separately identified endoscopic biopsies, skin lesions) are each appropriately assigned an individual code reflective of its proper level of service.

Service code 88300 is used for any specimen that in the opinion of the examining pathologist can be accurately diagnosed without microscopic examination. Service code 88302 is used when gross and microscopic examination is performed on a specimen to confirm identification and the absence of disease. Service codes 88304 through 88309 describe all other specimens requiring gross and microscopic examination, and represent additional ascending levels of physician work. Levels 88302 through 88309 are specifically defined by the assigned specimens.

Any unlisted specimen should be assigned to the code which most closely reflects the physician work involved when compared to other specimens assigned to that code.

▶(Do not report 88302-88309 on the same specimen as part of Mohs surgery)◀

88300   **Level I** - Surgical pathology, gross examination only

88302   **Level II** - Surgical pathology, gross and microscopic examination

Appendix, incidental

Fallopian tube, sterilization

Fingers/toes, amputation, traumatic

Foreskin, newborn

Hernia sac, any location

Hydrocele sac

Nerve

Skin, plastic repair

Sympathetic ganglion

Testis, castration

Vaginal mucosa, incidental

Vas deferens, sterilization

88304   **Level III** - Surgical pathology, gross and microscopic examination

Abortion, induced

Abscess

Aneurysm - arterial/ventricular

Anus, tag

Appendix, other than incidental

Artery, atheromatous plaque

Bartholin's gland cyst

Bone fragment(s), other than pathologic fracture

Pathology and Laboratory

Bursa/synovial cyst

Carpal tunnel tissue

Cartilage, shavings

Cholesteatoma

Colon, colostomy stoma

Conjunctiva - biopsy/pterygium

Cornea

Diverticulum - esophagus/small intestine

Dupuytren's contracture tissue

Femoral head, other than fracture

Fissure/fistula

Foreskin, other than newborn

Gallbladder

Ganglion cyst

Hematoma

Hemorrhoids

Hydatid of Morgagni

Intervertebral disc

Joint, loose body

Meniscus

Mucocele, salivary

Neuroma - Morton's/traumatic

Pilonidal cyst/sinus

Polyps, inflammatory - nasal/sinusoidal

Skin - cyst/tag/debridement

Soft tissue, debridement

Soft tissue,lipoma

Spermatocele

Tendon/tendon sheath

Testicular appendage

Thrombus or embolus

Tonsil and/or adenoids

Varicocele

Vas deferens, other than sterilization

Vein, varicosity

88305 **Level IV** - Surgical pathology, gross and microscopic examination

Abortion - spontaneous/missed

Artery, biopsy

Bone marrow, biopsy

Bone exostosis

Brain/meninges, other than for tumor resection

Breast, biopsy, not requiring microscopic evaluation of surgical margins

Breast, reduction mammoplasty

Bronchus, biopsy

Cell block, any source

Cervix, biopsy

Colon, biopsy

Duodenum, biopsy

Endocervix, curettings/biopsy

Endometrium, curettings/biopsy

Esophagus, biopsy

Extremity, amputation, traumatic

Fallopian tube, biopsy

Fallopian tube, ectopic pregnancy

Femoral head, fracture

Fingers/toes, amputation, non-traumatic

Gingiva/oral mucosa, biopsy

Heart valve

Joint, resection

Kidney, biopsy

Larynx, biopsy

Leiomyoma(s), uterine myomectomy - without uterus

Lip, biopsy/wedge resection

Lung, transbronchial biopsy

Lymph node, biopsy

Muscle, biopsy

Nasal mucosa, biopsy

Nasopharynx/oropharynx, biopsy

Nerve, biopsy

Odontogenic/dental cyst

Omentum, biopsy

Ovary with or without tube, non-neoplastic

Ovary, biopsy/wedge resection

Parathyroid gland

Peritoneum, biopsy

Pituitary tumor

Placenta, other than third trimester

Pleura/pericardium - biopsy/tissue

Polyp, cervical/endometrial

Polyp, colorectal

Polyp, stomach/small intestine

Prostate, needle biopsy

Prostate, TUR

Salivary gland, biopsy

Sinus, paranasal biopsy

Skin, other than cyst/tag/debridement/plastic repair

Small intestine, biopsy

Soft tissue, other than tumor/mass/lipoma/debridement

Spleen

Stomach, biopsy

Synovium

Testis, other than tumor/biopsy/castration

Thyroglossal duct/brachial cleft cyst

Tongue, biopsy

Tonsil, biopsy

Trachea, biopsy

Ureter, biopsy

Urethra, biopsy

Urinary bladder, biopsy

Uterus, with or without tubes and ovaries, for prolapse

Vagina, biopsy

Vulva/labia, biopsy

88307   **Level V** - Surgical pathology, gross and microscopic examination

Adrenal, resection

Bone - biopsy/curettings

Bone fragment(s), pathologic fracture

Brain, biopsy

Brain/meninges, tumor resection

Breast, excision of lesion, requiring microscopic evaluation of surgical margins

Breast, mastectomy - partial/simple

Cervix, conization

Colon, segmental resection, other than for tumor

Extremity, amputation, non-traumatic

Eye, enucleation

Kidney, partial/total nephrectomy

Larynx, partial/total resection

Liver, biopsy - needle/wedge

Liver, partial resection

Lung, wedge biopsy

Lymph nodes, regional resection

Mediastinum, mass

Myocardium, biopsy

Odontogenic tumor

Ovary with or without tube, neoplastic

Pancreas, biopsy

Placenta, third trimester

Prostate, except radical resection

Salivary gland

Sentinel lymph node

Small intestine, resection, other than for tumor

Soft tissue mass (except lipoma) - biopsy/simple excision

Stomach - subtotal/total resection, other than for tumor

Testis, biopsy

Thymus, tumor

Thyroid, total/lobe

Ureter, resection

Urinary bladder, TUR

Uterus, with or without tubes and ovaries, other than neoplastic/prolapse

88309   **Level VI** - Surgical pathology, gross and microscopic examination

Bone resection

Breast, mastectomy - with regional lymph nodes

Colon, segmental resection for tumor

Colon, total resection

Esophagus, partial/total resection

Extremity, disarticulation

Fetus, with dissection

Larynx, partial/total resection - with regional lymph nodes

Lung - total/lobe/segment resection

Pancreas, total/subtotal resection

Prostate, radical resection

Small intestine, resection for tumor

Soft tissue tumor, extensive resection

Stomach - subtotal/total resection for tumor

Testis, tumor

Tongue/tonsil -resection for tumor

Urinary bladder, partial/total resection

Uterus, with or without tubes and ovaries, neoplastic

Vulva, total/subtotal resection

(For fine needle aspiration, see 10021, 10022)

(For evaluation of fine needle aspirate, see 88172-88173)

▶(Do not report 88302-88309 on the same specimen as part of Mohs surgery◀

Pathology and Laboratory

+ 88311   Decalcification procedure (List separately in addition to code for surgical pathology examination)

+ 88312   Special stains (List separately in addition to code for primary service); Group I for microorganisms (eg, Gridley, acid fast, methenamine silver), each

+ 88313   Group II, all other, (eg, iron, trichrome), except immunocytochemistry and immunoperoxidase stains, each

(For immunocytochemistry and immunoperoxidase tissue studies, use 88342)

+ 88314   histochemical staining with frozen section(s)

▶(Do not report 88314 with 17311-17315 for routine frozen section stain (eg, hematoxylin and eosin, toluidine blue), performed during Mohs surgery. When a nonroutine histochemical stain on frozen tissue is utilized, report 88314 with modifier 59)◀

88318   Determinative histochemistry to identify chemical components (eg, copper, zinc)

88319   Determinative histochemistry or cytochemistry to identify enzyme constituents, each

88321   Consultation and report on referred slides prepared elsewhere

88323   Consultation and report on referred material requiring preparation of slides

88325   Consultation, comprehensive, with review of records and specimens, with report on referred material

88329   Pathology consultation during surgery;

88331   first tissue block, with frozen section(s), single specimen

88332   each additional tissue block with frozen section(s)

88333   cytologic examination (eg, touch prep, squash prep), initial site

88334   cytologic examination (eg, touch prep, squash prep), each additional site

(For intraoperative consultation on a specimen requiring both frozen section and cytologic evaluation, use 88331 and 88334)

(For percutaneous needle biopsy requiring intraprocedural cytologic examination, use 88333)

(Do not report 88333 and 88334 for non-intraoperative cytologic examination, see 88160-88162)

(Do not report 88333 and 88334 for intraprocedural cytologic evaluation of fine needle aspirate, see 88172)

88342   Immunohistochemistry (including tissue immunoperoxidase), each antibody

(Do not report 88342 in conjunction with 88360 or 88361 for the same antibody)

(For quantitative or semiquantitative immunohistochemistry, see 88360, 88361)

88346   Immunofluorescent study, each antibody; direct method

88347   indirect method

88348   Electron microscopy; diagnostic

88349   scanning

88355   Morphometric analysis; skeletal muscle

88356   nerve

88358   tumor (eg, DNA ploidy)

(Do not report 88358 with 88313 unless each procedure is for a different special stain)

88360   Morphometric analysis, tumor immunohistochemistry (eg, Her-2/neu, estrogen receptor/progesterone receptor), quantitative or semiquantitative, each antibody; manual

88361   using computer-assisted technology

(Do not report 88360, 88361 with 88342 unless each procedure is for a different antibody)

(For morphometric analysis using in situ hybridization techniques, see 88367, 88368)

(When semi-thin plastic-embedded sections are performed in conjunction with morphometric analysis, only the morphometric analysis should be reported; if performed as an independent procedure, see codes 88300-88309 for surgical pathology.)

88362   Nerve teasing preparations

88365   In situ hybridization (eg, FISH), each probe

(Do not report 88365 in conjunction with 88367, 88368 for the same probe)

88367   Morphometric analysis, in situ hybridization, (quantitative or semi-quantitative) each probe; using computer-assisted technology

88368   manual

88371   Protein analysis of tissue by Western Blot, with interpretation and report;

88372   immunological probe for band identification, each

88380   Microdissection (eg, mechanical, laser capture)

88384   Array-based evaluation of multiple molecular probes; 11 through 50 probes

88385   51 through 250 probes

88386   251 through 500 probes

(For preparation of array-based evaluation, see 83890-83892, 83898-83901)

(For preparation and analyses of less than 11 probes, see 83890-83914)

88399   Unlisted surgical pathology procedure

Transcutaneous Procedures

88400   Bilirubin, total, transcutaneous

Other Procedures

89049   Caffeine halothane contracture test (CHCT) for malignant hyperthermia susceptibility, including interpretation and report

89050   Cell count, miscellaneous body fluids (eg, cerebrospinal fluid, joint fluid), except blood;

89051   with differential count

89055   Leukocyte assessment, fecal, qualitative or semiquantitative

▲ **89060**   Crystal identification by light microscopy with or without polarizing lens analysis, tissue or any body fluid (except urine)

▶(Do not report 89060 for crystal identification on paraffin-embedded tissue)◀

89100   Duodenal intubation and aspiration; single specimen (eg, simple bile study or afferent loop culture) plus appropriate test procedure

89105   collection of multiple fractional specimens with pancreatic or gallbladder stimulation, single or double lumen tube

(For radiological localization, use 74340)

(For chemical analyses, see **Chemistry,** this section)

(Electrocardiogram, see 93000-93268)

(Esophagus acid perfusion test (Bernstein), see 91030)

89125   Fat stain, feces, urine, or respiratory secretions

89130   Gastric intubation and aspiration, diagnostic, each specimen, for chemical analyses or cytopathology;

89132   after stimulation

89135   Gastric intubation, aspiration, and fractional collections (eg, gastric secretory study); one hour

89136   two hours

89140   two hours including gastric stimulation (eg, histalog, pentagastrin)

89141   three hours, including gastric stimulation

(For gastric lavage, therapeutic, use 91105)

(For radiologic localization of gastric tube, use 74340)

(For chemical analyses, see 82926, 82928)

(Joint fluid chemistry, see **Chemistry,** this section)

89160   Meat fibers, feces

89190   Nasal smear for eosinophils

(Occult blood, feces, use 82270)

(Paternity tests, use 86910)

89220   Sputum, obtaining specimen, aerosol induced technique (separate procedure)

89225   Starch granules, feces

89230   Sweat collection by iontophoresis

89235   Water load test

89240   Unlisted miscellaneous pathology test

Reproductive Medicine Procedures

89250   Culture of oocyte(s)/embryo(s), less than 4 days;

89251   with co-culture of oocyte(s)/embryos

(For extended culture of oocyte(s)/embryo(s), see 89272)

89253   Assisted embryo hatching, microtechniques (any method)

89254   Oocyte identification from follicular fluid

89255   Preparation of embryo for transfer (any method)

89257   Sperm identification from aspiration (other than seminal fluid)

(For semen analysis, see 89300-89320)

(For sperm identification from testis tissue, use 89264)

89258   Cryopreservation; embryo(s)

89259   sperm

(For cryopreservation of reproductive tissue, testicular, use 89335)

(For cryopreservation of reproductive tissue, ovarian, use Category III code 0058T)

(For cryopreservation of oocyte(s), use Category III code 0059T)

89260   Sperm isolation; simple prep (eg, sperm wash and swim-up) for insemination or diagnosis with semen analysis

89261   complex prep (eg, Percoll gradient, albumin gradient) for insemination or diagnosis with semen analysis

(For semen analysis without sperm wash or swim-up, use 89320)

89264   Sperm identification from testis tissue, fresh or cryopreserved

(For biopsy of testis, see 54500, 54505)

(For sperm identification from aspiration, use 89257)

(For semen analysis, see 89300-89320)

89268   Insemination of oocytes

89272   Extended culture of oocyte(s)/embryo(s), 4-7 days

89280   Assisted oocyte fertilization, microtechnique; less than or equal to 10 oocytes

89281   greater than 10 oocytes

Pathology and Laboratory

89290   Biopsy, oocyte polar body or embryo blastomere, microtechnique (for pre-implantation genetic diagnosis); less than or equal to 5 embryos

89291   greater than 5 embryos

89300   Semen analysis; presence and/or motility of sperm including Huhner test (post coital)

89310   motility and count (not including Huhner test)

89320   complete (volume, count, motility, and differential)

(Skin tests, see 86485-86580 and 95010-95199)

89321   Semen analysis, presence and/or motility of sperm

(To report Hyaluronan binding assay (HBA), use Category III code 0087T)

89325   Sperm antibodies

(For medicolegal identification of sperm, use 88125)

89329   Sperm evaluation; hamster penetration test

89330   cervical mucus penetration test, with or without spinnbarkeit test

89335   Cryopreservation, reproductive tissue, testicular

(For cryopreservation of embryo(s), use 89258. For cryopreservation of sperm, use 89259)

(For cryopreservation of reproductive tissue, ovarian, use Category III code 0058T)

(For cryopreservation of oocyte, use Category III code 0059T)

89342   Storage, (per year); embryo(s)

89343   sperm/semen

89344   reproductive tissue, testicular/ovarian

89346   oocyte(s)

89352   Thawing of cryopreserved; embryo(s)

89353   sperm/semen, each aliquot

89354   reproductive tissue, testicular/ovarian

89356   oocytes, each aliquot

Pathology and Laboratory

Medicine Guidelines

In addition to the definitions and commonly used terms presented in the **Introduction**, several other items unique to this section on **Medicine** are defined or identified here.

Multiple Procedures

It is appropriate to designate multiple procedures that are rendered on the same date by separate entries. For example: If individual medical psychotherapy (90829) is rendered in addition to subsequent hospital care (eg, 99231), the psychotherapy would be reported separately from the hospital visit. In this instance, both 99231 and 90829 would be reported.

Add-on Codes

Some of the listed procedures are commonly carried out in addition to the primary procedure performed. All add-on codes found in the CPT codebook are exempt from the multiple procedure concept. They are exempt from the use of modifier 51, as these procedures are not reported as stand-alone codes. These additional or supplemental procedures are designated as "add-on" codes. Add-on codes in the CPT codebook can be readily identified by specific descriptor nomenclature which includes phrases such as "each additional" or "(List separately in addition to primary procedure)."

Separate Procedures

Some of the procedures or services listed in the CPT codebook that are commonly carried out as an integral component of a total service or procedure have been identified by the inclusion of the term "separate procedure." The codes designated as "separate procedure" should not be reported in addition to the code for the total procedure or service of which it is considered an integral component.

However, when a procedure or service that is designated as a "separate procedure" is carried out independently or considered to be unrelated or distinct from other procedures/services provided at that time, it may be reported by itself, or in addition to other procedures/services by appending modifier 59 to the specific "separate procedure" code to indicate that the procedure is not considered to be a component of another procedure, but is a distinct, independent procedure. This may represent a different session or patient encounter, different procedure or surgery, different site or organ system, separate incision/excision, separate lesion, or separate injury (or area of injury in extensive injuries).

Subsection Information

Several of the subheadings or subsections have special instructions unique to that section. These special instructions will be presented preceding those procedural terminology listings, referring to that subsection specifically. If there is an "Unlisted Procedure" code number (see section below) for the individual subsection, it will also be shown. Those subsections within the **Medicine** section that have special instructions are as follows:

Immune Globulins 90281-90399
Immunization Administration for
   Vaccines/Toxoids 90465-90474
Vaccines, Toxoids 90476-90749
Hydration, Therapeutic, Prophylactic,
   and Diagnostic Injections and
      Infusions 90760-90779
    ►Hydration 90760-90761
      Therapeutic, Prophylactic, and Diagnostic
        Injections and Infusions . . . . . 90765-90779◄
Psychiatry 90801-90899
Dialysis 90918-90999
   ►Hemodialysis 90935-90940
   Miscellaneous Dialysis Procedures 90945-90999◄
Ophthalmology 92002-92499
   ►**General Ophthalmological**
     Services 92002-92014
   Ophthalmoscopy . . . . 92225-92260◄
   Contact Lens Services 92310-92326
   Spectacle Services 92340-92371
Special Otorhinolaryngologic
   Services 92502-92700
   Audiologic Function Tests 92551-92597
   Evaluative and Therapeutic
     Services 92601-92633
Echocardiography 93303-93350
Cardiac Catheterization 93501-93581
Intracardiac Electrophysiological
   Procedures/Studies 93600-93662
Peripheral Arterial Disease
   Rehabilitation 93668
Noninvasive Vascular
   Diagnostic Studies 93875-93990
►**Cerebrovascular Arterial Studies** . . . 93875-93893◄
►**Pulmonary** . . . . 94002-94799◄
Allergy and Clinical Immunology . . . 95004-95199
Neurology and Neuromuscular 95805-95999
   ►Sleep Testing 95805-95811
Routine Electroencephalography
   (EEG) . . . . 95812-95830◄
Electromyography and Nerve Conduction
   Tests 95860-95904

Unlisted Service or Procedure

A service or procedure may be provided that is not listed in this edition of the CPT codebook. When reporting such a service, the appropriate "Unlisted Procedure" code may be used to indicate the service, identifying it by "Special Report" as discussed on this page. The "Unlisted Procedures" and accompanying codes for **Medicine** are as follows:

⊘ **90399** Unlisted immune globulin

⊘ **90749** Unlisted vaccine/toxoid

90779 Unlisted therapeutic, prophylactic or diagnostic intravenous or intra-arterial injection or infusion

90899 Unlisted psychiatric service or procedure

90999 Unlisted dialysis procedure, inpatient or outpatient

91299 Unlisted diagnostic gastroenterology procedure

92499 Unlisted ophthalmological service or procedure

92700 Unlisted otorhinolaryngological service or procedure

93799 Unlisted cardiovascular service or procedure

94799 Unlisted pulmonary service or procedure

95199 Unlisted allergy/clinical immunologic service or procedure

95999 Unlisted neurological or neuromuscular diagnostic procedure

96549 Unlisted chemotherapy procedure

96999 Unlisted special dermatological service or procedure

97039 Unlisted modality (specify type and time if constant attendance)

97139 Unlisted therapeutic procedure (specify)

97799 Unlisted physical medicine/rehabilitation service or procedure

99199 Unlisted special service, procedure or report

99600 Unlisted home visit service or procedure

►Results/Testing/Reports◄

►Results are the technical component of a service. Testing leads to results; results lead to interpretation. Reports are the work product of the interpretation of numerous test results.◄

Special Report

A service that is rarely provided, unusual, variable, or new may require a special report in determining medical appropriateness of the service. Pertinent information should include an adequate definition or description of the nature, extent, and need for the procedure; and the time, effort, and equipment necessary to provide the service. Additional items that may be included are:

- Complexity of symptoms
- Final diagnosis
- Pertinent physical findings
- Diagnostic and therapeutic procedures
- Concurrent problems
- Follow-up care

Materials Supplied by Physician

Supplies and materials provided by the physician (eg, sterile trays/drugs), over and above those usually included with the procedure(s) rendered are reported separately. List drugs, trays, supplies, and materials provided. Identify as 99070 or specific supply code.

Medicine Guidelines

Medicine

Immune Globulins

Codes 90281-90399 identify the immune globulin product only and must be reported in addition to the administration codes 90765-90768, 90772, 90774, 90775 as appropriate. Immune globulin products listed here include broad-spectrum and anti-infective immune globulins, antitoxins, and various isoantibodies.

⊘ **90281**   Immune globulin (Ig), human, for intramuscular use

⊘ **90283**   Immune globulin (IgIV), human, for intravenous use

⊘ **90287**   Botulinum antitoxin, equine, any route

⊘ **90288**   Botulism immune globulin, human, for intravenous use

⊘ **90291**   Cytomegalovirus immune globulin (CMV-IgIV), human, for intravenous use

⊘ **90296**   Diphtheria antitoxin, equine, any route

⊘ **90371**   Hepatitis B immune globulin (HBIg), human, for intramuscular use

⊘ **90375**   Rabies immune globulin (RIg), human, for intramuscular and/or subcutaneous use

⊘ **90376**   Rabies immune globulin, heat-treated (RIg-HT), human, for intramuscular and/or subcutaneous use

⊘ **90378**   Respiratory syncytial virus immune globulin (RSV-IgIM), for intramuscular use, 50 mg, each

⊘ **90379**   Respiratory syncytial virus immune globulin (RSV-IgIV), human, for intravenous use

⊘ **90384**   Rho(D) immune globulin (RhIg), human, full-dose, for intramuscular use

⊘ **90385**   Rho(D) immune globulin (RhIg), human, mini-dose, for intramuscular use

⊘ **90386**   Rho(D) immune globulin (RhIgIV), human, for intravenous use

⊘ **90389**   Tetanus immune globulin (TIg), human, for intramuscular use

⊘ **90393**   Vaccinia immune globulin, human, for intramuscular use

⊘ **90396**   Varicella-zoster immune globulin, human, for intramuscular use

⊘ **90399**   Unlisted immune globulin

Immunization Administration for Vaccines/Toxoids

Codes 90465-90474 must be reported in addition to the vaccine and toxoid code(s) 90476-90749.

Report codes 90465-90468 only when the physician provides face-to-face counseling of the patient and family during the administration of a vaccine. For immunization administration of any vaccine that is not accompanied by face-to-face physician counseling to the patient/family, report codes 90471-90474.

If a significant separately identifiable Evaluation and Management service (eg, office or other outpatient services, preventive medicine services) is performed, the appropriate E/M service code should be reported in addition to the vaccine and toxoid administration codes.

(For allergy testing, see 95004 et seq)

(For skin testing of bacterial, viral, fungal extracts, see 86485-86586)

(For therapeutic or diagnostic injections, see 90772-90779)

90465   Immunization administration younger than 8 years of age (includes percutaneous, intradermal, subcutaneous, or intramuscular injections) when the physician counsels the patient/family; first injection (single or combination vaccine/toxoid), per day

(Do not report 90465 in conjunction with 90467)

+ **90466**   each additional injection (single or combination vaccine/toxoid), per day (List separately in addition to code for primary procedure)

(Use 90466 in conjunction with 90465 or 90467)

90467   Immunization administration younger than age 8 years (includes intranasal or oral routes of administration) when the physician counsels the patient/family; first administration (single or combination vaccine/toxoid), per day

(Do not report 90467 in conjunction with 90465)

+ **90468**   each additional administration (single or combination vaccine/toxoid), per day (List separately in addition to code for primary procedure)

(Use 90468 in conjunction with 90465 or 90467)

90471   Immunization administration (includes percutaneous, intradermal, subcutaneous, or intramuscular injections); one vaccine (single or combination vaccine/toxoid)

(Do not report 90471 in conjunction with 90473)

+ **90472**   each additional vaccine (single or combination vaccine/toxoid) (List separately in addition to code for primary procedure)

(Use 90472 in conjunction with 90471 or 90473)

▶(For administration of immune globulins, see 90281-90399, 90760, 90761, 90765-90768, 90774)◀

(For intravesical administration of BCG vaccine, see 51720, 90586)

Medicine

90473   Immunization administration by intranasal or oral route; one vaccine (single or combination vaccine/toxoid)

(Do not report 90473 in conjunction with 90471)

+ 90474   each additional vaccine (single or combination vaccine/toxoid) (List separately in addition to code for primary procedure)

(Use 90474 in conjunction with 90471 or 90473)

Vaccines, Toxoids

To assist users to report the most recent new or revised vaccine product codes, the American Medical Association currently uses the CPT Web-site, which features updates of CPT Editorial Panel actions regarding these products. Once approved by the CPT Editorial Panel, these codes will be made available for release on a semi-annual (twice a year—July 1 and January 1) basis. As part of the electronic distribution, there is a 6-month implementation period from the initial release date (ie, codes released on January 1 are eligible for use on July 1 and codes released on July 1 are eligible for use January 1).

The CPT Editorial Panel, in recognition of the public health interest in vaccine products, has chosen to publish new vaccine product codes prior to FDA approval. These codes are indicated with the ∕ symbol and will be tracked by the AMA to monitor FDA approval status. Once the FDA status changes to approval, the ∕ symbol will be removed. CPT users should refer to the AMA Internet site (www.ama-assn.org/ama/pub/category/10902.html) for the most up-to-date information on codes with the ∕ symbol.

Codes 90476-90748 identify the vaccine product **only.** To report the administration of a vaccine/toxoid, the vaccine/toxoid product codes 90476-90749 must be used in addition to an immunization administration code(s) 90465-90474. Do not append modifier 51 to the vaccine/toxoid product codes 90476-90749.

If a significantly separately identifiable Evaluation and Management (E/M) service (eg, office or other outpatient services, preventive medicine services) is performed, the appropriate E/M service code should be reported in addition to the vaccine and toxoid administration codes.

To meet the reporting requirements of immunization registries, vaccine distribution programs, and reporting systems (eg, Vaccine Adverse Event Reporting System) the exact vaccine product administered needs to be reported. Multiple codes for a particular vaccine are provided in the CPT codebook when the schedule (number of doses or timing) differs for two or more products of the same vaccine type (eg, hepatitis A, Hib) or the vaccine product is available in more than one chemical formulation, dosage, or route of administration.

Separate codes are available for combination vaccines (eg, DTP-Hib, DtaP-Hib, HepB-Hib). It is inappropriate to code each component of a combination vaccine separately. If a specific vaccine code is not available, the unlisted procedure code should be reported, until a new code becomes available.

(For immune globulins, see codes 90281-90399, 90765-90768, 90772-90775 for administration of immune globulins)

⊘ **90476**   Adenovirus vaccine, type 4, live, for oral use

⊘ **90477**   Adenovirus vaccine, type 7, live, for oral use

⊘ **90581**   Anthrax vaccine, for subcutaneous use

⊘ **90585**   Bacillus Calmette-Guerin vaccine (BCG) for tuberculosis, live, for percutaneous use

⊘ **90586**   Bacillus Calmette-Guerin vaccine (BCG) for bladder cancer, live, for intravesical use

⊘ **90632**   Hepatitis A vaccine, adult dosage, for intramuscular use

⊘ **90633**   Hepatitis A vaccine, pediatric/adolescent dosage-2 dose schedule, for intramuscular use

⊘ **90634**   Hepatitis A vaccine, pediatric/adolescent dosage-3 dose schedule, for intramuscular use

⊘ **90636**   Hepatitis A and hepatitis B vaccine (HepA-HepB), adult dosage, for intramuscular use

⊘ **90645**   Hemophilus influenza b vaccine (Hib), HbOC conjugate (4 dose schedule), for intramuscular use

⊘ **90646**   Hemophilus influenza b vaccine (Hib), PRP-D conjugate, for booster use only, intramuscular use

⊘ **90647**   Hemophilus influenza b vaccine (Hib), PRP-OMP conjugate (3 dose schedule), for intramuscular use

⊘ **90648**   Hemophilus influenza b vaccine (Hib), PRP-T conjugate (4 dose schedule), for intramuscular use

⊘ **90649**   Human Papilloma virus (HPV) vaccine, types 6, 11, 16, 18 (quadrivalent), 3 dose schedule, for intramuscular use

⊘▲ **90655**   Influenza virus vaccine, split virus, preservative free, when administered to children 6-35 months of age, for intramuscular use

⊘▲ **90656**   Influenza virus vaccine, split virus, preservative free, when administered to 3 years and older, for intramuscular use

⊘▲ **90657**   Influenza virus vaccine, split virus, when administered to children 6-35 months of age, for intramuscular use

⊘▲ **90658**   Influenza virus vaccine, split virus, when administered to 3 years of age and older, for intramuscular use

⊘ **90660**   Influenza virus vaccine, live, for intranasal use

⊘ **90665**   Lyme disease vaccine, adult dosage, for intramuscular use

⊘▲ **90669**   Pneumococcal conjugate vaccine, polyvalent, when administered to children younger than 5 years, for intramuscular use

⊘ **90675**   Rabies vaccine, for intramuscular use

⊘ **90676**   Rabies vaccine, for intradermal use

⊘ **90680**   Rotavirus vaccine, pentavalent, 3 dose schedule, live, for oral use

⊘ **90690**   Typhoid vaccine, live, oral

⊘ **90691**   Typhoid vaccine, Vi capsular polysaccharide (ViCPs), for intramuscular use

⊘ **90692**   Typhoid vaccine, heat- and phenol-inactivated (H-P), for subcutaneous or intradermal use

⊘ **90693**   Typhoid vaccine, acetone-killed, dried (AKD), for subcutaneous use (U.S. military)

✎⊘ **90698**   Diphtheria, tetanus toxoids, acellular pertussis vaccine, haemophilus influenza Type B, and poliovirus vaccine, inactivated (DTaP - Hib - IPV), for intramuscular use

⊘▲ **90700**   Diphtheria, tetanus toxoids, and acellular pertussis vaccine (DTaP), when administered to younger than 7 years, for intramuscular use

⊘ **90701**   Diphtheria, tetanus toxoids, and whole cell pertussis vaccine (DTP), for intramuscular use

⊘▲ **90702**   Diphtheria and tetanus toxoids (DT) adsorbed when administered to younger than 7 years, for intramuscular use

⊘ **90703**   Tetanus toxoid adsorbed, for intramuscular use

⊘ **90704**   Mumps virus vaccine, live, for subcutaneous use

⊘ **90705**   Measles virus vaccine, live, for subcutaneous use

⊘ **90706**   Rubella virus vaccine, live, for subcutaneous use

⊘ **90707**   Measles, mumps and rubella virus vaccine (MMR), live, for subcutaneous use

⊘ **90708**   Measles and rubella virus vaccine, live, for subcutaneous use

⊘ **90710**   Measles, mumps, rubella, and varicella vaccine (MMRV), live, for subcutaneous use

⊘ **90712**   Poliovirus vaccine, (any type(s)) (OPV), live, for oral use

⊘ **90713**   Poliovirus vaccine, inactivated, (IPV), for subcutaneous or intramuscular use

⊘▲ **90714**   Tetanus and diphtheria toxoids (Td) adsorbed, preservative free, when administered to 7 years or older, for intramuscular use

⊘▲ **90715**   Tetanus, diphtheria toxoids and acellular pertussis vaccine (Tdap), when administered to 7 years or older, for intramuscular use

⊘ **90716**   Varicella virus vaccine, live, for subcutaneous use

⊘ **90717**   Yellow fever vaccine, live, for subcutaneous use

⊘▲ **90718**   Tetanus and diphtheria toxoids (Td) adsorbed when administered to 7 years or older, for intramuscular use

⊘ **90719**   Diphtheria toxoid, for intramuscular use

⊘ **90720**   Diphtheria, tetanus toxoids, and whole cell pertussis vaccine and Hemophilus influenza B vaccine (DTP-Hib), for intramuscular use

⊘ **90721**   Diphtheria, tetanus toxoids, and acellular pertussis vaccine and Hemophilus influenza B vaccine (DtaP-Hib), for intramuscular use

⊘ **90723**   Diphtheria, tetanus toxoids, acellular pertussis vaccine, Hepatitis B, and poliovirus vaccine, inactivated (DtaP-HepB-IPV), for intramuscular use

⊘ **90725**   Cholera vaccine for injectable use

⊘ **90727**   Plague vaccine, for intramuscular use

⊘▲ **90732**   Pneumococcal polysaccharide vaccine, 23-valent, adult or immunosuppressed patient dosage, when administered to 2 years or older, for subcutaneous or intramuscular use

⊘ **90733**   Meningococcal polysaccharide vaccine (any group(s)), for subcutaneous use

⊘ **90734**   Meningococcal conjugate vaccine, serogroups A, C, Y and W-135 (tetravalent), for intramuscular use

⊘ **90735**   Japanese encephalitis virus vaccine, for subcutaneous use

⊘ **90736**   Zoster (shingles) vaccine, live, for subcutaneous injection

⊘ **90740**   Hepatitis B vaccine, dialysis or immunosuppressed patient dosage (3 dose schedule), for intramuscular use

⊘ **90743**   Hepatitis B vaccine, adolescent (2 dose schedule), for intramuscular use

⊘ **90744**   Hepatitis B vaccine, pediatric/adolescent dosage (3 dose schedule), for intramuscular use

⊘ **90746**   Hepatitis B vaccine, adult dosage, for intramuscular use

⊘ **90747**   Hepatitis B vaccine, dialysis or immunosuppressed patient dosage (4 dose schedule), for intramuscular use

⊘ **90748**   Hepatitis B and Hemophilus influenza b vaccine (HepB-Hib), for intramuscular use

⊘ **90749**   Unlisted vaccine/toxoid

Hydration, Therapeutic, Prophylactic, and Diagnostic Injections and Infusions (Excludes Chemotherapy)

Physician work related to hydration, injection, and infusion services predominantly involves affirmation of treatment plan and direct supervision of staff.

If a significant separately identifiable Evaluation and Management service is performed, the appropriate E/M service code should be reported using modifier 25 in addition to 90760-90779. For same day E/M service a different diagnosis is not required.

If performed to facilitate the infusion or injection, the following services are included and are not reported separately:

Medicine

a. Use of local anesthesia

b. IV start

c. Access to indwelling IV, subcutaneous catheter or port

d. Flush at conclusion of infusion

e. Standard tubing, syringes, and supplies

(For declotting a catheter or port, see 36550)

When multiple drugs are administered, report the service(s) and the specific materials or drugs for each.

When administering multiple infusions, injections or combinations, only one "initial" service code should be reported, unless protocol requires that two separate IV sites must be used. The "initial" code that best describes the key or primary reason for the encounter should always be reported irrespective of the order in which the infusions or injections occur. If an injection or infusion is of a subsequent or concurrent nature, even if it is the first such service within that group of services, then a subsequent or concurrent code from the appropriate section should be reported (eg, the first IV push given subsequent to an initial one-hour infusion is reported using a subsequent IV push code).

When reporting codes for which infusion time is a factor, use the actual time over which the infusion is administered.

Hydration

Codes 90760-90761 are intended to report a hydration IV infusion to consist of a pre-packaged fluid and electrolytes (eg, normal saline, D5-Ω normal saline+30mEq KCl/liter), but are not used to report infusion of drugs or other substances. Hydration IV infusions typically require direct physician supervision for purposes of consent, safety oversight, or intraservice supervision of staff. Typically such infusions require little special handling to prepare or dispose of, and staff that administer these do not typically require advanced practice training. After initial set-up, infusion typically entails little patient risk and thus little monitoring.

90760   Intravenous infusion, hydration; initial, up to 1 hour

(Do not report 90760 if performed as a concurrent infusion service)

+▲ 90761   each additional hour (List separately in addition to code for primary procedure)

(Use 90761 in conjunction with 90760)

(Report 90761 for hydration infusion intervals of greater than 30 minutes beyond 1 hour increments)

(Report 90761 to identify hydration if provided as a secondary or subsequent service after a different initial service [90760, 90765, 90774, 96409, 96413] is provided)

Therapeutic, Prophylactic, and Diagnostic Injections and Infusions

►A therapeutic, prophylactic, or diagnostic IV infusion or injection (90765-90779) (other than hydration) is for the administration of substances/drugs. When fluids are used to administer the drug(s), the administration of the fluid is considered incidental hydration and is not separately reportable. These services typically require direct physician supervision for any or all purposes of patient assessment, provision of consent, safety oversight, and intra-service supervision of staff. Typically, such infusions require special consideration to prepare, dose or dispose of, require practice training and competency for staff who administer the infusions, and require periodic patient assessment with vital sign monitoring during the infusion.◄

Intravenous or intra-arterial push is defined as: a) an injection in which the health care professional who administers the substance/drug is continuously present to administer the injection and observe the patient, or b) an infusion of 15 minutes or less.

(Do not report 90765-90779 with codes for which IV push or infusion is an inherent part of the procedure (eg, administration of contrast material for a diagnostic imaging study))

90765   Intravenous infusion, for therapy, prophylaxis, or diagnosis (specify substance or drug); initial, up to 1 hour

+▲ 90766   each additional hour (List separately in addition to code for primary procedure)

(Report 90766 in conjunction with 90765, 90767)

(Report 90766 for additional hour(s) of sequential infusion)

(Report 90766 for infusion intervals of greater than 30 minutes beyond 1 hour increments)

+ 90767   additional sequential infusion, up to 1 hour (List separately in addition to code for primary procedure)

(Report 90767 in conjunction with 90765, 90774, 96409, 96413 if provided as a secondary or subsequent service after a different initial service. Report 90767 only once per sequential infusion of same infusate mix)

+ 90768   concurrent infusion (List separately in addition to code for primary procedure)

(Report 90768 only once per encounter)

►(Report 90768 in conjunction with 90765, 90766, 96413, 96415, 96416, 96422, 96423)◄

90772   Therapeutic, prophylactic or diagnostic injection (specify substance or drug); subcutaneous or intramuscular

(For administration of vaccines/toxoids, see 90465-90466, 90471-90472)

(Report 90772 for non-antineoplastic hormonal therapy injections)

(Report 96401 for anti-neoplastic nonhormonal injection therapy)

(Report 96402 for anti-neoplastic hormonal injection therapy)

(Do not report 90772 for injections given without direct physician supervision. To report, use 99211)

(90772 does not include injections for allergen immunotherapy. For allergen immunotherapy injections, see 95115-95117)

90773   intra-arterial

90774   intravenous push, single or initial substance/drug

+ 90775   each additional sequential intravenous push of a new substance/drug (List separately in addition to code for primary procedure)

(Use 90775 in conjunction with 90765, 90774, 96409, 96413)

(Report 90775 to identify intravenous push of a new substance/drug if provided as a secondary or subsequent service after a different initial service is provided)

90779   Unlisted therapeutic, prophylactic or diagnostic intravenous or intra-arterial injection or infusion

(For allergy immunizations, see 95004 et seq)

(90780 and 90781 have been deleted. To report, see 90760, 90761, 90765-90768)

(90782 has been deleted. To report, use 90772)

(90783 has been deleted. To report, use 90773)

(90784 has been deleted. To report, use 90774)

(90788 has been deleted. To report, use 90772)

(90799 has been deleted. To report, use 90779)

Psychiatry

Hospital care by the attending physician in treating a psychiatric inpatient or partial hospitalization may be initial or subsequent in nature (see 99221-99233) and may include exchanges with nursing and ancillary personnel. Hospital care services involve a variety of responsibilities unique to the medical management of inpatients, such as physician hospital orders, interpretation of laboratory or other medical diagnostic studies and observations.

Some patients receive hospital evaluation and management services only and others receive evaluation and management services and other procedures. If other procedures such as electroconvulsive therapy or psychotherapy are rendered in addition to hospital evaluation and management services, these should be listed separately (ie, hospital care service plus electroconvulsive therapy or when psychotherapy is done, an appropriate code defining psychotherapy with medical evaluation and management services). Modifier 22 may

be used to indicate a more extensive service. Modifier 52 may be used to signify a service that is reduced or less extensive than the usual procedure.

Other evaluation and management services, such as office medical service or other patient encounters, may be described as listed in the section on **Evaluation and Management,** if appropriate.

The evaluation and management services should not be reported separately, when reporting codes 90805, 90807, 90809, 90811, 90813, 90815, 90817, 90819, 90822, 90824, 90827, 90829.

Consultation for psychiatric evaluation of a patient includes examination of a patient and exchange of information with the primary physician and other informants such as nurses or family members, and preparation of a report. These consultation services (99241-99255) are limited to initial or follow-up evaluation and do not involve psychiatric treatment.

Psychiatric Diagnostic or Evaluative Interview Procedures

Psychiatric diagnostic interview examination includes a history, mental status, and a disposition, and may include communication with family or other sources, ordering and medical interpretation of laboratory or other medical diagnostic studies. In certain circumstances other informants will be seen in lieu of the patient.

Interactive psychiatric diagnostic interview examination is typically furnished to children. It involves the use of physical aids and non-verbal communication to overcome barriers to therapeutic interaction between the clinician and a patient who has not yet developed, or has lost, either the expressive language communication skills to explain his/her symptoms and response to treatment, or the receptive communication skills to understand the clinician if he/she were to use ordinary adult language for communication.

90801   Psychiatric diagnostic interview examination

90802   Interactive psychiatric diagnostic interview examination using play equipment, physical devices, language interpreter, or other mechanisms of communication

Psychiatric Therapeutic Procedures

Psychotherapy is the treatment for mental illness and behavioral disturbances in which the clinician establishes a professional contract with the patient and, through definitive therapeutic communication, attempts to alleviate the emotional disturbances, reverse or change maladaptive patterns of behavior, and encourage personality growth and development. The codes for reporting psychotherapy are divided into two broad categories: Interactive Psychotherapy; and Insight Oriented, Behavior Modifying and/or Supportive Psychotherapy.

Medicine

Interactive psychotherapy is typically furnished to children. It involves the use of physical aids and non-verbal communication to overcome barriers to therapeutic interaction between the clinician and a patient who has not yet developed, or has lost, either the expressive language communication skills to explain his/her symptoms and response to treatment, or the receptive communication skills to understand the clinician if he/she were to use ordinary adult language for communication.

Insight oriented, behavior modifying and/or supportive psychotherapy refers to the development of insight or affective understanding, the use of behavior modification techniques, the use of supportive interactions, the use of cognitive discussion of reality, or any combination of the above to provide therapeutic change.

Some patients receive psychotherapy only and others receive psychotherapy and medical evaluation and management services. These evaluation and management services involve a variety of responsibilities unique to the medical management of psychiatric patients, such as medical diagnostic evaluation (eg, evaluation of comorbid medical conditions, drug interactions, and physical examinations), drug management when indicated, physician orders, interpretation of laboratory or other medical diagnostic studies and observations.

In reporting psychotherapy, the appropriate code is chosen on the basis of the type of psychotherapy (interactive using non-verbal techniques versus insight oriented, behavior modifying and/or supportive using verbal techniques), the place of service (office versus inpatient), the face-to-face time spent with the patient during psychotherapy, and whether evaluation and management services are furnished on the same date of service as psychotherapy.

To report medical evaluation and management services furnished on a day when psychotherapy is not provided, select the appropriate code from the **Evaluation and Management Services Guidelines.**

Office or Other Outpatient Facility

Insight Oriented, Behavior Modifying and/or Supportive Psychotherapy

90804 Individual psychotherapy, insight oriented, behavior modifying and/or supportive, in an office or outpatient facility, approximately 20 to 30 minutes face-to-face with the patient;

90805 with medical evaluation and management services

90806 Individual psychotherapy, insight oriented, behavior modifying and/or supportive, in an office or outpatient facility, approximately 45 to 50 minutes face-to-face with the patient;

90807 with medical evaluation and management services

90808 Individual psychotherapy, insight oriented, behavior modifying and/or supportive, in an office or outpatient facility, approximately 75 to 80 minutes face-to-face with the patient;

90809 with medical evaluation and management services

Interactive Psychotherapy

90810 Individual psychotherapy, interactive, using play equipment, physical devices, language interpreter, or other mechanisms of non-verbal communication, in an office or outpatient facility, approximately 20 to 30 minutes face-to-face with the patient;

90811 with medical evaluation and management services

90812 Individual psychotherapy, interactive, using play equipment, physical devices, language interpreter, or other mechanisms of non-verbal communication, in an office or outpatient facility, approximately 45 to 50 minutes face-to-face with the patient;

90813 with medical evaluation and management services

90814 Individual psychotherapy, interactive, using play equipment, physical devices, language interpreter, or other mechanisms of non-verbal communication, in an office or outpatient facility, approximately 75 to 80 minutes face-to-face with the patient;

90815 with medical evaluation and management services

Inpatient Hospital, Partial Hospital or Residential Care Facility

Insight Oriented, Behavior Modifying and/or Supportive Psychotherapy

90816 Individual psychotherapy, insight oriented, behavior modifying and/or supportive, in an inpatient hospital, partial hospital or residential care setting, approximately 20 to 30 minutes face-to-face with the patient;

90817 with medical evaluation and management services

90818 Individual psychotherapy, insight oriented, behavior modifying and/or supportive, in an inpatient hospital, partial hospital or residential care setting, approximately 45 to 50 minutes face-to-face with the patient;

90819 with medical evaluation and management services

90821 Individual psychotherapy, insight oriented, behavior modifying and/or supportive, in an inpatient hospital, partial hospital or residential care setting, approximately 75 to 80 minutes face-to-face with the patient;

90822 with medical evaluation and management services

Medicine

Interactive Psychotherapy

90823   Individual psychotherapy, interactive, using play equipment, physical devices, language interpreter, or other mechanisms of non-verbal communication, in an inpatient hospital, partial hospital or residential care setting, approximately 20 to 30 minutes face-to-face with the patient;

90824   with medical evaluation and management services

90826   Individual psychotherapy, interactive, using play equipment, physical devices, language interpreter, or other mechanisms of non-verbal communication, in an inpatient hospital, partial hospital or residential care setting, approximately 45 to 50 minutes face-to-face with the patient;

90827   with medical evaluation and management services

90828   Individual psychotherapy, interactive, using play equipment, physical devices, language interpreter, or other mechanisms of non-verbal communication, in an inpatient hospital, partial hospital or residential care setting, approximately 75 to 80 minutes face-to-face with the patient;

90829   with medical evaluation and management services

Other Psychotherapy

90845   Psychoanalysis

90846   Family psychotherapy (without the patient present)

90847   Family psychotherapy (conjoint psychotherapy) (with patient present)

90849   Multiple-family group psychotherapy

90853   Group psychotherapy (other than of a multiple-family group)

90857   Interactive group psychotherapy

Other Psychiatric Services or Procedures

▶(For repetitive transcranial magnetic stimulation for treatment of clinical depression, see Category III codes 0160T, 0161T)◀

90862   Pharmacologic management, including prescription, use, and review of medication with no more than minimal medical psychotherapy

90865   Narcosynthesis for psychiatric diagnostic and therapeutic purposes (eg, sodium amobarbital (Amytal) interview)

90870   Electroconvulsive therapy (includes necessary monitoring)

(90871 has been deleted)

90875   Individual psychophysiological therapy incorporating biofeedback training by any modality (face-to-face with the patient), with psychotherapy (eg, insight oriented, behavior modifying or supportive psychotherapy); approximately 20-30 minutes

90876   approximately 45-50 minutes

90880   Hypnotherapy

90882   Environmental intervention for medical management purposes on a psychiatric patient's behalf with agencies, employers, or institutions

90885   Psychiatric evaluation of hospital records, other psychiatric reports, psychometric and/or projective tests, and other accumulated data for medical diagnostic purposes

90887   Interpretation or explanation of results of psychiatric, other medical examinations and procedures, or other accumulated data to family or other responsible persons, or advising them how to assist patient

90889   Preparation of report of patient's psychiatric status, history, treatment, or progress (other than for legal or consultative purposes) for other physicians, agencies, or insurance carriers

90899   Unlisted psychiatric service or procedure

Biofeedback

(For psychophysiological therapy incorporating biofeedback training, see 90875, 90876)

90901   Biofeedback training by any modality

90911   Biofeedback training, perineal muscles, anorectal or urethral sphincter, including EMG and/or manometry

(For incontinence treatment by pulsed magnetic neuromodulation, use Category III code 0029T)

(For testing of rectal sensation, tone and compliance, use 91120)

Dialysis

Codes 90918-90921 are reported ONCE per month to distinguish age-specific services related to the patient's end-stage renal disease (ESRD) performed in an outpatient setting. ESRD-related physician services include establishment of a dialyzing cycle, outpatient evaluation and management of the dialysis visits, telephone calls, and patient management during the dialysis, provided during a full month. These codes are not used if the physician also submits hospitalization codes during the month.

Codes 90918-90921 describe a full month of ESRD-related services provided in an outpatient setting. For ESRD and non-ESRD dialysis services performed in an inpatient setting, and for non-ESRD dialysis services performed in an outpatient setting, see 90935-90937 and 90945-90947.

Evaluation and management services unrelated to ESRD services that cannot be performed during the dialysis session may be reported separately.

Medicine

Codes 90922-90925 are reported when outpatient ESRD-related services are not performed consecutively during an entire full month (eg, when the patient spends part of the month as a hospital inpatient, or when the outpatient ESRD-related services are initiated after the first of the month). The appropriate age-related code from this series (90922-90925) is reported daily less the days of hospitalization. For reporting purposes, each month is considered 30 days.

Example:

Outpatient ESRD-related services are initiated on July 1 for a 57-year-old male. On July 11, he is admitted to the hospital as an inpatient and is discharged on July 27.

In this example, code 90925 should be reported for each day outside of the inpatient hospitalization (30 days/month less 17 days/hospitalization = 13 days). Report inpatient E/M services as appropriate. Dialysis procedures rendered during the hospitalization (July 11-27) should be reported as appropriate (90935-90937, 90945-90947).

End-Stage Renal Disease Services

90918 End-stage renal disease (ESRD) related services per full month; for patients younger than two years of age to include monitoring for the adequacy of nutrition, assessment of growth and development, and counseling of parents

90919 for patients between two and eleven years of age to include monitoring for the adequacy of nutrition, assessment of growth and development, and counseling of parents

90920 for patients between twelve and nineteen years of age to include monitoring for the adequacy of nutrition, assessment of growth and development, and counseling of parents

90921 for patients twenty years of age and older

90922 End-stage renal disease (ESRD) related services (less than full month), per day; for patients younger than two years of age

90923 for patients between two and eleven years of age

90924 for patients between twelve and nineteen years of age

90925 for patients twenty years of age and older

Hemodialysis

Codes 90935, 90937 are reported to describe the hemodialysis procedure with all evaluation and management services related to the patient's renal disease on the day of the hemodialysis procedure. These codes are used for inpatient ESRD and non-ESRD procedures or for outpatient non-ESRD dialysis services. Code 90935 is reported if only one evaluation of the patient is required related to that hemodialysis procedure. Code 90937 is

reported when patient re-evaluation(s) is required during a hemodialysis procedure. Use modifier 25 with Evaluation and Management codes for separately identifiable services unrelated to the dialysis procedure or renal failure which cannot be rendered during the dialysis session.

(For home visit hemodialysis services performed by a non-physician health care professional, use 99512)

(For cannula declotting, see 36831, 36833, 36860, 36861)

(For declotting of implanted vascular access device or catheter by thrombolytic agent, use 36550)

(For collection of blood specimen from a partially or completely implantable venous access device, use 36540)

(For prolonged physician attendance, see 99354-99360)

90935 Hemodialysis procedure with single physician evaluation

90937 Hemodialysis procedure requiring repeated evaluation(s) with or without substantial revision of dialysis prescription

(90939 has been deleted. To report, use 90940)

90940 Hemodialysis access flow study to determine blood flow in grafts and arteriovenous fistulae by an indicator method

(For duplex scan of hemodialysis access, use 93990)

Miscellaneous Dialysis Procedures

Codes 90945, 90947 describe dialysis procedures other than hemodialysis (eg, peritoneal dialysis, hemofiltration or continuous renal replacement therapies), and all evaluation and management services related to the patient's renal disease on the day of the procedure. Code 90945 is reported if only one evaluation of the patient is required related to that procedure. Code 90947 is reported when patient re-evaluation(s) is required during a procedure. Utilize modifier 25 with Evaluation and Management codes for separately identifiable services unrelated to the procedure or the renal failure which cannot be rendered during the dialysis session.

(For insertion of intraperitoneal cannula or catheter, see 49420, 49421)

(For prolonged physician attendance, see 99354-99360)

90945 Dialysis procedure other than hemodialysis (eg, peritoneal dialysis, hemofiltration, or other continuous renal replacement therapies), with single physician evaluation

(For home infusion of peritoneal dialysis, use 99601, 99602)

Medicine

90947   Dialysis procedure other than hemodialysis (eg, peritoneal dialysis, hemofiltration, or other continuous renal replacement therapies) requiring repeated physician evaluations, with or without substantial revision of dialysis prescription

90989   Dialysis training, patient, including helper where applicable, any mode, completed course

90993   Dialysis training, patient, including helper where applicable, any mode, course not completed, per training session

90997   Hemoperfusion (eg, with activated charcoal or resin)

90999   Unlisted dialysis procedure, inpatient or outpatient

Gastroenterology

(For duodenal intubation and aspiration, see 89100-89105)

(For gastrointestinal radiologic procedures, see 74210-74363)

(For esophagoscopy procedures, see 43200-43228; upper GI endoscopy 43234-43259; endoscopy, small intestine and stomal 44360-44393; proctosigmoidoscopy 45300-45321; sigmoidoscopy 45330-45339; colonoscopy 45355-45385; anoscopy 46600-46615)

91000   Esophageal intubation and collection of washings for cytology, including preparation of specimens (separate procedure)

91010   Esophageal motility (manometric study of the esophagus and/or gastroesophageal junction) study;

91011   with mecholyl or similar stimulant

91012   with acid perfusion studies

91020   Gastric motility (manometric) studies

91022   Duodenal motility (manometric) study

(If gastrointestinal endoscopy is performed, use 43235)

(If fluoroscopy is performed, use 76000)

(If gastric motility study is performed, use 91020)

91030   Esophagus, acid perfusion (Bernstein) test for esophagitis

(91032 and 91033 have been deleted. To report, see 91034, 91035)

91034   Esophagus, gastroesophageal reflux test; with nasal catheter pH electrode(s) placement, recording, analysis and interpretation

91035   with mucosal attached telemetry pH electrode placement, recording, analysis and interpretation

91037   Esophageal function test, gastroesophageal reflux test with nasal catheter intraluminal impedance electrode(s) placement, recording, analysis and interpretation;

91038   prolonged (greater than 1 hour, up to 24 hours)

91040   Esophageal balloon distension provocation study

(For balloon dilatation with endoscopy, see 43220, 43249, 43456, or 43458)

91052   Gastric analysis test with injection of stimulant of gastric secretion (eg, histamine, insulin, pentagastrin, calcium and secretin)

(For gastric biopsy by capsule, peroral, via tube, one or more specimens, use 43600)

(For gastric laboratory procedures, see also 89130-89141)

91055   Gastric intubation, washings, and preparing slides for cytology (separate procedure)

(For gastric lavage, therapeutic, use 91105)

▶(91060 has been deleted)◀

(For biopsy by capsule, small intestine, per oral, via tube [one or more specimens], use 44100)

91065   Breath hydrogen test (eg, for detection of lactase deficiency, fructose intolerance, bacterial overgrowth, or oro-cecal gastrointestinal transit)

(For H. pylori breath test analysis, use 83013 for non-radioactive (C-13) isotope or 78268 for radioactive (C-14) isotope)

91100   Intestinal bleeding tube, passage, positioning and monitoring

91105   Gastric intubation, and aspiration or lavage for treatment (eg, for ingested poisons)

(For cholangiography, see 47500, 74320)

(For abdominal paracentesis, see 49080, 49081; with instillation of medication, see 96440, 96445)

(For peritoneoscopy, use 49320; with biopsy, use 49321)

(For peritoneoscopy and guided transhepatic cholangiography, use 47560; with biopsy, use 47561)

(For splenoportography, see 38200, 75810)

91110   Gastrointestinal tract imaging, intraluminal (eg, capsule endoscopy), esophagus through ileum, with physician interpretation and report

(Visualization of the colon is not reported separately)

(Append modifier 52 if the ileum is not visualized)

● **91111**   Gastrointestinal tract imaging, intraluminal (eg, capsule endoscopy), esophagus with physician interpretation and report

▶(Do not report 91111 in conjunction with 91110)◀

Medicine

91120 Rectal sensation, tone, and compliance test (ie, response to graded balloon distention)

(For biofeedback training, use 90911)

(For anorectal manometry, use 91122)

91122 Anorectal manometry

91123 Pulsed irrigation of fecal impaction

Gastric Physiology

91132 Electrogastrography, diagnostic, transcutaneous;

91133 with provocative testing

Other Procedures

91299 Unlisted diagnostic gastroenterology procedure

Ophthalmology

(For surgical procedures, see **Surgery,** Eye and Ocular Adnexa, 65091 et seq)

Definitions

Intermediate ophthalmological services describes an evaluation of a new or existing condition complicated with a new diagnostic or management problem not necessarily relating to the primary diagnosis, including history, general medical observation, external ocular and adnexal examination and other diagnostic procedures as indicated; may include the use of mydriasis for ophthalmoscopy.

For example:

a. Review of history, external examination, ophthalmoscopy, biomicroscopy for an acute complicated condition (eg, iritis) not requiring comprehensive ophthalmological services.

b. Review of interval history, external examination, ophthalmoscopy, biomicroscopy and tonometry in established patient with known cataract not requiring comprehensive ophthalmological services.

Comprehensive ophthalmological services describes a general evaluation of the complete visual system. The comprehensive services constitute a single service entity but need not be performed at one session. The service includes history, general medical observation, external and ophthalmoscopic examinations, gross visual fields and basic sensorimotor examination. It often includes, as indicated: biomicroscopy, examination with cycloplegia or mydriasis and tonometry. It always includes initiation of diagnostic and treatment programs.

Intermediate and comprehensive ophthalmological services constitute integrated services in which medical decision making cannot be separated from the examining techniques used. Itemization of service components, such

as slit lamp examination, keratometry, routine ophthalmoscopy, retinoscopy, tonometry, or motor evaluation is not applicable.

For example:

The comprehensive services required for diagnosis and treatment of a patient with symptoms indicating possible disease of the visual system, such as glaucoma, cataract or retinal disease, or to rule out disease of the visual system, new or established patient.

Initiation of diagnostic and treatment program includes the prescription of medication, and arranging for special ophthalmological diagnostic or treatment services, consultations, laboratory procedures and radiological services.

Special ophthalmological services describes services in which a special evaluation of part of the visual system is made, which goes beyond the services included under general ophthalmological services, or in which special treatment is given. Special ophthalmological services may be reported in addition to the general ophthalmological services or evaluation and management services.

For example:

Fluorescein angioscopy, quantitative visual field examination, refraction or extended color vision examination (such as Nagel's anomaloscope) should be separately reported.

Prescription of lenses, when required, is included in 92015. It includes specification of lens type (monofocal, bifocal, other), lens power, axis, prism, absorptive factor, impact resistance, and other factors.

Interpretation and report by the physician is an integral part of special ophthalmological services where indicated. Technical procedures (which may or may not be performed by the physician personally) are often part of the service, but should not be mistaken to constitute the service itself.

General Ophthalmological Services

New Patient

Solely for the purposes of distinguishing between new and established patients, **professional services** are those face-to-face services rendered by a physician and reported by a specific code(s). A new patient is one who has not received any professional services from the physician or another physician of the same specialty who belongs to the same group practice within the past three years.

92002 Ophthalmological services: medical examination and evaluation with initiation of diagnostic and treatment program; intermediate, new patient

92004 comprehensive, new patient, one or more visits

Established Patient

Solely for the purposes of distinguishing between new and established patients, **professional services** are those face-to-face services rendered by a physician and reported by a specific code(s). An established patient is one who has received professional services from the physician or another physician of the same specialty who belongs to the same group practice within the past three years.

92012 Ophthalmological services: medical examination and evaluation, with initiation or continuation of diagnostic and treatment program; intermediate, established patient

92014 comprehensive, established patient, one or more visits

(For surgical procedures, see **Surgery,** Eye and Ocular Adnexa, 65091 et seq)

Special Ophthalmological Services

92015 Determination of refractive state

92018 Ophthalmological examination and evaluation, under general anesthesia, with or without manipulation of globe for passive range of motion or other manipulation to facilitate diagnostic examination; complete

92019 limited

92020 Gonioscopy (separate procedure)

(For gonioscopy under general anesthesia, use 92018)

● **92025** Computerized corneal topography, unilateral or bilateral, with interpretation and report

▶(Do not report 92025 in conjunction with 65710-65755)◀

▶(92025 is not used for manual keratoscopy, which is part of a single system Evaluation and Management or ophthalmological service)◀

92060 Sensorimotor examination with multiple measurements of ocular deviation (eg, restrictive or paretic muscle with diplopia) with interpretation and report (separate procedure)

92065 Orthoptic and/or pleoptic training, with continuing medical direction and evaluation

92070 Fitting of contact lens for treatment of disease, including supply of lens

92081 Visual field examination, unilateral or bilateral, with interpretation and report; limited examination (eg, tangent screen, Autoplot, arc perimeter, or single stimulus level automated test, such as Octopus 3 or 7 equivalent)

92082 intermediate examination (eg, at least 2 isopters on Goldmann perimeter, or semiquantitative, automated suprathreshold screening program, Humphrey suprathreshold automatic diagnostic test, Octopus program 33)

92083 extended examination (eg, Goldmann visual fields with at least 3 isopters plotted and static determination within the central 30°, or quantitative, automated threshold perimetry, Octopus program G-1, 32 or 42, Humphrey visual field analyzer full threshold programs 30-2, 24-2, or 30/60-2)

(Gross visual field testing (eg, confrontation testing) is a part of general ophthalmological services and is not reported separately)

92100 Serial tonometry (separate procedure) with multiple measurements of intraocular pressure over an extended time period with interpretation and report, same day (eg, diurnal curve or medical treatment of acute elevation of intraocular pressure)

92120 Tonography with interpretation and report, recording indentation tonometer method or perilimbal suction method

92130 Tonography with water provocation

92135 Scanning computerized ophthalmic diagnostic imaging (eg, scanning laser) with interpretation and report, unilateral

92136 Ophthalmic biometry by partial coherence interferometry with intraocular lens power calculation

92140 Provocative tests for glaucoma, with interpretation and report, without tonography

Ophthalmoscopy

Routine ophthalmoscopy is part of general and special ophthalmologic services whenever indicated. It is a non-itemized service and is not reported separately.

92225 Ophthalmoscopy, extended, with retinal drawing (eg, for retinal detachment, melanoma), with interpretation and report; initial

92226 subsequent

92230 Fluorescein angioscopy with interpretation and report

92235 Fluorescein angiography (includes multiframe imaging) with interpretation and report

92240 Indocyanine-green angiography (includes multiframe imaging) with interpretation and report

92250 Fundus photography with interpretation and report

92260 Ophthalmodynamometry

(For ophthalmoscopy under general anesthesia, use 92018)

Other Specialized Services

92265 Needle oculoelectromyography, one or more extraocular muscles, one or both eyes, with interpretation and report

92270 Electro-oculography with interpretation and report

Medicine

92275 Electroretinography with interpretation and report

(For electronystagmography for vestibular function studies, see 92541 et seq)

(For ophthalmic echography (diagnostic ultrasound), see 76511-76529)

92283 Color vision examination, extended, eg, anomaloscope or equivalent

(Color vision testing with pseudoisochromatic plates (such as HRR or Ishihara) is not reported separately. It is included in the appropriate general or ophthalmological service, or 99172)

92284 Dark adaptation examination with interpretation and report

92285 External ocular photography with interpretation and report for documentation of medical progress (eg, close-up photography, slit lamp photography, goniophotography, stereo-photography)

92286 Special anterior segment photography with interpretation and report; with specular endothelial microscopy and cell count

92287 with fluorescein angiography

Contact Lens Services

The prescription of contact lens includes specification of optical and physical characteristics (such as power, size, curvature, flexibility, gas-permeability). It is NOT a part of the general ophthalmological services.

The fitting of contact lens includes instruction and training of the wearer and incidental revision of the lens during the training period.

Follow-up of successfully fitted extended wear lenses is reported as part of a general ophthalmological service (92012 et seq).

The supply of contact lenses may be reported as part of the service of fitting. It may also be reported separately by using the appropriate supply codes.

(For therapeutic or surgical use of contact lens, see 68340, 92070)

92310 Prescription of optical and physical characteristics of and fitting of contact lens, with medical supervision of adaptation; corneal lens, both eyes, except for aphakia

(For prescription and fitting of one eye, add modifier 52)

92311 corneal lens for aphakia, one eye

92312 corneal lens for aphakia, both eyes

92313 corneoscleral lens

92314 Prescription of optical and physical characteristics of contact lens, with medical supervision of adaptation and direction of fitting by independent technician; corneal lens, both eyes except for aphakia

(For prescription and fitting of one eye, add modifier 52)

92315 corneal lens for aphakia, one eye

92316 corneal lens for aphakia, both eyes

92317 corneoscleral lens

92325 Modification of contact lens (separate procedure), with medical supervision of adaptation

92326 Replacement of contact lens

(92330, 92335 have been deleted)

(For prescription, fitting, and/or medical supervision of ocular prosthetic adaptation by a physician, see Evaluation and Management services or General Ophthalmological service codes 92002-92014)

Spectacle Services (Including Prosthesis for Aphakia)

Prescription of lenses, when required, is included in 92015 Determination of refractive state. It includes specification of lens type (monofocal, bifocal, other), lens power, axis, prism, absorptive factor, impact resistance, and other factors.

Fitting of spectacles is a separate service; when provided by the physician, it is reported as indicated by 92340-92371.

Fitting includes measurement of anatomical facial characteristics, the writing of laboratory specifications, and the final adjustment of the spectacles to the visual axes and anatomical topography. Presence of physician is not required.

Supply of materials is a separate service component; it is not part of the service of fitting spectacles.

92340 Fitting of spectacles, except for aphakia; monofocal

92341 bifocal

92342 multifocal, other than bifocal

92352 Fitting of spectacle prosthesis for aphakia; monofocal

92353 multifocal

92354 Fitting of spectacle mounted low vision aid; single element system

92355 telescopic or other compound lens system

92358 Prosthesis service for aphakia, temporary (disposable or loan, including materials)

92370 Repair and refitting spectacles; except for aphakia

92371 spectacle prosthesis for aphakia

(Codes 92390-92396 have been deleted. For supply of spectacles or contact lenses, use the appropriate supply codes)

Other Procedures

92499 Unlisted ophthalmological service or procedure

Special Otorhinolaryngologic Services

Diagnostic or treatment procedures usually included in a comprehensive otorhinolaryngologic evaluation or office visit, are reported as an integrated medical service, using appropriate descriptors from the 99201 series. Itemization of component procedures (eg, otoscopy, rhinoscopy, tuning fork test) does not apply.

Special otorhinolaryngologic services are those diagnostic and treatment services not usually included in a comprehensive otorhinolaryngologic evaluation or office visit. These services are reported separately, using codes 92502-92700.

All services include medical diagnostic evaluation. Technical procedures (which may or may not be performed by the physician personally) are often part of the service, but should not be mistaken to constitute the service itself.

Code 92506 is used to report evaluation of speech production, receptive language, and expressive language abilities. Tests may examine speech sound production, articulatory movements of oral musculature, the patient's ability to understand the meaning and intent of written and verbal expressions, and the appropriate formulation and utterance of expressive thought. In contrast, 92626 and 92627 are reported for an evaluation of auditory rehabilitation status determining the patient's ability to use residual hearing in order to identify the acoustic characteristics of sounds associated with speech communication.

> (For laryngoscopy with stroboscopy, use 31579)

92502   Otolaryngologic examination under general anesthesia

92504   Binocular microscopy (separate diagnostic procedure)

92506   Evaluation of speech, language, voice, communication, and/or auditory processing

92507   Treatment of speech, language, voice, communication, and/or auditory processing disorder; individual

92508   group, 2 or more individuals

> (92510 has been deleted)

> (For auditory rehabilitation, prelingual hearing loss, use 92630)

> (For auditory rehabilitation, postlingual hearing loss, use 92633)

> (For cochlear implant programming, see 92601-92604)

92511   Nasopharyngoscopy with endoscope (separate procedure)

92512   Nasal function studies (eg, rhinomanometry)

92516   Facial nerve function studies (eg, electroneuronography)

92520   Laryngeal function studies (ie, aerodynamic testing and acoustic testing)

> (For performance of a single test, use modifier 52)

> (To report flexible fiberoptic laryngeal evaluation of swallowing and laryngeal sensory testing, see 92611-92617)

> (To report other testing of laryngeal function (eg, electroglottography), use 92700)

92526   Treatment of swallowing dysfunction and/or oral function for feeding

Vestibular Function Tests, With Observation and Evaluation by Physician, Without Electrical Recording

92531   Spontaneous nystagmus, including gaze

92532   Positional nystagmus test

92533   Caloric vestibular test, each irrigation (binaural, bithermal stimulation constitutes four tests)

92534   Optokinetic nystagmus test

Vestibular Function Tests, With Recording (eg, ENG, PENG), and Medical Diagnostic Evaluation

92541   Spontaneous nystagmus test, including gaze and fixation nystagmus, with recording

92542   Positional nystagmus test, minimum of 4 positions, with recording

92543   Caloric vestibular test, each irrigation (binaural, bithermal stimulation constitutes four tests), with recording

92544   Optokinetic nystagmus test, bidirectional, foveal or peripheral stimulation, with recording

92545   Oscillating tracking test, with recording

92546   Sinusoidal vertical axis rotational testing

+ 92547   Use of vertical electrodes (List separately in addition to code for primary procedure)

> (Use 92547 in conjunction with 92541-92546)

> (For unlisted vestibular tests, use 92700)

92548   Computerized dynamic posturography

Audiologic Function Tests With Medical Diagnostic Evaluation

The audiometric tests listed below imply the use of calibrated electronic equipment. Other hearing tests (such as whispered voice, tuning fork) are considered part of the general otorhinolaryngologic services and are not reported separately. All services include testing of both ears. Use modifier 52 if a test is applied to one ear instead

Medicine

of to two ears. All codes (except 92559) apply to testing of individuals; for testing of groups, use 92559 and specify test(s) used.

(For evaluation of speech, language and/or hearing problems through observation and assessment of performance, use 92506)

92551	Screening test, pure tone, air only
92552	Pure tone audiometry (threshold); air only
92553	air and bone
92555	Speech audiometry threshold;
92556	with speech recognition
92557	Comprehensive audiometry threshold evaluation and speech recognition (92553 and 92556 combined)

(For hearing aid evaluation and selection, see 92590-92595)

92559	Audiometric testing of groups
92560	Bekesy audiometry; screening
92561	diagnostic
92562	Loudness balance test, alternate binaural or monaural
92563	Tone decay test
92564	Short increment sensitivity index (SISI)
92565	Stenger test, pure tone
92567	Tympanometry (impedance testing)
92568	Acoustic reflex testing; threshold
92569	decay
92571	Filtered speech test
92572	Staggered spondaic word test

▶(92573 has been deleted. To report the Lombard test, use 92700)◄

92575	Sensorineural acuity level test
92576	Synthetic sentence identification test
92577	Stenger test, speech
92579	Visual reinforcement audiometry (VRA)
92582	Conditioning play audiometry
92583	Select picture audiometry
92584	Electrocochleography
92585	Auditory evoked potentials for evoked response audiometry and/or testing of the central nervous system; comprehensive
92586	limited

92587	Evoked otoacoustic emissions; limited (single stimulus level, either transient or distortion products)
92588	comprehensive or diagnostic evaluation (comparison of transient and/or distortion product otoacoustic emissions at multiple levels and frequencies)

(92589 has been deleted)

(For central auditory function evaluation, see 92620, 92621)

92590	Hearing aid examination and selection; monaural
92591	binaural
92592	Hearing aid check; monaural
92593	binaural
92594	Electroacoustic evaluation for hearing aid; monaural
92595	binaural
92596	Ear protector attenuation measurements
92597	Evaluation for use and/or fitting of voice prosthetic device to supplement oral speech

(To report augmentative and alternative communication device services, see 92605, 92607, 92608)

Evaluative and Therapeutic Services

Codes 92601 and 92603 describe post-operative analysis and fitting of previously placed external devices, connection to the cochlear implant, and programming of the stimulator. Codes 92602 and 92604 describe subsequent sessions for measurements and adjustment of the external transmitter and re-programming of the internal stimulator.

(For placement of cochlear implant, use 69930)

92601	Diagnostic analysis of cochlear implant, patient younger than 7 years of age; with programming
92602	subsequent reprogramming

(Do not report 92602 in addition to 92601)

(For aural rehabilitation services following cochlear implant, including evaluation of rehabilitation status, see 92626-92627, 92630-92633)

92603	Diagnostic analysis of cochlear implant, age 7 years or older; with programming
92604	subsequent reprogramming

(Do not report 92604 in addition to 92603)

92605	Evaluation for prescription of non-speech-generating augmentative and alternative communication device
92606	Therapeutic service(s) for the use of non-speech-generating device, including programming and modification

Medicine

92607   Evaluation for prescription for speech-generating augmentative and alternative communication device, face-to-face with the patient; first hour

(For evaluation for prescription of a non-speech-generating device, use 92605)

+ **92608**   each additional 30 minutes (List separately in addition to code for primary procedure)

(Use 92608 in conjunction with 92607)

92609   Therapeutic services for the use of speech-generating device, including programming and modification

(For therapeutic service(s) for the use of a non-speech-generating device, use 92606)

92610   Evaluation of oral and pharyngeal swallowing function

(For motion fluoroscopic evaluation of swallowing function, use 92611)

(For flexible endoscopic examination, use 92612-92617)

92611   Motion fluoroscopic evaluation of swallowing function by cine or video recording

(For radiological supervision and interpretation, use 74230)

(For evaluation of oral and pharyngeal swallowing function, use 92610)

(For flexible fiberoptic diagnostic laryngoscopy, use 31575. Do not report 31575 in conjunction with 92612-92617)

92612   Flexible fiberoptic endoscopic evaluation of swallowing by cine or video recording;

(If flexible fiberoptic or endoscopic evaluation of swallowing is performed without cine or video recording, use 92700)

92613   physician interpretation and report only

(To report an evaluation of oral and pharyngeal swallowing function, use 92610)

(To report motion fluoroscopic evaluation of swallowing function, use 92611)

92614   Flexible fiberoptic endoscopic evaluation, laryngeal sensory testing by cine or video recording;

(If flexible fiberoptic or endoscopic evaluation of swallowing is performed without cine or video recording, use 92700)

92615   physician interpretation and report only

92616   Flexible fiberoptic endoscopic evaluation of swallowing and laryngeal sensory testing by cine or video recording;

(If flexible fiberoptic or endoscopic evaluation of swallowing is performed without cine or video recording, use 92700)

92617   physician interpretation and report only

92620   Evaluation of central auditory function, with report; initial 60 minutes

92621   each additional 15 minutes

(Do not report 92620, 92621 in conjunction with 92506)

92625   Assessment of tinnitus (includes pitch, loudness matching, and masking)

(Do not report 92625 in conjunction with 92562)

(For unilateral assessment, use modifier 52)

92626   Evaluation of auditory rehabilitation status; first hour

+ **92627**   each additional 15 minutes (List separately in addition to code for primary procedure)

(Use 92627 in conjunction with 92626)

(When reporting 92626, 92627, use the face-to-face time with the patient or family)

92630   Auditory rehabilitation; prelingual hearing loss

92633   postlingual hearing loss

►Special Diagnostic Procedures◄

● **92640**   Diagnostic analysis with programming of auditory brainstem implant, per hour

►(Report nonprogramming services separately [eg, cardiac monitoring])◄

Other Procedures

92700   Unlisted otorhinolaryngological service or procedure

Cardiovascular

►Therapeutic Services and Procedures◄

(For nonsurgical septal reduction therapy [eg, alcohol ablation], use Category III code 0024T)

92950   Cardiopulmonary resuscitation (eg, in cardiac arrest)

(See also critical care services, 99291, 99292)

⊙ **92953**   Temporary transcutaneous pacing

(For physician direction of ambulance or rescue personnel outside the hospital, use 99288)

⊙ **92960**   Cardioversion, elective, electrical conversion of arrhythmia; external

⊙ **92961**   internal (separate procedure)

(Do not report 92961 in addition to codes 93662, 93618-93624, 93631, 93640-93642, 93650-93652, 93741-93744)

Medicine

▲=Revised code   ●=New code   ►◄=Contains new or revised text   ⊘=Modifier 51 exempt

92970 Cardioassist-method of circulatory assist; internal

92971 external

(For balloon atrial-septostomy, use 92992)

(For placement of catheters for use in circulatory assist devices such as intra-aortic balloon pump, use 33970)

⊙+ **92973** Percutaneous transluminal coronary thrombectomy (List separately in addition to code for primary procedure)

(Use 92973 in conjunction with 92980, 92982)

⊙+ **92974** Transcatheter placement of radiation delivery device for subsequent coronary intravascular brachytherapy (List separately in addition to code for primary procedure)

(Use 92974 in conjunction with 92980, 92982, 92995, 93508)

(For intravascular radioelement application, see 77781-77784)

⊙ **92975** Thrombolysis, coronary; by intracoronary infusion, including selective coronary angiography

92977 by intravenous infusion

(For thrombolysis of vessels other than coronary, see 37201, 75896)

(For cerebral thrombolysis, use 37195)

⊙+ **92978** Intravascular ultrasound (coronary vessel or graft) during diagnostic evaluation and/or therapeutic intervention including imaging supervision, interpretation and report; initial vessel (List separately in addition to code for primary procedure)

⊙+ **92979** each additional vessel (List separately in addition to code for primary procedure)

(Use 92979 in conjunction with 92978)

(Intravascular ultrasound services include all transducer manipulations and repositioning within the specific vessel being examined, both before and after therapeutic intervention (eg, stent placement))

⊙ **92980** Transcatheter placement of an intracoronary stent(s), percutaneous, with or without other therapeutic intervention, any method; single vessel

⊙+ **92981** each additional vessel (List separately in addition to code for primary procedure)

(Use 92981 in conjunction with 92980)

(Codes 92980, 92981 are used to report coronary artery stenting. Coronary angioplasty (92982, 92984) or atherectomy (92995, 92996), in the same artery, is considered part of the stenting procedure and is not reported separately. Codes 92973 (percutaneous transluminal coronary thombectomy), 92974 (coronary brachytherapy) and 92978, 92979 (intravascular ultrasound) are add-on codes for reporting procedures performed in addition to coronary stenting, atherectomy, and angioplasty and are not included in the "therapeutic interventions" in 92980)

(To report additional vessels treated by angioplasty or atherectomy only during the same session, see 92984, 92996)

(To report transcatheter placement of radiation delivery device for coronary intravascular brachytherapy, use 92974)

(For intravascular radioelement application, see 77781-77784)

⊙ **92982** Percutaneous transluminal coronary balloon angioplasty; single vessel

⊙+ **92984** each additional vessel (List separately in addition to code for primary procedure)

(Use 92984 in conjunction with 92980, 92982, 92995)

(For stent placement following completion of angioplasty or atherectomy, see 92980, 92981)

(To report transcatheter placement of radiation delivery device for coronary intravascular brachytherapy, use 92974)

(For intravascular radioelement application, see 77781-77784)

⊙ **92986** Percutaneous balloon valvuloplasty; aortic valve

⊙ **92987** mitral valve

92990 pulmonary valve

92992 Atrial septectomy or septostomy; transvenous method, balloon (eg, Rashkind type) (includes cardiac catheterization)

92993 blade method (Park septostomy) (includes cardiac catheterization)

⊙ **92995** Percutaneous transluminal coronary atherectomy, by mechanical or other method, with or without balloon angioplasty; single vessel

⊙+ **92996** each additional vessel (List separately in addition to code for primary procedure)

(Use 92996 in conjunction with 92980, 92982, 92995)

(For stent placement following completion of angioplasty or atherectomy, see 92980, 92981)

(To report additional vessels treated by angioplasty only during the same session, use 92984)

92997 Percutaneous transluminal pulmonary artery balloon angioplasty; single vessel

+ **92998** each additional vessel (List separately in addition to code for primary procedure)

(Use 92998 in conjunction with 92997)

Medicine

Cardiography

(For echocardiography, see 93303-93350)

93000   Electrocardiogram, routine ECG with at least 12 leads; with interpretation and report

93005   tracing only, without interpretation and report

93010   interpretation and report only

(For ECG monitoring, see 99354-99360)

93012   Telephonic transmission of post-symptom electrocardiogram rhythm strip(s), 24-hour attended monitoring, per 30 day period of time; tracing only

93014   physician review with interpretation and report only

93015   Cardiovascular stress test using maximal or submaximal treadmill or bicycle exercise, continuous electrocardiographic monitoring, and/or pharmacological stress; with physician supervision, with interpretation and report

93016   physician supervision only, without interpretation and report

93017   tracing only, without interpretation and report

93018   interpretation and report only

(For inert gas rebreathing measurement, see Category III codes 0104T, 0105T)

93024   Ergonovine provocation test

93025   Microvolt T-wave alternans for assessment of ventricular arrhythmias

93040   Rhythm ECG, one to three leads; with interpretation and report

93041   tracing only without interpretation and report

93042   interpretation and report only

93224   Electrocardiographic monitoring for 24 hours by continuous original ECG waveform recording and storage, with visual superimposition scanning; includes recording, scanning analysis with report, physician review and interpretation

93225   recording (includes hook-up, recording, and disconnection)

93226   scanning analysis with report

93227   physician review and interpretation

93230   Electrocardiographic monitoring for 24 hours by continuous original ECG waveform recording and storage without superimposition scanning utilizing a device capable of producing a full miniaturized printout; includes recording, microprocessor-based analysis with report, physician review and interpretation

93231   recording (includes hook-up, recording, and disconnection)

93232   microprocessor-based analysis with report

93233   physician review and interpretation

93235   Electrocardiographic monitoring for 24 hours by continuous computerized monitoring and non-continuous recording, and real-time data analysis utilizing a device capable of producing intermittent full-sized waveform tracings, possibly patient activated; includes monitoring and real-time data analysis with report, physician review and interpretation

93236   monitoring and real-time data analysis with report

93237   physician review and interpretation

93268   Patient demand single or multiple event recording with presymptom memory loop, 24-hour attended monitoring, per 30 day period of time; includes transmission, physician review and interpretation

93270   recording (includes hook-up, recording, and disconnection)

93271   monitoring, receipt of transmissions, and analysis

93272   physician review and interpretation only

(For postsymptom recording, see 93012, 93014)

(For implanted patient activated cardiac event recording, see 33282, 93727)

93278   Signal-averaged electrocardiography (SAECG), with or without ECG

(For interpretation and report only, use 93278 with modifier 26)

(For unlisted cardiographic procedure, use 93799)

Echocardiography

Echocardiography includes obtaining ultrasonic signals from the heart and great arteries, with two-dimensional image and/or Doppler ultrasonic signal documentation, and interpretation and report. When interpretation is performed separately use modifier 26.

Echocardiography is an ultrasound examination of the cardiac chambers and valves, the adjacent great vessels, and the pericardium. A complete transthoracic echocardiogram (93307) is a comprehensive procedure that includes 2-dimensional and selected M-mode examination of the left and right atria, left and right ventricles, the aortic, mitral, and tricuspid valves, the pericardium, and adjacent portions of the aorta. These structures are assessed using multiple views as required to obtain a complete functional and anatomic evaluation, and appropriate measurements are obtained and recorded. Despite significant effort, identification and measurement of some structures may not always be possible. In such instances, the reason that an element could not be visualized must be documented. Additional structures that may be visualized (eg, pulmonary veins, pulmonary artery, pulmonic valve, inferior vena cava) would be included as part of the service.

Medicine

A follow-up or limited echocardiographic study (93308) is an examination that does not evaluate or document the attempt to evaluate all the structures that comprise the complete echocardiographic exam. This is typically performed in follow-up of a complete echocardiographic examination when a repeat complete exam is unnecessary due to the more focused clinical concern. In some emergent clinical situations, a limited echocardiographic study may be performed primarily.

Report of an echocardiographic study, whether complete or limited, includes an interpretation of all obtained information, documentation of all clinically relevant findings including quantitative measurements obtained, plus a description of any recognized abnormalities. Pertinent images, videotape, and/or digital data are archived for permanent storage and are available for subsequent review. Use of echocardiography not meeting these criteria is not separately reportable.

Use of ultrasound, without thorough evaluation of organ(s) or anatomic region, image documentation and final, written report, is not separately reportable.

(For fetal echocardiography, see 76825-76828)

93303 Transthoracic echocardiography for congenital cardiac anomalies; complete

93304 follow-up or limited study

93307 Echocardiography, transthoracic, real-time with image documentation (2D) with or without M-mode recording; complete

93308 follow-up or limited study

⊙ **93312** Echocardiography, transesophageal, real time with image documentation (2D) (with or without M-mode recording); including probe placement, image acquisition, interpretation and report

⊙ **93313** placement of transesophageal probe only

⊙ **93314** image acquisition, interpretation and report only

⊙ **93315** Transesophageal echocardiography for congenital cardiac anomalies; including probe placement, image acquisition, interpretation and report

⊙ **93316** placement of transesophageal probe only

⊙ **93317** image acquisition, interpretation and report only

⊙ **93318** Echocardiography, transesophageal (TEE) for monitoring purposes, including probe placement, real time 2-dimensional image acquisition and interpretation leading to ongoing (continuous) assessment of (dynamically changing) cardiac pumping function and to therapeutic measures on an immediate time basis

+ **93320** Doppler echocardiography, pulsed wave and/or continuous wave with spectral display (List separately in addition to codes for echocardiographic imaging); complete

(Use 93320 in conjunction with 93303, 93304, 93307, 93308, 93312, 93314, 93315, 93317, 93350)

+ **93321** follow-up or limited study (List separately in addition to codes for echocardiographic imaging)

(Use 93321 in conjunction with 93303, 93304, 93307, 93308, 93312, 93314, 93315, 93317, 93350)

+ **93325** Doppler echocardiography color flow velocity mapping (List separately in addition to codes for echocardiography)

(Use 93325 in conjunction with 76825, 76826, 76827, 76828, 93303, 93304, 93307, 93308, 93312, 93314, 93315, 93317, 93320, 93321, 93350)

93350 Echocardiography, transthoracic, real-time with image documentation (2D), with or without M-mode recording, during rest and cardiovascular stress test using treadmill, bicycle exercise and/or pharmacologically induced stress, with interpretation and report

(The appropriate stress testing code from the 93015-93018 series should be reported in addition to 93350 to capture the exercise stress portion of the study)

Cardiac Catheterization

Cardiac catheterization is a diagnostic medical procedure which includes introduction, positioning and repositioning of catheter(s), when necessary, recording of intracardiac and intravascular pressure, obtaining blood samples for measurement of blood gases or dilution curves and cardiac output measurements (Fick or other method, with or without rest and exercise and/or studies) with or without electrode catheter placement, final evaluation and report of procedure. When selective injection procedures are performed without a preceding cardiac catheterization, these services should be reported using codes in the Vascular Injection Procedures section, 36011-36015 and 36215-36218.

When coronary artery, arterial coronary conduit or venous bypass graft angiography is performed without concomitant left heart cardiac catheterization, use 93508. Injection procedures 93539, 93540, 93544, and 93545 represent separate identifiable services and may be reported in conjunction with one another in addition to 93508, as appropriate. To report imaging supervision, interpretation and report in conjunction with 93508, use 93556.

Modifier 51 should not be appended to 93501-93533, 93539-93556.

⊙⊘ **93501** Right heart catheterization

(For bundle of His recording, use 93600)

⊘ **93503** Insertion and placement of flow directed catheter (eg, Swan-Ganz) for monitoring purposes

(For subsequent monitoring, see 99356-99357)

⊙⊘ **93505** Endomyocardial biopsy

Medicine (vertical sidebar label)

⊙⊘ **93508**   Catheter placement in coronary artery(s), arterial coronary conduit(s), and/or venous coronary bypass graft(s) for coronary angiography without concomitant left heart catheterization

(93508 is to be used only when left heart catheterization 93510, 93511, 93524, 93526 is not performed)

(93508 is to be used only once per procedure)

(To report transcatheter placement of radiation delivery device for coronary intravascular brachytherapy, use 92974)

(For intravascular radioelement application, see 77781-77784)

⊙⊘ **93510**   Left heart catheterization, retrograde, from the brachial artery, axillary artery or femoral artery; percutaneous

⊙⊘ **93511**   by cutdown

⊙⊘ **93514**   Left heart catheterization by left ventricular puncture

⊙⊘ **93524**   Combined transseptal and retrograde left heart catheterization

⊙⊘ **93526**   Combined right heart catheterization and retrograde left heart catheterization

⊙⊘ **93527**   Combined right heart catheterization and transseptal left heart catheterization through intact septum (with or without retrograde left heart catheterization)

⊙⊘ **93528**   Combined right heart catheterization with left ventricular puncture (with or without retrograde left heart catheterization)

⊙⊘ **93529**   Combined right heart catheterization and left heart catheterization through existing septal opening (with or without retrograde left heart catheterization)

⊙⊘ **93530**   Right heart catheterization, for congenital cardiac anomalies

⊘ **93531**   Combined right heart catheterization and retrograde left heart catheterization, for congenital cardiac anomalies

⊘ **93532**   Combined right heart catheterization and transseptal left heart catheterization through intact septum with or without retrograde left heart catheterization, for congenital cardiac anomalies

⊘ **93533**   Combined right heart catheterization and transseptal left heart catheterization through existing septal opening, with or without retrograde left heart catheterization, for congenital cardiac anomalies

(When injection procedures are performed in conjunction with cardiac catheterization, these services do not include introduction of catheters but do include repositioning of catheters when necessary and use of automatic power injectors. Injection procedures 93539-93545 represent separate identifiable services and may be coded in conjunction with one another when appropriate. The technical details of angiography, supervision of filming and processing, interpretation and report are not included. To report imaging supervision, interpretation and report, use 93555 and/or 93556. Modifier 51 should not be appended to 93539-93556.)

⊙⊘ **93539**   Injection procedure during cardiac catheterization; for selective opacification of arterial conduits (eg, internal mammary), whether native or used for bypass

⊙⊘ **93540**   for selective opacification of aortocoronary venous bypass grafts, one or more coronary arteries

⊙⊘ **93541**   for pulmonary angiography

⊙⊘ **93542**   for selective right ventricular or right atrial angiography

⊙⊘ **93543**   for selective left ventricular or left atrial angiography

⊙⊘ **93544**   for aortography

⊙⊘ **93545**   for selective coronary angiography (injection of radiopaque material may be by hand)

(To report imaging supervision and interpretation, use 93555)

⊙⊘ **93555**   Imaging supervision, interpretation and report for injection procedure(s) during cardiac catheterization; ventricular and/or atrial angiography

⊙⊘ **93556**   pulmonary angiography, aortography, and/or selective coronary angiography including venous bypass grafts and arterial conduits (whether native or used in bypass)

(Codes 93561 and 93562 are not to be used with cardiac catheterization codes)

⊙ **93561**   Indicator dilution studies such as dye or thermal dilution, including arterial and/or venous catheterization; with cardiac output measurement (separate procedure)

⊙ **93562**   subsequent measurement of cardiac output

(For radioisotope method of cardiac output, see 78472, 78473, or 78481)

⊙+ **93571**   Intravascular Doppler velocity and/or pressure derived coronary flow reserve measurement (coronary vessel or graft) during coronary angiography including pharmacologically induced stress; initial vessel (List separately in addition to code for primary procedure)

⊙+ **93572**   each additional vessel (List separately in addition to code for primary procedure)

(Intravascular distal coronary blood flow velocity measurements include all Doppler transducer manipulations and repositioning within the specific vessel being examined, during coronary angiography or therapeutic intervention (eg, angioplasty))

(For unlisted cardiac catheterization procedure, use 93799)

Medicine

Repair of Septal Defect

93580   Percutaneous transcatheter closure of congenital interatrial communication (ie, Fontan fenestration, atrial septal defect) with implant

(Percutaneous transcatheter closure of atrial septal defect includes a right heart catheterization procedure. Code 93580 includes injection of contrast for atrial and ventricular angiograms. Codes 93501, 93529-93533, 93539, 93543, 93555 should not be reported separately in addition to code 93580)

93581   Percutaneous transcatheter closure of a congenital ventricular septal defect with implant

(Percutaneous transcatheter closure of ventricular septal defect includes a right heart catheterization procedure. Code 93581 includes injection of contrast for atrial and ventricular angiograms. Codes 93501, 93529-93533, 93539, 93543, 93555 should not be reported separately in addition to code 93581)

▶(For ventricular septal defect closure via transmyocardial implant delivery, see 0166T, 0167T)◄

(For echocardiographic services performed in addition to 93580, 93581, see 93303-93317, 93662 as appropriate)

Intracardiac Electrophysiological Procedures/Studies

Intracardiac electrophysiologic studies (EPS) are an invasive diagnostic medical procedure which include the insertion and repositioning of electrode catheters, recording of electrograms before and during pacing or programmed stimulation of multiple locations in the heart, analysis of recorded information, and report of the procedure. Electrophysiologic studies are most often performed with two or more electrode catheters. In many circumstances, patients with arrhythmias are evaluated and treated at the same encounter. In this situation, a diagnostic *electrophysiologic study* is performed, induced tachycardia(s) are *mapped*, and on the basis of the diagnostic and mapping information, the tissue is *ablated*. Electrophysiologic study(ies), mapping, and ablation represent distinctly different procedures, requiring individual reporting whether performed on the same or subsequent dates.

Definitions

Arrhythmia Induction: In most electrophysiologic studies, an attempt is made to induce arrhythmia(s) from single or multiple sites within the heart. Arrhythmia induction is achieved by performing pacing at different rates, programmed stimulation (introduction of critically timed electrical impulses), and other techniques. Because arrhythmia induction occurs via the same catheter(s) inserted for the electrophysiologic study(ies), catheter insertion and temporary pacemaker codes are not additionally reported. Codes 93600-93603, 93610-93612 and 93618 are used to describe unusual situations where there may be recording, pacing or an attempt at arrhythmia induction from only one site in the heart. Code 93619 describes only evaluation of the sinus node, atrioventricular node and His-Purkinje conduction system, without arrhythmia induction. Codes 93620-93624 and 93640-93642 all include recording, pacing and attempted arrhythmia induction from one or more site(s) in the heart.

Mapping: Mapping is a distinct procedure performed in addition to a diagnostic electrophysiologic procedure and should be separately reported using 93609 or 93613. Do not report standard mapping (93609) in addition to 3-D mapping (93613). When a tachycardia is induced, the site of tachycardia origination or its electrical path through the heart is often defined by mapping. Mapping creates a multidimensional depiction of a tachycardia by recording multiple electrograms obtained sequentially or simultaneously from multiple catheter sites in the heart. Depending upon the technique, certain types of mapping catheters may be repositioned from point-to-point within the heart, allowing sequential recording from the various sites to construct maps. Other types of mapping catheters allow mapping without a point-to-point technique by allowing simultaneous recording from many electrodes on the same catheter and computer-assisted three dimensional reconstruction of the tachycardia activation sequence.

Ablation: Once the part of the heart involved in the tachycardia is localized, the tachycardia may be treated by ablation (the delivery of a radiofrequency energy to the area to selectively destroy cardiac tissue). Ablation procedures (93651-93652) may be performed: independently on a date subsequent to a diagnostic electrophysiologic study and mapping; or, at the time a diagnostic electrophysiologic study, tachycardia(s) induction and mapping is performed. When an electrophysiologic study, mapping, and ablation are performed on the same date, each procedure should be separately reported. In reporting catheter ablation, 93651 and/or 93652 should be reported once to describe ablation of cardiac arrhythmias, regardless of the number of arrhythmias ablated.

Modifier 51 should not be appended to 93600-93660.

⊘ **93600**   Bundle of His recording

⊘ **93602**   Intra-atrial recording

⊘ **93603**   Right ventricular recording

⊙✚ **93609**   Intraventricular and/or intra-atrial mapping of tachycardia site(s) with catheter manipulation to record from multiple sites to identify origin of tachycardia (List separately in addition to code for primary procedure)

(Use 93609 in conjunction with 93620, 93651, 93652)

(Do not report 93609 in addition to 93613)

⊘ **93610**   Intra-atrial pacing

⊘ **93612**   Intraventricular pacing

(Do not report 93612 in conjunction with 93620-93622)

⊙**+ 93613**   Intracardiac electrophysiologic 3-dimensional mapping (List separately in addition to code for primary procedure)

(Use 93613 in conjunction with 93620, 93651, 93652)

(Do not report 93613 in addition to 93609)

⊙⊘ **93615**   Esophageal recording of atrial electrogram with or without ventricular electrogram(s);

⊙⊘ **93616**   with pacing

⊙⊘ **93618**   Induction of arrhythmia by electrical pacing

(For intracardiac phonocardiogram, use 93799)

⊙⊘ **93619**   Comprehensive electrophysiologic evaluation with right atrial pacing and recording, right ventricular pacing and recording, His bundle recording, including insertion and repositioning of multiple electrode catheters, without induction or attempted induction of arrhythmia

(Do not report 93619 in conjunction with 93600, 93602, 93610, 93612, 93618, or 93620-93622)

⊙⊘ **93620**   Comprehensive electrophysiologic evaluation including insertion and repositioning of multiple electrode catheters with induction or attempted induction of arrhythmia; with right atrial pacing and recording, right ventricular pacing and recording, His bundle recording

(Do not report 93620 in conjunction with 93600, 93602, 93610, 93612, 93618 or 93619)

⊙**+ 93621**   with left atrial pacing and recording from coronary sinus or left atrium (List separately in addition to code for primary procedure)

(Use 93621 in conjunction with 93620)

⊙**+ 93622**   with left ventricular pacing and recording (List separately in addition to code for primary procedure)

(Use 93622 in conjunction with 93620)

+ 93623   Programmed stimulation and pacing after intravenous drug infusion (List separately in addition to code for primary procedure)

(Use 93623 in conjunction with 93619, 93620)

⊙⊘ **93624**   Electrophysiologic follow-up study with pacing and recording to test effectiveness of therapy, including induction or attempted induction of arrhythmia

⊘ **93631**   Intra-operative epicardial and endocardial pacing and mapping to localize the site of tachycardia or zone of slow conduction for surgical correction

⊙⊘ **93640**   Electrophysiologic evaluation of single or dual chamber pacing cardioverter-defibrillator leads including defibrillation threshold evaluation (induction of arrhythmia, evaluation of sensing and pacing for arrhythmia termination) at time of initial implantation or replacement;

⊙⊘ **93641**   with testing of single or dual chamber pacing cardioverter-defibrillator pulse generator

(For subsequent or periodic electronic analysis and/or reprogramming of single or dual chamber pacing cardioverter-defibrillators, see 93642, 93741-93744)

⊙⊘ **93642**   Electrophysiologic evaluation of single or dual chamber pacing cardioverter-defibrillator (includes defibrillation threshold evaluation, induction of arrhythmia, evaluation of sensing and pacing for arrhythmia termination, and programming or reprogramming of sensing or therapeutic parameters)

⊙⊘ **93650**   Intracardiac catheter ablation of atrioventricular node function, atrioventricular conduction for creation of complete heart block, with or without temporary pacemaker placement

⊙⊘ **93651**   Intracardiac catheter ablation of arrhythmogenic focus; for treatment of supraventricular tachycardia by ablation of fast or slow atrioventricular pathways, accessory atrioventricular connections or other atrial foci, singly or in combination

⊙⊘ **93652**   for treatment of ventricular tachycardia

⊘ **93660**   Evaluation of cardiovascular function with tilt table evaluation, with continuous ECG monitoring and intermittent blood pressure monitoring, with or without pharmacological intervention

(For testing of autonomic nervous system function, see 95921-95923)

+ 93662   Intracardiac echocardiography during therapeutic/diagnostic intervention, including imaging supervision and interpretation (List separately in addition to code for primary procedure)

(Use 93662 in conjunction with 92987, 93527, 93532, 93580, 93581, 93621, 93622, 93651, or 93652, as appropriate)

(Do not report 92961 in addition to 93662)

Peripheral Arterial Disease Rehabilitation

Peripheral arterial disease (PAD) rehabilitative physical exercise consists of a series of sessions, lasting 45-60 minutes per session, involving use of either a motorized treadmill or a track to permit each patient to achieve symptom-limited claudication. Each session is supervised by an exercise physiologist or nurse. The supervising provider monitors the individual patient's claudication threshold and other cardiovascular limitations for adjustment of workload. During this supervised rehabilitation program, the development of new arrhythmias, symptoms that might suggest angina or the continued inability of the patient to progress to an adequate level of exercise may require physician review and examination of the patient. These physician services would be separately reported with an appropriate level E/M service code.

93668   Peripheral arterial disease (PAD) rehabilitation, per session

Medicine

►Noninvasive Physiologic Studies and Procedures◄

(For arterial cannulization and recording of direct arterial pressure, use 36620)

(For radiographic injection procedures, see 36000-36299)

(For vascular cannulization for hemodialysis, see 36800-36821)

►(For chemotherapy for malignant disease, see 96409-96549)◄

(For penile plethysmography, use 54240)

93701 Bioimpedance, thoracic, electrical

93720 Plethysmography, total body; with interpretation and report

93721 tracing only, without interpretation and report

93722 interpretation and report only

(For regional plethysmography, see 93875-93931)

93724 Electronic analysis of antitachycardia pacemaker system (includes electrocardiographic recording, programming of device, induction and termination of tachycardia via implanted pacemaker, and interpretation of recordings)

93727 Electronic analysis of implantable loop recorder (ILR) system (includes retrieval of recorded and stored ECG data, physician review and interpretation of retrieved ECG data and reprogramming)

93731 Electronic analysis of dual-chamber pacemaker system (includes evaluation of programmable parameters at rest and during activity where applicable, using electrocardiographic recording and interpretation of recordings at rest and during exercise, analysis of event markers and device response); without reprogramming

93732 with reprogramming

93733 Electronic analysis of dual chamber internal pacemaker system (may include rate, pulse amplitude and duration, configuration of wave form, and/or testing of sensory function of pacemaker), telephonic analysis

93734 Electronic analysis of single chamber pacemaker system (includes evaluation of programmable parameters at rest and during activity where applicable, using electrocardiographic recording and interpretation of recordings at rest and during exercise, analysis of event markers and device response); without reprogramming

93735 with reprogramming

93736 Electronic analysis of single chamber internal pacemaker system (may include rate, pulse amplitude and duration, configuration of wave form, and/or testing of sensory function of pacemaker), telephonic analysis

93740 Temperature gradient studies

93741 Electronic analysis of pacing cardioverter-defibrillator (includes interrogation, evaluation of pulse generator status, evaluation of programmable parameters at rest and during activity where applicable, using electrocardiographic recording and interpretation of recordings at rest and during exercise, analysis of event markers and device response); single chamber or wearable cardioverter-defibrillator system, without reprogramming

(Do not report 93741 in conjunction with 93745)

93742 single chamber or wearable cardioverter-defibrillator system, with reprogramming

(Do not report 93742 in conjunction with 93745)

93743 dual chamber, without reprogramming

93744 dual chamber, with reprogramming

93745 Initial set-up and programming by a physician of wearable cardioverter-defibrillator includes initial programming of system, establishing baseline electronic ECG, transmission of data to data repository, patient instruction in wearing system and patient reporting of problems or events

(Do not report 93745 in conjunction with 93741, 93742)

93760 Thermogram; cephalic

93762 peripheral

93770 Determination of venous pressure

(For central venous cannulization see 36555-36556, 36500)

93784 Ambulatory blood pressure monitoring, utilizing a system such as magnetic tape and/or computer disk, for 24 hours or longer; including recording, scanning analysis, interpretation and report

93786 recording only

93788 scanning analysis with report

93790 physician review with interpretation and report

Other Procedures

93797 Physician services for outpatient cardiac rehabilitation; without continuous ECG monitoring (per session)

93798 with continuous ECG monitoring (per session)

93799 Unlisted cardiovascular service or procedure

Noninvasive Vascular Diagnostic Studies

Vascular studies include patient care required to perform the studies, supervision of the studies and interpretation of study results with copies for patient records of hard copy output with analysis of all data, including bidirectional vascular flow or imaging when provided.

The use of a simple hand-held or other Doppler device that does not produce hard copy output, or that produces a record that does not permit analysis of bidirectional vascular flow, is considered to be part of the physical examination of the vascular system and is not separately reported.

Duplex scan (eg, 93880, 93882) describes an ultrasonic scanning procedure for characterizing the pattern and direction of blood flow in arteries or veins with the production of real time images integrating B-mode two-dimensional vascular structure with spectral and/or color flow Doppler mapping or imaging.

Noninvasive physiologic studies are performed using equipment separate and distinct from the duplex scanner. Codes 93875, 93965, 93922, 93923, and 93924 describe the evaluation of non-imaging physiologic recordings of pressures, Doppler analysis of bi-directional blood flow, plethysmography, and/or oxygen tension measurements appropriate for the anatomic area studied.

Cerebrovascular Arterial Studies

A complete transcranial Doppler (TCD) study (93886) includes ultrasound evaluation of the right and left anterior circulation territories and the posterior circulation territory (to include vertebral arteries and basilar artery). In a limited TCD study (93888) there is ultrasound evaluation of two or fewer of these territories. For TCD, ultrasound evaluation is a reasonable and concerted attempt to identify arterial signals through an acoustic window.

93875   Noninvasive physiologic studies of extracranial arteries, complete bilateral study (eg, periorbital flow direction with arterial compression, ocular pneumoplethysmography, Doppler ultrasound spectral analysis)

93880   Duplex scan of extracranial arteries; complete bilateral study

93882   unilateral or limited study

     (To report common carotid intima-media thickness (IMT) study for evaluation of atherosclerotic burden or coronary heart disease risk factor assessment, use Category III code 0126T)

93886   Transcranial Doppler study of the intracranial arteries; complete study

93888   limited study

93890   vasoreactivity study

93892   emboli detection without intravenous microbubble injection

93893   emboli detection with intravenous microbubble injection

     (Do not report 93890-93893 in conjunction with 93888)

Extremity Arterial Studies (Including Digits)

93922   Noninvasive physiologic studies of upper or lower extremity arteries, single level, bilateral (eg, ankle/brachial indices, Doppler waveform analysis, volume plethysmography, transcutaneous oxygen tension measurement)

93923   Noninvasive physiologic studies of upper or lower extremity arteries, multiple levels or with provocative functional maneuvers, complete bilateral study (eg, segmental blood pressure measurements, segmental Doppler waveform analysis, segmental volume plethysmography, segmental transcutaneous oxygen tension measurements, measurements with postural provocative tests, measurements with reactive hyperemia)

93924   Noninvasive physiologic studies of lower extremity arteries, at rest and following treadmill stress testing, complete bilateral study

93925   Duplex scan of lower extremity arteries or arterial bypass grafts; complete bilateral study

93926   unilateral or limited study

93930   Duplex scan of upper extremity arteries or arterial bypass grafts; complete bilateral study

93931   unilateral or limited study

Extremity Venous Studies (Including Digits)

93965   Noninvasive physiologic studies of extremity veins, complete bilateral study (eg, Doppler waveform analysis with responses to compression and other maneuvers, phleborheography, impedance plethysmography)

93970   Duplex scan of extremity veins including responses to compression and other maneuvers; complete bilateral study

93971   unilateral or limited study

Medicine

Visceral and Penile Vascular Studies

93975 Duplex scan of arterial inflow and venous outflow of abdominal, pelvic, scrotal contents and/or retroperitoneal organs; complete study

93976 limited study

93978 Duplex scan of aorta, inferior vena cava, iliac vasculature, or bypass grafts; complete study

93979 unilateral or limited study

93980 Duplex scan of arterial inflow and venous outflow of penile vessels; complete study

93981 follow-up or limited study

Extremity Arterial-Venous Studies

93990 Duplex scan of hemodialysis access (including arterial inflow, body of access and venous outflow)

(For measurement of hemodialysis access flow using indicator dilution methods, use 90940)

Pulmonary

►Ventilator Management◄

● **94002** Ventilation assist and management, initiation of pressure or volume preset ventilators for assisted or controlled breathing; hospital inpatient/observation, initial day

● **94003** hospital inpatient/observation, each subsequent day

● **94004** nursing facility, per day

►(Do not report 94002-94004 in conjunction with Evaluation and Management services 99201-99499)◄

● **94005** Home ventilator management care plan oversight of a patient (patient not present) in home, domiciliary or rest home (eg, assisted living) requiring review of status, review of laboratories and other studies and revision of orders and respiratory care plan (as appropriate), within a calendar month, 30 minutes or more

►(Do not report 94005 in conjunction with 99339-99340, 99374-99378)◄

►(Ventilator management care plan oversight is reported separately from home or domiciliary, rest home [eg, assisted living] services. A physician may report 94005, when performed, including when a different physician reports 99339-99340, 99374-99378 for the same 30 days)◄

►Other Procedures◄

Codes 94010-94799 include laboratory procedure(s) and interpretation of test results. If a separate identifiable Evaluation and Management service is performed, the appropriate E/M service code should be reported in addition to 94010-94799.

94010 Spirometry, including graphic record, total and timed vital capacity, expiratory flow rate measurement(s), with or without maximal voluntary ventilation

94014 Patient-initiated spirometric recording per 30-day period of time; includes reinforced education, transmission of spirometric tracing, data capture, analysis of transmitted data, periodic recalibration and physician review and interpretation

94015 recording (includes hook-up, reinforced education, data transmission, data capture, trend analysis, and periodic recalibration)

94016 physician review and interpretation only

94060 Bronchodilation responsiveness, spirometry as in 94010, pre- and post-bronchodilator administration

(Report bronchodilator supply separately with 99070 or appropriate supply code)

(For prolonged exercise test for bronchospasm with pre- and post-spirometry, use 94620)

94070 Bronchospasm provocation evaluation, multiple spirometric determinations as in 94010, with administered agents (eg, antigen(s), cold air, methacholine)

(Report antigen(s) administration separately with 99070 or appropriate supply code)

94150 Vital capacity, total (separate procedure)

94200 Maximum breathing capacity, maximal voluntary ventilation

94240 Functional residual capacity or residual volume: helium method, nitrogen open circuit method, or other method

94250 Expired gas collection, quantitative, single procedure (separate procedure)

94260 Thoracic gas volume

(For plethysmography, see 93720-93722)

94350 Determination of maldistribution of inspired gas: multiple breath nitrogen washout curve including alveolar nitrogen or helium equilibration time

94360 Determination of resistance to airflow, oscillatory or plethysmographic methods

94370 Determination of airway closing volume, single breath tests

94375 Respiratory flow volume loop

94400 Breathing response to CO_2 (CO_2 response curve)

94450   Breathing response to hypoxia (hypoxia response curve)

(For high altitude simulation test (HAST), see 94452, 94453)

94452   High altitude simulation test (HAST), with physician interpretation and report;

(For obtaining arterial blood gases, use 36600)

(Do not report 94452 in conjunction with 94453, 94760, 94761)

94453   with supplemental oxygen titration

(For obtaining arterial blood gases, use 36600)

(Do not report 94453 in conjunction with 94452, 94760, 94761)

⊘● **94610**   Intrapulmonary surfactant administration by a physician through endotracheal tube

►(Do not report 94610 in conjunction with 99293-99296)◄

►(For endotracheal intubation, use 31500)◄

►(Report 94610 once per dosing episode)◄

▲ **94620**   Pulmonary stress testing; simple (eg, 6-minute walk test, prolonged exercise test for bronchospasm with pre- and post-spirometry and oximetry)

94621   complex (including measurements of CO_2 production, O_2 uptake, and electrocardiographic recordings)

94640   Pressurized or nonpressurized inhalation treatment for acute airway obstruction or for sputum induction for diagnostic purposes (eg, with an aerosol generator, nebulizer, metered dose inhaler or intermittent positive pressure breathing [IPPB] device)

(For more than 1 inhalation treatment performed on the same date, append modifier 76)

►(For continuous inhalation treatment of 1 hour or more, see 94644, 94645)◄

94642   Aerosol inhalation of pentamidine for pneumocystis carinii pneumonia treatment or prophylaxis

● **94644**   Continuous inhalation treatment with aerosol medication for acute airway obstruction; first hour

►(For services of less than 1 hour, use 94640)◄

+● **94645**   each additional hour (List separately in addition to code for primary procedure)

►(Use 94645 in conjunction with 94644)◄

►(94656, 94657 have been deleted. To report, see 94002-94005)◄

94660   Continuous positive airway pressure ventilation (CPAP), initiation and management

94662   Continuous negative pressure ventilation (CNP), initiation and management

94664   Demonstration and/or evaluation of patient utilization of an aerosol generator, nebulizer, metered dose inhaler or IPPB device

(94664 can be reported one time only per day of service)

94667   Manipulation chest wall, such as cupping, percussing, and vibration to facilitate lung function; initial demonstration and/or evaluation

94668   subsequent

94680   Oxygen uptake, expired gas analysis; rest and exercise, direct, simple

94681   including CO_2 output, percentage oxygen extracted

94690   rest, indirect (separate procedure)

(For single arterial puncture, use 36600)

94720   Carbon monoxide diffusing capacity (eg, single breath, steady state)

94725   Membrane diffusion capacity

94750   Pulmonary compliance study (eg, plethysmography, volume and pressure measurements)

94760   Noninvasive ear or pulse oximetry for oxygen saturation; single determination

(For blood gases, see 82803-82810)

94761   multiple determinations (eg, during exercise)

94762   by continuous overnight monitoring (separate procedure)

94770   Carbon dioxide, expired gas determination by infrared analyzer

(For bronchoscopy, see 31622-31656)

(For placement of flow directed catheter, use 93503)

(For venipuncture, use 36410)

(For central venous catheter placement, see 36555-36556)

(For arterial puncture, use 36600)

(For arterial catheterization, use 36620)

(For thoracentesis, use 32000)

(For phlebotomy, therapeutic, use 99195)

(For lung biopsy, needle, use 32405)

(For intubation, orotracheal or nasotracheal, use 31500)

94772   Circadian respiratory pattern recording (pediatric pneumogram), 12-24 hour continuous recording, infant

(Separate procedure codes for electromyograms, EEG, ECG, and recordings of respiration are excluded when 94772 is reported)

Medicine

● **94774**   Pediatric home apnea monitoring event recording including respiratory rate, pattern and heart rate per 30-day period of time; includes monitor attachment, download of data, physician review, interpretation, and preparation of a report

►(Do not report 94774 in conjunction with 94775-94777 during the same reporting period)◄

● **94775**   monitor attachment only (includes hook-up, initiation of recording and disconnection)

● **94776**   monitoring, download of information, receipt of transmission(s) and analyses by computer only

● **94777**   physician review, interpretation and preparation of report only

►(When oxygen saturation monitoring is used in addition to heart rate and respiratory monitoring, it is not reported separately)◄

►(Do not report 94774-94777 in conjunction with 93224-93272)◄

►(Do not report apnea recording device separately)◄

►(For sleep study, see 95805-95811)◄

94799   Unlisted pulmonary service or procedure

Allergy and Clinical Immunology

Definitions

Immunotherapy (desensitization, hyposensitization) is the parenteral administration of allergenic extracts as antigens at periodic intervals, usually on an increasing dosage scale to a dosage which is maintained as maintenance therapy. Indications for immunotherapy are determined by appropriate diagnostic procedures coordinated with clinical judgment and knowledge of the natural history of allergic diseases.

Other therapy: for medical conferences on the use of mechanical and electronic devices (precipitators, air conditioners, air filters, humidifiers, dehumidifiers), climatotherapy, physical therapy, occupational and recreational therapy, see **Evaluation and Management** section.

Allergy Testing

►(For allergy laboratory tests, see 86000-86999)◄

►(For therapy for severe or intractable allergic disease, see 90765-90768, 90772, 90774, 90775)◄

95004   Percutaneous tests (scratch, puncture, prick) with allergenic extracts, immediate type reaction, specify number of tests

95010   Percutaneous tests (scratch, puncture, prick) sequential and incremental, with drugs, biologicals or venoms, immediate type reaction, specify number of tests

● **95012**   Nitric oxide expired gas determination

►(For nitric oxide determination by spectroscopy, use Category III code 0064T)◄

95015   Intracutaneous (intradermal) tests, sequential and incremental, with drugs, biologicals, or venoms, immediate type reaction, specify number of tests

95024   Intracutaneous (intradermal) tests with allergenic extracts, immediate type reaction, specify number of tests

95027   Intracutaneous (intradermal) tests, sequential and incremental, with allergenic extracts for airborne allergens, immediate type reaction, specify number of tests

95028   Intracutaneous (intradermal) tests with allergenic extracts, delayed type reaction, including reading, specify number of tests

95044   Patch or application test(s) (specify number of tests)

95052   Photo patch test(s) (specify number of tests)

95056   Photo tests

95060   Ophthalmic mucous membrane tests

95065   Direct nasal mucous membrane test

95070   Inhalation bronchial challenge testing (not including necessary pulmonary function tests); with histamine, methacholine, or similar compounds

95071   with antigens or gases, specify

(For pulmonary function tests, see 94060, 94070)

95075   Ingestion challenge test (sequential and incremental ingestion of test items, eg, food, drug or other substance such as metabisulfite)

►(95078 has been deleted)◄

Allergen Immunotherapy

Codes 95115-95199 include the professional services necessary for allergen immunotherapy. Office visit codes may be used in addition to allergen immunotherapy if other identifiable services are provided at that time.

95115   Professional services for allergen immunotherapy not including provision of allergenic extracts; single injection

95117   two or more injections

95120   Professional services for allergen immunotherapy in prescribing physicians office or institution, including provision of allergenic extract; single injection

95125   two or more injections

95130   single stinging insect venom

95131   two stinging insect venoms

Medicine

95132	three stinging insect venoms
95133	four stinging insect venoms
95134	five stinging insect venoms
95144	Professional services for the supervision of preparation and provision of antigens for allergen immunotherapy, single dose vial(s) (specify number of vials)

(A single dose vial contains a single dose of antigen administered in one injection)

95145	Professional services for the supervision of preparation and provision of antigens for allergen immunotherapy (specify number of doses); single stinging insect venom
95146	two single stinging insect venoms
95147	three single stinging insect venoms
95148	four single stinging insect venoms
95149	five single stinging insect venoms
95165	Professional services for the supervision of preparation and provision of antigens for allergen immunotherapy; single or multiple antigens (specify number of doses)
95170	whole body extract of biting insect or other arthropod (specify number of doses)

(For allergy immunotherapy reporting, a dose is the amount of antigen(s) administered in a single injection from a multiple dose vial)

95180	Rapid desensitization procedure, each hour (eg, insulin, penicillin, equine serum)
95199	Unlisted allergy/clinical immunologic service or procedure

(For skin testing of bacterial, viral, fungal extracts, see 95028, 86485-86586)

(For special reports on allergy patients, use 99080)

(For testing procedures such as radioallergosorbent testing (RAST), rat mast cell technique (RMCT), mast cell degranulation test (MCDT), lymphocytic transformation test (LTT), leukocyte histamine release (LHR), migration inhibitory factor test (MIF), transfer factor test (TFT), nitroblue tetrazolium dye test (NTD), see Immunology section in **Pathology** or use 95199)

Endocrinology

95250	Ambulatory continuous glucose monitoring of interstitial tissue fluid via a subcutaneous sensor for up to 72 hours; sensor placement, hook-up, calibration of monitor, patient training, removal of sensor, and printout of recording

(Do not report 95250 in conjunction with 99091)

95251	physician interpretation and report

(Do not report 95250, 95251 in conjunction with 99091)

Neurology and Neuromuscular Procedures

Neurologic services are typically consultative, and any of the levels of consultation (99241-99255) may be appropriate.

In addition, services and skills outlined under **Evaluation and Management** levels of service appropriate to neurologic illnesses should be reported similarly.

The EEG, autonomic function, evoked potential, reflex tests, EMG, NCV, and MEG services (95812-95829 and 95860-95967) include recording, interpretation by a physician, and report. For interpretation only, use modifier 26. For EMG guidance, see 95873, 95874.

►(For repetitive transcranial magnetic stimulation for treatment of clinical depression, see Category III codes 0160T, 0161T)◄

(Do not report codes 95860-95875 in addition to 96000-96004)

Sleep Testing

Sleep studies and polysomnography refer to the continuous and simultaneous monitoring and recording of various physiological and pathophysiological parameters of sleep for 6 or more hours with physician review, interpretation and report. The studies are performed to diagnose a variety of sleep disorders and to evaluate a patient's response to therapies such as nasal continuous positive airway pressure (NCPAP). Polysomnography is distinguished from sleep studies by the inclusion of sleep staging which is defined to include a 1-4 lead electroencephalogram (EEG), an electro-oculogram (EOG), and a submental electromyogram (EMG). Additional parameters of sleep include: 1) ECG; 2) airflow; 3) ventilation and respiratory effort; 4) gas exchange by oximetry, transcutaneous monitoring, or end tidal gas analysis; 5) extremity muscle activity, motor activity-movement; 6) extended EEG monitoring; 7) penile tumescence; 8) gastroesophageal reflux; 9) continuous blood pressure monitoring; 10) snoring; 11) body positions; etc.

The sleep services (95805-95811) include recording, interpretation and report. For interpretation only, use modifier 26.

For a study to be reported as polysomnography, sleep must be recorded and staged.

(Report with modifier 52 if less than 6 hours of recording or in other cases of reduced services as appropriate)

(For unattended sleep study, use 95806)

95805	Multiple sleep latency or maintenance of wakefulness testing, recording, analysis and interpretation of physiological measurements of sleep during multiple trials to assess sleepiness

Medicine

95806 Sleep study, simultaneous recording of ventilation, respiratory effort, ECG or heart rate, and oxygen saturation, unattended by a technologist

95807 Sleep study, simultaneous recording of ventilation, respiratory effort, ECG or heart rate, and oxygen saturation, attended by a technologist

95808 Polysomnography; sleep staging with 1-3 additional parameters of sleep, attended by a technologist

95810 sleep staging with 4 or more additional parameters of sleep, attended by a technologist

95811 sleep staging with 4 or more additional parameters of sleep, with initiation of continuous positive airway pressure therapy or bilevel ventilation, attended by a technologist

Routine Electroencephalography (EEG)

EEG codes 95812-95822 include hyperventilation and/or photic stimulation when appropriate. Routine EEG codes 95816-95822 include 20 to 40 minutes of recording. Extended EEG codes 95812-95813 include reporting times longer than 40 minutes.

95812 Electroencephalogram (EEG) extended monitoring; 41-60 minutes

95813 greater than one hour

95816 Electroencephalogram (EEG); including recording awake and drowsy

95819 including recording awake and asleep

95822 recording in coma or sleep only

95824 cerebral death evaluation only

95827 all night recording

(For 24-hour EEG monitoring, see 95950-95953 or 95956)

(For EEG during nonintracranial surgery, use 95955)

(For Wada test, use 95958)

(For digital analysis of EEG, use 95957)

95829 Electrocorticogram at surgery (separate procedure)

95830 Insertion by physician of sphenoidal electrodes for electroencephalographic (EEG) recording

Muscle and Range of Motion Testing

95831 Muscle testing, manual (separate procedure) with report; extremity (excluding hand) or trunk

95832 hand, with or without comparison with normal side

95833 total evaluation of body, excluding hands

95834 total evaluation of body, including hands

95851 Range of motion measurements and report (separate procedure); each extremity (excluding hand) or each trunk section (spine)

95852 hand, with or without comparison with normal side

95857 Tensilon test for myasthenia gravis

(95858 has been deleted)

Electromyography and Nerve Conduction Tests

Needle electromyographic procedures include the interpretation of electrical waveforms measured by equipment that produces both visible and audible components of electrical signals recorded from the muscle(s) studied by the needle electrode.

95860 Needle electromyography; one extremity with or without related paraspinal areas

95861 two extremities with or without related paraspinal areas

(For dynamic electromyography performed during motion analysis studies, see 96002-96003)

95863 three extremities with or without related paraspinal areas

95864 four extremities with or without related paraspinal areas

95865 larynx

(Do not report modifier 50 in conjunction with 95865)

(For unilateral procedure, report modifier 52 in conjunction with 95865)

95866 hemidiaphragm

95867 cranial nerve supplied muscle(s), unilateral

95868 cranial nerve supplied muscles, bilateral

95869 thoracic paraspinal muscles (excluding T1 or T12)

95870 limited study of muscles in one extremity or non-limb (axial) muscles (unilateral or bilateral), other than thoracic paraspinal, cranial nerve supplied muscles, or sphincters

(To report a complete study of the extremities, see 95860-95864)

(For anal or urethral sphincter, detrusor, urethra, perineum musculature, see 51785-51792)

(For eye muscles, use 92265)

95872 Needle electromyography using single fiber electrode, with quantitative measurement of jitter, blocking and/or fiber density, any/all sites of each muscle studied

+ 95873 Electrical stimulation for guidance in conjunction with chemodenervation (List separately in addition to code for primary procedure)

Medicine

+ 95874   Needle electromyography for guidance in conjunction with chemodenervation (List separately in addition to code for primary procedure)

(Use 95873, 95874 in conjunction with 64612-64614)

(Do not report 95874 in conjunction with 95873)

(Do not report 95873, 95874 in conjunction with 95860-95870)

95875   Ischemic limb exercise test with serial specimen(s) acquisition for muscle(s) metabolite(s)

(For listing of nerves considered for separate study, see Appendix J)

⊘ **95900**   Nerve conduction, amplitude and latency/velocity study, each nerve; motor, without F-wave study

⊘ **95903**   motor, with F-wave study

⊘ **95904**   sensory

(Report 95900, 95903, and/or 95904 only once when multiple sites on the same nerve are stimulated or recorded)

Intraoperative Neurophysiology

+ 95920   Intraoperative neurophysiology testing, per hour (List separately in addition to code for primary procedure)

(Use 95920 in conjunction with the study performed, 92585, 95822, 95860, 95861, 95867, 95868, 95870, 95900, 95904, 95925-95937)

(Code 95920 describes ongoing electrophysiologic testing and monitoring performed during surgical procedures. Code 95920 is reported per hour of service, and includes only the ongoing electrophysiologic monitoring time distinct from performance of specific type(s) of baseline electrophysiologic study(s) (95860, 95861, 95867, 95868, 95870, 95900, 95904, 95928, 95929, 95933-95937) or interpretation of specific type(s) of baseline electrophysiologic study(s) (92585, 95822, 95870, 95925-95928, 95929, 95930). The time spent performing or interpreting the baseline electrophysiologic study(s) should not be counted as intraoperative monitoring, but represents separately reportable procedures. Code 95920 should be used once per hour even if multiple electrophysiologic studies are performed. The baseline electrophysiologic study(s) should be used once per operative session.)

(For electrocorticography, use 95829)

(For intraoperative EEG during nonintracranial surgery, use 95955)

(For intraoperative functional cortical or subcortical mapping, see 95961-95962)

(For intraoperative neurostimulator programming and analysis, see 95970-95975)

Autonomic Function Tests

95921   Testing of autonomic nervous system function; cardiovagal innervation (parasympathetic function), including two or more of the following: heart rate response to deep breathing with recorded R-R interval, Valsalva ratio, and 30:15 ratio

95922   vasomotor adrenergic innervation (sympathetic adrenergic function), including beat-to-beat blood pressure and R-R interval changes during Valsalva maneuver and at least five minutes of passive tilt

95923   sudomotor, including one or more of the following: quantitative sudomotor axon reflex test (QSART), silastic sweat imprint, thermoregulatory sweat test, and changes in sympathetic skin potential

Evoked Potentials and Reflex Tests

95925   Short-latency somatosensory evoked potential study, stimulation of any/all peripheral nerves or skin sites, recording from the central nervous system; in upper limbs

95926   in lower limbs

95927   in the trunk or head

(To report a unilateral study, use modifier 52)

(For auditory evoked potentials, use 92585)

95928   Central motor evoked potential study (transcranial motor stimulation); upper limbs

95929   lower limbs

95930   Visual evoked potential (VEP) testing central nervous system, checkerboard or flash

95933   Orbicularis oculi (blink) reflex, by electrodiagnostic testing

95934   H-reflex, amplitude and latency study; record gastrocnemius/soleus muscle

95936   record muscle other than gastrocnemius/soleus muscle

(To report a bilateral study, use modifier 50)

95937   Neuromuscular junction testing (repetitive stimulation, paired stimuli), each nerve, any one method

Special EEG Tests

95950   Monitoring for identification and lateralization of cerebral seizure focus, electroencephalographic (eg, 8 channel EEG) recording and interpretation, each 24 hours

95951   Monitoring for localization of cerebral seizure focus by cable or radio, 16 or more channel telemetry, combined electroencephalographic (EEG) and video recording and interpretation (eg, for presurgical localization), each 24 hours

Medicine

95953 Monitoring for localization of cerebral seizure focus by computerized portable 16 or more channel EEG, electroencephalographic (EEG) recording and interpretation, each 24 hours

95954 Pharmacological or physical activation requiring physician attendance during EEG recording of activation phase (eg, thiopental activation test)

95955 Electroencephalogram (EEG) during nonintracranial surgery (eg, carotid surgery)

95956 Monitoring for localization of cerebral seizure focus by cable or radio, 16 or more channel telemetry, electroencephalographic (EEG) recording and interpretation, each 24 hours

95957 Digital analysis of electroencephalogram (EEG) (eg, for epileptic spike analysis)

95958 Wada activation test for hemispheric function, including electroencephalographic (EEG) monitoring

95961 Functional cortical and subcortical mapping by stimulation and/or recording of electrodes on brain surface, or of depth electrodes, to provoke seizures or identify vital brain structures; initial hour of physician attendance

+ 95962 each additional hour of physician attendance (List separately in addition to code for primary procedure)

(Use 95962 in conjunction with 95961)

95965 Magnetoencephalography (MEG), recording and analysis; for spontaneous brain magnetic activity (eg, epileptic cerebral cortex localization)

95966 for evoked magnetic fields, single modality (eg, sensory, motor, language, or visual cortex localization)

+ 95967 for evoked magnetic fields, each additional modality (eg, sensory, motor, language, or visual cortex localization) (List separately in addition to code for primary procedure)

(Use 95967 in conjunction with 95966)

(For electroencephalography performed in addition to magnetoencephalography, see 95812-95827)

(For somatosensory evoked potentials, auditory evoked potentials, and visual evoked potentials performed in addition to magnetic evoked field responses, see 92585, 95925, 95926, and/or 95930)

(For computerized tomography performed in addition to magnetoencephalography, see 70450-70470, 70496)

(For magnetic resonance imaging performed in addition to magnetoencephalography, see 70551-70553)

Neurostimulators, Analysis-Programming

A simple neurostimulator pulse generator/transmitter (95970, 95971) is one capable of affecting 3 or fewer of the following: pulse amplitude, pulse duration, pulse frequency, 8 or more electrode contacts, cycling, stimulation train duration, train spacing, number of programs, number of channels, alternating electrode polarities, dose time (stimulation parameters changing in time periods of minutes including dose lockout times), more than 1 clinical feature (eg, rigidity, dyskinesia, tremor). A complex neurostimulator pulse generator/transmitter (95970-95975) is one capable of affecting more than 3 of the above.

Code 95970 describes subsequent electronic analysis of a previously-implanted simple or complex brain, spinal cord, or peripheral neurostimulator pulse generator system, without reprogramming. Code 95971 describes intraoperative or subsequent electronic analysis of an implanted simple spinal cord, or peripheral (i.e., peripheral nerve, autonomic nerve, neuromuscular) neurostimulator pulse generator system, with programming. Codes 95972 and 95973 describe intraoperative (at initial insertion/revision) or subsequent electronic analysis of an implanted complex spinal cord or peripheral (except cranial nerve) neurostimulator pulse generator system, with programming. Codes 95974 and 95975 describe intraoperative (at initial insertion/revision) or subsequent electronic analysis of an implanted complex cranial nerve neurostimulator pulse generator system, with programming. Codes 95978 and 95979 describe initial or subsequent electronic analysis of an implanted brain neurostimulator pulse generator system, with programming.

►(For insertion of neurostimulator pulse generator, see 61885, 63685, 64590)◄

(For revision or removal of neurostimulator pulse generator or receiver, see 61888, 63688, 64595)

►(For implantation of neurostimulator electrodes, see 43647, 43881, 61850-61875, 63650-63655, 64553-64580, 0155T, 0157T. For revision or removal of neurostimulator electrodes, see 43648, 43882, 61880, 63660, 64585, 0156T, 0158T)◄

95970 Electronic analysis of implanted neurostimulator pulse generator system (eg, rate, pulse amplitude and duration, configuration of wave form, battery status, electrode selectability, output modulation, cycling, impedance and patient compliance measurements); simple or complex brain, spinal cord, or peripheral (ie, cranial nerve, peripheral nerve, autonomic nerve, neuromuscular) neurostimulator pulse generator/transmitter, without reprogramming

95971 simple spinal cord, or peripheral (ie, peripheral nerve, autonomic nerve, neuromuscular) neurostimulator pulse generator/transmitter, with intraoperative or subsequent programming

95972   complex spinal cord, or peripheral (except cranial nerve) neurostimulator pulse generator/transmitter, with intraoperative or subsequent programming, first hour

+ 95973   complex spinal cord, or peripheral (except cranial nerve) neurostimulator pulse generator/transmitter, with intraoperative or subsequent programming, each additional 30 minutes after first hour (List separately in addition to code for primary procedure)

(Use 95973 in conjunction with 95972)

95974   complex cranial nerve neurostimulator pulse generator/transmitter, with intraoperative or subsequent programming, with or without nerve interface testing, first hour

+ 95975   complex cranial nerve neurostimulator pulse generator/transmitter, with intraoperative or subsequent programming, each additional 30 minutes after first hour (List separately in addition to code for primary procedure)

(Use 95975 in conjunction with 95974)

►(For electronic analysis, programming, and reprogramming of gastric neurostimulator pulse generator, lesser curvature [morbid obesity], use Category III code 0162T)◄

95978   Electronic analysis of implanted neurostimulator pulse generator system (eg, rate, pulse amplitude and duration, battery status, electrode selectability and polarity, impedance and patient compliance measurements), complex deep brain neurostimulator pulse generator/transmitter, with initial or subsequent programming; first hour

+ 95979   each additional 30 minutes after first hour (List separately in addition to code for primary procedure)

(Use 95979 in conjunction with 95978)

Other Procedures

95990   Refilling and maintenance of implantable pump or reservoir for drug delivery, spinal (intrathecal, epidural) or brain (intraventricular);

(For analysis and/or reprogramming of implantable infusion pump, see 62367-62368)

►(For refill and maintenance of implanted infusion pump or reservoir for systemic drug therapy [eg, chemotherapy or insulin], use 96522)◄

95991   administered by physician

95999   Unlisted neurological or neuromuscular diagnostic procedure

Motion Analysis

Codes 96000-96004 describe services performed as part of a major therapeutic or diagnostic decision making process. Motion analysis is performed in a dedicated motion analysis laboratory (ie, a facility capable of performing videotaping from the front, back and both sides, computerized 3-D kinematics, 3-D kinetics, and dynamic electromyography). Code 96000 may include 3-D kinetics and stride characteristics. Codes 96002-96003 describe dynamic electromyography.

Code 96004 should only be reported once regardless of the number of study(ies) reviewed/interpreted.

(For performance of needle electromyography procedures, see 95860-95875)

(For gait training, use 97116)

96000   Comprehensive computer-based motion analysis by video-taping and 3-D kinematics;

96001   with dynamic plantar pressure measurements during walking

96002   Dynamic surface electromyography, during walking or other functional activities, 1-12 muscles

96003   Dynamic fine wire electromyography, during walking or other functional activities, 1 muscle

(Do not report 96002, 96003 in conjunction with 95860-95864, 95869-95872)

96004   Physician review and interpretation of comprehensive computer-based motion analysis, dynamic plantar pressure measurements, dynamic surface electromyography during walking or other functional activities, and dynamic fine wire electromyography, with written report

►Functional Brain Mapping◄

►Code 96020 includes selection and administration of testing of language, memory, cognition, movement, sensation, and other neurological functions when conducted in association with functional neuroimaging, monitoring of performance of this testing, and determination of validity of neurofunctional testing relative to separately interpreted functional magnetic resonance images.◄

● **96020**   Neurofunctional testing selection and administration during noninvasive imaging functional brain mapping, with test administered entirely by a physician or psychologist, with review of test results and report

►(For functional magnetic resonance imaging [fMRI], brain, use 70555)◄

►(Do not report 96020 in conjunction with 96101-96103, 96116-96120)◄

►(Do not report 96020 in conjunction with 70554)◄

►(Evaluation and Management services codes should not be reported on the same day as 96020)◄

Medicine

►Medical Genetics and Genetic Counseling Services◄

►These services are provided by trained genetic counselors and may include obtaining a structured family genetic history, pedigree construction, analysis for genetic risk assessment, and counseling of the patient and family. These activities may be provided during one or more sessions and may include review of medical data and family information, face-to-face interviews, and counseling services.◄

● **96040**   Medical genetics and genetic counseling services, each 30 minutes face-to-face with patient/family

►(For genetic counseling and education provided by a physician to an individual, see the appropriate Evaluation and Management codes)◄

►(For genetic counseling and education provided by a physician to a group, use 99078)◄

►(For education regarding genetic risks by a nonphysician to a group, see 98961, 98962)◄

►(For genetic counseling and/or risk factor reduction intervention provided by a physician to patient(s) without symptoms or established disease, see 99401-99412)◄

Central Nervous System Assessments/Tests (eg, Neuro-Cognitive, Mental Status, Speech Testing)

The following codes are used to report the services provided during testing of the cognitive function of the central nervous system. The testing of cognitive processes, visual motor responses, and abstractive abilities is accomplished by the combination of several types of testing procedures. It is expected that the administration of these tests will generate material that will be formulated into a report.

(96100 has been deleted. To report, see 96101, 96102, 96103)

(For development of cognitive skills, see 97532, 97533)

(For mini-mental status examination performed by a physician, see **Evaluation and Management** services codes)

96101   Psychological testing (includes psychodiagnostic assessment of emotionality, intellectual abilities, personality and psychopathology, eg, MMPI, Rorschach, WAIS), per hour of the psychologist's or physician's time, both face-to-face time with the patient and time interpreting test results and preparing the report

96102   Psychological testing (includes psychodiagnostic assessment of emotionality, intellectual abilities, personality and psychopathology, eg, MMPI and WAIS), with qualified health care professional interpretation and report, administered by technician, per hour of technician time, face-to-face

96103   Psychological testing (includes psychodiagnostic assessment of emotionality, intellectual abilities, personality and psychopathology, eg, MMPI), administered by a computer, with qualified health care professional interpretation and report

96105   Assessment of aphasia (includes assessment of expressive and receptive speech and language function, language comprehension, speech production ability, reading, spelling, writing, eg, by Boston Diagnostic Aphasia Examination) with interpretation and report, per hour

96110   Developmental testing; limited (eg, Developmental Screening Test II, Early Language Milestone Screen), with interpretation and report

96111   extended (includes assessment of motor, language, social, adaptive and/or cognitive functioning by standardized developmental instruments) with interpretation and report

(96115 has been deleted. To report, use 96116)

96116   Neurobehavioral status exam (clinical assessment of thinking, reasoning and judgment, eg, acquired knowledge, attention, language, memory, planning and problem solving, and visual spatial abilities), per hour of the psychologist's or physician's time, both face-to-face time with the patient and time interpreting test results and preparing the report

(96117 has been deleted. To report, see 96118, 96119, 96120)

96118   Neuropsychological testing (eg, Halstead-Reitan Neuropsychological Battery, Wechsler Memory Scales and Wisconsin Card Sorting Test), per hour of the psychologist's or physician's time, both face-to-face time with the patient and time interpreting test results and preparing the report

96119   Neuropsychological testing (eg, Halstead-Reitan Neuropsychological Battery, Wechsler Memory Scales and Wisconsin Card Sorting Test), with qualified health care professional interpretation and report, administered by technician, per hour of technician time, face-to-face

96120   Neuropsychological testing (eg, Wisconsin Card Sorting Test), administered by a computer, with qualified health care professional interpretation and report

Medicine

Health and Behavior Assessment/Intervention

Health and behavior assessment procedures are used to identify the psychological, behavioral, emotional, cognitive, and social factors important to the prevention, treatment, or management of physical health problems.

The focus of the assessment is not on mental health but on the biopsychosocial factors important to physical health problems and treatments. The focus of the intervention is to improve the patient's health and well-being utilizing cognitive, behavioral, social, and/or psychophysiological procedures designed to ameliorate specific disease-related problems.

Codes 96150-96155 describe services offered to patients who present with primary physical illnesses, diagnoses, or symptoms and may benefit from assessments and interventions that focus on the biopsychosocial factors related to the patient's health status. These services do not represent preventive medicine counseling and risk factor reduction interventions.

For patients that require psychiatric services (90801-90899) as well as health and behavior assessment/intervention (96150-96155), report the predominant service performed. Do not report 96150-96155 in conjunction with 90801-90899 on the same date.

Evaluation and Management services codes (including **Preventive Medicine, Individual Counseling** codes 99401-99404, and **Preventive Medicine, Group Counseling** codes 99411-99412), should not be reported on the same day.

> (For health and behavior assessment and/or intervention performed by a physician, see **Evaluation and Management** or **Preventive Medicine** services codes)

96150   Health and behavior assessment (eg, health-focused clinical interview, behavioral observations, psychophysiological monitoring, health-oriented questionnaires), each 15 minutes face-to-face with the patient; initial assessment

96151   re-assessment

96152   Health and behavior intervention, each 15 minutes, face-to-face; individual

96153   group (2 or more patients)

96154   family (with the patient present)

96155   family (without the patient present)

Chemotherapy Administration

Chemotherapy administration codes 96401-96549 apply to parenteral administration of non-radionuclide anti-neoplastic drugs; and also to anti-neoplastic agents provided for treatment of noncancer diagnoses (eg, cyclophosphamide for auto-immune conditions) or to substances such as monoclonal antibody agents, and other biologic response modifiers. These services can be provided by any physician. Chemotherapy services are typically highly complex and require direct physician supervision for any or all purposes of patient assessment, provision of consent, safety oversight and intra-service supervision of staff. Typically, such chemotherapy services require advanced practice training and competency for staff who provide these services; special considerations for preparation, dosage or disposal; and commonly, these services entail significant patient risk and frequent monitoring. Examples are frequent changes in the infusion rate, prolonged presence of nurse administering the solution for patient monitoring and infusion adjustments, and frequent conferring with the physician about these issues.

If performed to facilitate the infusion or injection, the following services are included and are not reported separately:

a. Use of local anesthesia

b. IV start

c. Access to indwelling IV, subcutaneous catheter or port

d. Flush at conclusion of infusion

e. Standard tubing, syringes and supplies

f. Preparation of chemotherapy agent(s)

> (For declotting a catheter or port, use 36550)

Report separate codes for each parenteral method of administration employed when chemotherapy is administered by different techniques. The administration of medications (eg, antibiotics, steroidal agents, antiemetics, narcotics, analgesics) administered independently or sequentially as supportive management of chemotherapy administration, should be separately reported using 90760, 90761, 90765, 90779 as appropriate.

Report both the specific service as well as code(s) for the specific substance(s) or drug(s) provided. The fluid used to administer the drug(s) is considered incidental hydration and is not separately reportable.

When administering multiple infusions, injections or combinations, only one "initial" service code should be reported, unless protocol requires that two separate IV sites must be used. The "initial" code that best describes the key or primary reason for the encounter should always be reported irrespective of the order in which the infusions or injections occur. If an injection or infusion is

Medicine

of a subsequent or concurrent nature, even if it is the first such service within that group of services, then a subsequent or concurrent code from the appropriate section should be reported (eg, the first IV push given subsequent to an initial one-hour infusion is reported using a subsequent IV push code).

When reporting codes for which infusion time is a factor, use the actual time over which the infusion is administered.

If a significant separately identifiable Evaluation and Management service is performed, the appropriate E/M service code should be reported using modifier 25 in addition to 96401-96549. For same day E/M service, a different diagnosis is not required.

Regional (isolation) chemotherapy perfusion should be reported using the codes for arterial infusion (96420-96425). Placement of the intra-arterial catheter should be reported using the appropriate code from the **Cardiovascular Surgery** section. Placement of arterial and venous cannula(s) for extracorporeal circulation via a membrane oxygenator perfusion pump should be reported using 36823. Code 36823 includes dose calculation and administration of the chemotherapy agent by injection into the perfusate. Do not report 96409-96425 in conjunction with 36823.

(For home infusion services, see 99601-99602)

Injection and Intravenous Infusion Chemotherapy

Intravenous or intra-arterial push is defined as: a) an injection in which the healthcare professional who administers the substance/drug is continuously present to administer the injection and observe the patient, or b) an infusion of 15 minutes or less.

(96400 has been deleted. To report, see 96401, 96402)

96401 Chemotherapy administration, subcutaneous or intramuscular; non-hormonal anti-neoplastic

96402 hormonal anti-neoplastic

96405 Chemotherapy administration; intralesional, up to and including 7 lesions

96406 intralesional, more than 7 lesions

(96408 has been deleted. To report, use 96409)

96409 intravenous, push technique, single or initial substance/drug

(96410 has been deleted. To report, use 96413)

+ 96411 intravenous, push technique, each additional substance/drug (List separately in addition to code for primary procedure)

(Use 96411 in conjunction with 96409, 96413)

(96412 has been deleted. To report, use 96415)

96413 Chemotherapy administration, intravenous infusion technique; up to 1 hour, single or initial substance/drug

(96414 has been deleted. To report, use 96416)

+▲ 96415 each additional hour (List separately in addition to code for primary procedure)

(Use 96415 in conjunction with 96413)

(Report 96415 for infusion intervals of greater than 30 minutes beyond 1-hour increments)

(Report 90761 to identify hydration, or 90766, 90767, 90775 to identify therapeutic, prophylactic, or diagnostic drug infusion or injection, if provided as a secondary or subsequent service in association with 96413)

96416 initiation of prolonged chemotherapy infusion (more than 8 hours), requiring use of a portable or implantable pump

(For refilling and maintenance of a portable pump or an implantable infusion pump or reservoir for drug delivery, see 96521-96523)

+ 96417 each additional sequential infusion (different substance/drug), up to 1 hour (List separately in addition to code for primary procedure)

(Use 96417 in conjunction with 96413)

(Report only once per sequential infusion. Report 96415 for additional hour(s) of sequential infusion)

Intra-Arterial Chemotherapy

96420 Chemotherapy administration, intra-arterial; push technique

96422 infusion technique, up to one hour

+▲ 96423 infusion technique, each additional hour (List separately in addition to code for primary procedure)

(Use 96423 in conjunction with 96422)

(Report 96423 for infusion intervals of greater than 30 minutes beyond 1-hour increments)

(For regional chemotherapy perfusion via membrane oxygenator perfusion pump to an extremity, use 36823)

96425 infusion technique, initiation of prolonged infusion (more than 8 hours), requiring the use of a portable or implantable pump

(For refilling and maintenance of a portable pump or an implantable infusion pump or reservoir for drug delivery, see 96521-96523)

Other Chemotherapy

Code 96523 does not require direct physician supervision. Codes 96521-96523 may be reported when these devices are used for therapeutic drugs other than chemotherapy.

(For collection of blood specimen from a completely implantable venous access device, use 36540)

Medicine

96440   Chemotherapy administration into pleural cavity, requiring and including thoracentesis

96445   Chemotherapy administration into peritoneal cavity, requiring and including peritoneocentesis

96450   Chemotherapy administration, into CNS (eg, intrathecal), requiring and including spinal puncture

(For intravesical (bladder) chemotherapy administration, use 51720)

(For insertion of subarachnoid catheter and reservoir for infusion of drug, see 62350, 62351, 62360-62362; for insertion of intraventricular catheter and reservoir, see 61210, 61215)

(96520 has been deleted. To report, use 96521)

96521   Refilling and maintenance of portable pump

96522   Refilling and maintenance of implantable pump or reservoir for drug delivery, systemic (eg, intravenous, intra-arterial)

(For refilling and maintenance of an implantable infusion pump for spinal or brain drug infusion, use 95990-95991)

96523   Irrigation of implanted venous access device for drug delivery systems

(Do not report 96523 if an injection or infusion is provided on the same day)

(96530 has been deleted. To report, use 96522)

96542   Chemotherapy injection, subarachnoid or intraventricular via subcutaneous reservoir, single or multiple agents

(96545 has been deleted)

(For radioactive isotope therapy, use 79005)

96549   Unlisted chemotherapy procedure

Photodynamic Therapy

(To report ocular photodynamic therapy, use 67221)

96567   Photodynamic therapy by external application of light to destroy premalignant and/or malignant lesions of the skin and adjacent mucosa (eg, lip) by activation of photosensitive drug(s), each phototherapy exposure session

+ 96570   Photodynamic therapy by endoscopic application of light to ablate abnormal tissue via activation of photosensitive drug(s); first 30 minutes (List separately in addition to code for endoscopy or bronchoscopy procedures of lung and esophagus)

+ 96571   each additional 15 minutes (List separately in addition to code for endoscopy or bronchoscopy procedures of lung and esophagus)

(96570, 96571 are to be used in addition to bronchoscopy, endoscopy codes)

(Use 96570, 96571 in conjunction with 31641, 43228 as appropriate)

Special Dermatological Procedures

Dermatologic services are typically consultative, and any of the five levels of consultation (99241-99255) may be appropriate.

In addition, services and skills outlined under **Evaluation and Management** levels of service appropriate to dermatologic illnesses should be coded similarly.

▶(For whole body photography, use 96904)◀

(For intralesional injections, see 11900, 11901)

▶(For Tzanck smear, see 88160-88161)◀

96900   Actinotherapy (ultraviolet light)

96902   Microscopic examination of hairs plucked or clipped by the examiner (excluding hair collected by the patient) to determine telogen and anagen counts, or structural hair shaft abnormality

● **96904**   Whole body integumentary photography, for monitoring of high risk patients with dysplastic nevus syndrome or a history of dysplastic nevi, or patients with a personal or familial history of melanoma

96910   Photochemotherapy; tar and ultraviolet B (Goeckerman treatment) or petrolatum and ultraviolet B

96912   psoralens and ultraviolet A (PUVA)

96913   Photochemotherapy (Goeckerman and/or PUVA) for severe photoresponsive dermatoses requiring at least four to eight hours of care under direct supervision of the physician (includes application of medication and dressings)

96920   Laser treatment for inflammatory skin disease (psoriasis); total area less than 250 sq cm

96921   250 sq cm to 500 sq cm

96922   over 500 sq cm

96999   Unlisted special dermatological service or procedure

Physical Medicine and Rehabilitation

Codes 97001-97755 should be used to report each distinct procedure performed. Do not append modifier 51 to 97001-97755.

(For muscle testing, range of joint motion, electromyography, see 95831 et seq)

(For biofeedback training by EMG, use 90901)

(For transcutaneous nerve stimulation (TNS), use 64550)

97001   Physical therapy evaluation

97002   Physical therapy re-evaluation

97003   Occupational therapy evaluation

Medicine

97004   Occupational therapy re-evaluation

97005   Athletic training evaluation

97006   Athletic training re-evaluation

Modalities

Any physical agent applied to produce therapeutic changes to biologic tissue; includes but not limited to thermal, acoustic, light, mechanical, or electric energy.

Supervised

The application of a modality that does not require direct (one-on-one) patient contact by the provider.

97010   Application of a modality to one or more areas; hot or cold packs

97012   traction, mechanical

97014   electrical stimulation (unattended)

(For acupuncture with electrical stimulation, see 97813, 97814)

97016   vasopneumatic devices

97018   paraffin bath

(97020 has been deleted. To report, use 97024)

97022   whirlpool

97024   diathermy (eg, microwave)

97026   infrared

97028   ultraviolet

Constant Attendance

The application of a modality that requires direct (one-on-one) patient contact by the provider.

97032   Application of a modality to one or more areas; electrical stimulation (manual), each 15 minutes

97033   iontophoresis, each 15 minutes

97034   contrast baths, each 15 minutes

97035   ultrasound, each 15 minutes

97036   Hubbard tank, each 15 minutes

97039   Unlisted modality (specify type and time if constant attendance)

Therapeutic Procedures

A manner of effecting change through the application of clinical skills and/or services that attempt to improve function.

Physician or therapist required to have direct (one-on-one) patient contact.

97110   Therapeutic procedure, one or more areas, each 15 minutes; therapeutic exercises to develop strength and endurance, range of motion and flexibility

97112   neuromuscular reeducation of movement, balance, coordination, kinesthetic sense, posture, and/or proprioception for sitting and/or standing activities

97113   aquatic therapy with therapeutic exercises

97116   gait training (includes stair climbing)

(Use 96000-96003 to report comprehensive gait and motion analysis procedures)

97124   massage, including effleurage, petrissage and/or tapotement (stroking, compression, percussion)

(For myofascial release, use 97140)

97139   Unlisted therapeutic procedure (specify)

97140   Manual therapy techniques (eg, mobilization/manipulation, manual lymphatic drainage, manual traction), one or more regions, each 15 minutes

97150   Therapeutic procedure(s), group (2 or more individuals)

(Report 97150 for each member of group)

(Group therapy procedures involve constant attendance of the physician or therapist, but by definition do not require one-on-one patient contact by the physician or therapist)

(For manipulation under general anesthesia, see appropriate anatomic section in **Musculoskeletal System**)

(For osteopathic manipulative treatment (OMT), see 98925-98929)

(97504 has been deleted. To report, use 97760)

(97520 has been deleted. To report, use 97761)

97530   Therapeutic activities, direct (one-on-one) patient contact by the provider (use of dynamic activities to improve functional performance), each 15 minutes

97532   Development of cognitive skills to improve attention, memory, problem solving, (includes compensatory training), direct (one-on-one) patient contact by the provider, each 15 minutes

97533   Sensory integrative techniques to enhance sensory processing and promote adaptive responses to environmental demands, direct (one-on-one) patient contact by the provider, each 15 minutes

97535   Self-care/home management training (eg, activities of daily living (ADL) and compensatory training, meal preparation, safety procedures, and instructions in use of assistive technology devices/adaptive equipment) direct one-on-one contact by provider, each 15 minutes

Medicine

97537   Community/work reintegration training (eg, shopping, transportation, money management, avocational activities and/or work environment/modification analysis, work task analysis, use of assistive technology device/adaptive equipment), direct one-on-one contact by provider, each 15 minutes

(For wheelchair management/propulsion training, use 97542)

97542   Wheelchair management (eg, assessment, fitting, training), each 15 minutes

97545   Work hardening/conditioning; initial 2 hours

+ 97546   each additional hour (List separately in addition to code for primary procedure)

(Use 97546 in conjunction with 97545)

Active Wound Care Management

Active wound care procedures are performed to remove devitalized and/or necrotic tissue and promote healing. Provider is required to have direct (one-on-one) patient contact.

(Do not report 97597-97602 in conjunction with 11040-11044)

97597   Removal of devitalized tissue from wound(s), selective debridement, without anesthesia (eg, high pressure waterjet with/without suction, sharp selective debridement with scissors, scalpel and forceps), with or without topical application(s), wound assessment, and instruction(s) for ongoing care, may include use of a whirlpool, per session; total wound(s) surface area less than or equal to 20 square centimeters

97598   total wound(s) surface area greater than 20 square centimeters

(97601 has been deleted. To report, use 97597, 97598)

97602   Removal of devitalized tissue from wound(s), non-selective debridement, without anesthesia (eg, wet-to-moist dressings, enzymatic, abrasion), including topical application(s), wound assessment, and instruction(s) for ongoing care, per session

97605   Negative pressure wound therapy (eg, vacuum assisted drainage collection), including topical application(s), wound assessment, and instruction(s) for ongoing care, per session; total wound(s) surface area less than or equal to 50 square centimeters

97606   total wound(s) surface area greater than 50 square centimeters

Tests and Measurements

Requires direct one-on-one patient contact.

(For muscle testing, manual or electrical, joint range of motion, electromyography or nerve velocity determination, see 95831-95904)

(97703 has been deleted. To report, use 97762)

97750   Physical performance test or measurement (eg, musculoskeletal, functional capacity), with written report, each 15 minutes

97755   Assistive technology assessment (eg, to restore, augment or compensate for existing function, optimize functional tasks and/or maximize environmental accessibility), direct one-on-one contact by provider, with written report, each 15 minutes

(To report augmentative and alternative communication devices, see 92605, 92607)

Orthotic Management and Prosthetic Management

97760   Orthotic(s) management and training (including assessment and fitting when not otherwise reported), upper extremity(s), lower extremity(s) and/or trunk, each 15 minutes

(Code 97760 should not be reported with 97116 for the same extremity)

97761   Prosthetic training, upper and/or lower extremity(s), each 15 minutes

97762   Checkout for orthotic/prosthetic use, established patient, each 15 minutes

Other Procedures

(For extracorporeal shock wave musculoskeletal therapy, see Category III codes 0019T, 0101T, 0102T)

(97780 has been deleted. To report, see 97810, 97811)

(97781 has been deleted. To report, see 97813, 97814)

97799   Unlisted physical medicine/rehabilitation service or procedure

Medical Nutrition Therapy

97802   Medical nutrition therapy; initial assessment and intervention, individual, face-to-face with the patient, each 15 minutes

97803   re-assessment and intervention, individual, face-to-face with the patient, each 15 minutes

97804   group (2 or more individual(s)), each 30 minutes

(For medical nutrition therapy assessment and/or intervention performed by a physician, see **Evaluation and Management** or **Preventive Medicine** service codes)

Medicine

Acupuncture

Acupuncture is reported based on 15-minute increments of personal (face-to-face) contact with the patient, not the duration of acupuncture needle(s) placement.

If no electrical stimulation is used during a 15-minute increment, use 97810, 97811. If electrical stimulation of any needle is used during a 15-minute increment, use 97813, 97814.

Only one code may be reported for each 15-minute increment. Use either 97810 or 97813 for the initial 15-minute increment. Only one initial code is reported per day.

Evaluation and Management services may be reported separately, using modifier 25, if the patient's condition requires a significant separately identifiable E/M service, above and beyond the usual preservice and postservice work associated with the acupuncture services. The time of the E/M service is not included in the time of the acupuncture service.

97810   Acupuncture, 1 or more needles; without electrical stimulation, initial 15 minutes of personal one-on-one contact with the patient

(Do not report 97810 in conjunction with 97813)

+ 97811   without electrical stimulation, each additional 15 minutes of personal one-on-one contact with the patient, with re-insertion of needle(s) (List separately in addition to code for primary procedure)

(Use 97811 in conjunction with 97810, 97813)

97813   with electrical stimulation, initial 15 minutes of personal one-on-one contact with the patient

(Do not report 97813 in conjunction with 97810)

+ 97814   with electrical stimulation, each additional 15 minutes of personal one-on-one contact with the patient, with re-insertion of needle(s) (List separately in addition to code for primary procedure)

(Use 97814 in conjunction with 97810, 97813)

Osteopathic Manipulative Treatment

Osteopathic manipulative treatment (OMT) is a form of manual treatment applied by a physician to eliminate or alleviate somatic dysfunction and related disorders. This treatment may be accomplished by a variety of techniques.

Evaluation and Management services may be reported separately if, using modifier 25, the patient's condition requires a significant separately identifiable E/M service, above and beyond the usual preservice and postservice work associated with the procedure. The E/M service may be caused or prompted by the same symptoms or

condition for which the OMT service was provided. As such, different diagnoses are not required for the reporting of the OMT and E/M service on the same date.

Body regions referred to are: head region; cervical region; thoracic region; lumbar region; sacral region; pelvic region; lower extremities; upper extremities; rib cage region; abdomen and viscera region.

98925   Osteopathic manipulative treatment (OMT); one to two body regions involved

98926   three to four body regions involved

98927   five to six body regions involved

98928   seven to eight body regions involved

98929   nine to ten body regions involved

Chiropractic Manipulative Treatment

Chiropractic manipulative treatment (CMT) is a form of manual treatment to influence joint and neurophysiological function. This treatment may be accomplished using a variety of techniques.

The chiropractic manipulative treatment codes include a pre-manipulation patient assessment. Additional Evaluation and Management services may be reported separately using modifier 25, if the patient's condition requires a significant separately identifiable E/M service, above and beyond the usual preservice and postservice work associated with the procedure. The E/M service may be caused or prompted by the same symptoms or condition for which the CMT service was provided. As such, different diagnoses are not required for the reporting of the CMT and E/M service on the same date.

For purposes of CMT, the five spinal regions referred to are: cervical region (includes atlanto-occipital joint); thoracic region (includes costovertebral and costotransverse joints); lumbar region; sacral region; and pelvic (sacro-iliac joint) region. The five extraspinal regions referred to are: head (including temporomandibular joint, excluding atlanto-occipital) region; lower extremities; upper extremities; rib cage (excluding costotransverse and costovertebral joints) and abdomen.

98940   Chiropractic manipulative treatment (CMT); spinal, one to two regions

98941   spinal, three to four regions

98942   spinal, five regions

98943   extraspinal, one or more regions

Medicine

Education and Training for Patient Self-Management

The following codes are used to report educational and training services prescribed by a physician and provided by a qualified, nonphysician healthcare professional using a standardized curriculum to an individual or a group of patients for the treatment of established illness(s)/disease(s) or to delay comorbidity(s). Education and training for patient self-management may be reported with these codes only when using a standardized curriculum as described below. This curriculum may be modified as necessary for the clinical needs, cultural norms and health literacy of the individual patient(s).

The purpose of the educational and training services is to teach the patient (may include caregiver(s)) how to effectively self-manage the patient's illness(s)/disease(s) or delay disease comorbidity(s) in conjunction with the patient's professional healthcare team. Education and training related to subsequent reinforcement or due to changes in the patient's condition or treatment plan are reported in the same manner as the original education and training. The type of education and training provided for the patient's clinical condition will be identified by the appropriate diagnosis code(s) reported.

The qualifications of the nonphysician healthcare professionals and the content of the educational and training program must be consistent with guidelines or standards established or recognized by a physician society, nonphysician healthcare professional society/association, or other appropriate source.

> (For counseling and education provided by a physician to an individual, see the appropriate Evaluation and Management codes)
>
> (For counseling and education provided by a physician to a group, use 99078)
>
> (For counseling and/or risk factor reduction intervention provided by a physician to patient(s) without symptoms or established disease, see 99401-99412)
>
> (For medical nutrition therapy, see 97802-97804)
>
> (For health and behavior assessment/intervention that is not part of a standardized curriculum, see 96150-96155)
>
> ▶(For education provided as genetic counseling services, use 96040. For education to a group regarding genetic risks, see 98961, 98962)◀

98960   Education and training for patient self-management by a qualified, nonphysician health care professional using a standardized curriculum, face-to-face with the patient (could include caregiver/family) each 30 minutes; individual patient

98961   2-4 patients

98962   5-8 patients

Special Services, Procedures and Reports

The procedures with code numbers 99000 through 99091 provide the reporting physician or other qualified healthcare professional with the means of identifying the completion of special reports and services that are an adjunct to the basic services rendered. The specific number assigned indicates the special circumstances under which a basic procedure is performed.

Code 99091 should be reported no more than once in a 30-day period to include the physician or health care provider time involved with data accession, review and interpretation, modification of care plan as necessary (including communication to patient and/or caregiver), and associated documentation.

If the services described by 99091 are provided on the same day the patient presents for an E/M service, these services should be considered part of the E/M service and not separately reported.

Do not report 99091 if it occurs within 30 days of care plan oversight services 99374-99380. Do not report 99091 if other more specific CPT codes exist (eg, 93014, 93227, 93233, 93272 for cardiographic services; 95250 for continuous glucose monitoring). Do not report 99091 for transfer and interpretation of data from hospital or clinical laboratory computers.

Codes 99050-99060 are reported in addition to an associated basic service. Typically only a single adjunct code from among 99050-99060 would be reported per patient encounter. However, there may be circumstances in which reporting multiple adjunct codes per patient encounter may be appropriate.

Miscellaneous Services

99000   Handling and/or conveyance of specimen for transfer from the physician's office to a laboratory

99001   Handling and/or conveyance of specimen for transfer from the patient in other than a physician's office to a laboratory (distance may be indicated)

99002   Handling, conveyance, and/or any other service in connection with the implementation of an order involving devices (eg, designing, fitting, packaging, handling, delivery or mailing) when devices such as orthotics, protectives, prosthetics are fabricated by an outside laboratory or shop but which items have been designed, and are to be fitted and adjusted by the attending physician

> (For routine collection of venous blood, use 36415)

Medicine

99024 Postoperative follow-up visit, normally included in the surgical package, to indicate that an evaluation and management service was performed during a postoperative period for a reason(s) related to the original procedure

(As a component of a surgical "package," see **Surgery Guidelines**)

99026 Hospital mandated on call service; in-hospital, each hour

99027   out-of-hospital, each hour

(For physician standby services requiring prolonged physician attendance, use 99360, as appropriate. Time spent performing separately reportable procedure(s) or service(s) should not be included in the time reported as mandated on call service)

99050 Services provided in the office at times other than regularly scheduled office hours, or days when the office is normally closed (eg, holidays, Saturday or Sunday), in addition to basic service

99051 Service(s) provided in the office during regularly scheduled evening, weekend, or holiday office hours, in addition to basic service

(99052 has been deleted)

99053 Service(s) provided between 10:00 PM and 8:00 AM at 24-hour facility, in addition to basic service

(99054 has been deleted)

99056 Service(s) typically provided in the office, provided out of the office at request of patient, in addition to basic service

99058 Service(s) provided on an emergency basis in the office, which disrupts other scheduled office services, in addition to basic service

99060 Service(s) provided on an emergency basis, out of the office, which disrupts other scheduled office services, in addition to basic service

99070 Supplies and materials (except spectacles), provided by the physician over and above those usually included with the office visit or other services rendered (list drugs, trays, supplies, or materials provided)

(For supply of spectacles, use the appropriate supply codes)

99071 Educational supplies, such as books, tapes, and pamphlets, provided by the physician for the patient's education at cost to physician

99075 Medical testimony

99078 Physician educational services rendered to patients in a group setting (eg, prenatal, obesity, or diabetic instructions)

99080 Special reports such as insurance forms, more than the information conveyed in the usual medical communications or standard reporting form

(Do not report 99080 in conjunction with 99455, 99456 for the completion of Workmen's Compensation forms)

99082 Unusual travel (eg, transportation and escort of patient)

99090 Analysis of clinical data stored in computers (eg, ECGs, blood pressures, hematologic data)

(For physician/health care professional collection and interpretation of physiologic data stored/transmitted by patient/caregiver, see 99091)

(Do not report 99090 if other more specific CPT codes exist, eg, 93014, 93227, 93233, 93272 for cardiographic services; 95250 for continuous glucose monitoring, 97750 for musculoskeletal function testing)

99091 Collection and interpretation of physiologic data (eg, ECG, blood pressure, glucose monitoring) digitally stored and/or transmitted by the patient and/or caregiver to the physician or other qualified health care professional, requiring a minimum of 30 minutes of time

Qualifying Circumstances for Anesthesia

(For explanation of these services, see **Anesthesia Guidelines**)

+ 99100 Anesthesia for patient of extreme age, younger than 1 year and older than 70 (List separately in addition to code for primary anesthesia procedure)

(For procedure performed on infants younger than 1 year of age at time of surgery, see 00326, 00561, 00834, 00836)

+ 99116 Anesthesia complicated by utilization of total body hypothermia (List separately in addition to code for primary anesthesia procedure)

+ 99135 Anesthesia complicated by utilization of controlled hypotension (List separately in addition to code for primary anesthesia procedure)

+ 99140 Anesthesia complicated by emergency conditions (specify) (List separately in addition to code for primary anesthesia procedure)

(An emergency is defined as existing when delay in treatment of the patient would lead to a significant increase in the threat to life or body part.)

Moderate (Conscious) Sedation

Moderate (conscious) sedation is a drug induced depression of consciousness during which patients respond purposefully to verbal commands, either alone or accompanied by light tactile stimulation. No interventions are required to maintain a patent airway, and spontaneous ventilation is adequate. Cardiovascular function is usually maintained.

Medicine

Moderate sedation does not include minimal sedation (anxiolysis), deep sedation or monitored anesthesia care (00100-01999).

When providing moderate sedation, the following services are included and NOT reported separately:

- Assessment of the patient (not included in intraservice time);

- Establishment of IV access and fluids to maintain patency, when performed;

- Administration of agent(s);

- Maintenance of sedation;

- Monitoring of oxygen saturation, heart rate and blood pressure; and

- Recovery (not included in intraservice time).

Intraservice time starts with the administration of the sedation agent(s), requires continuous face-to-face attendance, and ends at the conclusion of personal contact by the physician providing the sedation.

Do not report 99143-99150 in conjunction with 94760-94762.

Do not report 99143-99145 in conjunction with codes listed in Appendix G. Do not report 99148-99150 in conjunction with codes listed in Appendix G when performed in the nonfacility setting.

When a second physician other than the healthcare professional performing the diagnostic or therapeutic services provides moderate sedation in the facility setting (eg, hospital, outpatient hospital/ambulatory surgery center, skilled nursing facility) for the procedures listed in Appendix G, the second physician reports 99148-99150. However, for the circumstance in which these services are performed by the second physician in the nonfacility setting (eg, physician office, freestanding imaging center), codes 99148-99150 are not reported.

(99141, 99142 have been deleted. To report, see 99143-99145)

⊘ **99143**   Moderate sedation services (other than those services described by codes 00100-01999) provided by the same physician performing the diagnostic or therapeutic service that the sedation supports, requiring the presence of an independent trained observer to assist in the monitoring of the patient's level of consciousness and physiological status; younger than 5 years of age, first 30 minutes intra-service time

⊘ **99144**   age 5 years or older, first 30 minutes intra-service time

+ **99145**   each additional 15 minutes intra-service time (List separately in addition to code for primary service)

(Use 99145 in conjunction with 99143, 99144)

⊘ **99148**   Moderate sedation services (other than those services described by codes 00100-01999), provided by a physician other than the health care professional performing the diagnostic or therapeutic service that the sedation supports; younger than 5 years of age, first 30 minutes intra-service time

⊘ **99149**   age 5 years or older, first 30 minutes intra-service time

+ **99150**   each additional 15 minutes intra-service time (List separately in addition to code for primary service)

(Use 99150 in conjunction with 99148, 99149)

Other Services and Procedures

99170   Anogenital examination with colposcopic magnification in childhood for suspected trauma

(For conscious sedation, use 99143-99150)

99172   Visual function screening, automated or semi-automated bilateral quantitative determination of visual acuity, ocular alignment, color vision by pseudoisochromatic plates, and field of vision (may include all or some screening of the determination(s) for contrast sensitivity, vision under glare)

(This service must employ graduated visual acuity stimuli that allow a quantitative determination of visual acuity (eg, Snellen chart). This service may not be used in addition to a general ophthalmological service or an E/M service)

(Do not report 99172 in conjunction with 99173)

99173   Screening test of visual acuity, quantitative, bilateral

(The screening test used must employ graduated visual acuity stimuli that allow a quantitative estimate of visual acuity (eg, Snellen chart). Other identifiable services unrelated to this screening test provided at the same time may be reported separately (eg, preventive medicine services). When acuity is measured as part of a general ophthalmological service or of an E/M service of the eye, it is a diagnostic examination and not a screening test.)

(Do not report 99173 in conjunction with 99172)

99175   Ipecac or similar administration for individual emesis and continued observation until stomach adequately emptied of poison

(For diagnostic intubation, see 82926-82928, 89130-89141)

(For gastric lavage for diagnostic purposes, see 91055)

99183   Physician attendance and supervision of hyperbaric oxygen therapy, per session

(Evaluation and Management services and/or procedures (eg, wound debridement) provided in a hyperbaric oxygen treatment facility in conjunction with a hyperbaric oxygen therapy session should be reported separately)

Medicine

99185	Hypothermia; regional
99186	total body
99190	Assembly and operation of pump with oxygenator or heat exchanger (with or without ECG and/or pressure monitoring); each hour
99191	45 minutes
99192	30 minutes
99195	Phlebotomy, therapeutic (separate procedure)
99199	Unlisted special service, procedure or report

Home Health Procedures/Services

These codes are used by non-physician health care professionals. Physicians should utilize the home visit codes 99341-99350, and utilize CPT codes other than 99500-99600 for any additional procedure/service provided to a patient living in a residence.

The following codes are used to report services provided in a patient's residence (including assisted living apartments, group homes, non-traditional private homes, custodial care facilities, or schools).

Health care professionals who are authorized to use Evaluation and Management Home Visit codes (99341-99350) may report 99500-99600 in addition to 99341-99350 if both services are performed. Evaluation and Management services may be reported separately, using modifier 25, if the patient's condition requires a significant separately identifiable E/M service, above and beyond the home health service(s)/procedure(s) codes 99500-99600.

99500	Home visit for prenatal monitoring and assessment to include fetal heart rate, non-stress test, uterine monitoring, and gestational diabetes monitoring
99501	Home visit for postnatal assessment and follow-up care
99502	Home visit for newborn care and assessment
99503	Home visit for respiratory therapy care (eg, bronchodilator, oxygen therapy, respiratory assessment, apnea evaluation)
99504	Home visit for mechanical ventilation care
99505	Home visit for stoma care and maintenance including colostomy and cystostomy
99506	Home visit for intramuscular injections
99507	Home visit for care and maintenance of catheter(s) (eg, urinary, drainage, and enteral)

| 99509 | Home visit for assistance with activities of daily living and personal care |

(To report self-care/home management training, see 97535)

(To report home medical nutrition assessment and intervention services, see 97802-97804)

(To report home speech therapy services, see 92507-92508)

99510	Home visit for individual, family, or marriage counseling
99511	Home visit for fecal impaction management and enema administration
99512	Home visit for hemodialysis

(For home infusion of peritoneal dialysis, use 99601, 99602)

| 99600 | Unlisted home visit service or procedure |

Home Infusion Procedures/Services

| 99601 | Home infusion/specialty drug administration, per visit (up to 2 hours); |
| + 99602 | each additional hour (List separately in addition to code for primary procedure) |

(Use 99602 in conjunction with 99601)

Medicine

Category II Codes

The following section of *Current Procedural Terminology (CPT)* contains a set of supplemental tracking codes that can be used for performance measurement. It is anticipated that the use of Category II codes for performance measurement will decrease the need for record abstraction and chart review, and thereby minimize administrative burden on physicians, other health care professionals, hospitals, and entities seeking to measure the quality of patient care. These codes are intended to facilitate data collection about the quality of care rendered by coding certain services and test results that support nationally established performance measures and that have an evidence base as contributing to quality patient care.

The use of these codes is optional. The codes are not required for correct coding and may not be used as a substitute for Category I codes.

These codes describe clinical components that may be typically included in evaluation and management services or clinical services and, therefore, do not have a relative value associated with them. Category II codes may also describe results from clinical laboratory or radiology tests and other procedures, identified processes intended to address patient safety practices, or services reflecting compliance with state or federal law.

Category II codes described in this section make use of alphabetical characters as the 5th character in the string (ie, 4 digits followed by the letter **F**). These digits are not intended to reflect the placement of the code in the regular (Category I) part of the CPT codebook. To promote understanding of these codes and their associated measures, users are referred to Appendix H, which contains information about performance measurement exclusion modifiers, measures, and their source.

CPT Category II codes are arranged according to the following categories derived from standard clinical documentation format:

Composite Measures 0001F

Patient Management 0500F

Patient History 1000F

Physical Examination. 2000F

Diagnostic/Screening Processes
or Results. 3000F

Therapeutic, Preventive or Other
Interventions 4000F

Follow-up or Other Outcomes
. . . . 5000F (no codes at this time)

►Patient Safety. . . . . 6005F◄

►Cross-references to the measures associated with each Category II code and their source are included for reference in Appendix H. In addition, acronyms for the related diseases or clinical condition(s) have been added at the end of each code descriptor to identify the topic or clinical category in which that code is included. A complete listing of the diseases/clinical conditions, and their acronyms are provided in alphabetical order in Appendix H. Users should review the complete measure(s) associated with each code prior to implementation.◄

Category II codes are reviewed by the Performance Measures Advisory Group (PMAG), an advisory body to the CPT Editorial Panel and the CPT/HCPAC Advisory Committee. The PMAG is comprised of performance measurement experts representing the Agency for Healthcare Research and Quality (AHRQ), the American Medical Association (AMA), the Centers for Medicare and Medicaid Services (CMS), the Joint Commission on Accreditation of Healthcare Organizations (JCAHO), the National Committee for Quality Assurance (NCQA), and the Physician Consortium for Performance Improvement (PCPI). The PMAG may seek additional expertise and/or input from other national health care organizations, as necessary, for the development of tracking codes. These may include national medical specialty societies, other national health care professional associations, accrediting bodies, and federal regulatory agencies.

►The most current listing of Category II codes, including guidelines, Code Change Proposal forms, and release and implementation dates for Category II codes may be accessed at www.ama-assn.org/go/cpt.◄

(For blood pressure measured, use 2000F)

(0002F has been deleted. To report, use 1000F)

►(0003F has been deleted. To report, see 1034F-1036F)◄

(0004F has been deleted. To report, use 4000F)

(For tobacco use cessation intervention, pharmacologic therapy, use 4001F)

(0006F has been deleted. To report, use 4002F)

(0007F has been deleted. To report, use 4006F)

(0008F has been deleted. To report, use 4009F)

(0009F has been deleted. To report, use 1002F)

(0010F has been deleted)

(0011F has been deleted. To report, use 4011F)

Modifiers

►The following performance measurement modifiers may be used for Category II codes to indicate that a service specified in the associated measure(s) was considered but, due to either medical, patient, or system circumstance(s) documented in the medical record, the service was not provided. These modifiers serve as denominator exclusions from the performance measure. The user should note that not all listed measures provide for exclusions (see Appendix H for more discussion regarding exclusion criteria).

Category II modifiers should only be reported with Category II codes—they should not be reported with Category I or Category III codes. In addition, the modifiers in the Category II section should only be used where specified in the guidelines, reporting instructions, parenthetic notes, or code descriptor language listed in the Category II section (code listing and Appendix H).◄

1P Performance Measure Exclusion Modifier due to Medical Reasons:

►Includes:

- Not indicated (absence of organ/limb, already received/performed, other)

- Contraindicated (patient allergic history, potential adverse drug interaction, other)

2P Performance Measure Exclusion Modifier due to Patient Reasons:

Includes:

- Patient declined

- Economic, social, or religious reasons

- Other patient reasons

3P Performance Measure Exclusion Modifier due to System Reasons:

Includes:

- Resources to perform the services not available

- Insurance coverage/payor-related limitations

- Other reasons attributable to health care delivery system◄

►Composite Codes◄

►Composite codes combine several measures grouped within a single code descriptor to facilitate reporting for a clinical condition when all components are met. If only some of the components are met or if services are provided in addition to those included in the composite code, they may be reported individually using the corresponding CPT Category II codes for those services.◄

▲ **0001F** Heart failure assessed (includes assessment of all the following components)(CAD, HF)[1]:

Blood pressure measured (2000F)[1]

Level of activity assessed (1003F)[1]

Clinical symptoms of volume overload (excess) assessed (1004F)[1]

Weight, recorded (2001F)[1]

Clinical signs of volume overload (excess) assessed (2002F)[1]

(To report blood pressure measured, use 2000F)

0005F Osteoarthritis assessed (OA)[1]

Includes assessment of all the following components:

Osteoarthritis symptoms and functional status assessed (1006F)[1]

Use of anti-inflammatory or over-the-counter (OTC) analgesic medications assessed (1007F)[1]

Initial examination of the involved joint(s) (includes visual inspection, palpation, range of motion) (2004F)[1]

(To report tobacco use cessation intervention, use 4001F)

● **0012F** Community-acquired bacterial pneumonia assessment (includes all of the following components) (CAP)[1]:

Co-morbid conditions assessed (1026F)[1]

Vital signs recorded (2010F)[1]

Mental status assessed (2014F)[1]

Hydration status assessed (2018F)[1]

Patient Management

Patient management codes describe utilization measures or measures of patient care provided for specific clinical purposes (eg, prenatal care, pre- and post-surgical care).

0500F Initial prenatal care visit (report at first prenatal encounter with health care professional providing obstetrical care. Report also date of visit and, in a separate field, the date of the last menstrual period - LMP) (Prenatal)[2]

Footnotes

[1] Physician Consortium for Performance Improvement, www.ama-assn.org/go/quality

[2] National Committee on Quality Assurance (NCQA), Health Employer Data Information Set (HEDIS®), www.ncqa.org

[3] Joint Commission on Accreditation of Healthcare Organizations (JCAHO), ORYX Initiative Performance Measures, www.jcaho.org/pms

[4] National Diabetes Quality Improvement Alliance (NDQIA), www.nationaldiabetesalliance.org

Category II Codes

0501F   Prenatal flow sheet documented in medical record by first prenatal visit (documentation includes at minimum blood pressure, weight, urine protein, uterine size, fetal heart tones, and estimated date of delivery). Report also: date of visit and, in a separate field, the date of the last menstrual period - LMP (Note: If reporting 0501F Prenatal flow sheet, it is not necessary to report 0500F Initial prenatal care visit) (Prenatal)[1]

0502F   Subsequent prenatal care visit (Prenatal)[2]

[Excludes: patients who are seen for a condition unrelated to pregnancy or prenatal care (eg, an upper respiratory infection; patients seen for consultation only, not for continuing care)]

0503F   Postpartum care visit (Prenatal)[2]

Patient History

Patient history codes describe measures for select aspects of patient history or review of systems.

▲ **1000F**   Tobacco use assessed (CAD, CAP, COPD, PV)[1] (DM)[4]

►(1001F has been deleted. To report smoking use, tobacco use, or non-use of tobacco products, see 1034F-1036F)◄

1002F   Anginal symptoms and level of activity assessed (CAD)[1]

1003F   Level of activity assessed (HF)[1]

1004F   Clinical symptoms of volume overload (excess) assessed (HF)[1]

1005F   Asthma symptoms evaluated (includes physician documentation of numeric frequency of symptoms or patient completion of an asthma assessment tool/survey/questionnaire) (Asthma)[1]

1006F   Osteoarthritis symptoms and functional status assessed (may include the use of a standardized scale or the completion of an assessment questionnaire, such as the SF-36, AAOS Hip & Knee Questionnaire) (OA)[1]

[Instructions: Report when osteoarthritis is addressed during the patient encounter]

1007F   Use of anti-inflammatory or analgesic over-the-counter (OTC) medications for symptom relief assessed (OA)[1]

1008F   Gastrointestinal and renal risk factors assessed for patients on prescribed or OTC non-steroidal anti-inflammatory drug (NSAID) (OA)[1]

● **1015F**   Chronic obstructive pulmonary disease (COPD) symptoms assessed (Includes assessment of at least one of the following: dyspnea, cough/sputum, wheezing), or respiratory symptom assessment tool completed (COPD)[1]

● **1018F**   Dyspnea assessed, not present (COPD)[1]

● **1019F**   Dyspnea assessed, present (COPD)[1]

● **1022F**   Pneumococcus immunization status assessed (CAP, COPD)[1]

● **1026F**   Co-morbid conditions assessed (eg, includes assessment for presence or absence of: malignancy, liver disease, congestive heart failure, cerebrovascular disease, renal disease, chronic obstructive pulmonary disease, asthma, diabetes, other co-morbid conditions) (CAP)[1]

● **1030F**   Influenza immunization status assessed (CAP)[1]

● **1034F**   Current tobacco smoker (CAD, CAP, COPD, PV)[1] (DM)[4]

● **1035F**   Current smokeless tobacco user (eg, chew, snuff) (PV)[1]

● **1036F**   Current tobacco non-user (CAD, CAP, COPD, PV)[1] (DM)[4]

● **1038F**   Persistent asthma (mild, moderate or severe) (Asthma)[1]

● **1039F**   Intermittent asthma (Asthma)[1]

Physical Examination

Physical examination codes describe aspects of physical examination or clinical assessment.

2000F   Blood pressure, measured (HF, CAD, HTN)[1]

2001F   Weight recorded (HF)[1]

2002F   Clinical signs of volume overload (excess) assessed (HF)[1]

►(Code 2003F has been deleted. For performance measurement coding information regarding heart failure, see the Heart Failure Clinical Topic listing in Appendix H)◄

2004F   Initial examination of the involved joint(s) (includes visual inspection, palpation, range of motion) (OA)[1]

[Instructions: Report only for initial osteoarthritis visit or for visits for new joint involvement]

● **2010F**   Vital signs recorded (includes at minimum: temperature, pulse, respiration, and blood pressure)(CAP)[1]

● **2014F**   Mental status assessed (normal/mildly impaired/severely impaired) (CAP)[1]

● **2018F**   Hydration status assessed (normal/mildly dehydrated/severely dehydrated) (CAP)[1]

● **2022F**   Dilated retinal eye exam with interpretation by an ophthalmologist or optometrist documented and reviewed (DM)[4]

● **2024F**   Seven standard field stereoscopic photos with interpretation by an ophthalmologist or optometrist documented and reviewed (DM)[4]

Footnotes.

[1] Physician Consortium for Performance Improvement, www.ama-assn.org/go/quality

[2] National Committee on Quality Assurance (NCQA), Health Employer Data Information Set (HEDIS®), www.ncqa.org

[3] Joint Commission on Accreditation of Healthcare Organizations (JCAHO), ORYX Initiative Performance Measures, www.jcaho.org/pms

[4] National Diabetes Quality Improvement Alliance (NDQIA), www.nationaldiabetesalliance.org

Category II Codes

▲=Revised code   ●=New code   ►◄=Contains new or revised text   ⊘=Modifier 51 exempt   American Medical Association   **341**

● **2026F** Eye imaging validated to match diagnosis from seven standard field stereoscopic photos results documented and reviewed (DM)[4]

● **2028F** Foot examination performed (includes examination through visual inspection, sensory exam with monofilament, and pulse exam – report when any of the three components are completed) (DM)[4]

Diagnostic/Screening Processes or Results

Diagnostic/screening processes or results codes describe results of tests ordered (clinical laboratory tests, radiological or other procedural examinations).

▶(Code 3000F has been deleted. To report blood pressure use the corresponding systolic codes (3076F and 3077F) and diastolic codes (3078F, 3079F, 3080F)◀

▶(Code 3002F has been deleted. To report blood pressure use the corresponding systolic codes (3076F and 3077F) and diastolic codes (3078F, 3079F, 3080F)◀

● **3006F** Chest X-ray results documented and reviewed (CAP)[1]

● **3011F** Lipid panel results documented and reviewed (must include total cholesterol, HDL-C, triglycerides and calculated LDL-C) (CAD)[1]

● **3014F** Screening mammography results documented and reviewed (PV)[1]

● **3017F** Colorectal cancer screening results documented and reviewed (PV)[1]

(Includes: fecal occult blood testing annually, flexible sigmoidoscopy every 5 years, annual fecal occult blood testing plus flexible sigmoidoscopy every 5 years, double-contrast barium enema every 5 years, or colonoscopy every 10 years)

● **3020F** Left ventricular function (LVF) assessment (eg, echocardiography, nuclear test, or ventriculography) documented in the medical record (Includes quantitative or qualitative assessment results)(CHF)[1]

● **3021F** Left ventricular ejection fraction (LVEF) <40% or documentation of moderately or severely depressed left ventricular systolic function (CAD, HF)[1]

● **3022F** Left ventricular ejection fraction (LVEF) ≥40% or documentation as normal or mildly depressed left ventricular systolic function (CAD, HF)[1]

● **3023F** Spirometry results documented and reviewed (COPD)[1]

● **3025F** Spirometry test results demonstrate FEV_1/FVC<70% with COPD symptoms (eg, dyspnea, cough/sputum, wheezing) (CAP, COPD)[1]

● **3027F** Spirometry test results demonstrate FEV_1/FVC≥70% or patient does not have COPD symptoms (COPD)[1]

● **3028F** Oxygen saturation results documented and reviewed (Includes assessment through pulse oximetry or arterial blood gas measurement) (CAP, COPD)[1]

● **3035F** Oxygen saturation ≤ 88 % or a PaO2 ≤ 55 mm Hg (COPD)[1]

● **3037F** Oxygen saturation > 88% or PaO_2 > 55 mmHg (COPD)[1]

● **3040F** Functional expiratory volume (FEV_1) < 40% of predicted value (COPD)[1]

● **3042F** Functional expiratory volume (FEV_1) ≥ 40% of predicted value (COPD)[1]

● **3046F** Most recent hemoglobin A1c level > 9.0% (DM)[4]

● **3047F** Most recent hemoglobin A1c level ≤ 9.0% (DM)[4]

● **3048F** Most recent LDL-C <100 mg/dL (DM)[4]

● **3049F** Most recent LDL-C 100-129 mg/dL (DM)[4]

● **3050F** Most recent LDL-C ≥130 mg/dL (DM)[4]

● **3060F** Positive microalbuminuria test result documented and reviewed (DM)[4]

● **3061F** Negative microalbuminuria test result documented and reviewed (DM)[4]

● **3062F** Positive macroalbuminuria test result documented and reviewed (DM)[4]

● **3066F** Documentation of treatment for nephropathy (eg, patient receiving dialysis, patient being treated for ESRD, CRF, ARF, or renal insufficiency, any visit to a nephrologist) (DM)[4]

● **3072F** Low risk for retinopathy (no evidence of retinopathy in the prior year) (DM)[4]

● **3076F** Most recent systolic blood pressure < 140 mm Hg (HTN)[1] (DM)[4]

● **3077F** Most recent systolic blood pressure ≥ 140 mm Hg (HTN)[1] (DM)[4]

● **3078F** Most recent diastolic blood pressure < 80 mm Hg (HTN)[1] (DM)[4]

● **3079F** Most recent diastolic blood pressure 80-89 mm Hg (HTN)[1] (DM)[4]

● **3080F** Most recent diastolic blood pressure ≥ 90 mm Hg (HTN)[1] (DM)[4]

Footnotes

[1] Physician Consortium for Performance Improvement, www.ama-assn.org/go/quality

[2] National Committee on Quality Assurance (NCQA), Health Employer Data Information Set (HEDIS®), www.ncqa.org

[3] Joint Commission on Accreditation of Healthcare Organizations (JCAHO), ORYX Initiative Performance Measures, www.jcaho.org/pms

[4] National Diabetes Quality Improvement Alliance (NDQIA), www.nationaldiabetesalliance.org

Category II Codes

Therapeutic, Preventive or Other Interventions

Therapeutic, preventive or other interventions codes describe pharmacologic, procedural, or behavioral therapies, including preventive services such as patient education and counseling.

4000F Tobacco use cessation intervention, counseling (COPD, CAP, CAD)[1]

4001F Tobacco use cessation intervention, pharmacologic therapy (COPD, CAD, CAP, PV)[1] (DM)[4]

4002F Statin therapy, prescribed (CAD)[1]

4003F Patient education, written/oral, appropriate for patients with heart failure, performed (HF)[1]

4006F Beta-blocker therapy, prescribed (CAD, HF)[1]

▲ **4009F** Angiotensin converting enzyme (ACE) inhibitor or Angiotensin Receptor Blocker (ARB) therapy, prescribed (HF, CAD)[1]

4011F Oral antiplatelet therapy prescribed (eg, aspirin, clopidogrel/Plavix, or combination of aspirin and dipyridamole/Aggrenox) (CAD)[1]

4012F Warfarin therapy prescribed (CHF)[1]

4014F Written discharge instructions provided to heart failure patients discharged home. (Instructions include all of the following components: activity level, diet, discharge medications, follow-up appointment, weight monitoring, what to do if symptoms worsen)[3]

(Excludes patients < 18 years of age)

▲ **4015F** Persistent asthma, preferred long term control medication or an acceptable alternative treatment, prescribed (Asthma)[1]

(Note: There are no medical exclusion criteria)

(Do not report modifier 1P with 4015F)

(To report patient reasons for not prescribing, use modifier 2P)

4016F Anti-inflammatory/analgesic agent prescribed (OA)[1]

(Use for prescribed or continued medication[s], including over-the-counter medication[s])

4017F Gastrointestinal prophylaxis for NSAID use prescribed (OA)[1]

4018F Therapeutic exercise for the involved joint(s) instructed or physical or occupational therapy prescribed (OA)[1]

● **4025F** Inhaled bronchodilator prescribed (COPD)[1]

● **4030F** Long term oxygen therapy prescribed (more than fifteen hours per day) (COPD)[1]

● **4033F** Pulmonary rehabilitation exercise training recommended (COPD)[1]

▶(Report 4033F with 1019F)◀

● **4035F** Influenza immunization recommended (COPD)[1]

● **4037F** Influenza immunization ordered or administered (COPD, PV)[1]

● **4040F** Pneumococcal immunization ordered or administered (COPD)[1]

● **4045F** Appropriate empiric antibiotic prescribed (See measure developer's Web site for definition of appropriate antibiotic) (CAP)[1]

● **4050F** Hypertension plan of care documented as appropriate (HTN)[1]

Follow-up or Other Outcomes

Follow-up or other outcomes codes describe review and communication of test results to patients, patient satisfaction or experience with care, patient functional status, and patient morbidity and mortality.

Patient Safety

Patient safety codes that describe patient safety practices.

● **6005F** Rationale (eg, severity of illness and safety) for level of care (eg, home, hospital) documented (CAP)[1]

Footnotes

[1] Physician Consortium for Performance Improvement, www.ama-assn.org/go/quality

[2] National Committee on Quality Assurance (NCQA), Health Employer Data Information Set (HEDIS®), www.ncqa.org

[3] Joint Commission on Accreditation of Healthcare Organizations (JCAHO), ORYX Initiative Performance Measures, www.jcaho.org/pms

[4] National Diabetes Quality Improvement Alliance (NDQIA), www.nationaldiabetesalliance.org

Category II Codes

Notes

Category III Codes

The following section contains a set of temporary codes for emerging technology, services, and procedures. Category III codes allow data collection for these services/procedures. Use of unlisted codes does not offer the opportunity for the collection of specific data. If a Category III code is available, this code must be reported instead of a Category I unlisted code. This is an activity that is critically important in the evaluation of health care delivery and the formation of public and private policy. The use of the codes in this section allow physicians and other qualified health care professionals, insurers, health services researchers, and health policy experts to identify emerging technology, services, and procedures for clinical efficacy, utilization and outcomes.

The inclusion of a service or procedure in this section neither implies nor endorses clinical efficacy, safety or the applicability to clinical practice. The codes in this section may not conform to the usual requirements for CPT Category I codes established by the Editorial Panel. For Category I codes, the Panel requires that the service/procedure be performed by many health care professionals in clinical practice in multiple locations and that FDA approval, as appropriate, has already been received. The nature of emerging technology, services, and procedures is such that these requirements may not be met. For these reasons, temporary codes for emerging technology, services, and procedures have been placed in a separate section of the CPT codebook and the codes are differentiated from Category I CPT codes by the use of alphanumeric characters.

►Services/procedures described in this section make use of alphanumeric characters. These codes have an alpha character as the 5th character in the string, preceded by four digits. The digits are not intended to reflect the placement of the code in the Category I section of CPT nomenclature. Codes in this section may or may not eventually receive a Category I CPT code. In either case, a given Category III code will be archived five years from its date of publication or revision in the CPT code book unless it is demonstrated that a temporary code is still needed. New codes in this section are released semi-annually via the AMA/CPT internet site, to expedite dissemination for reporting. The full set of temporary codes for emerging technology, services, and procedures are published annually in the CPT codebook. Go to www.ama-assn.org/go/cpt for the most current listing.◄

(0001T has been deleted. To report, use 34803)

►(0003T has been deleted)◄

(0005T-0007T have been deleted. To report, see 0075T, 0076T)

►(0008T has been deleted)◄

(0009T has been deleted. To report, use 58356)

(0010T has been deleted. To report, use 86480)

(0012T has been deleted. To report, use 29866)

(0013T has been deleted. To report, see 29867, 27415)

(0014T has been deleted. To report, use 29868)

0016T   Destruction of localized lesion of choroid (eg, choroidal neovascularization), transpupillary thermotherapy

0017T   Destruction of macular drusen, photocoagulation

►(0018T has been deleted. To report, see 0160T, 0161T)◄

0019T   Extracorporeal shock wave involving musculoskeletal system, not otherwise specified, low energy

(For application of high energy extracorporeal shock wave involving musculoskeletal system not otherwise specified, use 0101T)

(For application of high energy extracorporeal shock wave involving lateral humeral epicondyle, use 0102T)

(0020T has been deleted. To report, use 28890)

►(0021T has been deleted)◄

(0023T has been deleted. To report, use 87900)

0024T   Non-surgical septal reduction therapy (eg, alcohol ablation), for hypertrophic obstructive cardiomyopathy, with coronary arteriograms, with or without temporary pacemaker

0026T   Lipoprotein, direct measurement, intermediate density lipoproteins (IDL) (remnant lipoproteins)

0027T   Endoscopic lysis of epidural adhesions with direct visualization using mechanical means (eg, spinal endoscopic catheter system) or solution injection (eg, normal saline) including radiologic localization and epidurography

(For diagnostic epidurography, use 64999)

0028T   Dual energy x-ray absorptiometry (DEXA) body composition study, one or more sites

0029T   Treatment(s) for incontinence, pulsed magnetic neuromodulation, per day

0030T   Antiprothrombin (phospholipid cofactor) antibody, each Ig class

---

▲=Revised code   ●=New code   ►◄=Contains new or revised text   ⊘=Modifier 51 exempt

0031T   Speculoscopy;

0032T   with directed sampling

(0033T has been deleted. For endovascular repair of descending thoracic aorta, involving coverage of left subclavian artery origin, use 33880)

(0034T has been deleted. For endovascular repair of descending thoracic aorta, not involving coverage of left subclavian artery origin, use 33881)

(0035T has been deleted. For proximal extension during endovascular repair of descending thoracic aorta, use 33883. Distal extensions are included in 33880, 33881. Distal extensions performed after endovascular repair of descending thoracic aorta are reported with 33886)

(0036T has been deleted. For additional proximal extensions use 33884. Additional distal extensions during endovascular repair of descending thoracic aorta are included in 33880, 33881. Additional distal extensions placed after endovascular repair of thoracic aorta are included in 33886)

(0037T has been deleted. For open subclavian to carotid artery transposition performed in conjunction with endovascular thoracic aortic repair by neck incision, use 33889)

(0038T has been deleted. For endovascular repair of descending thoracic aorta, involving coverage of left subclavian artery origin, radiological supervision and interpretation, use 75956)

(0039T has been deleted. For endovascular repair of descending thoracic aorta, not involving coverage of left subclavian artery origin, radiological supervision and interpretation, use 75957)

(0040T has been deleted. For placement of proximal extension prosthesis for endovascular repair of descending thoracic aorta, radiological supervision and interpretation, use 75958. For placement of distal extension prosthesis after thoracic endovascular repair of descending thoracic aorta, radiological supervision and interpretation, use 75959)

0041T   Urinalysis infectious agent detection, semi-quantitative analysis of volatile compounds

0042T   Cerebral perfusion analysis using computed tomography with contrast administration, including post-processing of parametric maps with determination of cerebral blood flow, cerebral blood volume, and mean transit time

0043T   Carbon monoxide, expired gas analysis (eg, $ETCO_c$/hemolysis breath test)

►(0044T and 0045T have been deleted. To report, use 96904)◄

0046T   Catheter lavage of a mammary duct(s) for collection of cytology specimen(s), in high risk individuals (GAIL risk scoring or prior personal history of breast cancer), each breast; single duct

0047T   each additional duct

0048T   Implantation of a ventricular assist device, extracorporeal, percutaneous transseptal access, single or dual cannulation

+ 0049T   Prolonged extracorporeal percutaneous transseptal ventricular assist device, greater than 24 hours, each subsequent 24 hour period (List separately in addition to code for primary procedure)

(Use 0049T in conjunction with 0048T)

0050T   Removal of a ventricular assist device, extracorporeal, percutaneous transseptal access, single or dual cannulation

0051T   Implantation of a total replacement heart system (artificial heart) with recipient cardiectomy

(For implantation of heart assist or ventricular assist device, see 33975, 33976)

0052T   Replacement or repair of thoracic unit of a total replacement heart system (artificial heart)

(For replacement or repair of other implantable components in a total replacement heart system (artificial heart), use 0053T)

0053T   Replacement or repair of implantable component or components of total replacement heart system (artificial heart), excluding thoracic unit

(For replacement or repair of a thoracic unit of a total replacement heart system (artificial heart), use 0052T)

+ 0054T   Computer-assisted musculoskeletal surgical navigational orthopedic procedure, with image-guidance based on fluoroscopic images (List separately in addition to code for primary procedure)

+ 0055T   Computer-assisted musculoskeletal surgical navigational orthopedic procedure, with image-guidance based on CT/MRI images (List separately in addition to code for primary procedure)

(When CT and MRI are both performed, report 0055T only once)

+ 0056T   Computer-assisted musculoskeletal surgical navigational orthopedic procedure, image-less (List separately in addition to code for primary procedure)

(0057T has been deleted. To report, use 43257)

0058T   Cryopreservation; reproductive tissue, ovarian

0059T   oocyte(s)

(For cryopreservation of embryo(s), sperm and testicular reproductive tissue, see 89258, 89259, 89335)

0060T   Electrical impedance scan of the breast, bilateral (risk assessment device for breast cancer)

Category III Codes

0061T Destruction/reduction of malignant breast tumor including breast carcinoma cells in the margins, microwave phased array thermotherapy, disposable catheter with combined temperature monitoring probe and microwave sensor, externally applied microwave energy, including interstitial placement of sensor

▶(For imaging guidance performed in conjunction with 0061T, see 76942, 76998)◀

▲ **0062T** Percutaneous intradiscal annuloplasty, any method except electrothermal, unilateral or bilateral including fluoroscopic guidance; single level

+ **0063T** 1 or more additional levels (List separately in addition to 0062T for primary procedure)

▶(For CT or MRI guidance and localization for needle placement and annuloplasty in conjunction with 0062T, 0063T, see 77012, 77021)◀

▶(For intradiscal electrothermal annuloplasty see 22526-22527)◀

0064T Spectroscopy, expired gas analysis (eg, nitric oxide/carbon dioxide test)

0065T Ocular photoscreening, with interpretation and report, bilateral

(Do not report 0065T in conjunction with 99172 or 99173)

0066T Computed tomographic (CT) colonography (ie, virtual colonoscopy); screening

0067T diagnostic

(Do not report 0066T or 0067T in conjunction with 72192-72194, 74150-74170)

+ **0068T** Acoustic heart sound recording and computer analysis; with interpretation and report (List separately in addition to codes for electrocardiography)

(Use 0068T in conjunction with 93000)

+ **0069T** acoustic heart sound recording and computer analysis only (List separately in addition to codes for electrocardiography)

(Use 0069T in conjunction with 93005)

+ **0070T** interpretation and report only (List separately in addition to codes for electrocardiography)

(Use 0070T in conjunction with 93010)

0071T Focused ultrasound ablation of uterine leiomyomata, including MR guidance; total leiomyomata volume less than 200 cc of tissue

0072T total leiomyomata volume greater or equal to 200 cc of tissue

▶(Do not report 0071T, 0072T in conjunction with 51702 or 77022)◀

0073T Compensator-based beam modulation treatment delivery of inverse planned treatment using three or more high resolution (milled or cast) compensator convergent beam modulated fields, per treatment session

(For treatment planning, use 77301)

(Do not report 0073T in conjunction with 77401-77416, 77418)

Online Medical Evaluation

An online medical evaluation is a type of Evaluation and Management (E/M) service provided by a physician or qualified health care professional to a patient using internet resources in response to the patient's online inquiry. Reportable services involve the physician's personal timely response to the patient's inquiry and must involve permanent storage (electronic or hard copy) of the encounter. This service should not be reported for patient contacts (eg, telephone calls) considered to be pre-service or post-service work for other E/M or non E/M services. A reportable service would encompass the sum of communication (eg, related telephone calls, prescription provision, laboratory orders) pertaining to the online patient encounter or problem(s).

0074T Online evaluation and management service, per encounter, provided by a physician, using the Internet or similar electronic communications network, in response to a patient's request, established patient

0075T Transcatheter placement of extracranial vertebral or intrathoracic carotid artery stent(s), including radiologic supervision and interpretation, percutaneous; initial vessel

+ **0076T** each additional vessel (List separately in addition to code for primary procedure)

(Use 0076T in conjunction with 0075T)

(When the ipsilateral extracranial vertebral or intrathoracic carotid arteriogram (including imaging and selective catheterization) confirms the need for stenting, then 0075T and 0076T include all ipsilateral extracranial vertebral or intrathoracic selective carotid catheterization, all diagnostic imaging for ipsilateral extracranial vertebral or intrathoracic carotid artery stenting, and all related radiologic supervision and interpretation. If stenting is not indicated, then the appropriate codes for selective catheterization and imaging should be reported in lieu of code 0075T or 0076T.)

0077T Implanting and securing cerebral thermal perfusion probe, including twist drill or burr hole, to measure absolute cerebral tissue perfusion

(0078T-0081T should be reported in accordance with the Endovascular Abdominal Aneurysm Repair guidelines established for 34800-34826)

0078T   Endovascular repair using prosthesis of abdominal aortic aneurysm, pseudoaneurysm or dissection, abdominal aorta involving visceral branches (superior mesenteric, celiac and/or renal artery(s))

(Do not report 0078T in conjunction with 34800-34805, 35081, 35102, 35452, 35454, 35472, 37205-37208)

(Report 0078T in conjunction with 35454, 37205-37208 when these procedures are performed outside the target zone of the endoprosthesis)

+ 0079T   Placement of visceral extension prosthesis for endovascular repair of abdominal aortic aneurysm involving visceral vessels, each visceral branch (List separately in addition to code for primary procedure)

(Use 0079T in conjunction with 0078T)

(Do not report 0079T in conjunction with 34800-34805, 35081, 35102, 35452, 35454, 35472, 37205-37208)

(Report 0079T in conjunction with 35454, 37205-37208 when these procedures are performed outside the target zone of the endoprosthesis)

0080T   Endovascular repair of abdominal aortic aneurysm, pseudoaneurysm or dissection, abdominal aorta involving visceral vessels (superior mesenteric, celiac or renal), using fenestrated modular bifurcated prosthesis (two docking limbs), radiological supervision and interpretation

(Do not report 0080T in conjunction with 34800-34805, 35081, 35102, 35452, 35454, 35472, 37205-37208)

(Report 0080T in conjunction with 35454, 37205-37208 when these procedures are performed outside the target zone of the endoprosthesis)

+ 0081T   Placement of visceral extension prosthesis for endovascular repair of abdominal aortic aneurysm involving visceral vessels, each visceral branch, radiological supervision and interpretation (List separately in addition to code for primary procedure)

(Use 0081T in conjunction with 0080T)

(Do not report 0081T in conjunction with 34800-34805, 35081, 35102, 35452, 35454, 35472, 37205-37208)

(Report 0081T in conjunction with 35454, 37205-37208 when these procedures are performed outside the target zone of the endoprosthesis)

►(0082T, 0083T have been deleted. To report, see 77373-77435)◄

0084T   Insertion of a temporary prostatic urethral stent

0085T   Breath test for heart transplant rejection

0086T   Left ventricular filling pressure indirect measurement by computerized calibration of the arterial waveform response to Valsalva maneuver

0087T   Sperm evaluation, Hyaluronan binding assay

0088T   Submucosal radiofrequency tissue volume reduction of tongue base, one or more sites, per session (ie, for treatment of obstructive sleep apnea syndrome)

0089T   Actigraphy testing, recording, analysis and interpretation (minimum of three-day recording)

▲ 0090T   Total disc arthroplasty (artificial disc), anterior approach, including discectomy to prepare interspace (other than for decompression) cervical; single interspace

►(0091T has been deleted)◄

►(To report total disc lumbar arthroplasty, use 22857)◄

+ 0092T   each additional interspace (List separately in addition to code for primary procedure)

►(Use 0092T in conjunction with 0090T)◄

►(For total disc lumbar arthroplasty of additional interspaces, use 0163T)◄

►(Do not report 0092T in conjunction with 22857)◄

▲ 0093T   Removal of total disc arthroplasty, anterior approach cervical; single interspace

►(0094T has been deleted)◄

►(To report removal of total disc lumbar arthroplasty, use 22865)◄

+ 0095T   each additional interspace (List separately in addition to code for primary procedure)

►(Use 0095T in conjunction with 0093T)◄

►(For removal of total disc lumbar arthroplasty additional interspaces, use 0164T)◄

►(Do not report 0095T in conjunction with 22865)◄

▲ 0096T   Revision of total disc arthroplasty, anterior approach cervical; single interspace

(Do not report 0096T in conjunction with 0093T)

►(0097T has been deleted)◄

►(To report revision of total disc lumbar arthroplasty, use 22862)◄

+ 0098T   each additional interspace (List separately in addition to code for primary procedure)

►(Use 0098T in conjunction with 0096T)◄

►(0090T-0098T include fluoroscopy when performed)◄

(Do not report 0090T-0098T in conjunction with 22851, 49010, when performed at the same level)

►(Do not report 0098T in conjunction with 22862, 0095T)◄

►(For revision of total disc lumbar arthroplasty additional interspaces, use 0165T)◄

►(For decompression, see 63001-63048)◄

0099T   Implantation of intrastromal corneal ring segments

0100T   Placement of a subconjunctival retinal prosthesis receiver and pulse generator, and implantation of intra-ocular retinal electrode array, with vitrectomy

Category III Codes

0101T Extracorporeal shock wave involving musculoskeletal system, not otherwise specified, high energy

(For application of low energy musculoskeletal system extracorporeal shock wave, use 0019T)

0102T Extracorporeal shock wave, high energy, performed by a physician, requiring anesthesia other than local, involving lateral humeral epicondyle

(For application of low energy musculoskeletal system extracorporeal shock wave, use 0019T)

0103T Holotranscobalamin, quantitative

0104T Inert gas rebreathing for cardiac output measurement; during rest

0105T   during exercise

0106T Quantitative sensory testing (QST), testing and interpretation per extremity; using touch pressure stimuli to assess large diameter sensation

0107T   using vibration stimuli to assess large diameter fiber sensation

0108T   using cooling stimuli to assess small nerve fiber sensation and hyperalgesia

0109T   using heat-pain stimuli to assess small nerve fiber sensation and hyperalgesia

0110T   using other stimuli to assess sensation

0111T Long-chain (C20-22) omega-3 fatty acids in red blood cell (RBC) membranes

(For very long chain fatty acids, use 82726)

Medication Therapy Management

Medication Therapy Management Service(s) (MTMS) describe face-to-face patient assessment and intervention as appropriate, by a pharmacist. MTMS is provided to optimize the response to medications or to manage treatment-related medication interactions or complications.

MTMS includes the following documented elements: review of the pertinent patient history, medication profile (prescription and non-prescription), and recommendations for improving health outcomes and treatment compliance. These codes are not to be used to describe the provision of product-specific information at the point of dispensing or any other routine dispensing-related activities.

0115T Medication therapy management service(s) provided by a pharmacist, individual, face-to-face with patient, initial 15 minutes, with assessment, and intervention if provided; initial encounter

0116T   subsequent encounter

+ 0117T   each additional 15 minutes (List separately in addition to code for primary service)

(Use 0117T in conjunction with 0115T, 0116T)

▶(0120T has been deleted. To report, use 19105)◀

0123T Fistulization of sclera for glaucoma, through ciliary body

0124T Conjunctival incision with posterior juxtascleral placement of pharmacological agent (does not include supply of medication)

0126T Common carotid intima-media thickness (IMT) study for evaluation of atherosclerotic burden or coronary heart disease risk factor assessment

0130T Validated, statistically reliable, randomized, controlled, single-patient clinical investigation of FDA approved chronic care drugs, provided by a pharmacist, interpretation and report to the prescribing health care professional

0133T Upper gastrointestinal endoscopy, including esophagus, stomach, and either the duodenum and/or jejunum as appropriate, with injection of implant material into and along the muscle of the lower esophageal sphincter (eg, for treatment of gastroesophageal reflux disease)

0135T Ablation, renal tumor(s), unilateral, percutaneous, cryotherapy

0137T Biopsy, prostate, needle, saturation sampling for prostate mapping

(Do not report 0137T in conjunction with 76942)

0140T Exhaled breath condensate pH

▶Pancreatic islet cells are transplanted by infusion into the portal vein. The portal vein may be cannulated percutaneously with imaging guidance, by laparoscopy, or by laparotomy. Codes 0141T-0143T include infusion of islet cells with monitoring and management of portal and systemic hemodynamics, monitoring and management of blood glucose and insulin therapy, immunotherapy infusion, antibiotic infusion, analgesic and sedative administration and monitoring, and all other therapeutic injections and infusions administered during the islet infusion. Codes 0141T-0143T also include typical postprocedural care. When reporting 0141T, percutaneous portal vein catheterization is reported separately (see codes 36481, 75887). Code 0142T includes diagnostic laparotomy (49000, 49002). Code 0143T includes diagnostic laparoscopy (49320).◀

● **0141T** Pancreatic islet cell transplantation through portal vein, percutaneous

▶(For open approach, use 0142T)◀

▶(For laparoscopic approach, use 0143T)◀

▶(For percutaneous portal vein catheterization, use 36481)◀

▶(For radiological supervision and interpretation, use 75887)◀

● **0142T** Pancreatic islet cell transplantation through portal vein, open

▶(For percutaneous approach, use 0141T)◀

▶(For laparoscopic approach, use 0143T)◀

▶(Do not report 0142T in conjunction with 49000, 49002)◀

● **0143T** Laparoscopy, surgical, pancreatic islet cell transplantation through portal vein

►(For percutaneous approach, use 0141T)◄

►(For open approach, use 0142T)◄

►(Do not report 0143T in conjunction with 49320)◄

● **0144T** Computed tomography, heart, without contrast material, including image postprocessing and quantitative evaluation of coronary calcium

►(Do not report 0144T in conjunction with 0145T-0151T)◄

● **0145T** Computed tomography, heart, without contrast material followed by contrast material(s) and further sections, including cardiac gating and 3D image postprocessing; cardiac structure and morphology

►(For cardiac structure and morphology in congenital heart disease, use 0150T)◄

● **0146T** computed tomographic angiography of coronary arteries (including native and anomalous coronary arteries, coronary bypass grafts), without quantitative evaluation of coronary calcium

● **0147T** computed tomographic angiography of coronary arteries (including native and anomalous coronary arteries, coronary bypass grafts), with quantitative evaluation of coronary calcium

►(Do not report 0147T in conjunction with 0144T)◄

● **0148T** cardiac structure and morphology and computed tomographic angiography of coronary arteries (including native and anomalous coronary arteries, coronary bypass grafts), without quantitative evaluation of coronary calcium

● **0149T** cardiac structure and morphology and computed tomographic angiography of coronary arteries (including native and anomalous coronary arteries, coronary bypass grafts), with quantitative evaluation of coronary calcium

►(Do not report 0149T in conjunction with 0144T)◄

● **0150T** cardiac structure and morphology in congenital heart disease

+● **0151T** Computed tomography, heart, without contrast material followed by contrast material(s) and further sections, including cardiac gating and 3D image postprocessing, function evaluation (left and right ventricular function, ejection-fraction and segmental wall motion) (List separately in addition to code for primary procedure)

►(Use 0151T in conjunction with 0145T-0150T)◄

+● **0153T** Transcatheter placement of wireless physiologic sensor in aneurysmal sac during endovascular repair, including radiological supervision and interpretation and instrument calibration (List separately in addition to code for primary procedure)

►(Use 0153T in conjunction with 34800, 34802, 34803, 34804, 34805, 34900)◄

►(0153T includes deployment of the sensor, repositioning if required, and intraoperative calibration)◄

● **0154T** Noninvasive physiologic study of implanted wireless pressure sensor in aneurysmal sac following endovascular repair, complete study including recording, analysis of pressure and waveform tracings, interpretation and report

►(Do not report 0154T in conjunction with 0153T)◄

● **0155T** Laparoscopy, surgical; implantation or replacement of gastric stimulation electrodes, lesser curvature (ie, morbid obesity)

● **0156T** revision or removal of gastric stimulation electrodes, lesser curvature (ie, morbid obesity)

►(For open approach, see 0157T, 0158T)◄

►(For insertion of gastric neurostimulator pulse generator, use 64590)◄

►(For revision or removal of gastric neurostimulator pulse generator, use 64595)◄

►(For electronic analysis and programming of gastric neurostimulator pulse generator, see 95999)◄

● **0157T** Laparotomy, implantation or replacement of gastric stimulation electrodes, lesser curvature (ie, morbid obesity)

● **0158T** Laparotomy, revision or removal of gastric stimulation electrodes, lesser curvature (ie, morbid obesity)

►(For laparoscopic approach, see 0155T, 0156T)◄

►(For insertion of gastric neurostimulator pulse generator, use 64590)◄

►(For revision or removal of gastric neurostimulator pulse generator, use 64595)◄

►(For electronic analysis and programming of gastric neurostimulator pulse generator, see 95999)◄

►(For electronic analysis, programming and reprogramming of gastric neurostimulator, use 0162T)◄

+● **0159T** Computer-aided detection, including computer algorithm analysis of MRI image data for lesion detection/characterization, pharmacokinetic analysis, with further physician review for interpretation, breast MRI (List separately in addition to code for primary procedure)

►(Use 0159T in conjunction with 77058, 77059)◄

Category III Codes

● **0160T**   Therapeutic repetitive transcranial magnetic stimulation treatment planning

▶(Pre-treatment determination of optimal magnetic field strength via titration, treatment location determination and stimulation parameter and protocol programming in the therapeutic use of high power, focal magnetic pulses for the direct, noninvasive modulation of cortical neurons)◀

● **0161T**   Therapeutic repetitive transcranial magnetic stimulation treatment delivery and management, per session

▶(Treatment session using high power, focal magnetic pulses for the direct, noninvasive modulation of cortical neurons. Clinical evaluation, safety monitoring and treatment parameter review in the therapeutic use of high power, focal magnetic pulses for the direct, noninvasive modulation of cortical neurons)◀

● **0162T**   Electronic analysis and programming, reprogramming of gastric neurostimulator (ie, morbid obesity)

+● **0163T**   Total disc arthroplasty (artificial disc), anterior approach, including discectomy to prepare interspace (other than for decompression), lumbar, each additional interspace

▶(Use 0163T in conjunction with 22857)◀

+● **0164T**   Removal of total disc arthroplasty, anterior approach, lumbar, each additional interspace

▶(Use 0164T in conjunction with 22865)◀

+● **0165T**   Revision of total disc arthroplasty, anterior approach, lumbar, each additional interspace

▶(Use 0165T in conjunction with 22862)◀

▶(0163T-0165T include fluoroscopy when performed)◀

▶(Do not report 0163T-0165T in conjunction with 22851, 49010, when performed at the same level)◀

▶(For cervical total disc arthroplasty procedures, see 0090T-0098T)◀

▶(For decompression, see 63001-63048)◀

● **0166T**   Transmyocardial transcatheter closure of ventricular septal defect, with implant; without cardiopulmonary bypass

● **0167T**   with cardiopulmonary bypass

▶(Do not report 0166T, 0167T in conjunction with 32020, 33210, 33211)◀

▶(For ventricular septal defect closure via percutaneous transcatheter implant delivery, use 93581)◀

● **0168T**   Rhinophototherapy, intranasal application of ultraviolet and visible light, bilateral

● **0169T**   Stereotactic placement of infusion catheter(s) in the brain for delivery of therapeutic agent(s), including computerized stereotactic planning and burr hole(s)

▶(Do not report code 0169T in conjunction with 20660, 61107, 61795)◀

● **0170T**   Repair of anorectal fistula with plug (eg, porcine small intestine submucosa [SIS])

▶(For repair of anal fistula using fibrin glue, use 46706)◀

▶(Do not report 0170T in conjunction with 15430, 15431)◀

Category III Codes

Notes

⊙=Moderate sedation   ✚=Add-on code   ⟋=FDA approval pending

Appendix A

Modifiers

This list includes all of the modifiers applicable to *CPT 2007* codes.

21 Prolonged Evaluation and Management Services: When the face-to-face or floor/unit service(s) provided is prolonged or otherwise greater than that usually required for the highest level of evaluation and management service within a given category, it may be identified by adding modifier 21 to the evaluation and management code number. A report may also be appropriate.

22 Unusual Procedural Services: When the service(s) provided is greater than that usually required for the listed procedure, it may be identified by adding modifier 22 to the usual procedure number. A report may also be appropriate.

23 Unusual Anesthesia: Occasionally, a procedure, which usually requires either no anesthesia or local anesthesia, because of unusual circumstances must be done under general anesthesia. This circumstance may be reported by adding modifier 23 to the procedure code of the basic service.

24 Unrelated Evaluation and Management Service by the Same Physician During a Postoperative Period: The physician may need to indicate that an evaluation and management service was performed during a postoperative period for a reason(s) unrelated to the original procedure. This circumstance may be reported by adding modifier 24 to the appropriate level of E/M service.

25 Significant, Separately Identifiable Evaluation and Management Service by the Same Physician on the Same Day of the Procedure or Other Service: The physician may need to indicate that on the day a procedure or service identified by a CPT code was performed, the patient's condition required a significant, separately identifiable E/M service above and beyond the other service provided or beyond the usual preoperative and postoperative care associated with the procedure that was performed. A significant, separately identifiable E/M service is defined or substantiated by documentation that satisfies the relevant criteria for the respective E/M service to be reported (see **Evaluation and Management Services Guidelines** for instructions on determining level of E/M service). The E/M service may be prompted by the symptom or condition for which the procedure and/or service was provided. As such, different diagnoses are not required for reporting of the E/M services on the same date. This circumstance may be reported by adding modifier 25 to the appropriate level of E/M service. **Note:** This modifier is not used to report an E/M service that resulted in a decision to perform surgery. See modifier 57.

26 Professional Component: Certain procedures are a combination of a physician component and a technical component. When the physician component is reported separately, the service may be identified by adding modifier 26 to the usual procedure number.

32 Mandated Services: Services related to *mandated* consultation and/or related services (eg, PRO, third party payer, governmental, legislative or regulatory requirement) may be identified by adding modifier 32 to the basic procedure.

47 Anesthesia by Surgeon: Regional or general anesthesia provided by the surgeon may be reported by adding modifier 47 to the basic service. (This does not include local anesthesia.) **Note:** Modifier 47 would not be used as a modifier for the anesthesia procedures.

50 Bilateral Procedure: Unless otherwise identified in the listings, bilateral procedures that are performed at the same operative session should be identified by adding modifier 50 to the appropriate five digit code.

51 Multiple Procedures: When multiple procedures, other than E/M services, are performed at the same session by the same provider, the primary procedure or service may be reported as listed. The additional procedure(s) or service(s) may be identified by appending modifier 51 to the additional procedure or service code(s). **Note:** This modifier should not be appended to designated "add-on" codes (see Appendix D).

52 Reduced Services: Under certain circumstances a service or procedure is partially reduced or eliminated at the physician's discretion. Under these circumstances the service provided can be identified by its usual procedure number and the addition of modifier 52, signifying that the service is reduced. This provides a means of reporting reduced services without disturbing the identification of the basic service. **Note:** For hospital outpatient reporting of a previously scheduled procedure/service that is partially reduced or cancelled as a result of extenuating circumstances or those that threaten the well-being of the patient prior to or after administration of anesthesia, see modifiers 73 and 74 (see modifiers approved for ASC hospital outpatient use).

53 Discontinued Procedure: Under certain circumstances, the physician may elect to terminate a surgical or diagnostic procedure. Due to extenuating circumstances or those that threaten the well being of the patient, it may be necessary to indicate that a surgical or diagnostic procedure was started but discontinued. This circumstance may be reported by adding modifier 53 to the code reported by the physician for the discontinued procedure. **Note:** This modifier is not used to report the elective cancellation of a procedure prior to the patient's anesthesia induction and/or surgical preparation in the operating suite. For outpatient hospital/ambulatory surgery center (ASC) reporting of a previously scheduled procedure/service that is partially reduced or cancelled as a result of extenuating circumstances or those that threaten the well being of the patient prior to or after administration of anesthesia, see modifiers 73 and 74 (see modifiers approved for ASC hospital outpatient use).

54   Surgical Care Only: When one physician performs a surgical procedure and another provides preoperative and/or postoperative management, surgical services may be identified by adding modifier 54 to the usual procedure number.

55   Postoperative Management Only: When one physician performed the postoperative management and another physician performed the surgical procedure, the postoperative component may be identified by adding modifier 55 to the usual procedure number.

56   Preoperative Management Only: When one physician performed the preoperative care and evaluation and another physician performed the surgical procedure, the preoperative component may be identified by adding modifier 56 to the usual procedure number.

57   Decision for Surgery: An evaluation and management service that resulted in the initial decision to perform the surgery may be identified by adding modifier 57 to the appropriate level of E/M service.

58   Staged or Related Procedure or Service by the Same Physician During the Postoperative Period: The physician may need to indicate that the performance of a procedure or service during the postoperative period was: a) planned prospectively at the time of the original procedure (staged); b) more extensive than the original procedure; or c) for therapy following a diagnostic surgical procedure. This circumstance may be reported by adding modifier 58 to the staged or related procedure. **Note:** This modifier is not used to report the treatment of a problem that requires a return to the operating room. See modifier 78.

59   Distinct Procedural Service: Under certain circumstances, the physician may need to indicate that a procedure or service was distinct or independent from other services performed on the same day. Modifier 59 is used to identify procedures/services that are not normally reported together, but are appropriate under the circumstances. This may represent a different session or patient encounter, different procedure or surgery, different site or organ system, separate incision/excision, separate lesion, or separate injury (or area of injury in extensive injuries) not ordinarily encountered or performed on the same day by the same physician. However, when another already established modifier is appropriate it should be used rather than modifier 59. Only if no more descriptive modifier is available, and the use of modifier 59 best explains the circumstances, should modifier 59 be used.

62   Two Surgeons: When two surgeons work together as primary surgeons performing distinct part(s) of a procedure, each surgeon should report his/her distinct operative work by adding modifier 62 to the procedure code and any associated add-on code(s) for that procedure as long as both surgeons continue to work together as primary surgeons. Each surgeon should report the co-surgery once using the same procedure code. If additional procedure(s) (including add-on procedure(s) are performed during the same surgical session, separate code(s) may also be reported with modifier 62 added. **Note:** If a co-surgeon acts as an assistant in the performance of additional procedure(s) during the same surgical session, those services may be reported using separate procedure code(s) with modifier 80 or modifier 82 added, as appropriate.

63   Procedure Performed on Infants less than 4 kg: Procedures performed on neonates and infants up to a present body weight of 4 kg may involve significantly increased complexity and physician work commonly associated with these patients. This circumstance may be reported by adding modifier 63 to the procedure number. **Note:** Unless otherwise designated, this modifier may only be appended to procedures/services listed in the 20000-69990 code series. Modifier 63 should not be appended to any CPT codes listed in the **Evaluation and Management Services, Anesthesia, Radiology, Pathology/Laboratory, or Medicine** sections.

66   Surgical Team: Under some circumstances, highly complex procedures (requiring the concomitant services of several physicians, often of different specialties, plus other highly skilled, specially trained personnel, various types of complex equipment) are carried out under the "surgical team" concept. Such circumstances may be identified by each participating physician with the addition of modifier 66 to the basic procedure number used for reporting services.

76   Repeat Procedure by Same Physician: The physician may need to indicate that a procedure or service was repeated subsequent to the original procedure or service. This circumstance may be reported by adding modifier 76 to the repeated procedure/service.

77   Repeat Procedure by Another Physician: The physician may need to indicate that a basic procedure or service performed by another physician had to be repeated. This situation may be reported by adding modifier 77 to the repeated procedure/service.

78   Return to the Operating Room for a Related Procedure During the Postoperative Period: The physician may need to indicate that another procedure was performed during the postoperative period of the initial procedure. When this subsequent procedure is related to the first, and requires the use of the operating room, it may be reported by adding modifier 78 to the related procedure. (For repeat procedures on the same day, see modifier 76.)

79   Unrelated Procedure or Service by the Same Physician During the Postoperative Period: The physician may need to indicate that the performance of a procedure or service during the postoperative period was unrelated to the original procedure. This circumstance may be reported by using modifier 79. (For repeat procedures on the same day, see modifier 76.)

80   Assistant Surgeon: Surgical assistant services may be identified by adding modifier 80 to the usual procedure number(s).

81 Minimum Assistant Surgeon: Minimum surgical assistant services are identified by adding modifier 81 to the usual procedure number.

82 Assistant Surgeon (when qualified resident surgeon not available): The unavailability of a qualified resident surgeon is a prerequisite for use of modifier 82 appended to the usual procedure code number(s).

90 Reference (Outside) Laboratory: When laboratory procedures are performed by a party other than the treating or reporting physician, the procedure may be identified by adding modifier 90 to the usual procedure number.

91 Repeat Clinical Diagnostic Laboratory Test: In the course of treatment of the patient, it may be necessary to repeat the same laboratory test on the same day to obtain subsequent (multiple) test results. Under these circumstances, the laboratory test performed can be identified by its usual procedure number and the addition of modifier 91. **Note:** This modifier may not be used when tests are rerun to confirm initial results; due to testing problems with specimens or equipment; or for any other reason when a normal, one-time, reportable result is all that is required. This modifier may not be used when other code(s) describe a series of test results (eg, glucose tolerance tests, evocative/suppression testing). This modifier may only be used for laboratory test(s) performed more than once on the same day on the same patient.

99 Multiple Modifiers: Under certain circumstances two or more modifiers may be necessary to completely delineate a service. In such situations modifier 99 should be added to the basic procedure, and other applicable modifiers may be listed as part of the description of the service.

Anesthesia Physical Status Modifiers

The Physical Status modifiers are consistent with the American Society of Anesthesiologists ranking of patient physical status, and distinguishing various levels of complexity of the anesthesia service provided. All anesthesia services are reported by use of the anesthesia five-digit procedure code (00100-01999) with the appropriate physical status modifier appended.

Example: 00100-P1

Under certain circumstances, when another established modifier(s) is appropriate, it should be used in addition to the physical status modifier.

Example: 00100-P4-53

Physical Status Modifier P1: A normal healthy patient

Physical Status Modifier P2: A patient with mild systemic disease

Physical Status Modifier P3: A patient with severe systemic disease

Physical Status Modifier P4: A patient with severe systemic disease that is a constant threat to life

Physical Status Modifier P5: A moribund patient who is not expected to survive without the operation

Physical Status Modifier P6: A declared brain-dead patient whose organs are being removed for donor purposes

Modifiers Approved for Ambulatory Surgery Center (ASC) Hospital Outpatient Use

CPT Level I Modifiers

25 Significant, Separately Identifiable Evaluation and Management Service by the Same Physician on the Same Day of the Procedure or Other Service: The physician may need to indicate that on the day a procedure or service identified by a CPT code was performed, the patient's condition required a significant, separately identifiable E/M service above and beyond the other service provided or beyond the usual preoperative and postoperative care associated with the procedure that was performed. A significant, separately identifiable E/M service is defined or substantiated by documentation that satisfies the relevant criteria for the respective E/M service to be reported (see **Evaluation and Management Services Guidelines** for instructions on determining level of E/M service). The E/M service may be prompted by the symptom or condition for which the procedure and/or service was provided. As such, different diagnoses are not required for reporting of the E/M services on the same date. This circumstance may be reported by adding modifier 25 to the appropriate level of E/M service. **Note:** This modifier is not used to report an E/M service that resulted in a decision to perform surgery (see modifier 57).

27 Multiple Outpatient Hospital E/M Encounters on the Same Date: For hospital outpatient reporting purposes, utilization of hospital resources related to separate and distinct E/M encounters performed in multiple outpatient hospital settings on the same date may be reported by adding modifier 27 to each appropriate level outpatient and/or emergency department E/M code(s). This modifier provides a means of reporting circumstances involving evaluation and management services provided by physician(s) in more than one (multiple) outpatient hospital setting(s) (eg, hospital emergency department, clinic). **Note:** This modifier is not to be used for physician reporting of multiple E/M services performed by the same physician on the same date. For physician reporting of all outpatient evaluation and management services provided by the same physician on the same date and performed in multiple outpatient setting(s) (eg, hospital emergency department, clinic), see **Evaluation and Management, Emergency Department, or Preventive Medicine Services** codes.

50 Bilateral Procedure: Unless otherwise identified in the listings, bilateral procedures that are performed at the same operative session should be identified by adding modifier 50 to the appropriate five digit code.

52 **Reduced Services:** Under certain circumstances a service or procedure is partially reduced or eliminated at the physician's discretion. Under these circumstances the service provided can be identified by its usual procedure number and the addition of modifier 52, signifying that the service is reduced. This provides a means of reporting reduced services without disturbing the identification of the basic service. **Note:** For hospital outpatient reporting of a previously scheduled procedure/service that is partially reduced or cancelled as a result of extenuating circumstances or those that threaten the well-being of the patient prior to or after administration of anesthesia, see modifiers 73 and 74.

58 **Staged or Related Procedure or Service by the Same Physician During the Postoperative Period:** The physician may need to indicate that the performance of a procedure or service during the postoperative period was: a) planned prospectively at the time of the original procedure (staged); b) more extensive than the original procedure; or c) for therapy following a diagnostic surgical procedure. This circumstance may be reported by adding modifier 58 to the staged or related procedure. **Note:** This modifier is not used to report the treatment of a problem that requires a return to the operating room (see modifier 78).

59 **Distinct Procedural Service:** Under certain circumstances, the physician may need to indicate that a procedure or service was distinct or independent from other services performed on the same day. Modifier 59 is used to identify procedures/services that are not normally reported together, but are appropriate under the circumstances. This may represent a different session or patient encounter, different procedure or surgery, different site or organ system, separate incision/excision, separate lesion, or separate injury (or area of injury in extensive injuries) not ordinarily encountered or performed on the same day by the same physician. However, when another already established modifier is appropriate it should be used rather than modifier 59. Only if no more descriptive modifier is available, and the use of modifier 59 best explains the circumstances, should modifier 59 be used.

73 **Discontinued Out-Patient Hospital/Ambulatory Surgery Center (ASC) Procedure Prior to the Administration of Anesthesia:** Due to extenuating circumstances or those that threaten the well being of the patient, the physician may cancel a surgical or diagnostic procedure subsequent to the patient's surgical preparation (including sedation when provided, and being taken to the room where the procedure is to be performed), but prior to the administration of anesthesia (local, regional block(s) or general). Under these circumstances, the intended service that is prepared for but cancelled can be reported by its usual procedure number and the addition of modifier 73. **Note:** The elective cancellation of a service prior to the administration of anesthesia and/or surgical preparation of the patient should not be reported. For physician reporting of a discontinued procedure, see modifier 53.

74 **Discontinued Out-Patient Hospital/Ambulatory Surgery Center (ASC) Procedure After Administration of Anesthesia:** Due to extenuating circumstances or those that threaten the well being of the patient, the physician may terminate a surgical or diagnostic procedure after the administration of anesthesia (local, regional block(s), general) or after the procedure was started (incision made, intubation started, scope inserted, etc). Under these circumstances, the procedure started but terminated can be reported by its usual procedure number and the addition of modifier 74. **Note:** The elective cancellation of a service prior to the administration of anesthesia and/or surgical preparation of the patient should not be reported. For physician reporting of a discontinued procedure, see modifier 53.

76 **Repeat Procedure by Same Physician:** The physician may need to indicate that a procedure or service was repeated subsequent to the original procedure or service. This circumstance may be reported by adding modifier 76 to the repeated procedure/service.

77 **Repeat Procedure by Another Physician:** The physician may need to indicate that a basic procedure or service performed by another physician had to be repeated. This situation may be reported by adding modifier 77 to the repeated procedure/service.

78 **Return to the Operating Room for a Related Procedure During the Postoperative Period:** The physician may need to indicate that another procedure was performed during the postoperative period of the initial procedure. When this subsequent procedure is related to the first, and requires the use of the operating room, it may be reported by adding modifier 78 to the related procedure. (For repeat procedures on the same day, see 76.)

79 **Unrelated Procedure or Service by the Same Physician During the Postoperative Period:** The physician may need to indicate that the performance of a procedure or service during the postoperative period was unrelated to the original procedure. This circumstance may be reported by using modifier 79. (For repeat procedures on the same day, see 76.)

91 **Repeat Clinical Diagnostic Laboratory Test:** In the course of treatment of the patient, it may be necessary to repeat the same laboratory test on the same day to obtain subsequent (multiple) test results. Under these circumstances, the laboratory test performed can be identified by its usual procedure number and the addition of modifier 91. **Note:** This modifier may not be used when tests are rerun to confirm initial results; due to testing problems with specimens or equipment; or for any other reason when a normal, one-time, reportable result is all that is required. This modifier may not be used when other code(s) describe a series of test results (eg, glucose tolerance tests, evocative/suppression testing). This modifier may only be used for laboratory test(s) performed more than once on the same day on the same patient.

Level II (HCPCS/National) Modifiers

E1 Upper left, eyelid

E2 Lower left, eyelid

E3 Upper right, eyelid

E4 Lower right, eyelid

F1 Left hand, second digit

F2 Left hand, third digit

F3 Left hand, fourth digit

F4 Left hand, fifth digit

F5 Right hand, thumb

F6 Right hand, second digit

F7 Right hand, third digit

F8 Right hand, fourth digit

F9 Right hand, fifth digit

FA Left hand, thumb

GG Performance and payment of a screening mammogram and diagnostic mammogram on the same patient, same day

GH Diagnostic mammogram converted from screening mammogram on same day

LC Left circumflex coronary artery (Hospitals use with codes 92980-92984, 92995, 92996)

LD Left anterior descending coronary artery (Hospitals use with codes 92980-92984, 92995, 92996)

LT Left side (used to identify procedures performed on the left side of the body)

QM Ambulance service provided under arrangement by a provider of services

QN Ambulance service furnished directly by a provider of services

RC Right coronary artery (Hospitals use with codes 92980-92984, 92995, 92996)

RT Right side (used to identify procedures performed on the right side of the body)

T1 Left foot, second digit

T2 Left foot, third digit

T3 Left foot, fourth digit

T4 Left foot, fifth digit

T5 Right foot, great toe

T6 Right foot, second digit

T7 Right foot, third digit

T8 Right foot, fourth digit

T9 Right foot, fifth digit

TA Left foot, great toe

Appendix B

Summary of Additions, Deletions, and Revisions

Appendix B shows the actual changes that were made to the code descriptors. New codes appear with a bullet (●) and are indicated as "Code Added." Revised codes are preceded with a triangle (▲). Within revised codes, the deleted language appears with a ~~strikethrough~~, while new text appears <u>underlined</u>. Codes with which conscious sedation would not be separately reported when performed at the same session by the same provider are denoted with the bullseye (⊙). The symbol ⚡ is used to identify codes for vaccines that are pending FDA approval (see **Appendix K**).

Revisions to the headings, notes, introductory paragraphs, and cross-references are not included in this Appendix, but are identified in the main text of the book with the "► ◄" symbols and presented in green.

Evaluation and Management

▲ 99251 ~~Initial i~~<u>I</u>npatient consultation for a new or established patient, which requires these three key components:

- A problem focused history;
- A problem focused examination; and
- Straightforward medical decision making.

Counseling and/or coordination of care with other providers or agencies are provided consistent with the nature of the problem(s) and the patient's and/or family's needs.

Usually, the presenting problem(s) are self limited or minor. Physicians typically spend 20 minutes at the bedside and on the patient's hospital floor or unit.

▲ 99252 ~~Initial i~~<u>I</u>npatient consultation for a new or established patient, which requires these three key components:

- An expanded problem focused history;
- An expanded problem focused examination; and
- Straightforward medical decision making.

Counseling and/or coordination of care with other providers or agencies are provided consistent with the nature of the problem(s) and the patient's and/or family's needs.

Usually, the presenting problem(s) are of low severity. Physicians typically spend 40 minutes at the bedside and on the patient's hospital floor or unit.

▲ 99253 ~~Initial i~~<u>I</u>npatient consultation for a new or established patient, which requires these three key components:

- A detailed history;
- A detailed examination; and
- Medical decision making of low complexity.

Counseling and/or coordination of care with other providers or agencies are provided consistent with the nature of the problem(s) and the patient's and/or family's needs.

Usually, the presenting problem(s) are of moderate severity. Physicians typically spend 55 minutes at the bedside and on the patient's hospital floor or unit.

▲ 99254 ~~Initial i~~<u>I</u>npatient consultation for a new or established patient, which requires these three key components:

- A comprehensive history;
- A comprehensive examination; and
- Medical decision making of moderate complexity.

Counseling and/or coordination of care with other providers or agencies are provided consistent with the nature of the problem(s) and the patient's and/or family's needs.

Usually, the presenting problem(s) are of moderate to high severity. Physicians typically spend 80 minutes at the bedside and on the patient's hospital floor or unit.

▲ 99255 ~~Initial i~~<u>I</u>npatient consultation for a new or established patient, which requires these three key components:

- A comprehensive history;
- A comprehensive examination; and
- Medical decision making of high complexity.

Counseling and/or coordination of care with other providers or agencies are provided consistent with the nature of the problem(s) and the patient's and/or family's needs.

Usually, the presenting problem(s) are of moderate to high severity. Physicians typically spend 110 minutes at the bedside and on the patient's hospital floor or unit.

● 99363 Code added

● 99364 Code added

Anesthesia

● 00625 Code added

● 00626 Code added

~~01995~~ ~~Regional intravenous administration of local anesthetic agent or other medication (upper or lower extremity)~~

Surgery

~~15000~~ ~~Surgical preparation or creation of recipient site by excision of open wounds, burn eschar, or scar (including subcutaneous tissues), or incisional release of scar contracture; first 100 sq cm or one percent of body area of infants and children~~

+ ~~15001~~ ~~each additional 100 sq cm or each additional one percent of body area of infants and children (List separately in addition to code for primary procedure)~~

● 15002 Code added

+● 15003 Code added

● 15004   Code added

+● 15005   Code added

● 15731   Code added

● 15830   Code added

~~15831~~   ~~abdomen (eg, abdominoplasty) (includes umbilical transposition, fascial plication and undermining) (List separately in addition to code for primary procedure)~~

+● 15847   Code added

▲ 17000   Destruction (eg, laser surgery, electrosurgery, cryosurgery, chemosurgery, surgical curettement), ~~all benign or~~ premalignant lesions (eg, actinic keratoses) ~~other than skin tags or cutaneous vascular proliferative lesions~~; first lesion

⊘▲ 17004   Destruction (eg, laser surgery, electrosurgery, cryosurgery, chemosurgery, surgical curettement), ~~all benign or~~ premalignant lesions (eg, actinic keratoses), ~~other than skin tags or cutaneous vascular proliferative lesions,~~ 15 or more lesions

▲ 17110   Destruction (eg, laser surgery, electrosurgery, cryosurgery, chemosurgery, surgical curettement), of benign lesions other than skin tags or cutaneous vascular lesions~~flat warts, molluscum contagiosum, or milia~~; up to 14 lesions

⊘ ~~17304~~   ~~Chemosurgery (Mohs micrographic technique), including removal of all gross tumor, surgical excision of tissue specimens, mapping, color coding of specimens, microscopic examination of specimens by the surgeon, and complete histopathologic preparation including the first routine stain (eg, hematoxylin and eosin, toluidine blue); first stage, fresh tissue technique, up to 5 specimens~~

~~17305~~   ~~second stage, fixed or fresh tissue, up to 5 specimens~~

~~17306~~   ~~third stage, fixed or fresh tissue, up to 5 specimens~~

~~17307~~   ~~additional stage(s), up to 5 specimens, each stage~~

+ ~~17310~~   ~~each additional specimen, after the first 5 specimens, fixed or fresh tissue, any stage (List separately in addition to code for primary procedure)~~

● 17311   Code added

+● 17312   Code added

● 17313   Code added

+● 17314   Code added

+● 17315   Code added

● 19105   Code added

▲ 19120   Excision of cyst, fibroadenoma, or other benign or malignant tumor, aberrant breast tissue, duct lesion, nipple or areolar lesion (except ~~19140~~ 19300), open, male or female, one or more lesions

~~19140~~   ~~Mastectomy for gynecomastia~~

~~19160~~   ~~Mastectomy, partial (eg, lumpectomy, tylectomy, quadrantectomy, segmentectomy);~~

~~19162~~   ~~with axillary lymphadenectomy~~

~~19180~~   ~~Mastectomy, simple, complete~~

~~19182~~   ~~Mastectomy, subcutaneous~~

~~19200~~   ~~Mastectomy, radical, including pectoral muscles, axillary lymph nodes~~

~~19220~~   ~~Mastectomy, radical, including pectoral muscles, axillary and internal mammary lymph nodes (Urban type operation)~~

~~19240~~   ~~Mastectomy, modified radical, including axillary lymph nodes, with or without pectoralis minor muscle, but excluding pectoralis major muscle~~

● 19300   Code added

● 19301   Code added

● 19302   Code added

● 19303   Code added

● 19304   Code added

● 19305   Code added

● 19306   Code added

● 19307   Code added

▲ 19361   Breast reconstruction with latissimus dorsi flap, ~~with or~~ without prosthetic implant

~~21300~~   ~~Closed treatment of skull fracture without operation~~

⊙● 22526   Code added

+⊙● 22527   Code added

● 22857   Code added

● 22862   Code added

● 22865   Code added

● 25109   Code added

▲ 25600   Closed treatment of distal radial fracture (eg, Colles or Smith type) or epiphyseal separation, ~~with or without~~ includes closed treatment of fracture of ulnar styloid, when performed; without manipulation

● 25606   Code added

● 25607   Code added

● 25608   Code added

● 25609   Code added

~~25611~~   ~~Percutaneous skeletal fixation of distal radial fracture (eg, Colles or Smith type) or epiphyseal separation, with or without fracture of ulnar styloid, requiring manipulation, with or without external fixation~~

~~25620~~   ~~Open treatment of distal radial fracture (eg, Colles or Smith type) or epiphyseal separation, with or without fracture of ulnar styloid, with or without internal or external fixation~~

▲ 26170   Excision of tendon, palm, flexor or extensor, single ~~(separate procedure)~~, each tendon

▲ 26180   Excision of tendon, finger, flexor or extensor ~~(separate procedure)~~, each tendon

~~26504~~   ~~with tendon prosthesis (separate procedure)~~

~~27315~~   ~~Neurectomy, hamstring muscle~~

~~27320~~   ~~Neurectomy, popliteal (gastrocnemius)~~

● 27325   Code added

● 27326   Code added

~~28030~~ ~~Neurectomy, intrinsic musculature of foot~~

● 28055 Code added

~~31700~~ ~~Catheterization, transglottic (separate procedure)~~

~~31708~~ ~~Instillation of contrast material for laryngography or~~
~~bronchography, without catheterization~~

~~31710~~ ~~Catheterization for bronchography, with or without instillation of~~
~~contrast material~~

● 32998 Code added

~~33200~~ ~~Insertion of permanent pacemaker with epicardial electrode(s);~~
~~by thoracotomy~~

~~33201~~ ~~by xiphoid approach~~

● 33202 Code added

● 33203 Code added

~~33245~~ ~~Insertion of epicardial single or dual chamber pacing~~
~~cardioverter defibrillator electrodes by thoracotomy;~~

~~33246~~ ~~with insertion of pulse generator~~

~~33253~~ ~~Operative incisions and reconstruction of atria for treatment of~~
~~atrial fibrillation or atrial flutter (eg, maze procedure)~~

● 33254 Code added

● 33255 Code added

● 33256 Code added

● 33265 Code added

● 33266 Code added

● 33675 Code added

● 33676 Code added

● 33677 Code added

▲ 33681 Closure of <u>single</u> ventricular septal defect, with or without patch;

● 33724 Code added

● 33726 Code added

▲ 35301 Thromboendarterectomy, ~~with or without~~<u>including</u> patch graft<u>, if
performed</u>; carotid, vertebral, subclavian, by neck incision

● 35302 Code added

● 35303 Code added

● 35304 Code added

● 35305 Code added

+● 35306 Code added

~~35381~~ ~~femoral and/or popliteal, and/or tibioperoneal~~

▲ 35501 Bypass graft, with vein; <u>common</u> carotid-<u>ipsilateral internal</u>
carotid

▲ 35506 carotid-subclavian <u>or subclavian-carotid</u>

~~35507~~ ~~subclavian-carotid~~

▲ 35509 carotid-<u>contralateral</u> carotid

● 35537 Code added

● 35538 Code added

● 35539 Code added

● 35540 Code added

~~35541~~ ~~aortoiliac or bi-iliac~~

~~35546~~ ~~aortofemoral or bifemoral~~

▲ 35601 Bypass graft, with other than vein; <u>common</u> carotid-<u>ipsilateral
internal carotid</u>

● 35637 Code added

● 35638 Code added

~~35641~~ ~~aortoiliac or bi-iliac~~

● 35883 Code added

● 35884 Code added

⊙● 37210 Code added

● 43647 Code added

● 43648 Code added

● 43881 Code added

● 43882 Code added

~~44152~~ ~~with rectal mucosectomy, ileoanal anastomosis, with or without~~
~~loop ileostomy~~

~~44153~~ ~~with rectal mucosectomy, ileoanal anastomosis, creation of ileal~~
~~reservoir (S or J), with or without loop ileostomy~~

● 44157 Code added

● 44158 Code added

▲ 44211 colectomy, total, abdominal, with proctectomy, with ileoanal
anastomosis, creation of ileal reservoir (S or J), with loop
ileostomy, ~~with or without~~<u>includes</u> rectal mucosectomy<u>, when
performed</u>

~~47716~~ ~~Anastomosis, choledochal cyst, without excision~~

● 47719 Code added

~~48005~~ ~~Resection or debridement of pancreas and peripancreatic tissue~~
~~for acute necrotizing pancreatitis~~

● 48105 Code added

~~48180~~ ~~Pancreaticojejunostomy, side-to-side anastomosis (Puestow-type~~
~~operation)~~

● 48548 Code added

~~49085~~ ~~Removal of peritoneal foreign body from peritoneal cavity~~

● 49324 Code added

● 49325 Code added

+● 49326 Code added

● 49402 Code added

+● 49435 Code added

● 49436 Code added

▲ 51720 Bladder instillation of anticarcinogenic agent (including
~~detention~~<u>retention</u> time)

▲ 52204 Cystourethroscopy, with biopsy<u>(s)</u>

▲ 54150 Circumcision, using clamp or other device<u> with regional dorsal
penile or ring block</u>;~~ newborn~~

~~54152~~ ~~older than 28 days of age~~

▲ 54160 Circumcision, surgical excision other than clamp, device, or dorsal slit; ~~newborn~~neonate (28 days of age or less)

▲ 54161 ~~except newborn~~older than 28 days of age

~~54820~~ ~~Exploration of epididymis, with or without biopsy~~

● 54865 Code added

~~55859~~ ~~Transperineal placement of needles or catheters into prostate for interstitial radioelement application, with or without cystoscopy~~

● 55875 Code added

● 55876 Code added

● 56442 Code added

~~56720~~ ~~Hymenotomy, simple incision~~

● 57296 Code added

● 57558 Code added

~~57820~~ ~~Dilation and curettage of cervical stump~~

● 58541 Code added

● 58542 Code added

● 58543 Code added

● 58544 Code added

● 58548 Code added

▲ 58950 Resection (initial) of ovarian, tubal or primary peritoneal malignancy with bilateral salpingo-oophorectomy and omentectomy;

● 58957 Code added

● 58958 Code added

⊘▲ 61107 Twist drill hole(s) for subdural, intracerebral, or ventricular puncture; for implanting ventricular catheter, ~~or~~pressure recording device, or other intracerebral monitoring device

⊘▲ 61210 for implanting ventricular catheter, reservoir, EEG electrode(s), ~~or~~ pressure recording device, or other cerebral monitoring device (separate procedure)

▲ 64590 Insertion or replacement of peripheral or gastric neurostimulator pulse generator or receiver, direct or inductive coupling

▲ 64595 Revision or removal of peripheral or gastric neurostimulator pulse generator or receiver

● 64910 Code added

● 64911 Code added

● 67346 Code added

~~67350~~ ~~Biopsy of extraocular muscle~~

Radiology

▲ 70540 Magnetic resonance (eg, proton) imaging, orbit, face, and/or neck; without contrast material(s)

● 70554 Code added

● 70555 Code added

▲ 71275 Computed tomographic angiography, chest (noncoronary), without contrast material(s), followed by contrast material(s) and further sections, including image postprocessing

● 72291 Code added

● 72292 Code added

+ ~~75998~~ ~~Fluoroscopic guidance for central venous access device placement, replacement (catheter only or complete), or removal (includes fluoroscopic guidance for vascular access and catheter manipulation, any necessary contrast injections through access site or catheter with related venography radiologic supervision and interpretation, and radiographic documentation of final catheter position) (List separately in addition to code for primary procedure)~~

~~76003~~ ~~Fluoroscopic guidance for needle placement (eg, biopsy, aspiration, injection, localization device)~~

~~76005~~ ~~Fluoroscopic guidance and localization of needle or catheter tip for spine or paraspinous diagnostic or therapeutic injection procedures (epidural, transforaminal epidural, subarachnoid, paravertebral facet joint, paravertebral facet joint nerve or sacroiliac joint), including neurolytic agent destruction~~

~~76006~~ ~~Manual application of stress performed by physician for joint radiography, including contralateral joint if indicated~~

~~76012~~ ~~Radiological supervision and interpretation, percutaneous vertebroplasty or vertebral augmentation including cavity creation, per vertebral body; under fluoroscopic guidance~~

~~76013~~ ~~under CT guidance~~

~~76020~~ ~~Bone age studies~~

~~76040~~ ~~Bone length studies (orthoroentgenogram, scanogram)~~

~~76061~~ ~~Radiologic examination, osseous survey; limited (eg, for metastases)~~

~~76062~~ ~~complete (axial and appendicular skeleton)~~

~~76065~~ ~~Radiologic examination, osseous survey, infant~~

~~76066~~ ~~Joint survey, single view, two or more joints (specify)~~

~~76070~~ ~~Computed tomography, bone mineral density study, one or more sites; axial skeleton (eg, hips, pelvis, spine)~~

~~76071~~ ~~appendicular skeleton (peripheral) (eg, radius, wrist, heel)~~

~~76075~~ ~~Dual energy X-ray absorptiometry (DXA), bone density study, one or more sites; axial skeleton (eg, hips, pelvis, spine)~~

~~76076~~ ~~appendicular skeleton (peripheral) (eg, radius, wrist, heel)~~

~~76077~~ ~~vertebral fracture assessment~~

~~76078~~ ~~Radiographic absorptiometry (eg, photodensitometry, radiogrammetry), one or more sites~~

+ ~~76082~~ ~~Computer-aided detection (computer algorithm analysis of digital image data for lesion detection) with further physician review for interpretation, with or without digitization of film radiographic images; diagnostic mammography (List separately in addition to code for primary procedure)~~

+ ~~76083~~ ~~screening mammography (List separately in addition to code for primary procedure)~~

~~76086~~ ~~Mammary ductogram or galactogram, single duct, radiological supervision and interpretation~~

~~76088~~ ~~Mammary ductogram or galactogram, multiple ducts, radiological supervision and interpretation~~

~~76090~~ ~~Mammography; unilateral~~

~~76091~~ ~~bilateral~~

~~76092~~ ~~Screening mammography, bilateral (two view film study of each breast)~~

76093 ~~Magnetic resonance imaging, breast, without and/or with contract material(s); unilateral~~

76094 ~~bilateral~~

76095 ~~Stereotactic localization guidance for breast biopsy or needle placement (eg, for wire localization or for injection), each lesion, radiological supervision and interpretation~~

76096 ~~Mammographic guidance for needle placement, breast (eg, for wire localization or for injection), each lesion, radiological supervision and interpretation~~

76355 ~~Computed tomography guidance for stereotactic localization~~

76360 ~~Computed tomography guidance for needle placement (eg, biopsy, aspiration, injection, localization device), radiological supervision and interpretation~~

76362 ~~Computed tomography guidance for, and monitoring of, visceral tissue ablation~~

76370 ~~Computed tomography guidance for placement of radiation therapy fields~~

76393 ~~Magnetic resonance guidance for needle placement (eg, for biopsy, needle aspiration, injection, or placement of localization device) radiological supervision and interpretation~~

76394 ~~Magnetic resonance guidance for, and monitoring of, visceral tissue ablation~~

76400 ~~Magnetic resonance (eg, proton) imaging, bone marrow blood supply~~

▲ 76536 Ultrasound, soft tissues of head and neck (eg, thyroid, parathyroid, parotid), ~~B-scan and/or~~ real time with image documentation

▲ 76604 Ultrasound, chest ~~B-scan~~ (includes mediastinum), ~~and/or~~ real time with image documentation

▲ 76645 Ultrasound, breast(s) (unilateral or bilateral), ~~B-scan and/or~~ real time with image documentation

▲ 76700 Ultrasound, abdominal, ~~B-scan and/or~~ real time with image documentation; complete

▲ 76770 Ultrasound, retroperitoneal (eg, renal, aorta, nodes), ~~B-scan and/or~~ real time with image documentation; complete

● 76776 Code added

76778 ~~Ultrasound, transplanted kidney, B-scan and/or real time with image documentation, with or without duplex Doppler study~~

● 76813 Code added

+● 76814 Code added

▲ 76856 Ultrasound, pelvic (nonobstetric), ~~B-scan and/or~~ real time with image documentation; complete

▲ 76880 Ultrasound, extremity, nonvascular, ~~B-scan and/or~~ real time with image documentation

▲ 76940 Ultrasound guidance for, and monitoring of, ~~visceral~~parenchymal tissue ablation

76986 ~~Ultrasonic guidance, intraoperative~~

● 76998 Code added

+● 77001 Code added

● 77002 Code added

● 77003 Code added

● 77011 Code added

● 77012 Code added

● 77013 Code added

● 77014 Code added

● 77021 Code added

● 77022 Code added

● 77031 Code added

● 77032 Code added

+● 77051 Code added

+● 77052 Code added

● 77053 Code added

● 77054 Code added

● 77055 Code added

● 77056 Code added

● 77057 Code added

● 77058 Code added

● 77059 Code added

● 77071 Code added

● 77072 Code added

● 77073 Code added

● 77074 Code added

● 77075 Code added

● 77076 Code added

● 77077 Code added

● 77078 Code added

● 77079 Code added

● 77080 Code added

● 77081 Code added

● 77082 Code added

● 77083 Code added

● 77084 Code added

● 77371 Code added

● 77372 Code added

● 77373 Code added

● 77435 Code added

▲ 78700 Kidney imaging~~; static only~~morphology;

78704 ~~with function study (ie, imaging renogram)~~

▲ 78707 ~~Kidney imaging~~ with vascular flow and function~~;~~, single study without pharmacological intervention

▲ 78708 with vascular flow and function, single study, with pharmacological intervention (eg, angiotensin converting enzyme inhibitor and/or diuretic)

▲ 78709 with vascular flow and function, multiple studies, with and without pharmacological intervention (eg, angiotensin converting enzyme inhibitor and/or diuretic)

▲ 78710 ~~Kidney imaging,~~ tomographic (SPECT)

78715   ~~Kidney vascular flow only~~

+▲ 78730   Urinary bladder residual study (List separately in addition to code for primary procedure)

78760   ~~Testicular imaging;~~

▲ 78761   Testicular imaging with vascular flow

Pathology and Laboratory

● 82107   Code added

● 83698   Code added

● 83913   Code added

● 86788   Code added

● 86789   Code added

▲ 87088   with isolation and presumptive identification of ~~isolates~~each isolate, urine

● 87305   Code added

● 87498   Code added

● 87640   Code added

● 87641   Code added

● 87653   Code added

● 87808   Code added

▲ 88106   simple filter method ~~only~~with interpretation

▲ 88107   smears and simple filter preparation with interpretation

▲ 89060   Crystal identification by light microscopy with or without polarizing lens analysis, tissue or any body fluid (except urine)

Medicine

⊘▲ 90655   Influenza virus vaccine, split virus, preservative free, ~~for~~when administered to children 6-35 months of age, for intramuscular use

⊘▲ 90656   Influenza virus vaccine, split virus, preservative free, ~~for use in individuals~~when administered to 3 years and older, for intramuscular use

⊘▲ 90657   Influenza virus vaccine, split virus, ~~for~~when administered to children 6-35 months of age, for intramuscular use

⊘▲ 90658   Influenza virus vaccine, split virus, ~~for use in individuals~~when administered to 3 years of age and older, for intramuscular use

⊘▲ 90669   Pneumococcal conjugate vaccine, polyvalent, ~~for~~when administered to children younger than 5 years, for intramuscular use

⊘▲ 90700   Diphtheria, tetanus toxoids, and acellular pertussis vaccine (DTaP), ~~for use in individuals~~when administered to younger than 7 years, for intramuscular use

⊘▲ 90702   Diphtheria and tetanus toxoids (DT) adsorbed ~~for use in individuals~~when administered to younger than 7 years, for intramuscular use

⊘▲ 90714   Tetanus and diphtheria toxoids (Td) adsorbed, preservative free, ~~for use in individuals~~when administered to 7 years or older, for intramuscular use

⊘▲ 90715   Tetanus, diphtheria toxoids and acellular pertussis vaccine (Tdap), ~~for use in individuals~~when administered to 7 years or older, for intramuscular use

⊘▲ 90718   Tetanus and diphtheria toxoids (Td) adsorbed ~~for use in individuals~~when administered to 7 years or older, for intramuscular use

⊘▲ 90732   Pneumococcal polysaccharide vaccine, 23-valent, adult or immunosuppressed patient dosage, ~~for use in individuals~~when administered to 2 years or older, for subcutaneous or intramuscular use

+▲ 90761   each additional hour~~, up to 8 hours~~ (List separately in addition to code for primary procedure)

+▲ 90766   each additional hour~~, up to 8 hours~~ (List separately in addition to code for primary procedure)

91060   ~~Gastric saline load test~~

● 91111   Code added

● 92025   Code added

92573   ~~Lombard test~~

● 92640   Code added

● 94002   Code added

● 94003   Code added

● 94004   Code added

● 94005   Code added

⊘● 94610   Code added

▲ 94620   Pulmonary stress testing; simple (eg, 6-minute walk test, prolonged exercise test for bronchospasm with pre- and post-spirometry and oximetry)

● 94644   Code added

+● 94645   Code added

94656   ~~Ventilation assist and management, initiation of pressure or volume preset ventilators for assisted or controlled breathing; first day~~

94657   ~~subsequent days~~

● 94774   Code added

● 94775   Code added

● 94776   Code added

● 94777   Code added

● 95012   Code added

95078   ~~Provocative testing (eg, Rinkel test)~~

● 96020   Code added

● 96040   Code added

+▲ 96415   each additional hour~~, 1 to 8 hours~~ (List separately in addition to code for primary procedure)

+▲ 96423   infusion technique, each additional hour ~~up to 8 hours~~ (List separately in addition to code for primary procedure)

● 96904   Code added

Category II Codes

▲ 0001F   ~~Auscultation of heart performed (2003F)¹~~

● 0012F   Code added

▲ 1000F   Tobacco use~~, smoking,~~ assessed (CAD, CAP, COPD, PV)[1] (DM)[4]

1001F   ~~Tobacco use, non-smoking, assessed¹ (CAD)~~

● **1015F**   Code added

● **1018F**   Code added

● **1019F**   Code added

● **1022F**   Code added

● **1026F**   Code added

● **1030F**   Code added

● **1034F**   Code added

● **1035F**   Code added

● **1036F**   Code added

● **1038F**   Code added

● **1039F**   Code added

~~2003F~~   ~~Auscultation of the heart performed⁺~~

● **2010F**   Code added

● **2014F**   Code added

● **2018F**   Code added

● **2022F**   Code added

● **2024F**   Code added

● **2026F**   Code added

● **2028F**   Code added

~~3000F~~   ~~Blood pressure ≤ 140/90 mm Hg²~~

~~3002F~~   ~~Blood pressure > 140/90 mm Hg²~~

● **3006F**   Code added

● **3011F**   Code added

● **3014F**   Code added

● **3017F**   Code added

● **3020F**   Code added

● **3021F**   Code added

● **3022F**   Code added

● **3023F**   Code added

● **3025F**   Code added

● **3027F**   Code added

● **3028F**   Code added

● **3035F**   Code added

● **3037F**   Code added

● **3040F**   Code added

● **3042F**   Code added

● **3046F**   Code added

● **3047F**   Code added

● **3048F**   Code added

● **3049F**   Code added

● **3050F**   Code added

● **3060F**   Code added

● **3061F**   Code added

● **3062F**   Code added

● **3066F**   Code added

● **3072F**   Code added

● **3076F**   Code added

● **3077F**   Code added

● **3078F**   Code added

● **3079F**   Code added

● **3080F**   Code added

▲ **4009F**   Angiotensin converting enzyme (ACE) inhibitor <u>or angiotensin receptor blocker (ARB)</u> therapy, prescribed (HF[1], CAD[1])

▲ **4015F**   Persistent asthma, <u>preferred</u> long-term control medication [~~inhaled corticosteroids~~ or an acceptable alternative treatment, ~~(cromolyn sodium, leukotriene modifier, nedocromil, OR sustained release theophylline)~~] prescribed (Asthma[1])

● **4025F**   Code added

● **4030F**   Code added

● **4033F**   Code added

● **4035F**   Code added

● **4037F**   Code added

● **4040F**   Code added

● **4045F**   Code added

● **4050F**   Code added

● **6005F**   Code added

Category III Codes

0003T   Code added

0008T   Code added

~~0018T~~   ~~Delivery of high power, focal magnetic pulses for direct stimulation to cortical neurons~~

0021T   Code added

~~0044T~~   ~~Whole body integumentary photography, at request of a physician, for monitoring of high risk patients; with dysplastic nevus syndrome or familial melanoma~~

~~0045T~~   ~~with history of dysplastic nevi or personal history of melanoma~~

▲ **0062T**   Percutaneous intradiscal annuloplasty, any method <u>except electrothermal</u>, unilateral or bilateral including fluoroscopic guidance; single level

~~0082T~~   ~~Stereotactic body radiation therapy, treatment delivery, one or more treatment areas, per day~~

~~0083T~~   ~~Stereotactic body radiation therapy, treatment management, per day~~

▲ **0090T**   Total disc arthroplasty (artificial disc), anterior approach, including discectomy to prepare interspace (other than for decompression)~~;~~ <u>cervical;</u> single interspace~~, cervical~~

~~0091T~~   ~~single interspace, lumbar~~

▲ **0093T**   Removal of total disc arthroplasty, anterior approach~~;~~ <u>cervical;</u> single interspace~~, cervical~~

~~0094T~~   ~~single interspace, lumbar~~

▲ **0096T**   Revision of total disc arthroplasty, anterior approach~~;~~ <u>cervical;</u> single interspace~~, cervical~~

~~0097T~~   ~~single interspace, lumbar~~

~~0120T~~   ~~Ablation, cryosurgical, of fibroadenoma, including ultrasound~~
         ~~guidance, each fibroadenoma~~

● 0141T   Code added

● 0142T   Code added

● 0143T   Code added

● 0144T   Code added

● 0145T   Code added

● 0146T   Code added

● 0147T   Code added

● 0148T   Code added

● 0149T   Code added

● 0150T   Code added

+● 0151T   Code added

+● 0152T   Code added

+● 0153T   Code added

● 0154T   Code added

● 0155T   Code added

● 0156T   Code added

● 0157T   Code added

● 0158T   Code added

+● 0159T   Code added

● 0160T   Code added

● 0161T   Code added

● 0162T   Code added

+● 0163T   Code added

+● 0164T   Code added

+● 0165T   Code added

● 0166T   Code added

● 0167T   Code added

● 0168T   Code added

● 0169T   Code added

● 0170T   Code added

Appendix C

Clinical Examples

As described in *CPT 2007*, clinical examples of the CPT codes for Evaluation and Management (E/M) services are intended to be an important element of the coding system. The clinical examples, when used with the E/M descriptors contained in the full text of *CPT*, provide a comprehensive and powerful tool for physicians to report the services provided to their patients.

The American Medical Association is pleased to provide you with these clinical examples for *CPT 2007*. The clinical examples that are provided in this supplement are limited to Office or Other Outpatient Services, Hospital Inpatient Services, Consultations, Critical Care, Prolonged Services and Care Plan Oversight.

These clinical examples do not encompass the entire scope of medical practice. Inclusion or exclusion of any particular specialty group does not infer any judgment of importance or lack thereof; nor does it limit the applicability of the example to any particular specialty.

Of utmost importance is that these clinical examples are just that: examples. A particular patient encounter, depending on the specific circumstances, must be judged by the services provided by the physician for that particular patient. Simply because the patient's complaints, symptoms, or diagnoses match those of a particular clinical example, does not automatically assign that patient encounter to that particular level of service. The three components (history, examination, and medical decision making) must be met and documented in the medical record to report a particular level of service.

New Patient

Office or Other Outpatient Service

99201   Initial office visit for a 50-year-old male from out-of-town who needs a prescription refill for a nonsteroidal anti-inflammatory drug. (Anesthesiology)

Initial office visit for a 40-year-old female, new patient, requesting information about local pain clinics. (Anesthesiology/Pain Medicine)

Initial office visit for a 10-year-old girl for determination of visual acuity as part of a summer camp physical (does not include determination of refractive error). (Ophthalmology)

Initial office visit for an out-of-town patient requiring topical refill. (Dermatology)

Initial office visit for a 65-year-old male for reassurance about an isolated seborrheic keratosis on upper back. (Plastic Surgery)

Initial office visit for an out-of-state visitor who needs refill of topical steroid to treat lichen planus. (Dermatology)

Initial office visit for an 86-year-old male, out-of-town visitor, who needs prescription refilled for an anal skin preparation that he forgot. (General Surgery/Colon & Rectal Surgery)

Initial office visit for a patient with alveolar osteitis for repacking. (Oral & Maxillofacial Surgery)

Initial office visit for a patient with a pedunculated lesion of the neck which is unsightly. (Dermatology)

Initial office visit for a 10-year-old male for limited subungual hematoma not requiring drainage. (Internal Medicine)

Initial office visit with an out-of-town visitor who needs a prescription refilled because she forgot her hay fever medication. (Allergy & Immunology/Internal Medicine)

Initial office visit with a 9-month-old female with diaper rash. (Pediatrics)

Initial office visit with a 10-year-old male with severe rash and itching for the past 24 hours, positive history for contact with poison oak 48 hours prior to the visit. (Family Medicine)

Initial office visit with a 5-year-old female to remove sutures from simple wound placed by another physician. (Plastic Surgery)

Initial office visit for a 22-year-old male with a small area of sunburn requiring first aid. (Dermatology/Family Medicine/Internal Medicine)

Initial office visit for the evaluation and management of a contusion of a finger. (Orthopaedic Surgery)

99202   Initial office visit for a 13-year-old patient with comedopapular acne of the face unresponsive to over-the-counter medications. (Family Medicine)

Initial office visit for a patient with a clinically benign lesion or nodule of the lower leg which has been present for many years. (Dermatology)

Initial office visit for a patient with a circumscribed patch of dermatitis of the leg. (Dermatology)

Initial office visit for a patient with papulosquamous eruption of elbows. (Dermatology)

Initial office visit for a 9-year-old patient with erythematous grouped, vesicular eruption of the lip of three day's duration. (Pediatrics)

Initial office visit for an 18-year-old male referred by an orthodontist for advice regarding removal of four wisdom teeth. (Oral & Maxillofacial Surgery)

Initial office visit for a 14-year-old male, who was referred by his orthodontist, for advice on the exposure of impacted maxillary cuspids. (Oral & Maxillofacial Surgery)

Initial office visit for a patient presenting with itching patches on the wrists and ankles. (Dermatology)

Initial office visit for a 30-year-old male for evaluation and discussion of treatment of rhinophyma. (Plastic Surgery)

Initial office visit for a 16-year-old male with severe cystic acne, new patient. (Dermatology)

Initial office evaluation for gradual hearing loss, 58-year-old male, history and physical examination, with interpretation of complete audiogram, air bone, etc. (Otolaryngology)

Initial evaluation and management of recurrent urinary infection in female. (Internal Medicine)

Initial office visit with a 10-year-old girl with history of chronic otitis media and a draining ear. (Pediatrics)

Initial office visit for a 10-year-old female with acute maxillary sinusitis. (Family Medicine)

Initial office visit for a patient with recurring episodes of herpes simplex who has developed a clustering of vesicles on the upper lip. (Internal Medicine)

Initial office visit for a 25-year-old patient with a single season allergic rhinitis. (Allergy & Immunology)

99203 Initial office visit of a 76-year-old male with a stasis ulcer of three month's duration. (Dermatology)

Initial office visit for a 30-year-old female with pain in the lateral aspect of the forearm. (Physical Medicine & Rehabilitation)

Initial office visit for a 15-year-old patient with a four-year history of moderate comedopapular acne of the face, chest, and back with early scarring. Discussion of use of systemic medication. (Dermatology)

Initial office visit for a patient with papulosquamous eruption of the elbow with pitting of nails and itchy scalp. (Dermatology)

Initial office visit for a 57-year-old female who complains of painful parotid swelling for one week's duration. (Oral & Maxillofacial Surgery)

Initial office visit for a patient with an ulcerated non-healing lesion or nodule on the tip of the nose. (Dermatology)

Initial office visit for a patient with dermatitis of the antecubital and popliteal fossae. (Dermatology)

Initial office visit for a 22-year-old female with irregular menses. (Family Medicine)

Initial office visit for a 50-year-old female with dyspepsia and nausea. (Family Medicine)

Initial office visit for a 53-year-old laborer with degenerative joint disease of the knee with no prior treatment. (Orthopaedic Surgery)

Initial office visit for a 60-year-old male with Dupuytren's contracture of one hand with multiple digit involvement. (Orthopaedic Surgery)

Initial office visit for a 33-year-old male with painless gross hematuria without cystoscopy. (Internal Medicine)

Initial office visit for a 55-year-old female with chronic blepharitis. There is a history of use of many medications. (Ophthalmology)

Initial office visit for an 18-year-old female with a two-day history of acute conjunctivitis. Extensive history of possible exposures, prior normal ocular history, and medication use is obtained. (Ophthalmology)

Initial office visit for a 14-year-old male with unilateral anterior knee pain. (Physical Medicine & Rehabilitation)

Initial office visit of an adult who presents with symptoms of an upper-respiratory infection that has progressed to unilateral purulent nasal discharge and discomfort in the right maxillary teeth. (Otolaryngology, Head & Neck Surgery)

Initial office visit of a 40-year-old female with symptoms of atopic allergies including eye and sinus congestion, often associated with infections. She would like to be tested for allergies. (Otolaryngology, Head & Neck Surgery)

Initial office visit of a 65-year-old with nasal stuffiness. (Otolaryngology, Head & Neck Surgery)

Initial office visit for initial evaluation of a 48-year-old man with recurrent low back pain radiating to the leg. (General Surgery)

Initial office visit for evaluation, diagnosis, and management of painless gross hematuria in a new patient, without cystoscopy. (Internal Medicine)

Initial office visit with couple for counseling concerning voluntary vasectomy for sterility. Spent 30 minutes discussing procedure, risks and benefits, and answering questions. (Urology)

Initial office visit of a 49-year-old male with nasal obstruction. Detailed exam with topical anesthesia. (Plastic Surgery)

Initial office visit for evaluation of a 13-year-old female with progressive scoliosis. (Physical Medicine & Rehabilitation)

Initial office visit for a 21-year-old female desiring counseling and evaluation of initiation of contraception. (Family Practice/Internal Medicine/Obstetrics & Gynecology)

Initial office visit for a 49-year-old male presenting with painless blood per rectum associated with bowel movement. (Colon & Rectal Surgery)

Initial office visit for a 19-year-old football player with three-day-old acute knee injury; now with swelling and pain. (Orthopaedic Surgery)

99204 Initial office visit for a 13-year-old female with progressive scoliosis. (Orthopaedic Surgery)

Initial office visit for a 34-year-old female with primary infertility for evaluation and counseling. (Obstetrics & Gynecology)

Initial office visit for a 6-year-old male with multiple upper respiratory infections. (Allergy & Immunology)

Initial office visit for a patient with generalized dermatitis of 80 percent of the body surface area. (Dermatology)

Initial office visit for an adolescent who was referred by school counselor because of repeated skipping school. (Psychiatry)

Initial office visit for a 50-year-old machinist with a generalized eruption. (Dermatology)

Initial office visit for a 45-year-old female who has been abstinent from alcohol and benzodiazepines for three months but complains of headaches, insomnia, and anxiety. (Psychiatry)

Initial office visit for a 60-year-old male with recent change in bowel habits, weight loss, and abdominal pain. (Abdominal Surgery/General Surgery)

Initial office visit for a 50-year-old male with an aortic aneurysm who is considering surgery. (General Surgery)

Initial office visit for a 17-year-old female with depression. (Internal Medicine)

Initial office visit of a 40-year-old with chronic draining ear, imbalance, and probable cholesteatoma. (Otolaryngology, Head & Neck Surgery)

Initial office visit for initial evaluation of a 63-year-old male with chest pain on exertion. (Cardiology/Internal Medicine)

Initial office visit for evaluation of a 70-year-old patient with recent onset of episodic confusion. (Internal Medicine)

Initial office visit for a 7-year-old female with juvenile diabetes mellitus, new to area, past history of hospitalization times three. (Pediatrics)

Initial office visit of a 50-year-old female with progressive solid food dysphagia. (Gastroenterology)

Initial office visit for a 34-year-old patient with primary infertility, including counseling. (Obstetrics & Gynecology)

Initial office visit for evaluation of a 70-year-old female with polyarthralgia. (Rheumatology)

Initial office visit for a patient with papulosquamous eruption involving 60 percent of the cutaneous surface with joint pain. Combinations of topical and systemic treatments discussed. (Dermatology)

99205   Initial office visit for a patient with disseminated lupus erythematosus with kidney disease, edema, purpura, and scarring lesions on the extremities plus cardiac symptoms. (Dermatology/General Surgery/Internal Medicine)

Initial office visit for a 25-year-old female with systemic lupus erythematosus, fever, seizures, and profound thrombocytopenia. (Rheumatology/Allergy & Immunology)

Initial office visit for an adult with multiple cutaneous blisters, denuded secondarily infected ulcerations, oral lesions, weight loss, and increasing weakness refractory to high dose corticosteroid. Initiation of new immunosuppressive therapy. (Dermatology)

Initial office visit for a 28-year-old male with systemic vasculitis and compromised circulation to the limbs. (Rheumatology)

Initial office visit for a 41-year-old female new to the area requesting rheumatologic care, on disability due to scleroderma and recent hospitalization for malignant hypertension. (Rheumatology)

Initial office visit for a 52-year-old female with acute four extremity weakness and shortness of breath one week post-flu vaccination. (Physical Medicine & Rehabilitation)

Initial office visit for a 60-year-old male with previous back surgery; now presents with back and pelvic pain, two-month history of bilateral progressive calf and thigh tightness and weakness when walking, causing several falls. (Orthopaedic Surgery)

Initial office visit for an adolescent referred from ER after making suicide gesture. (Psychiatry)

Initial office visit for a 49-year-old female with a history of headaches and dependence on opioids. She reports weight loss, progressive headache, and depression. (Psychiatry)

Initial office visit for a 50-year-old female with symptoms of rash, swellings, recurrent arthritic complaints, and diarrhea and lymphadenopathy. Patient has had a 25 lb. weight loss and was recently camping in the Amazon. (Allergy & Immunology)

Initial office visit for a 34-year-old uremic Type I diabetic patient referred for ESRD modality assessment and planning. (Nephrology)

Initial office visit for a 75-year-old female with neck and bilateral shoulder pain, brisk deep tendon reflexes, and stress incontinence. (Physical Medicine & Rehabilitation)

Initial office visit for an 8-year-old male with cerebral palsy and spastic quadriparesis. (Physical Medicine & Rehabilitation)

Initial office visit for a 73-year-old male with known prostate malignancy, who presents with severe back pain and a recent onset of lower extremity weakness. (Physical Medicine & Rehabilitation)

Initial office visit for a 38-year-old male with paranoid delusions and a history of alcohol abuse. (Psychiatry)

Initial office visit for a 12-week-old with bilateral hip dislocations and bilateral club feet. (Orthopaedic Surgery)

Initial office visit for a 29-year-old female with acute orbital congestion, eyelid retraction, and bilateral visual loss from optic neuropathy. (Ophthalmology)

Initial office visit for a 70-year-old diabetic patient with progressive visual field loss, advanced optic disc cupping and neovascularization of retina. (Ophthalmology)

Initial office visit for a newly diagnosed Type I diabetic patient. (Endocrinology)

Initial office evaluation of a 65-year-old female with exertional chest pain, intermittent claudication, syncope and a murmur of aortic stenosis. (Cardiology)

Initial office visit for a 73-year-old male with an unexplained 20 lb. weight loss. (Hematology/Oncology)

Initial office evaluatin, patient with systemic lupus erythematosus, fever, seizures and profound thrombocytopenia. (Allergy & Immunology/Internal Medicine/Rheumatology)

Initial office evaluaton and management of patient with systemic vasculitis and compromised circulation to the limbs. (Rheumatology)

Initial office visit for a 24-year-old homosexual male who has a fever, a cough, and shortness of breath. (Infectious Disease)

Initial outpatient evaluation of a 69-year-old male with severe chronic obstructive pulmonary disease, congestive heart failure, and hypertension. (Family Medicine)

Initial office visit for a 17-year-old female who is having school problems and has told a friend that she is considering suicide. The patient and her family are consulted in regard to treatment options. (Psychiatry)

Initial office visit for a female with severe hirsutism, amenorrhea, weight loss and a desire to have children. (Endocrinology/Obstetrics & Gynecology)

Initial office visit for a 42-year-old male on hypertensive medication, newly arrived to the area, with diastolic blood pressure of 110, history of recurrent calculi, episodic headaches, intermittent chest pain and orthopnea. (Internal Medicine)

Established Patient

99211   Office visit for an 82-year-old female, established patient, for a monthly B12 injection with documented Vitamin B12 deficiency. (Geriatrics/Internal Medicine/Family Medicine)

Office visit for a 50-year-old male, established patient, for removal of uncomplicated facial sutures. (Plastic Surgery)

Office visit for an established patient who lost prescription for lichen planus. Returned for new copy. (Dermatology)

Office visit for an established patient undergoing orthodontics who complains of a wire which is irritating his/her cheek and asks you to check it. (Oral & Maxillofacial Surgery)

Office visit for a 50-year-old female, established patient, seen for her gold injection by the nurse. (Rheumatology)

Office visit for a 73-year-old female, established patient, with pernicious anemia for weekly B12 injection. (Gastroenterology)

Office visit for an established patient for dressing change on a skin biopsy. (Dermatology)

Office visit for a 19-year-old, established patient, for removal of sutures from a two cm. laceration of forehead, which you placed four days ago in ER. (Plastic Surgery)

Office visit of a 20-year-old female, established patient, who receives an allergy vaccine injection and is observed for a reaction by the nurse. (Otolaryngology, Head & Neck Surgery)

Office visit for a 45-year-old male, established patient, with chronic renal failure for the administration of erythropoietin. (Nephrology)

Office visit for an established patient, a Peace Corps enlistee, who requests documentation that third molars have been removed. (Oral & Maxillofacial Surgery)

Office visit for a 69-year-old female, established patient, for partial removal of antibiotic gauze from an infected wound site. (Plastic Surgery)

Office visit for a 9-year-old, established patient, successfully treated for impetigo, requiring release to return to school. (Dermatology/Pediatrics)

Office visit for an established patient requesting a return-to-work certificate for resolving contact dermatitis. (Dermatology)

Office visit for an established patient who is performing glucose monitoring and wants to check accuracy of machine with lab blood glucose by technician who checks accuracy and function of patient machine. (Endocrinology)

Follow-up office visit for a 65-year-old female with a chronic indwelling percutaneous nephrostomy catheter seen for routine pericatheter skin care and dressing change. (Interventional Radiology)

Outpatient visit with 19-year-old male, established patient, for supervised drug screen. (Addiction Medicine)

Office visit with 12-year-old male, established patient, for cursory check of hematoma one day after venipuncture. (Internal Medicine)

Office visit with 31-year-old female, established patient, for return to work certificate. (Anesthesiology)

Office visit for a 42-year-old, established patient, to read tuberculin test results. (Allergy & Immunology)

Office visit for 14-year-old, established patient, to re-dress an abrasion. (Orthopaedic Surgery)

Office visit for a 45-year-old female, established patient, for a blood pressure check. (Obstetrics & Gynecology)

Office visit for a 23-year-old, established patient, for instruction in use of peak flow meter. (Allergy & Immunology)

Office visit for prescription refill for a 35-year-old female, established patient, with schizophrenia who is stable but has run out of neuroleptic and is scheduled to be seen in a week. (Psychiatry)

99212 Office visit for an 11-year-old, established patient, seen in follow-up for mild comedonal acne of the cheeks on topical desquamating agents. (Dermatology/Family Medicine/Pediatrics)

Office visit for a 10-year-old female, established patient, who has been swimming in a lake, now presents with a one-day history of left ear pain with purulent drainage. (Family Medicine)

Office visit for a child, established patient, with chronic secretory otitis media. (Otolaryngology, Head & Neck Surgery)

Office visit for an established patient seen in follow-up of clearing patch of localized contact dermatitis. (Family Medicine/Dermatology)

Office visit for an established patient returning for evaluation of response to treatment of lichen planus on wrists and ankles. (Dermatology)

Office visit for an established patient with tinea pedis being treated with topical therapy. (Dermatology)

Office visit for an established patient with localized erythematous plaque of psoriasis with topical hydration. (Dermatology)

Office visit for a 50-year-old male, established patient, recently seen for acute neck pain, diagnosis of spondylosis, responding to physical therapy and intermittent cervical traction. Returns for evaluation for return to work. (Neurology)

Office visit for an established patient with recurring episodes of herpes simplex who has developed a clustering of vesicles on the upper lip. (Oral & Maxillofacial Surgery)

Evaluation of a 50-year-old male, established patient, who has experienced a recurrence of knee pain after he discontinued NSAID. (Anesthesiology/Pain Medicine)

Office visit for an established patient with an irritated skin tag for reassurance. (Dermatology)

Office visit for a 40-year-old, established patient, who has experienced a systemic allergic reaction following administration of immunotherapy. The dose must be readjusted. (Allergy & Immunology)

Office visit for a 33-year-old, established patient, for contusion and abrasion of lower extremity. (Orthopaedic Surgery)

Office visit for a 22-year-old male, established patient, one month after I & D of "wrestler's ear". (Plastic Surgery)

Office visit for a 21-year-old, established patient, who is seen in follow-up after antibiotic therapy for acute bacterial tonsilitis. (Otolaryngology, Head & Neck Surgery)

Office visit for a 4-year-old, established patient, with tympanostomy tubes, check-up. (Otolaryngology, Head & Neck Surgery)

Office visit for an established patient who has had needle aspiration of a peritonsillar abscess. (Otolaryngology, Head & Neck Surgery)

Follow-up office examination for evaluation and treatment of acute draining ear in a 5-year-old with tympanotomy tubes. (Otolaryngology, Head & Neck Surgery)

Office visit, established patient, 6-year-old with sore throat and headache. (Family Medicine/Pediatrics)

Office evaluation for possible purulent bacterial conjunctivitis with one- to two-day history of redness and discharge, 16-year-old female, established patient. (Pediatrics/Internal Medicine/Family Medicine)

Office visit for a 65-year-old female, established patient, returns for three-week follow-up for resolving severe ankle sprain. (Orthopaedic Surgery)

Office visit, sore throat, fever and fatigue in a 19-year-old college student, established patient. (Internal Medicine)

Office visit with a 33-year-old female, established patient, recently started on treatment for hemorrhoidal complaints, for re-evaluation. (Colon & Rectal Surgery)

Office visit with a 36-year-old male, established patient, for follow-up on effectiveness of medicine management of oral candidiasis. (Oral & Maxillofacial Surgery)

Office visit for a 27-year-old female, established patient, with complaints of vaginal itching. (Obstetrics & Gynecology)

Office visit for a 65-year-old, established patient, with eruptions on both arms from poison oak exposure. (Allergy & Immunology/Internal Medicine)

99213   Office visit for an established patient with new lesions of lichen planus in spite of topical therapies. (Dermatology)

Office visit for the quarterly follow-up of a 45-year-old male with stable chronic asthma requiring regular drug therapy. (Allergy & Immunology)

Office visit for a 13-year-old, established patient, with comedopapular acne of the face which has shown poor response to topical medication. Discussion of use of systemic medication. (Dermatology)

Office visit for a 62-year-old female, established patient, for follow-up for stable cirrhosis of the liver. (Internal Medicine/Family Medicine)

Office visit for a 3-year-old, established patient, with atopic dermatitis and food hypersensitivity for quarterly follow-up evaluation. The patient is on topical lotions and steroid creams as well as oral antihistamines. (Allergy & Immunology)

Office visit for an 80-year-old female, established patient, to evaluate medical management of osteoarthritis of the temporomandibular joint. (Rheumatology)

Office visit for a 70-year-old female, established patient, one year post excision of basal cell carcinoma of nose with nasolabial flap. Now presents with new suspicious recurrent lesion and suspicious lesion of the back. (Plastic Surgery)

Office visit for a 68-year-old female, established patient, with polymyalgia rheumatic, maintained on chronic low-dose corticosteroid, with no new complaints. (Rheumatology)

Office visit for a 3-year-old female, established patient, for earache and dyshidrosis of feet. (Pediatrics/Family Medicine)

Office visit for an established patient for 18-months post-operative follow-up of TMJ repair. (Oral & Maxillofacial Surgery)

Office visit for a 45-year-old male, established patient, being re-evaluated for recurrent acute prostatitis. (Urology)

Office visit for a 43-year-old male, established patient, with known reflex sympathetic dystrophy. (Anesthesiology)

Office visit for an established patient with an evenly pigmented superficial nodule of leg which is symptomatic. (Dermatology)

Office visit for an established patient with psoriasis involvement of the elbows, pitting of the nails, and itchy scalp. (Dermatology)

Office visit for a 27-year-old male, established patient, with deep follicular and perifollicular inflammation unable to tolerate systemic antibiotics due to GI upset, requires change of systemic medication. (Dermatology)

Office visit for a 16-year-old male, established patient, who is on medication for exercise-induced bronchospasm. (Allergy & Immunology)

Office visit for a 60-year-old, established patient, with chronic essential hypertension on multiple drug regimen, for blood pressure check. (Family Medicine)

Office visit for a 20-year-old male, established patient, for removal of sutures in hand. (Family Medicine)

Office visit for a 58-year-old female, established patient, with unilateral painful bunion. (Orthopaedic Surgery)

Office visit for a 45-year-old female, established patient, with known osteoarthritis and painful swollen knees. (Rheumatology)

Office visit for a 25-year-old female, established patient, complaining of bleeding and heavy menses. (Obstetrics & Gynecology)

Office visit for a 55-year-old male, established patient, with hypertension managed by a beta blocker/thiazide regime; now experiencing mild fatigue. (Nephrology)

Office visit for a 65-year-old female, established patient, with primary glaucoma for interval determination of intraocular pressure and possible adjustment of medication. (Ophthalmology)

Office visit for a 56-year-old man, established patient, with stable exertional angina who complains of new onset of calf pain while walking. (Cardiology)

Office visit for a 63-year-old female, established patient, with rheumatoid arthritis on auranofin and ibuprofen, seen for routine follow-up visit. (Rheumatology)

Office visit for an established patient with Graves' disease, three months post I-131 therapy, who presents with lassitude and malaise. (Endocrinology)

Office visit for the quarterly follow-up of a 63-year-old male, established patient, with chronic myofascial pain syndrome, effectively managed by doxepin, who presents with new onset urinary hesitancy. (Pain Medicine)

Office visit for the biannual follow-up of an established patient with migraine variant having infrequent, intermittent, moderate to severe headaches with nausea and vomiting, which are sometimes effectively managed by ergotamine tartrate and an antiemetic, but occasionally requiring visits to an emergency department. (Pain Medicine)

Office visit for an established patient after discharge from a pain rehabilitation program to review and adjust medication dosage. (Pain Medicine)

Office visit with 55-year-old male, established patient, for management of hypertension, mild fatigue, on beta blocker/thiazide regimen. (Family Medicine/Internal Medicine)

Outpatient visit with 37-year-old male, established patient, who is three years post total colectomy for chronic ulcerative colitis, presents for increased irritation at his stoma. (General Surgery)

Office visit for a 70-year-old diabetic hypertensive established patient with recent change in insulin requirement. (Internal Medicine/Nephrology)

Office visit with 80-year-old female, established patient, for follow-up osteoporosis, status-post compression fractures. (Rheumatology)

Office visit for an established patient with stable cirrhosis of the liver. (Gastroenterology)

Routine, follow-up office evaluation at a three-month interval for a 77-year-old female, established patient, with nodular small cleaved-cell lymphoma. (Hematology/Oncology)

Quarterly follow-up office visit for a 45-year-old male, established patient, with stable chronic asthma, on steroid and bronchodilator therapy. (Pulmonary Medicine)

Office visit for a 50-year-old female, established patient, with insulin-dependent diabetes mellitus and stable coronary artery disease, for monitoring. (Family Medicine/Internal Medicine)

99214 Office visit for an established patient now presenting with generalized dermatitis of 80 percent of the body surface area. (Dermatology)

Office visit for a 32-year-old female, established patient, with new onset right lower quadrant pain. (Family Medicine)

Office visit for reassessment and reassurance/counseling of a 40-year-old female, established patient, who is experiencing increased symptoms while on a pain management treatment program. (Pain Medicine)

Office visit for a 30-year-old, established patient, under management for intractable low back pain, who now presents with new onset right posterior thigh pain. (Pain Medicine)

Office visit for an established patient with frequent intermittent, moderate to severe headaches requiring beta blocker or tricyclic antidepressant prophylaxis, as well as four symptomatic treatments, but who is still experiencing headaches at a frequency of several times a month that are unresponsive to treatment. (Pain Medicine)

Office visit for an established patient with psoriasis with extensive involvement of scalp, trunk, palms, and soles with joint pain. Combinations of topical and systemic treatments discussed and instituted. (Dermatology)

Office visit for a 55-year-old male, established patient, with increasing night pain, limp, and progressive varus of both knees. (Orthopaedic Surgery)

Follow-up visit for a 15-year-old withdrawn patient with four-year history of papulocystic acne of the face, chest, and back with early scarring and poor response to past treatment. Discussion of use of systemic medication. (Dermatology)

Office visit for a 28-year-old male, established patient, with regional enteritis, diarrhea, and low-grade fever. (Internal Medicine)

Office visit for a 25-year-old female, established patient, following recent arthrogram and MR imaging for TMJ pain. (Oral & Maxillofacial Surgery)

Office visit for a 32-year-old female, established patient, with large obstructing stone in left mid-ureter, to discuss management options including urethroscopy with extraction or ESWL. (Urology)

Evaluation for a 28-year-old male, established patient, with new onset of low back pain. (Anesthesiology/Pain Medicine)

Office visit for a 28-year-old female, established patient, with right lower quadrant abdominal pain, fever, and anorexia. (Internal Medicine/Family Medicine)

Office visit for a 45-year-old male, established patient, four months follow-up of L4-5 diskectomy, with persistent incapacitating low back and leg pain. (Orthopaedic Surgery)

Outpatient visit for a 77-year-old male, established patient, with hypertension, presenting with a three-month history of episodic substernal chest pain on exertion. (Cardiology)

Office visit for a 25-year-old female, established patient, for evaluation of progressive saddle nose deformity of unknown etiology. (Plastic Surgery)

Office visit for a 65-year-old male, established patient, with BPH and severe bladder outlet obstruction, to discuss management options such as TURP. (Urology)

Office visit for an adult diabetic established patient with a past history of recurrent sinusitis who presents with a one-week history of double vision. (Otolaryngology, Head & Neck Surgery)

Office visit for an established patient with lichen planus and 60 percent of the cutaneous surface involved, not responsive to systemic steroids, as well as developing symptoms of progressive heartburn and paranoid ideation. (Dermatology)

Office visit for a 52-year-old male, established patient, with a 12-year history of bipolar disorder responding to lithium carbonate and brief psychotherapy. Psychotherapy and prescription provided. (Psychiatry)

Office visit for a 63-year-old female, established patient, with a history of familial polyposis, status post-colectomy with sphincter sparing procedure, who now presents with rectal bleeding and increase in stooling frequency. (General Surgery)

Office visit for a 68-year-old male, established patient, with the sudden onset of multiple flashes and floaters in the right eye due to a posterior vitreous detachment. (Ophthalmology)

Office visit for a 55-year-old female, established patient, on cyclosporin for treatment of resistant, small vessel vasculitis. (Rheumatology)

Follow-up office visit for a 55-year-old male, two months after iliac angioplasty with new onset of contralateral extremity claudication. (Interventional Radiology)

Office visit for a 68-year-old male, established patient, with stable angina, two months post myocardial infarction, who is not tolerating one of his medications. (Cardiology)

Weekly office visit for 5FU therapy for an ambulatory established patient with metastatic colon cancer and increasing shortness of breath. (Hematology/Oncology)

Follow-up office visit for a 60-year-old male, established patient, whose post-traumatic seizures have disappeared on medication and who now raises the question of stopping the medication. (Neurology)

Office evaluation on new onset RLQ pain in a 32-year-old woman, established patient. (Urology/General Surgery/Internal Medicine/Family Medicine)

Office evaluation of 28-year-old, established patient, with regional enteritis, diarrhea and low-grade fever. (Family Medicine/Internal Medicine)

Office visit with 50-year-old female, established patient, diabetic, blood sugar controlled by diet. She now complains of frequency of urination and weight loss, blood sugar of 320 and negative ketones on dipstick. (Internal Medicine)

Follow-up office visit for a 45-year-old, established patient, with rheumatoid arthritis on gold, methotrexate, or immunosuppressive therapy. (Rheumatology)

Office visit for a 60-year-old male, established patient, two years post-removal of intracranial meningioma, now with new headaches and visual disturbance. (Neurosurgery)

Office visit for a 68-year-old female, established patient, for routine review and follow-up of non-insulin dependent diabetes, obesity, hypertension and congestive heart failure. Complains of vision difficulties and admits dietary noncompliance. Patient is counseled concerning diet and current medications adjusted. (Family Medicine)

99215 Office visit for an established patient who developed persistent cough, rectal bleeding, weakness, and diarrhea plus pustular infection on skin. Patient on immunosuppressive therapy. (Dermatology)

Office visit for an established patient with disseminated lupus erythematosus, extensive edema of extremities, kidney disease, and weakness requiring monitored course on azathioprene, corticosteroid and complicated by acute depression. (Dermatology/Internal Medicine/Rheumatology)

Office visit for an established patient with progressive dermatomyositis and recent onset of fever, nasal speech, and regurgitation of fluids through the nose. (Dermatology)

Office visit for a 28-year-old female, established patient, who is abstinent from previous cocaine dependence, but reports progressive panic attacks and chest pains. (Psychiatry)

Office visit for an established adolescent patient with history of bipolar disorder treated with lithium; seen on urgent basis at family's request because of severe depressive symptoms. (Psychiatry)

Office visit for an established patient having acute migraine with new onset neurological symptoms and whose headaches are unresponsive to previous attempts at management with a combination of preventive and abortive medication. (Pain Medicine)

Office visit for an established patient with exfoliative lichen planus with daily fever spikes, disorientation, and shortness of breath. (Dermatology)

Office visit for a 25-year-old, established patient, two years post-burn with bilateral ectropion, hypertrophic facial burn scars, near absence of left breast, and burn syndactyly of both hands. Discussion of treatment options following examination. (Plastic Surgery)

Office visit for a 6-year-old, established patient, to review newly diagnosed immune deficiency with recommendations for therapy including IV immunoglobulin and chronic antibiotics. (Allergy & Immunology)

Office visit for a 36-year-old, established patient, three months status post-transplant, with new onset of peripheral edema, increased blood pressure, and progressive fatigue. (Nephrology)

Office visit for an established patient with Kaposi's sarcoma who presents with fever and widespread vesicles. (Dermatology)

Office visit for a 27-year-old female, established patient, with bipolar disorder who was stable on lithium carbonate and monthly supportive psychotherapy but now has developed symptoms of hypomania. (Psychiatry)

Office visit for a 25-year-old male, established patient with a history of schizophrenia who has been seen bi-monthly but is complaining of auditory hallucinations. (Psychiatry)

Office visit for a 62-year-old male, established patient, three years post-op abdominal perineal resection, now with a rising carcinoembryonic antigen, weight loss, and pelvic pain. (Abdominal Surgery)

Office visit for a 42-year-old male, established patient, nine months post-op emergency vena cava shunt for variceal bleeding, now presents with complaints of one episode of "dark" bowel movement, weight gain, tightness in abdomen, whites of eyes seem "yellow" and occasional drowsiness after eating hamburgers. (Abdominal Surgery)

Office visit for a 68-year-old male, established patient, with biopsy-proven rectal carcinoma, for evaluation and discussion of treatment options. (General Surgery)

Office visit for a 60-year-old, established patient, with diabetic nephropathy with increasing edema and dyspnea. (Endocrinology)

Office visit with 30-year-old male, established patient for three-month history of fatigue, weight loss, intermittent fever, and presenting with diffuse adenopathy and splenomegaly. (Family Medicine)

Office visit for restaging of an established patient with new lymphadenopathy one year post-therapy for lymphoma. (Hematology/Oncology)

Office visit for evaluation of recent onset syncopal attacks in a 70-year-old woman, established patient. (Internal Medicine)

Follow-up visit, 40-year-old mother of three, established patient, with acute rheumatoid arthritis, anatomical Stage 3, ARA function Class 3 rheumatoid arthritis, and deteriorating function. (Rheumatology)

Follow-up office visit for a 65-year-old male, established patient, with a fever of recent onset while on outpatient antibiotic therapy for endocarditis. (Infectious Disease)

Office visit for a 75-year-old, established patient, with ALS (amyotrophic lateral sclerosis), who is no longer able to swallow. (Neurology)

Office visit for a 70-year-old female, established patient, with diabetes mellitus and hypertension, presenting with a two-month history of increasing confusion, agitation and short-term memory loss. (Family Medicine/Internal Medicine)

Hospital Inpatient Services

Initial Hospital Care

New or Established Patient

99221 Initial hospital visit following admission for a 42-year-old male for observation following an uncomplicated mandible fracture. (Plastic Surgery/Oral & Maxillofacial Surgery)

Initial hospital visit for a 40-year-old patient with a thrombosed synthetic arteriovenous conduit. (Nephrology)

Initial hospital visit for a healthy 24-year-old male with an acute onset of low back pain following a lifting injury. (Internal Medicine/Anesthesiology/Pain Medicine)

Initial hospital visit for a 69-year-old female with controlled hypertension, scheduled for surgery. (Internal Medicine/Cardiology)

Initial hospital visit for a 24-year-old healthy female with benign tumor of palate. (Oral & Maxillofacial Surgery)

Initial hospital visit for a 14-year-old female with infectious mononucleosis and dehydration. (Internal Medicine)

Initial hospital visit for a 62-year-old female with stable rheumatoid arthritis, admitted for total joint replacement. (Rheumatology)

Initial hospital visit for a 12-year-old patient with a laceration of the upper eyelid, involving the lid margin and superior canaliculus, admitted prior to surgery for IV antibiotic therapy. (Plastic Surgery)

Initial hospital visit for a 69-year-old female with controlled hypertension, scheduled for surgery. (Cardiology)

Hospital admission, examination, and initiation of treatment program for a 67-year-old male with uncomplicated pneumonia who requires IV antibiotic therapy. (Internal Medicine)

Hospital admission for an 18-month-old with 10 percent dehydration. (Pediatrics)

Hospital admission for a 12-year-old with a laceration of the upper eyelid involving the lid margin and superior canaliculus, admitted prior to surgery for IV antibiotic therapy. (Ophthalmology)

Hospital admission for a 32-year-old female with severe flank pain, hematuria and presumed diagnosis of ureteral calculus as determined by Emergency Department physician. (Urology)

Initial hospital visit for a patient with several large venous stasis ulcers not responding to outpatient therapy. (Dermatology)

Initial hospital visit for 21-year-old pregnant patient (nine weeks gestation) with hyperemesis gravidarum. (Obstetrics & Gynecology)

Initial hospital visit for a 73-year-old female with acute pyelonephritis who is otherwise generally healthy. (Geriatrics)

Initial hospital visit for 62-year-old patient with cellulitis of the foot requiring bedrest and intravenous antibiotics. (Orthopaedic Surgery)

99222 Initial hospital visit for a 50-year-old patient with lower quadrant abdominal pain and increased temperature, but without septic picture. (General Surgery/Abdominal Surgery/Colon & Rectal Surgery)

Initial hospital visit for airway management, due to a benign laryngeal mass. (Otolaryngology, Head & Neck Surgery)

Initial hospital visit for a 66-year-old female with an L-2 vertebral compression fracture with acute onset of paralytic ileus; seen in the office two days previously. (Orthopaedic Surgery)

Initial hospital visit and evaluation of a 15-year-old male admitted with peritonsillar abscess or cellulitis requiring intravenous antibiotic therapy. (Otolaryngology, Head & Neck Surgery)

Initial hospital visit for a 42-year-old male with vertebral compression fracture following a motor vehicle accident. (Orthopaedic Surgery)

Initial hospital visit for a patient with generalized atopic dermatitis and secondary infection. (Dermatology)

Initial hospital visit for a 3-year-old patient with high temperature, limp, and painful hip motion of 18 hours' duration. (Pediatrics/Orthopaedic Surgery)

Initial hospital visit for a young adult, presenting with an acute asthma attack unresponsive to outpatient therapy. (Allergy & Immunology)

Initial hospital visit for an 18-year-old male who has suppurative sialoadenitis and dehydration. (Oral & Maxillofacial Surgery)

Initial hospital visit for a 65-year-old female for acute onset of thrombotic cerebrovascular accident with contralateral paralysis and aphasia. (Neurology)

Initial hospital visit for a 50-year-old male chronic paraplegic patient with pain and spasm below the lesion. (Anesthesiology)

Partial hospital admission for an adolescent patient from chaotic blended family, transferred from inpatient setting, for continued treatment to control symptomatic expressions of hostility and depression. (Psychiatry)

Initial hospital visit for a 15-year-old male with acute status asthmaticus, unresponsive to outpatient therapy. (Internal Medicine)

Initial hospital visit for a 61-year-old male with history of previous myocardial infarction, who now complains of chest pain. (Internal Medicine)

Initial hospital visit of a 15-year-old on medications for a sore throat over the last two weeks. The sore throat has worsened and patient now has dysphagia. The exam shows large necrotic tonsils with an adequate airway and small palpable nodes. The initial mono test was negative. (Otolaryngology, Head & Neck Surgery)

Initial hospital evaluation of a 23-year-old allergy patient admitted with eyelid edema and pain on fifth day of oral antibiotic therapy. (Otolaryngology, Head & Neck Surgery)

Hospital admission, young adult patient, failed previous therapy and now presents in acute asthmatic attack. (Family Medicine/Allergy & Immunology)

Hospital admission of a 62-year-old smoker, established patient, with bronchitis in acute respiratory distress. (Internal Medicine/Pulmonary Medicine)

Hospital admission, examination, and initiation of a treatment program for a 65-year-old female with new onset of right-sided paralysis and aphasia. (Neurology)

Hospital admission, examination, and initiation of treatment program for a 66-year-old chronic hemodialysis patient with fever and a new pulmonary infiltrate. (Nephrology)

Hospital admission for an 8-year-old febrile patient with chronic sinusitis and severe headache, unresponsive to oral antibiotics. (Allergy & Immunology)

Hospital admission for a 40-year-old male with submaxillary cellulitis and trismus from infected lower molar. (Oral & Maxillofacial Surgery)

99223 Initial hospital visit for a 45-year-old female, who has a history of rheumatic fever as a child and now has anemia, fever, and congestive heart failure. (Cardiology)

Initial hospital visit for a 50-year-old male with acute chest pain and diagnostic electrocardiographic changes of an acute anterior myocardial infarction. (Cardiology/Family Medicine/Internal Medicine)

Initial hospital visit of a 75-year-old with progressive stridor and dysphagia with history of cancer of the larynx treated by radiation therapy in the past. Exam shows a large recurrent tumor of the glottis with a mass in the neck. (Otolaryngology, Head & Neck Surgery)

Initial hospital visit for a 70-year-old male admitted with chest pain, complete heart block, and congestive heart failure. (Cardiology)

Initial hospital visit for an 82-year-old male who presents with syncope, chest pain, and ventricular arrhythmias. (Cardiology)

Initial hospital visit for a 75-year-old male with history of arteriosclerotic coronary vascular disease, who is severely dehydrated, disoriented, and experiencing auditory hallucinations. (Psychiatry)

Initial hospital visit for a 70-year-old male with alcohol and sedative-hypnotic dependence, admitted by family for severe withdrawal, hypertension, and diabetes mellitus. (Psychiatry)

Initial hospital visit for a persistently suicidal latency-aged child whose parents have requested admission to provide safety during evaluation, but are anxious about separation from her. (Psychiatry)

Initial psychiatric visit for an adolescent patient without previous psychiatric history, who was transferred from the medical ICU after a significant overdose. (Psychiatry)

Initial hospital visit for a 35-year-old female with severe systemic lupus erythematosus on corticosteroid and cyclophosphamide, with new onset of fever, chills, rash, and chest pain. (Rheumatology)

Initial hospital visit for a 52-year-old male with known rheumatic heart disease who presents with anasarca, hypertension, and history of alcohol abuse. (Cardiology)

Initial hospital visit for a 55-year-old female with a history of congenital heart disease; now presents with cyanosis. (Cardiology)

Initial hospital visit for a psychotic, hostile, violently combative adolescent, involuntarily committed, for seclusion and restraint in order to provide safety on unit. (Psychiatry)

Initial hospital visit for a now subdued and sullen teenage male with six-month history of declining school performance, increasing self-endangerment, and resistance of parental expectations, including running away past weekend after physical fight with father. (Psychiatry)

Initial partial hospital admission for a 17-year-old female with history of borderline mental retardation who has developed auditory hallucinations. Parents are known to abuse alcohol, and Child Protective Services is investigating allegations of sexual abuse of a younger sibling. (Psychiatry)

Initial hospital visit of a 67-year-old male admitted with a large neck mass, dysphagia, and history of myocardial infarction three months before. (Otolaryngology, Head & Neck Surgery)

Initial hospital visit for a patient with suspected cerebrospinal fluid rhinorrhea which developed two weeks after head injury. (Otolaryngology, Head & Neck Surgery)

Initial hospital visit for a 25-year-old female with history of poly-substance abuse and psychiatric disorder. The patient appears to be psychotic with markedly elevated vital signs. (Psychiatry)

Initial hospital visit for a 70-year-old male with cutaneous T-cell lymphoma who has developed fever and lymphadenopathy. (Internal Medicine)

Initial hospital visit for a 62-year-old female with known coronary artery disease, for evaluation of increasing edema, dyspnea on exertion, confusion, and sudden onset of fever with productive cough. (Internal Medicine)

Initial hospital visit for a 3-year-old female with 36-hour history of sore throat and high fever; now with sudden onset of lethargy, irritability, photophobia, and nuchal rigidity. (Pediatrics)

Initial hospital visit for a 26-year-old female for evaluation of severe facial fractures (LeFort's II/III). (Plastic Surgery)

Initial hospital visit for a 55-year-old female for bilateral mandibular fractures resulting in flail mandible and airway obstruction. (Plastic Surgery)

Initial hospital visit for a 71-year-old patient with a red painful eye four days following uncomplicated cataract surgery due to endophthalmitis. (Ophthalmology)

Initial hospital visit for a 45-year-old patient involved in a motor vehicle accident who suffered a perforating corneoscleral laceration with loss of vision. (Ophthalmology)

Initial hospital visit for a 58-year-old male who has Ludwig's angina and progressive airway compromise. (Oral & Maxillofacial Surgery)

Initial hospital visit for a patient with generalized systemic sclerosis, receiving immunosuppressive therapy because of recent onset of cough, fever, and inability to swallow. (Dermatology)

Initial hospital visit for an 82-year-old male who presents with syncope, chest pain, and ventricular arrhythmias. (Cardiology)

Initial hospital visit for a 62-year-old male with history of previous myocardial infarction, comes in with recurrent, sustained ventricular tachycardia. (Cardiology)

Initial hospital visit for a chronic dialysis patient with infected PTFE fistula, septicemia, and shock. (Nephrology)

Initial hospital visit for a 1-year-old male, victim of child abuse, with central nervous system depression, skull fracture, and retinal hemorrhage. (Family Medicine/Neurology)

Initial hospital visit for a 25-year-old female with recent C4-5 quadriplegia, admitted for rehabilitation. (Physical Medicine & Rehabilitation)

Initial hospital visit for an 18-year-old male, post-traumatic brain injury with multiple impairment. (Physical Medicine & Rehabilitation)

Initial partial hospital admission for 16-year-old male, sullen and subdued, with six-month history of declining school performance, increasing self-endangerment, and resistance to parental expectations. (Psychiatry)

Initial hospital visit for a 16-year-old primigravida at 32 weeks gestation with severe hypertension (200/110), thrombocytopenia, and headache. (Obstetrics & Gynecology)

Initial hospital visit for a 49-year-old male with cirrhosis of liver with hematemesis, hepatic encephalopathy, and fever. (Gastroenterology)

Initial hospital visit for a 55-year-old female in chronic pain who has attempted suicide. (Psychiatry)

Initial hospital visit for a 70-year-old male with multiple organ system disease, admitted with history of being aneuric and septic for 24 hours prior to admission. (Urology)

Initial hospital visit for a 3-year-old female with 36-hour history of sore throat and high fever, now with sudden onset of lethargy, irritability, photophobia, and nuchal rigidity. (Internal Medicine)

Initial hospital visit for a 78-year-old male, transfers from nursing home with dysuria and pyuria, increasing confusion, and high fever. (Internal Medicine)

Initial hospital visit for a 1-day-old male with cyanosis, respiratory distress, and tachypnea. (Cardiology)

Initial hospital visit for a 3-year-old female with recurrent tachycardia and syncope. (Cardiology)

Initial hospital visit for a thyrotoxic patient who presents with fever, atrial fibrillation, and delirium. (Endocrinology)

Initial hospital visit for a 50-year-old Type I diabetic who presents with diabetic ketoacidosis with fever and obtundation. (Endocrinology)

Initial hospital visit for a 40-year-old female with anatomical stage 3, ARA functional class 3 rheumatoid arthritis on methotrexate, corticosteroid, and nonsteroidal anti-inflammatory drugs. Patient presents with severe arthritis flare, new oral ulcers, abdominal pain, and leukopenia. (Rheumatology)

Initial hospital exam of a pediatric patient with high fever and proptosis. (Otolaryngology, Head & Neck Surgery)

Initial hospital visit for a 25-year-old patient admitted for the first time to the rehab unit, with recent C-4-5 quadriplegia. (Physical Medicine & Rehabilitation)

Hospital admission, examination, and initiation of treatment program for a previously unknown 58-year-old male who presents with acute chest pain. (Cardiology)

Hospital admission, examination, and initiation of induction chemotherapy for a 42-year-old patient with newly diagnosed acute myelogenous leukemia. (Hematology/Oncology)

Hospital admission following a motor vehicle accident of a 24-year-old male with fracture dislocation of C5-6; neurologically intact. (Neurosurgery)

Hospital admission for a 78-year-old female with left lower lobe pneumonia and a history of coronary artery disease, congestive heart failure, osteoarthritis and gout. (Family Medicine)

Hospital admission, examination, and initiation of treatment program for a 65-year-old immunosuppressed male with confusion, fever, and a headache. (Infectious Disease)

Hospital admission for a 9-year-old with vomiting, dehydration, fever, tachypnea and an admitting diagnosis of diabetic ketoacidosis. (Pediatrics)

Initial hospital visit for a 65-year-old male who presents with acute myocardial infarction, oliguria, hypotension, and altered state of consciousness. (Cardiology)

Initial hospital visit for a hostile/resistant adolescent patient who is severely depressed and involved in poly-substance abuse. Patient is experiencing significant conflict in his chaotic family situation and was suspended from school following an attack on a teacher with a baseball bat. (Psychiatry)

Initial hospital visit for 89-year-old female with fulminant hepatic failure and encephalopathy. (Gastroenterology)

Initial hospital visit for a 42-year-old female with rapidly progressing scleroderma, malignant hypertension, digital infarcts, and oligurea. (Rheumatology)

Subsequent Hospital Care

99231 Subsequent hospital visit for a 65-year-old female, post-open reduction and internal fixation of a fracture. (Physical Medicine & Rehabilitation)

Subsequent hospital visit for a 33-year-old patient with pelvic pain who is responding to pain medication and observation. (Obstetrics & Gynecology)

Subsequent hospital visit for a 21-year-old female with hyperemesis who has responded well to intravenous fluids. (Obstetrics & Gynecology)

Subsequent hospital visit to re-evaluate post-op pain and titrate patient-controlled analgesia for a 27-year-old female. (Anesthesiology)

Follow-up hospital visit for a 35-year-old female, status post-epidural analgesia. (Anesthesiology/Pain Medicine)

Subsequent hospital visit for a 56-year-old male, post-gastrectomy, for maintenance of analgesia using an intravenous dilaudid infusion. (Anesthesiology)

Subsequent hospital visit for a 4-year-old on day three receiving medication for uncomplicated pneumonia. (Allergy & Immunology)

Subsequent hospital visit for a 30-year-old female with urticaria which has stabilized with medication. (Allergy & Immunology)

Subsequent hospital visit for a 76-year-old male with venous stasis ulcers. (Dermatology)

Subsequent hospital visit for a 24-year-old female with otitis externa, seen two days before in consultation, now to have otic wick removal. (Otolaryngology, Head & Neck Surgery)

Subsequent hospital visit for a 27-year-old with acute labyrinthitis. (Otolaryngology, Head & Neck Surgery)

Subsequent hospital visit for a 10-year-old male admitted for lobar pneumonia with vomiting and dehydration; is becoming afebrile and tolerating oral fluids. (Family Medicine/Pediatrics)

Subsequent hospital visit for a 62-year-old patient with resolving cellulitis of the foot. (Orthopaedic Surgery)

Subsequent hospital visit for a 25-year-old male admitted for supra-ventricular tachycardia and converted on medical therapy. (Cardiology)

Subsequent hospital visit for a 27-year-old male two days after open reduction and internal fixation for malar complex fracture. (Plastic Surgery)

Subsequent hospital visit for a 76-year-old male with venous stasis ulcers. (Geriatrics)

Subsequent hospital visit for a 67-year-old female admitted three days ago with bleeding gastric ulcer; now stable. (Gastroenterology)

Subsequent hospital visit for stable 33-year-old male, status post-lower gastrointestinal bleeding. (General Surgery/Gastroenterology)

Subsequent hospital visit for a 29-year-old auto mechanic with effort thrombosis of left upper extremity. (General Surgery)

Subsequent hospital visit for a 14-year-old female in middle phase of inpatient treatment, who is now behaviorally stable and making satisfactory progress in treatment. (Psychiatry)

Subsequent hospital visit for an 18-year-old male with uncomplicated asthma who is clinically stable. (Allergy & Immunology)

Subsequent hospital visit for a 55-year-old male with rheumatoid arthritis, two days following an uncomplicated total joint replacement. (Rheumatology)

Subsequent hospital visit for a 60-year-old dialysis patient with an access infection, now afebrile on antibiotic. (Nephrology)

Subsequent hospital visit for a 36-year-old female with stable post-rhinoplasty epistaxis. (Plastic Surgery)

Subsequent hospital visit for a 66-year-old female with L-2 vertebral compression fracture with resolving ileus. (Orthopaedic Surgery)

Subsequent hospital visit for a patient with peritonsillar abscess. (Otolaryngology, Head & Neck Surgery)

Subsequent hospital visit for an 18-year-old female responding to intravenous antibiotic therapy for ear or sinus infection. (Otolaryngology, Head & Neck Surgery)

Subsequent hospital visit for a 70-year-old male admitted with congestive heart failure who has responded to therapy. (Cardiology)

Follow-up hospital visit for a 32-year-old female with left ureteral calculus; being followed in anticipation of spontaneous passage. (Urology)

Subsequent hospital visit for a 50-year-old Type II diabetic who is clinically stable and without complications requiring regulation of a single dose of insulin daily. (Endocrinology)

Subsequent hospital visit to reassesses the status of a 65-year-old patient post-open reduction and internal fixation of hip fracture, on the rehab unit. (Physical Medicine & Rehabilitation)

Subsequent hospital visit for a 78-year-old male with cholangiocarcinoma managed by biliary drainage. (Interventional Radiology)

Subsequent hospital visit for a 50-year-old male with uncomplicated myocardial infarction who is clinically stable and without chest pain. (Family Medicine/Cardiology/Internal Medicine)

Subsequent hospital visit for a stable 72-year-old lung cancer patient undergoing a five-day course of infusion chemotherapy. (Hematology/Oncology)

Subsequent hospital visit, two days post admission for a 65-year-old male with a CVA (cerebral vascular accident) and left hemiparesis, who is clinically stable. (Neurology/Physical Medicine and Rehabilitation)

Subsequent hospital visit for now stable, 33-year-old male, status post lower gastrointestinal bleeding. (General Surgery)

Subsequent visit on third day of hospitalization for a 60-year-old female recovering from an uncomplicated pneumonia. (Infectious Disease/Internal Medicine/Pulmonary Medicine)

Subsequent hospital visit for a 3-year-old patient in traction for a congenital dislocation of the hip. (Orthopaedic Surgery)

Subsequent hospital visit for a 4-year-old female, admitted for acute gastroenteritis and dehydration, requiring IV hydration; now stable. (Family Medicine/Internal Medicine)

Subsequent hospital visit for 50-year-old female with resolving uncomplicated acute pancreatitis. (Gastroenterology)

99232 Subsequent hospital visit for a patient with venous stasis ulcers who developed fever and red streaks adjacent to the ulcer. (Dermatology/Internal Medicine/Family Medicine)

Subsequent hospital visit for a 66-year-old male for dressing changes and observation. Patient has had a myocutaneous flap to close a pharyngeal fistula and now has a low-grade fever. (Plastic Surgery)

Subsequent hospital visit for a 54-year-old female admitted for myocardial infarction, but who is now having frequent premature ventricular contractions. (Internal Medicine)

Subsequent hospital visit for an 80-year-old patient with a pelvic rim fracture, inability to walk, and severe pain; now 36 hours post-injury, experiencing urinary retention. (Orthopaedic Surgery)

Subsequent hospital visit for a 17-year-old female with fever, pharyngitis, and airway obstruction, who after 48 hours develops a maculopapular rash. (Pediatrics/Family Medicine)

Follow-up hospital visit for a 32-year-old patient admitted the previous day for corneal ulcer. (Dermatology)

Follow-up visit for a 67-year-old male with congestive heart failure who has responded to antibiotics and diuretics, and has now developed a monoarthropathy. (Internal Medicine)

Follow-up hospital visit for a 58-year-old male receiving continuous opioids who is experiencing severe nausea and vomiting. (Pain Medicine)

Subsequent hospital visit for a patient after an auto accident who is slow to respond to ambulation training. (Physical Medicine & Rehabilitation)

Subsequent hospital visit for a 14-year-old with unstable bronchial asthma complicated by pneumonia. (Allergy & Immunology)

Subsequent hospital visit for a 50-year-old diabetic, hypertensive male with back pain not responding to conservative inpatient management with continued radiation of pain to the lower left extremity. (Orthopaedic Surgery)

Subsequent hospital visit for a 37-year-old female on day five of antibiotics for bacterial endocarditis, who still has low-grade fever. (Cardiology)

Subsequent hospital visit for a 54-year-old patient, post MI (myocardial infarction), who is out of the CCU (coronary care unit) but is now having frequent premature ventricular contractions on telemetry. (Cardiology/Internal Medicine)

Subsequent hospital visit for a patient with neutropenia, a fever responding to antibiotics, and continued slow gastrointestinal bleeding on platelet support. (Hematology/Oncology)

Subsequent hospital visit for a 50-year-old male admitted two days ago for sub-acute renal allograft rejection. (Nephrology)

Subsequent hospital visit for a 35-year-old drug addict, not responding to initial antibiotic therapy for pyelonephritis. (Urology)

Subsequent hospital visit of an 81-year-old male with abdominal distention, nausea, and vomiting. (General Surgery)

Subsequent hospital care for a 62-year-old female with congestive heart failure, who remains dyspneic and febrile. (Internal Medicine)

Subsequent hospital visit for a 73-year-old female with recently diagnosed lung cancer, who complains of unsteady gait. (Pulmonary Medicine)

Subsequent hospital visit for a 20-month-old male with bacterial meningitis treated one week with antibiotic therapy; has now developed a temperature of 101.0. (Pediatrics)

Subsequent hospital visit for 13-year-old male admitted with left lower quadrant abdominal pain and fever, not responding to therapy. (General Surgery)

Subsequent hospital visit for a 65-year-old male with hemiplegia and painful paretic shoulder. (Physical Medicine & Rehabilitation)

99233 Subsequent hospital visit for a 38-year-old male, quadriplegic with acute autonomic hyperreflexia, who is not responsive to initial care. (Physical Medicine & Rehabilitation)

Follow-up hospital visit for a teenage female who continues to experience severely disruptive, violent and life-threatening symptoms in a complicated multi-system illness. Family/social circumstances also a contributing factor. (Psychiatry)

Subsequent hospital visit for a 42-year-old female with progressive systemic sclerosis (scleroderma), renal failure on dialysis, congestive heart failure, cardiac arrhythmias, and digital ulcers. (Allergy & Immunology)

Subsequent hospital visit for a 50-year-old diabetic, hypertensive male with nonresponding back pain and radiating pain to the lower left extremity, who develops chest pain, cough, and bloody sputum. (Orthopaedic Surgery)

Subsequent hospital visit for a 64-year-old female, status post-abdominal aortic aneurysm resection, with non-responsive coagulopathy, who has now developed lower GI bleeding. (Abdominal Surgery/Colon & Rectal Surgery/General Surgery) Follow-up hospital care of a patient with pansinusitis infection complicated by a brain abscess and asthma; no response to current treatment. (Otolaryngology, Head & Neck Surgery)

Subsequent hospital visit for a patient with a laryngeal neoplasm who develops airway compromise, suspected metastasis. (Otolaryngology, Head & Neck Surgery)

Subsequent hospital visit for a 49-year-old male with significant rectal bleeding, etiology undetermined, not responding to treatment. (Abdominal Surgery/General Surgery/Colon & Rectal Surgery)

Subsequent hospital visit for a 50-year-old male, post-aortocoronary bypass surgery; now develops hypotension and oliguria. (Cardiology)

Subsequent hospital visit for an adolescent patient who is violent, unsafe, and noncompliant, with multiple expectations for participation in treatment plan and behavior on the treatment unit. (Psychiatry)

Subsequent hospital visit for an 18-year-old male being treated for presumed PCP psychosis. Patient is still moderately symptomatic with auditory hallucinations and is insisting on signing out against medical advice. (Psychiatry)

Subsequent hospital visit for an 8-year-old female with caustic ingestion, who now has fever, dyspnea, and dropping hemoglobin. (Gastroenterology)

Follow-up hospital visit for a chronic renal failure patient on dialysis who develops chest pain and shortness of breath and a new onset pericardial friction rub. (Nephrology)

Subsequent hospital visit for a 44-year-old patient with electrical burns to the left arm with ascending infection. (Orthopaedic Surgery)

Subsequent hospital visit for a patient with systemic sclerosis who has aspirated and is short of breath. (Dermatology)

Subsequent hospital visit for a 65-year-old female, status post-op resection of abdominal aortic aneurysm, with suspected ischemic bowel. (General Surgery)

Subsequent hospital visit for a 50-year-old male, post-aortocoronary bypass surgery, now develops hypotension and oliguria. (Cardiology)

Subsequent hospital visit for a 65-year-old male, following an acute myocardial infarction, who complains of shortness of breath and new chest pain. (Cardiology)

Subsequent hospital visit for a 65-year-old female with rheumatoid arthritis (stage 3, class 3) admitted for urosepsis. On the third hospital day, chest pain, dyspnea and fever develop. (Rheumatology)

Follow-up hospital care of a pediatric case with stridor, laryngomalacia, established tracheostomy, complicated by multiple medical problems in PICU. (Otolaryngology, Head & Neck Surgery)

Subsequent hospital visit for a 60-year-old female, four days post uncomplicated inferior myocardial infarction who has developed severe chest pain, dyspnea, diaphoresis and nausea. (Family Medicine)

Subsequent hospital visit for a patient with AML (acute myelogenous leukemia), fever, elevated white count and uric acid undergoing induction chemotherapy. (Hematology/Oncology)

Subsequent hospital visit for a 38-year-old quadriplegic male with acute autonomic hyperreflexia, who is not responsive to initial care. (Physical Medicine & Rehabilitation)

Subsequent hospital visit for a 65-year-old female post-op resection of abdominal aortic aneurysm, with suspected ischemic bowel. (General Surgery)

Subsequent hospital visit for a 60-year-old female with persistent leukocytosis and a fever seven days after a sigmoid colon resection for carcinoma. (Infectious Disease)

Subsequent hospital visit for a chronic renal failure patient on dialysis, who develops chest pain, shortness of breath and new onset of pericardial friction rub. (Nephrology)

Subsequent hospital visit for a 65-year-old male with acute myocardial infarction who now demonstrates complete heart block and congestive heart failure. (Cardiology)

Subsequent hospital visit for a 25-year-old female with hypertension and systemic lupus erythematosus, admitted for fever and respiratory distress. On the third hospital day, the patient presented with purpuric skin lesions and acute renal failure. (Allergy & Immunology)

Subsequent hospital visit for a 55-year-old male with severe chronic obstructive pulmonary disease and bronchospasm; initially admitted for acute respiratory distress requiring ventilatory support in the ICU. The patient was stabilized, extubated and transferred to the floor, but has now developed acute fever, dyspnea, left lower lobe rhonchi and laboratory evidence of carbon dioxide retention and hypoxemia. (Family Medicine/Internal Medicine)

Subsequent hospital visit for 46-year-old female, known liver cirrhosis patient, with recent upper gastrointestinal hemorrhage from varices; now with worsening ascites and encephalopathy. (Gastroenterology)

Subsequent hospital visit for 62-year-old female admitted with acute subarachnoid hemorrhage, negative cerebral arteriogram, increased lethargy and hemiparesis with fever. (Neurosurgery)

Consultations

Office or Other Outpatient Consultations

New or Established Patient

99241   Initial office consultation for a 40-year-old female in pain from blister on lip following a cold. (Oral & Maxillofacial Surgery)

Initial office consultation for a 62-year-old construction worker with olecranon bursitis. (Orthopaedic Surgery)

Office consultation with 25-year-old postpartum female with severe symptomatic hemorrhoids. (Colon & Rectal Surgery)

Office consultation with 58-year-old male, referred for follow-up of creatinine level and evaluation of obstructive uropathy, relieved two months ago. (Nephrology)

Office consultation for 30-year-old female tennis player with sprain or contusion of the forearm. (Orthopaedic Surgery)

Office consultation for a 45-year-old male, requested by his internist, with asymptomatic torus palatinus requiring no further treatment. (Oral & Maxillofacial Surgery)

99242   Initial office consultation for a 20-year-old male with acute upper respiratory tract symptoms. (Allergy & Immunology)

Initial office consultation for a 29-year-old soccer player with painful proximal thigh/groin injury. (Orthopaedic Surgery)

Initial office consultation for a 66-year-old female with wrist and hand pain, numbness of finger tips, suspected median nerve compression by carpal tunnel syndrome. (Plastic Surgery)

Initial office consultation for a patient with a solitary lesion of discoid lupus erythematosus on left cheek to rule out malignancy or self-induced lesion. (Dermatology)

Office consultation for management of systolic hypertension in a 70-year-old male scheduled for elective prostate resection. (Geriatrics)

Office consultation with 27-year-old female, with old amputation, for evaluation of existing above-knee prosthesis. (Physical Medicine & Rehabilitation)

Office consultation with 66-year-old female with wrist and hand pain, and finger numbness, secondary to suspected carpal tunnel syndrome. (Orthopaedic Surgery)

Office consultation for 61-year-old female, recently on antibiotic therapy, now with diarrhea and leukocytosis. (Abdominal Surgery)

Office consultation for a patient with papulosquamous eruption of elbow with pitting of nails and itchy scalp. (Dermatology)

Office consultation for a 30-year-old female with single season allergic rhinitis. (Allergy & Immunology)

99243   Initial office consultation for a 60-year-old male with avascular necrosis of the left femoral head with increasing pain. (Orthopaedic Surgery)

Office consultation for a 31-year-old woman complaining of palpitations and chest pains. Her internist had described a mild systolic click. (Cardiology)

Office consultation for a 65-year-old female with persistent bronchitis. (Infectious Disease)

Office consultation for a 65-year-old man with chronic low-back pain radiating to the leg. (Neurosurgery)

Office consultation for 23-year-old female with Crohn's disease not responding to therapy. (Abdominal Surgery/Colon & Rectal Surgery)

Office consultation for 25-year-old patient with symptomatic knee pain and swelling, with torn anterior cruciate ligament and/or torn meniscus. (Orthopaedic Surgery)

Office consultation for a 67-year-old patient with osteoporosis and mandibular atrophy with regard to reconstructive alternatives. (Oral & Maxillofacial Surgery)

Office consultation for 39-year-old patient referred at a perimenopausal age for irregular menses and menopausal symptoms. (Obstetrics & Gynecology)

99244   Initial office consultation for a 28-year-old male, HIV+, with a recent change in visual acuity. (Ophthalmology)

Initial office consultation for a 15-year-old male with failing grades, suspected drug abuse. (Pediatrics)

Initial office consultation for a 36-year-old factory worker, status four months post-occupational low back injury and requires management of intractable low back pain. (Pain Medicine)

Initial office consultation for a 45-year-old female with a history of chronic arthralgia of TMJ and associated myalgia and sudden progressive symptomatology over last two to three months. (Oral & Maxillofacial Surgery)

Initial office consultation for evaluation of a 70-year-old male with appetite loss and diminished energy. (Psychiatry)

Initial office consultation for an elementary school-aged patient, referred by pediatrician, with multiple systematic complaints and recent onset of behavioral discontrol. (Psychiatry)

Initial office consultation for a 23-year-old female with developmental facial skeletal anomaly and subsequent abnormal relationship of jaw(s) to cranial base. (Oral & Maxillofacial Surgery)

Initial office consultation for a 45-year-old myopic patient with a one-week history of floaters and a partial retinal detachment. (Ophthalmology)

Initial office consultation for a 65-year-old female with moderate dementia, mild unsteadiness, back pain fatigue on ambulation, intermittent urinary incontinence. (Neurosurgery)

Initial office consultation for a 33-year-old female referred by endocrinologist with amenorrhea and galactorrhea, for evaluation of pituitary tumor. (Neurosurgery)

Initial office consultation for a 34-year-old male with new onset nephrotic syndrome. (Nephrology)

Initial office consultation for a 39-year-old female with intractable chest wall pain secondary to metastatic breast cancer. (Anesthesiology/Pain Medicine)

Initial office consultation for a patient with multiple giant tumors of jaws. (Oral & Maxillofacial Surgery)

Initial office consultation for a patient with a failed total hip replacement with loosening and pain upon walking. (Orthopaedic Surgery)

Initial office consultation for a 60-year-old female with three-year history of intermittent tic-like unilateral facial pain; now constant pain for six weeks without relief by adequate carbamazepine dosage. (Neurosurgery)

Initial office consultation for a 45-year-old male heavy construction worker with prior lumbar disk surgery two years earlier; now gradually recurring low back and unilateral leg pain for three months, unable to work for two weeks. (Neurosurgery)

Initial office consultation of a patient who presents with a 30-year history of smoking and right neck mass. (Otolaryngology, Head & Neck Surgery)

Office consultation with 38-year-old female, with inflammatory bowel disease, who now presents with right lower quadrant pain and suspected intra-abdominal abscess. (General Surgery/Colon & Rectal Surgery)

Office consultation with 72-year-old male with esophageal carcinoma, symptoms of dysphagia and reflux. (Thoracic Surgery)

Office consultation for discussion of treatment options for a 40-year-old female with a two-centimeter adenocarcinoma of the breast. (Radiation Oncology)

Office consultation for young patient referred by pediatrician because of patient's short attention span, easy distractibility and hyperactivity. (Psychiatry)

Office consultation for 66-year-old female, history of colon resection for adenocarcinoma six years earlier, now with severe mid-back pain; x-rays showing osteoporosis and multiple vertebral compression fractures. (Neurosurgery)

Office consultation for a patient with chronic pelvic inflammatory disease who now has left lower quadrant pain with a palpable pelvic mass. (Obstetrics & Gynecology)

Office consultation for a patient with long-standing psoriasis with acute onset of erythroderma, pustular lesions, chills and fever. Combinations of topical and systemic treatments discussed and instituted. (Dermatology)

99245 Initial office consultation for a 35-year-old multiple-trauma male patient with complex pelvic fractures, for evaluation and formulation of management plan. (Orthopaedic Surgery)

Initial emergency room consultation for 10-year-old male in status epilepticus, recent closed head injury, information about medication not available. (Neurosurgery)

Initial emergency room consultation for a 23-year-old patient with severe abdominal pain, guarding, febrile, and unstable vital signs. (Obstetrics & Gynecology)

Office consultation for a 67-year-old female longstanding uncontrolled diabetic who presents with retinopathy, nephropathy, and a foot ulcer. (Endocrinology)

Office consultation for a 37-year-old male for initial evaluation and management of Cushing's disease. (Endocrinology)

Office consultation for a 60-year-old male who presents with thyrotoxicosis, exophthalmos, frequent premature ventricular contractions and congestive heart failure. (Endocrinology)

Initial office consultation for a 36-year-old patient, one year status post occupational herniated cervical disk treated by laminectomy, requiring management of multiple sites of intractable pain, depression, and narcotic dependence. (Pain Medicine)

Office consultation for a 58-year-old man with a history of MI and CHF who complains of the recent onset of rest angina and shortness of breath. The patient has a systolic blood pressure of 90mmHG and is in Class IV heart failure. (Cardiology)

Emergency room consultation for a 1-year-old with a three-day history of fever with increasing respiratory distress who is thought to have cardiac tamponade by the ER physician. (Cardiology)

Office consultation in the emergency room for a 25-year-old male with severe, acute, closed head injury. (Neurosurgery)

Office consultation for a 23-year-old female with Stage II A Hodgkins disease with positive supraclavicular and mediastinal nodes. (Radiation Oncology)

Office consultation for a 27-year-old juvenile diabetic patient with severe diabetic retinopathy, gastric atony, nephrotic syndrome and progressive renal failure, now with a serum creatinine of 2.7, and a blood pressure of 170/114. (Nephrology)

Office consultation for independent medical evaluation of a patient with a history of complicated low back and neck problems with previous multiple failed back surgeries. (Orthopaedic Surgery)

Office consultation for an adolescent referred by pediatrician for recent onset of violent and self-injurious behavior. (Psychiatry)

Office consultation for a 6-year-old male for evaluation of severe muscle and joint pain and a diffuse rash. Patient well until 4-6 weeks earlier, when he developed arthralgia, myalgias, and a fever of 102 for one week. (Rheumatology)

Inpatient Consultations

New or Established Patient

99251 Initial hospital consultation for a 27-year-old female with fractured incisor post-intubation. (Oral & Maxillofacial Surgery)

Initial hospital consultation for an orthopaedic patient on IV antibiotics who has developed an apparent candida infection of the oral cavity. (Oral & Maxillofacial Surgery)

Initial inpatient consultation for a 30-year-old female complaining of vaginal itching, post orthopaedic surgery. (Obstetrics & Gynecology)

Initial inpatient consultation for a 36-year-old male on orthopaedic service with complaint of localized dental pain. (Oral & Maxillofacial Surgery)

99252 Initial hospital consultation for a 45-year-old male, previously abstinent alcoholic, who relapsed and was admitted for management of gastritis. The patient readily accepts the need for further treatment. (Addiction Medicine)

Initial hospital consultation for a 35-year-old dialysis patient with episodic oral ulcerations. (Oral & Maxillofacial Surgery)

Initial inpatient preoperative consultation for a 43-year-old woman with cholecystitis and well-controlled hypertension. (Cardiology)

Initial inpatient consultation for recommendation of antibiotic prophylaxis for a patient with a synthetic heart valve who will undergo urologic surgery. (Internal Medicine)

Initial inpatient consultation for possible drug induced skin eruption in 50-year-old male. (Dermatology)

Preoperative inpatient consultation for evaluation of hypertension in a 60-year-old male who will undergo a cholecystectomy. Patient had a normal annual check-up in your office four months ago. (Internal Medicine)

Initial inpatient consultation for 66-year-old patient with wrist and hand pain and finger numbness, secondary to carpal tunnel syndrome. (Orthopaedic Surgery/Plastic Surgery)

Initial inpatient consultation for a 66-year-old male smoker referred for pain management immediately status post-biliary tract surgery done via sub-costal incision. (Anesthesiology/Pain Medicine)

99253 Initial hospital consultation for a 50-year-old female with incapacitating knee pain due to generalized rheumatoid arthritis. (Orthopaedic Surgery)

Initial hospital consultation for a 60-year-old male with avascular necrosis of the left femoral heel with increasing pain. (Orthopaedic Surgery)

Initial hospital consultation for a 45-year-old female with compound mandibular fracture and concurrent head, abdominal and/or orthopaedic injuries. (Oral & Maxillofacial Surgery)

Initial hospital consultation for a 22-year-old female, paraplegic, to evaluate wrist and hand pain. (Orthopaedic Surgery)

Initial hospital consultation for a 40-year-old male with 10-day history of incapacitating unilateral sciatica, unable to walk now, not improved by bed rest. (Neurosurgery)

Initial hospital consultation, requested by pediatrician, for treatment recommendations for a patient admitted with persistent inability to walk following soft tissue injury to ankle. (Physiatry)

Initial hospital consultation for a 27-year-old previously healthy male who vomited during IV sedation and may have aspirated gastric contents. (Anesthesiology)

Initial hospital consultation for a 33-year-old female, post-abdominal surgery, who now has a fever. (Internal Medicine)

Initial inpatient consultation for a 57-year-old male, post lower endoscopy, for evaluation of abdominal pain and fever. (General Surgery)

Initial inpatient consultation for rehabilitation of a 73-year-old female one week after surgical management of a hip fracture. (Physical Medicine & Rehabilitation)

Initial inpatient consultation for diagnosis/management of fever following abdominal surgery. (Internal Medicine)

Initial inpatient consultation for a 35-year-old female with a fever and pulmonary infiltrate following cesarean section. (Pulmonary Medicine)

Initial inpatient consultation for a 42-year-old non-diabetic patient, post-op cholecystectomy, now with an acute urinary tract infection. (Nephrology)

Initial inpatient consultation for 53-year-old female with moderate uncomplicated pancreatitis. (Gastroenterology)

Initial inpatient consultation for 45-year-old patient with chronic neck pain with radicular pain of the left arm. (Orthopaedic Surgery)

Initial inpatient consultation for 8-year-old patient with new onset of seizures who has a normal examination and previous history. (Neurology)

99254 Initial hospital consultation for a 15-year-old patient with painless swelling of proximal humerus with lytic lesion by x-ray. (Orthopaedic Surgery)

Initial hospital consultation for evaluation of a 29-year-old female with a diffusely positive medical review of systems and history of multiple surgeries. (Psychiatry)

Initial hospital consultation for a 70-year-old diabetic female with gangrene of the foot. (Orthopaedic Surgery)

Initial inpatient consultation for a 47-year-old female with progressive pulmonary infiltrate, hypoxemia, and diminished urine output. (Anesthesiology)

Initial hospital consultation for a 13-month-old with spasmodic cough, respiratory distress, and fever. (Allergy & Immunology)

Initial hospital consultation for a patient with failed total hip replacement with loosening and pain upon walking. (Orthopaedic Surgery)

Initial hospital consultation for a 62-year-old female with metastatic breast cancer to the femoral neck and thoracic vertebra. (Orthopaedic Surgery)

Initial hospital consultation for a 39-year-old female with nephrolithiasis requiring extensive opioid analgesics, whose vital signs are now elevated. She initially denied any drug use, but today gives history of multiple substance abuse, including opioids and prior treatment for a personality disorder. (Psychiatry)

Initial hospital consultation for a 70-year-old female without previous psychiatric history, who is now experiencing nocturnal confusion and visual hallucinations following hip replacement surgery. (Psychiatry)

Initial inpatient consultation for evaluation of a 63-year-old in the ICU with diabetes and chronic renal failure who develops acute respiratory distress syndrome 36 hours after a mitral valve replacement. (Anesthesiology)

Initial inpatient consultation for a 66-year-old female with enlarged supraclavicular lymph nodes, found on biopsy to be malignant. (Hematology/Oncology)

Initial inpatient consultation for a 43-year-old female for evaluation of sudden painful visual loss, optic neuritis and episodic paresthesia. (Ophthalmology)

Initial inpatient consultation for evaluation of a 71-year-old male with hyponatremia (serum sodium 114) who was admitted to the hospital with pneumonia. (Nephrology)

Initial inpatient consultation for a 72-year-old male with emergency admission for possible bowel obstruction. (Internal Medicine/General Surgery)

Initial inpatient consultation for a 35-year-old female with fever, swollen joints, and rash of one-week duration. (Rheumatology)

99255 Initial inpatient consultation for a 76-year-old female with massive, life-threatening gastrointestinal hemorrhage and chest pain. (Gastroenterology)

Initial inpatient consultation for a 75-year-old female, admitted to intensive care with acute respiratory distress syndrome, who is hypersensitive, has a moderate metabolic acidosis, and a rising serum creatinine. (Nephrology)

Initial hospital consultation for patient with a history of complicated low back pain and neck problems with previous multiple failed back surgeries. (Orthopaedic Surgery/Neurosurgery)

Initial hospital consultation for a 66-year-old female, two days post-abdominal aneurysm repair, with oliguria and hypertension of one-day duration. (Nephrology/Internal Medicine)

Initial hospital consultation for a patient with shotgun wound to face with massive facial trauma and airway obstruction. (Oral & Maxillofacial Surgery)

Initial hospital consultation for patient with severe pancreatitis complicated by respiratory insufficiency, acute renal failure, and abscess formation. (General Surgery/Colon & Rectal Surgery)

Initial hospital consultation for a 35-year-old multiple-trauma male patient with complex pelvic fractures to evaluate and formulate management plan. (Orthopaedic Surgery)

Initial inpatient consultation for adolescent patient with fractured femur and pelvis who pulled out IVs and disconnected traction in attempt to elope from hospital. (Psychiatry)

Initial hospital consultation for a 16-year-old primigravida at 32 weeks gestation requested by a family practitioner for evaluation of severe hypertension, thrombocytopenia, and headache. (Obstetrics & Gynecology)

Initial hospital consultation for a 58-year-old insulin-dependent diabetic with multiple antibiotic allergies, now with multiple fascial plane abscesses and airway obstruction. (Oral & Maxillofacial Surgery)

Initial inpatient consultation for a 55-year-old male with known cirrhosis and ascites, now with jaundice, encephalopathy, and massive hematemesis. (Gastroenterology)

Initial hospital consultation for a 25-year-old male, seen in emergency room with severe, closed head injury. (Neurosurgery)

Initial hospital consultation for a 2-day-old male with single ventricle physiology and subaortic obstruction. Family counseling following evaluation for multiple, staged surgical procedures. (Thoracic Surgery)

Initial hospital consultation for a 45-year-old male admitted with subarachnoid hemorrhage and intracranial aneurysm on angiogram. (Neurosurgery)

Initial inpatient consultation for myxedematous patient who is hypoventilating and obtunded. (Endocrinology)

Initial hospital consultation for a 45-year-old patient with widely metastatic lung carcinoma, intractable back pain, and a history that includes substance dependence, NSAID allergy, and two prior laminectomies with fusion for low back pain. (Pain Medicine)

Initial hospital consultation for evaluation of treatment options in a 50-year-old patient with cirrhosis, known peptic ulcer disease, hypotension, encephalopathy, and massive acute upper gastrointestinal bleeding which cannot be localized by endoscopy. (Interventional Radiology)

Initial inpatient consultation in the ICU for a 70-year-old male who experienced a cardiac arrest during surgery and was resuscitated. (Cardiology)

Initial inpatient consultation for a patient with severe pancreatitis complicated by respiratory insufficiency, acute renal failure and abscess formation. (Gastroenterology)

Initial inpatient consultation for a 70-year-old cirrhotic male admitted with ascites, jaundice, encephalopathy, and massive hematemesis. (Gastroenterology)

Initial inpatient consultation in the ICU for a 51-year-old patient who is on a ventilator and has a fever two weeks after a renal transplantation. (Infectious Disease)

Initial inpatient consultation for evaluation and formulation of plan for management of multiple trauma patient with complex pelvic fracture, 35-year-old male. (General Surgery/Orthopaedic Surgery)

Initial inpatient consultation for a 50-year-old male with a history of previous myocardial infarction, now with acute pulmonary edema and hypotension. (Cardiology)

Initial inpatient consultation for 45-year-old male with recent, acute subarachnoid hemorrhage, hesitant speech, mildly confused, drowsy. High risk group for HIV+ status. (Neurosurgery)

Initial inpatient consultation for 36-year-old female referred by her internist to evaluate a patient being followed for abdominal pain and fever. The patient has developed diffuse abdominal pain, guarding, rigidity and increased fever. (Obstetrics & Gynecology)

Emergency Department Services

New or Established Patient

99281 Emergency department visit for a patient for removal of sutures from a well-healed, uncomplicated laceration. (Emergency Medicine)

Emergency department visit for a patient for tetanus toxoid immunization. (Emergency Medicine)

Emergency department visit for a patient with several uncomplicated insect bites. (Emergency Medicine)

99282 Emergency department visit for a 20-year-old student who presents with a painful sunburn with blister formation on the back. (Emergency Medicine)

Emergency department visit for a child presenting with impetigo localized to the face. (Emergency Medicine)

Emergency department visit for a patient with a minor traumatic injury of an extremity with localized pain, swelling, and bruising. (Emergency Medicine)

Emergency department visit for an otherwise healthy patient whose chief complaint is a red, swollen cystic lesion on his/her back. (Emergency Medicine)

Emergency department visit for a patient presenting with a rash on both legs after exposure to poison ivy. (Emergency Medicine)

Emergency department visit for a young adult patient with infected sclera and purulent discharge from both eyes without pain, visual disturbance or history of foreign body in either eye. (Emergency Medicine)

99283 Emergency department visit for a sexually active female complaining of vaginal discharge who is afebrile and denies experiencing abdominal or back pain. (Emergency Medicine)

Emergency department visit for a well-appearing 8-year-old who has a fever, diarrhea and abdominal cramps, is tolerating oral fluids and is not vomiting. (Emergency Medicine)

Emergency department visit for a patient with an inversion ankle injury, who is unable to bear weight on the injured foot and ankle. (Emergency Medicine)

Emergency department visit for a patient who has a complaint of acute pain associated with a suspected foreign body in the painful eye. (Emergency Medicine)

Emergency department visit for a healthy, young adult patient who sustained a blunt head injury with local swelling and bruising without subsequent confusion, loss of consciousness or memory deficit. (Emergency Medicine)

99284 Emergency department visit for a 4-year-old who fell off a bike sustaining a head injury with brief loss of consciousness. (Emergency Medicine)

Emergency department visit for an elderly female who has fallen and is now complaining of pain in her right hip and is unable to walk. (Emergency Medicine)

Emergency department visit for a patient with flank pain and hematuria. (Emergency Medicine)

Emergency department visit for a female presenting with lower abdominal pain and a vaginal discharge. (Emergency Medicine)

99285 Emergency department visit for a patient with a complicated overdose requiring aggressive management to prevent side effects from the ingested materials. (Emergency Medicine)

Emergency department visit for a patient with a new onset of rapid heart rate requiring IV drugs. (Emergency Medicine)

Emergency department visit for a patient exhibiting active, upper gastrointestinal bleeding. (Emergency Medicine)

Emergency department visit for a previously healthy young adult patient who is injured in an automobile accident and is brought to the emergency department immobilized and has symptoms compatible with intra-abdominal injuries or multiple extremity injuries. (Emergency Medicine)

Emergency department visit for a patient with an acute onset of chest pain compatible with symptoms of cardiac ischemia and/or pulmonary embolus. (Emergency Medicine)

Emergency department visit for a patient who presents with a sudden onset of "the worst headache of her life," and complains of a stiff neck, nausea, and inability to concentrate. (Emergency Medicine)

Emergency department visit for a patient with a new onset of a cerebral vascular accident. (Emergency Medicine)

Emergency department visit for acute febrile illness in an adult, associated with shortness of breath and an altered level of alertness. (Emergency Medicine)

Critical Care Services

99291 First hour of critical care of a 65-year-old man with septic shock following relief of ureteral obstruction caused by a stone.

First hour of critical care of a 15-year-old with acute respiratory failure from asthma.

First hour of critical care of a 45-year-old who sustained a liver laceration, cerebral hematoma, flailed chest, and pulmonary contusion after being struck by an automobile.

First hour of critical care of a 65-year-old woman who, following a hysterectomy, suffered a cardiac arrest associated with a pulmonary embolus.

First hour of critical care of a 6-month-old with hypovolemic shock secondary to diarrhea and dehydration.

First hour of critical care of a 3-year-old with respiratory failure secondary to pneumocystis carinii pneumonia.

Prolonged Services

Prolonged Physician Service With Direct (Face-to-Face) Patient Contact

Office or Other Outpatient

99354/ 99355 A 20-year-old female with history of asthma presents with acute bronchospasm and moderate respiratory distress. Initial evaluation shows respiratory rate 30, labored breathing and wheezing heard in all lung fields. Office treatment is initiated which includes intermittent bronchial dilation and subcutaneous epinephrine. Requires intermittent physician face-to-face time with patient over a period of 2-3 hours. (Family Medicine/Internal Medicine)

Inpatient

99356 A 34-year-old primigravida presents to hospital in early labor. Admission history and physical reveals severe preeclampsia. Physician supervises management of preeclampsia, IV magnesium initiation and maintenance, labor augmentation with pitocin, and close maternal-fetal monitoring. Physician face-to-face involvement includes 40 minutes of continuous bedside care until the patient is stable, then is intermittent over several hours until the delivery. (Family Medicine/Internal Medicine/Obstetrics & Gynecology)

Prolonged Physician Service Without Direct Patient (Face-to-Face) Contact

99358/ 99359 A 65-year-old new patient with multiple problems is seen and evaluated. After the visit, the physician requires extensive time to talk with the patient's daughter, to review complex, detailed medical records transferred from previous physicians and to complete a comprehensive treatment plan. This plan also requires the physician to personally initiate and coordinate the care plan with a local home health agency and a dietician. (Family Medicine/Internal Medicine)

Physician Standby Services

99360   A 24-year-old patient is admitted to OB unit attempting VBAC. Fetal monitoring shows increasing fetal distress. Patient's blood pressure is rising and labor progressing slowly. A primary care physician is requested by the OB/GYN to standby in the unit for possible cesarean delivery and neonatal resuscitation. (Family Medicine/Internal Medicine)

Care Plan Oversight Services

99375   First month of care plan oversight for terminal care of a 58-year-old woman with advanced intraabdominal ovarian cancer. Care plan includes home oxygen, diuretics IV for edema and ascites control and pain control management involving IV morphine infusion when progressive ileus occurred. Physician phone contacts with nurse, family, and MSW. Discussion with MSW concerning plans to withdraw supportive measures per patient wishes. Documentation includes review and modification of care plan and certifications from nursing, MSW, pharmacy, and DME. (Family Medicine/Internal Medicine)

Appendix D

Summary of CPT Add-on Codes

This listing is a summary of CPT add-on codes for *CPT 2007*. The codes listed below are identified in *CPT 2007* with a **+** symbol.

				63035	75996	93572
				63043	76125	93609
				63044	76802	93613
				63048	76810	93621
				63057	76812	93622
				63066	76814	93623
				63076	76937	93662
				63078	77001	94645
				63082	77051	95873
				63086	77052	95874
				63088	78020	95920
01953	15366	31637	38746	63091	78478	95962
01968	15401	32501	38747	63103	78480	95967
01969	15421	33141	43635	63295	78496	95973
11001	15431	33225	44015	63308	78730	95975
11008	15787	33508	44121	64472	83901	95979
11101	15831	33530	44128	64476	87187	96411
11201	15847	33572	44139	64480	87904	96415
11732	16036	33768	44203	64484	88155	96417
11922	17003	33884	44213	64623	88185	96423
13102	17312	33924	44701	64627	88311	96570
13122	17314	33961	44955	64727	88312	96571
13133	17315	34808	47001	64778	88313	97546
13153	19001	34813	47550	64783	88314	97811
15003	19126	34826	48400	64787	90466	97814
15005	19291	35306	49326	64832	90468	99100
15101	19295	35390	49435	64837	90472	99116
15111	19297	35400	49568	64859	90474	99135
15116	22103	35500	49905	64872	90761	99140
15121	22116	35572	56606	64874	90766	99145
15131	22216	35681	57267	64876	90767	99150
15136	22226	35682	58110	64901	90768	99290
15151	22328	35683	58611	64902	90775	99292
15152	22522	35685	59525	66990	92547	99354
15156	22525	35686	60512	67225	92608	99355
15157	22527	35697	61316	67320	92627	99356
15171	22534	35700	61517	67331	92973	99357
15176	22585	36218	61609	67332	92974	99358
15201	22614	36248	61610	67334	92978	99359
15221	22632	36476	61611	67335	92979	99602
15241	26125	36479	61612	67340	92981	0049T
15261	26861	37185	61641	69990	92984	0054T
15301	26863	37186	61642	74301	92996	0055T
15321	27358	37206	61795	75774	92998	0056T
15331	27692	37208	61864	75946	93320	0063T
15336	31620	37250	61868	75964	93321	0068T
15341	31632	37251	62148	75968	93325	0069T
15361	31633	38102	62160	75993	93571	0070T

0076T

0079T

0081T

0092T

0095T

0098T

0117T

0151T

0153T

0159T

0163T

0164T

0165T

Appendix E

Summary of CPT Codes Exempt From Modifier 51

This listing is a summary of CPT codes that are exempt from the use of modifier 51 but have NOT been designated as CPT add-on procedures/services. The codes listed below are identified in *CPT 2007* with a ⊘ symbol.

17004	33521	90634	90716
20660	33522	90636	90717
20690	33523	90645	90718
20692	35600	90646	90719
20900	36620	90647	90720
20902	36660	90648	90721
20910	38792	90649	90723
20912	44500	90655	90725
20920	61107	90656	90727
20922	61210	90657	90732
20924	62284	90658	90733
20926	90281	90660	90734
20930	90283	90665	90735
20931	90287	90669	90736
20936	90288	90675	90740
20937	90291	90676	90743
20938	90296	90680	90744
20974	90371	90690	90746
20975	90375	90691	90747
22840	90376	90692	90748
22841	90378	90693	90749
22842	90379	90698	93501
22843	90384	90700	93503
22844	90385	90701	93505
22845	90386	90702	93508
22846	90389	90703	93510
22847	90393	90704	93511
22848	90396	90705	93514
22851	90399	90706	93524
31500	90476	90707	93526
32000	90477	90708	93527
32002	90581	90710	93528
32020	90585	90712	93529
33517	90586	90713	93530
33518	90632	90714	93531
33519	90633	90715	93532

93533
93539
93540
93541
93542
93543
93544
93545
93555
93556
93600
93602
93603
93610
93612
93615
93616
93618
93619
93620
93624
93631
93640
93641
93642
93650
93651
93652
93660
94610
95900
95903
95904
99143
99144
99148
99149

Appendix F

Summary of CPT Codes Exempt From Modifier 63

The listing is a summary of CPT codes that are exempt from the use of modifier 63. The codes listed below are additionally identified in *CPT 2007* with the parenthetical instruction "(Do not report modifier 63 in conjunction with…)"

30540	36660	63700
30545	39503	63702
31520	43313	63704
33401	43314	63706
33403	43520	65820
33470	43831	
33472	44055	
33502	44126	
33503	44127	
33505	44128	
33506	46070	
33610	46705	
33611	46715	
33619	46716	
33647	46730	
33670	46735	
33690	46740	
33694	46742	
33730	46744	
33732	47700	
33735	47701	
33736	49215	
33750	49491	
33755	49492	
33762	49495	
33778	49496	
33786	49600	
33922	49605	
33960	49606	
33961	49610	
36415	49611	
36420	53025	
36450	54000	
36460	54150	
36510	54160	

Appendix G

Summary of CPT Codes That Include Moderate (Conscious) Sedation

The following list of procedures includes conscious sedation as an inherent part of providing the procedure. These codes are identified in the CPT codebook with a ⊙ symbol.

Since these services include moderate sedation, it is not appropriate for the same physician to report both the service and the sedation codes 99143-99145. It is expected that if conscious sedation is provided to the patient as part of one of these services, it is provided by the same physician who is providing the service.

In the unusual event when a second physician other than the health care professional performing the diagnostic or therapeutic services provides moderate sedation in the facility setting (eg, hospital, outpatient hospital/ambulatory surgery center, skilled nursing facility) for the procedures listed in Appendix G, the second physician can report 99148-99150. However, for the circumstance in which these services are performed by the second physician in the nonfacility setting (eg, physician office, freestanding imaging center), codes 99148-99150 would not be reported. Moderate sedation does not include minimal sedation (anxiolysis), deep sedation, or monitored anesthesia care (00100-01999).

The inclusion of a procedure on this list does not prevent separate reporting of an associated anesthesia procedure/service (CPT codes 00100-01999) when performed by a physician other than the health care professional performing the diagnostic or therapeutic procedure. In such cases the person providing anesthesia services shall be present for the purpose of continuously monitoring the patient and shall not act as a surgical assistant. When clinical conditions of the patient require such anesthesia services, or in the circumstances when the patient does not require sedation, the operating physician is not required to report the procedure as a reduced service using modifier 52.

19298	31624	31725	33208	33218	43202	43456
20982	31625	32019	33210	33220	43204	43458
22526	31628	32020	33211	33222	43205	43750
22527	31629	32201	33212	33223	43215	44360
31615	31635	33010	33213	33233	43216	44361
31620	31645	33011	33214	33234	43217	44363
31622	31646	33206	33216	33235	43219	44364
31623	31656	33207	33217	33240	43220	44365
				33241	43226	44366
				33244	43227	44369
				33249	43228	44370
				35470	43231	44372
				35471	43232	44373
				35472	43234	44376
				35473	43235	44377
				35474	43236	44378
				35475	43237	44379
				35476	43238	44380
				36555	43239	44382
				36557	43240	44383
				36558	43241	44385
				36560	43242	44386
				36561	43243	44388
				36563	43244	44389
				36565	43245	44390
				36566	43246	44391
				36568	43247	44392
				36570	43248	44393
				36571	43249	44394
				36576	43250	44397
				36578	43251	44500
				36581	43255	44901
				36582	43256	45303
				36583	43257	45305
				36585	43258	45307
				36590	43259	45308
				36870	43260	45309
				37184	43261	45315
				37185	43262	45317
				37186	43263	45320
				37187	43264	45321
				37188	43265	45327
				37203	43267	45332
				37210	43268	45333
				37215	43269	45334
				37216	43271	45335
				43200	43272	45337
				43201	43453	45338

45339	92987	93650
45340	92995	93651
45341	92996	93652
45342	93312	
45345	93313	
45355	93314	
45378	93315	
45379	93316	
45380	93317	
45381	93318	
45382	93501	
45383	93505	
45384	93508	
45385	93510	
45386	93511	
45387	93514	
45391	93524	
45392	93526	
47011	93527	
48511	93528	
49021	93529	
49041	93530	
49061	93539	
50021	93540	
50382	93541	
50384	93542	
50387	93543	
50592	93544	
58823	93545	
66720	93555	
69300	93556	
77600	93561	
77605	93562	
77610	93571	
77615	93572	
92953	93609	
92960	93613	
92961	93615	
92973	93616	
92974	93618	
92975	93619	
92978	93620	
92979	93621	
92980	93622	
92981	93624	
92982	93640	
92984	93641	
92986	93642	

Appendix H

Alphabetic Index of Performance Measures by Clinical Condition or Topic

Appendix H is an alphabetical listing of the diseases with which the measures and codes are associated. It provides an overview of the performance measures, a listing of the CPT Category II codes that may be used with each measure, as well as any applicable reporting instructions. It is intended to be used as a crosswalk to the Category II codes section allowing users an overview of the measures and the Category II codes that should be used with each measure, linking the Category II codes to the specific measures and measure sets from which these codes were derived. The clinical conditions or topics are listed in alphabetic order within the appendix to allow rapid access to the conditions/topics currently included in the coding manual. For the latest Appendix H information, visit the website at www.ama-assn.org/go/cpt.

In order for a patient to be included in the numerator for a particular performance measure, a patient must meet the denominator inclusion criteria for that measure. Prior to coding, users must review (1) the complete description of the code in the Category II section of the CPT codebook and Web site and (2) the specification documents of its associated performance measure as found on the measure developer's Website. Symbols proceeding the specific performance measure direct users to footnotes at the bottom of each page of this appendix. The footnotes identify the measure developer and the developer's Web address.

In addition, the modifiers included within the Category II code section and Appendix H are only intended to be used when parenthetic notes, guidelines, or reporting language specifically allow use.

Performance measurement exclusion modifiers may be used to indicate that a service specified by a performance measure was considered but, due to either medical, patient, or sytems reason(s) documented in the medical record, the service was not provided. These modifiers serve as denominator exclusions from the performance measure. *Not all listed measures provide for exclusions*. The three modifiers currently in effect include the following:

Performance Measure Exclusion Modifiers

1P Performance measure exclusion modifier due to medical reasons

Reasons include:
- not indicated (absence of organ/limb, already received/performed, other)
- contraindicated (patient allergic history, potential adverse drug interaction, other)
- other medical reasons

2P Performance measure exclusion modifier due to patient reasons

Reasons include:
- Patient declined
- Economic, social, or religious reasons
- Other patient reasons

3P Performance measure exclusion modifier due to system reasons

Reasons include:
- Resources to perform the services not available (eg, equipment, supplies)
- Insurance coverage or payer-related limitations
- Other reasons attributable to health care delivery system

[1] Physician Consortium for Performance Improvement: www.physicianconsortium.org
[2] National Committee on Quality Assurance (NCQA): Health Employer Data Information Set (HEDIS®): www.ncqa.org
[3] Joint Commission on Accreditation of Healthcare Organizations (JCAHO), ORYX Initiative Performance Measures: www.jcaho.org/pms
[4] National Diabetes Quality Improvement Alliance (NDQIA): www.nationaldiabetesalliance.org

Brief Description of Performance Measure & Source and Reporting Instructions	CPT Code(s)	Short Code Descriptor
Asthma		
Asthma Assessment[1]—Whether or not patient was evaluated during at least one office visit during the reporting year for the frequency (numeric) of daytime and nocturnal asthma symptoms **Numerator:** Patients who were evaluated during at least one office visit during the reporting year for the frequency (numeric) of daytime and nocturnal asthma symptoms **Denominator:** All patients aged 5-40 years with asthma **Percentage** of patients aged 5-40 years with asthma who were evaluated during at least one office visit during the reporting year for the frequency (numeric) of daytime and nocturnal asthma symptoms **Reporting Instructions:** To be counted in calculations of this measure, symptom frequency must be numerically quantified. Measure may also be met by physician documentation or patient completion of an asthma assessment tool/survey/questionnaire. Assessment tool may include the Quality Metric Asthma Control Test™, National Asthma Education & Prevention Program (NAEPP) Asthma Symptoms and Peak Flow Diary	**1005F**	Asthma symptoms evaluated
Asthma Pharmacologic Therapy[1]—Whether or not patient with mild, moderate, or severe *persistent* asthma was prescribed *either* the preferred long-term control medication (inhaled corticosteroid) or an acceptable alternative treatment **Numerator:** Patients who were prescribed *either* the preferred[a] long-term control medication (inhaled corticosteroids) or an acceptable alternative treatment[b] (cromolyn sodium, leukotriene modifier, nedocromil, OR sustained release theophylline) **Denominator:** All patients aged 5-40 years with mild, moderate or severe persistent asthma **Exclusion(s):** Documentation of patient reason(s) (eg economic, social, religious) for not prescribing either the preferred long-term control medication (inhaled corticosteroids) or an acceptable alternative treatment. (There are no medical exclusion criteria.) **Percentage** of all patients with mild, moderate, or severe *persistent* asthma who were prescribed *either* the preferred long-term control medication (inhaled corticosteroids) or an acceptable alternative treatment **Reporting Instructions:** Report 1038F or 1039F for each asthma patient. If long-term control medication (or acceptable alternative treatment) prescribed, report 4015F. Report 4015F with 1038F. Report modifier 2P for patient who meets exclusion criteria. Modifier 1P may not be reported with 4015F. [a, b]Refer to complete description of measure developer's Web site for list of medications, treatment recommendations, dosages	**4015F** **Denominator Codes:** **1038F** **1039F**	Persist asthma medicine ctrl Persistent asthma Intermittent asthma
Chronic Obstructive Pulmonary Disease (COPD)		
Smoking Assessment[1]—Whether or not patient with COPD was queried about smoking **Numerator:** All patients who were queried about smoking during one or more office visits each year **Denominator:** All patients with the diagnosis of COPD **Percentage** of patients who were queried about smoking at least annually **Reporting Instructions:** When reporting 1000F, it is required to report 1034F, and/or 1035F, or 1036F	**1000F** **1034F** **1035F** **1036F**	Tobacco use assessed Current tobacco smoker Smokeless tobacco user Tobacco non-user
Assessment of Symptoms[1]—Whether or not patient had COPD symptoms assessed at least annually **Numerator:** All patients with COPD symptoms assessed during one or more office visits each year **Denominator:** All patients with the diagnosis of COPD **Percentage** of patients who were assessed for COPD symptoms at least annually	**1015F**	COPD symptoms assess

[1]Physician Consortium for Performance Improvement: www.physicianconsortium.org
[2]National Committee on Quality Assurance (NCQA): Health Employer Data Information Set (HEDIS®): www.ncqa.org
[3]Joint Commission on Accreditation of Healthcare Organizations (JCAHO), ORYX Initiative Performance Measures: www.jcaho.org/pms
[4]National Diabetes Quality Improvement Alliance (NDQIA): www.nationaldiabetesalliance.org

Brief Description of Performance Measure & Source and Reporting Instructions	CPT Code(s)	Short Code Descriptor
Chronic Obstructive Pulmonary Disease (COPD), cont'd		
Spirometry Evaluation[1]—Whether or not patient spirometry results were documented **Numerator:** All patients with documented spirometry results on the medical record **Denominator:** All patients with the diagnosis of COPD **Exclusion Criteria:** Documentation of medical reason(s) for no spirometry evaluation OR Documentation of patient reason(s) for no spirometry evaluation Documentation of system reason(s) for no spirometry evaluation **Percentage** of patients with COPD who had a spirometry evaluation documented **Reporting Instructions:** For patients with appropriate exclusion criteria, report 3023F with modifier 1P, 2P, or 3P	3023F	Spirom doc rev
Smoking Cessation Intervention[1]—Whether or not the patient who is a smoker received a smoking cessation intervention **Numerator:** All smokers who received a smoking cessation intervention during one or more office visits each year **Denominator:** All patients with the diagnosis of COPD identified as smokers **Percentage** of smokers with COPD who received a smoking cessation intervention at least annually **Reporting Instructions:** Report 1034F for each cigarette smoker. Report either 1034F, 1035F, or 1036 for each patient. If patient is a smoker and received cessation intervention, report 4000F or 4001F, or both. Report 4000F or 4001F only if 1034F has been reported	4000F 4001F **Denominator codes:** 1034F 1035F 1036F	Tobacco use txmnt, counseling Tobacco use txmnt, pharmacol Current tobacco smoker Smokeless tobacco user Tobacco non-user
Inhaled Bronchodilator[1]—Whether or not the symptomatic patient was prescribed an inhaled bronchodilator **Numerator:** All symptomatic patients who were prescribed an inhaled bronchodilator **Denominator:** All patients with the diagnosis of COPD who have an $FEV_1/FVC < 70\%$ and have symptoms **Denominator Inclusions:** Documentation of COPD symptoms; Documentation of $FEV_1/FVC < 70\%$ **Denominator Exclusions:** Documentation of medical reason(s) for not prescribing an inhaled bronchodilator or Documentation of patient reason(s) for not prescribing an inhaled bronchodilator or Documentation of system reason(s) for not prescribing an inhaled bronchodilator **Percentage** of symptomatic patients with COPD who were prescribed an inhaled bronchodilator **Reporting Instructions:** Report either 3025F or 3027F for all COPD patients. For patients with appropriate exclusion criteria, report 4025F with modifier 1P, 2P, or 3P	4025F **Denominator codes:** 3025F 3027F	Inhaled bronchodilator RX Spirom FEV/FVC<70% w COPD Spirom FEV/FVC≥70%/ w/o COPD
Assessment of Oxygen Saturation[1]—Whether or not oxygen saturation was assessed at least annually **Numerator:** All patients with oxygen saturation assessed and documented **Denominator:** All patients with the diagnosis of COPD and a FEV_1 40% of predicted value **Denominator Inclusion:** Documentation of $FEV_1 < 40\%$ of predicted value **Denominator Exclusions:** Documentation of medical reason(s) for not assessing oxygen saturation Documentation of patient reason(s) for not assessing oxygen saturation Documentation of systems reason(s) for not assessing oxygen saturation **Percentage** of COPD patients with oxygen saturation assessed at least annually **Reporting Instructions:** Report 3040F or 3042F for all COPD patients. If oxygen saturation assessed, also report 3028F. For patients with appropriate exclusion criteria, report 3028F with modifier 1P, 2P, or 3P	3028F **Denominator codes:** 3040F 3042F	O_2 saturation doc rev FEV<40% predicted value FEV≥ 40% predicted value

[1]Physician Consortium for Performance Improvement: www.physicianconsortium.org
[2]National Committee on Quality Assurance (NCQA): Health Employer Data Information Set (HEDIS®): www.ncqa.org
[3]Joint Commission on Accreditation of Healthcare Organizations (JCAHO), ORYX Initiative Performance Measures: www.jcaho.org/pms
[4]National Diabetes Quality Improvement Alliance (NDQIA): www.nationaldiabetesalliance.org

Brief Description of Performance Measure & Source and Reporting Instructions	CPT Code(s)	Short Code Descriptor
Chronic Obstructive Pulmonary Disease (COPD), cont'd		
Long-Term Oxygen Therapy[1]—Whether or not patient with COPD was prescribed long-term oxygen therapy **Numerator:** All patients who were prescribed long term oxygen therapy **Denominator:** All patients with a diagnosis of COPD and an oxygen saturation ≤ 88 % or a $PaO_2 \leq 55$ mm Hg **Denominator Inclusion:** $PaO_2 \leq 55$ mm Hg or oxygen saturation $\leq 88\%$ **Denominator Exclusion:** Documentation of medical reason(s) for not prescribing long term oxygen therapy. Documentation of patient reason(s) for not prescribing long term oxygen therapy Documentation of system reason(s) for not prescribing long term oxygen therapy **Percentage** of patients with COPD that were prescribed long term oxygen therapy **Reporting Instructions:** Report 3035F or 3037F for all COPD patients. Report 4030F with 3035F if long term oxygen therapy prescribed For patients with appropriate exclusion criteria, report 4030F with modifier 1P, 2P, or 3P	**4030F** **Denominator codes:** **3035F** **3037F**	Oxygen therapy RX O_2 saturation $\leq 88\%$ /PAO ≤ 55 O_2 saturation $> 88\%$ /PAO > 55
Recommendation of Influenza Immunization[1]—Whether or not COPD patient received recommendation for influenza immunization annually **Numerator:** All patients who were recommended to receive an influenza immunization during one or more office visits every year **Denominator:** All patients with the diagnosis of COPD **Denominator Exclusion:** Documentation of immunization given during the current flu season; documentation of medical reason(s) for not recommending an influenza immunization; documentation of system reason(s) for not recommending an influenza immunization **Percentage** of patients with COPD who were recommended to receive an influenza immunization annually **Reporting Instructions:** Report only one code (4035F) for immunization recommended **or** immunization ordered or administrated (4037F) For patients with appropriate exclusion criteria, report 4035F with modifier 1P or 3P	**4035F** **4037F** **Category I Codes:** **90656** **90658** **90660**	Influenza imm rec Influenza imm order/admin Flu vaccine no preserv 3 & > Flu vaccine age 3 & over, im Flu vaccine, nasal
Influenza Immunization Administered[1]—Whether or not influenza immunization was received during a current flu season **Numerator:** All patients who are administered an influenza immunization during the visit or who have already received an influenza immunization during the current flu season **Denominator:** All patients with the diagnosis of COPD **Denominator Inclusion:** Documentation of visit during flu season **Denominator Exclusion:** Documentation that patient is planning to receive influenza immunization during current flu season; documentation of medical reason(s) for not administering the influenza immunization; documentation of patient reason(s) for not administering the influenza immunization; documentation of system reason(s) for not administering the influenza immunization **Percentage** of patients who received influenza immunization during the current flu season **Reporting Instructions:** Use 4037F with appropriate exclusion criteria (medical, patient, or system use 4037F with modifier 1P, 2P, or 3P) If patient planning to receive immunization use 1P modifier with order code (4037F) Report only one code	**4037F** **Category I Codes:** **90656** **90658** **90660**	influenza imm order/admin Flu vaccine no preserv 3 & > Flu vaccine age 3 & over, im Flu vaccine, nasal
Assessment of Pneumococcus Immunization Status[1]—Whether or not pneumococcus immunization status was assessed **Numerator:** All patients who were assessed for pneumococcus immunization status **Denominator:** All patients with the diagnosis of COPD (continued)	**1022F**	Pneunmo imm status assess

[1]Physician Consortium for Performance Improvement: www.physicianconsortium.org
[2]National Committee on Quality Assurance (NCQA): Health Employer Data Information Set (HEDIS®): www.ncqa.org
[3]Joint Commission on Accreditation of Healthcare Organizations (JCAHO), ORYX Initiative Performance Measures: www.jcaho.org/pms
[4]National Diabetes Quality Improvement Alliance (NDQIA): www.nationaldiabetesalliance.org

Brief Description of Performance Measure & Source and Reporting Instructions	CPT Code(s)	Short Code Descriptor
Chronic Obstructive Pulmonary Disease (COPD), cont'd		
Denominator Exclusion: Documentation of medical reason(s) for not recommending pneumococcus immunization Documentation of patient reason(s) for not recommending pneumococcus immunization Documentation of system reason(s) for not recommending pneumococcus immunization **Percentage** of patients with COPD that were assessed for pneumococcus immunization status **Reporting Instructions:** For patients with appropriate exclusion criteria documented for not assessing pneumococcus immunization status, report 1022F with modifier 1P, 2P, or 3P		
Pneumococcus Immunization Administered[1]—Whether or not the patient was administered a pneumococcus immunization during a visit or had already received a pneumococcus immunization **Numerator:** All patients who are administered a pneumococcus immunization during a visit or who have already received a pneumococcus immunization status **Denominator:** All patients with the diagnosis of COPD **Denominator Exclusions:** Pneumococcus immunization recommended but not administered; documentation of medical reason(s) for not administering the pneumococcus immunization; documentation of patient reason(s) for not administering the pneumococcus immunization; documentation of system reason(s) for not administering the pneumococcus immunization **Percentage** of patients who were administered a pneumococcus immunization during a visit or who had already received a pneumcoccus immunization **Reporting Instructions:** Report only one code for ordered or administered For patients with appropriate exclusion criteria, report 4040F with modifier 1P, 2P, or 3P If patient planning to receive immunization use 1P modifier with order code (4040F). Report only one code	**4040F** **Category I Codes:** **90669** **90732**	Pneumoc imm order/admin Pneumococcal vacc, ped <5 Pneumococcal vaccine
Pulmonary Rehabilitation: Exercise Training Recommended[1]—Whether or not patient exercise training was recommended **Numerator:** All patients for whom exercise training was recommended **Denominator:** All patients with the diagnosis of COPD and dyspnea **Denominator Inclusion:** Documentation of dyspnea (1019F) **Denominator Exclusion:** Documentation of medical reason(s) for not recommending exercise training Documentation of system reason(s) for not recommending exercise training **Percentage** of patients for whom exercise training was recommended **Reporting Instructions:** Report 1018F or 1019F for all COPD patients For patients with appropriate exclusion criteria, report 4033F with modifier 1P or 3P. Report 4033F with 1019F	**4033F** **Denominator Codes:** **1018F** **1019F**	Pulmonary rehab rec Assess dyspnea not present Assess dyspnea present
Community-Acquired Bacterial Pneumonia (CAP)		
Chest Radiograph[1]—Whether or not patient had a chest x-ray performed **Numerator:** All patients with a chest x-ray performed **Denominator:** All patients with the diagnosis of community-acquired bacterial pneumonia **Denominator Exclusion:** Documentation of medical reason(s) for not performing a chest x-ray; documentation of patient reason(s) for not performing a chest x-ray (eg, economic, social, religious, other patient reasons); documentation of system reason(s) for not performing a chest x-ray (eg, chest x-ray equipment not accessible) (continued)	**3006F**	Cxr doc rev

[1]Physician Consortium for Performance Improvement: www.physicianconsortium.org
[2]National Committee on Quality Assurance (NCQA): Health Employer Data Information Set (HEDIS®): www.ncqa.org
[3]Joint Commission on Accreditation of Healthcare Organizations (JCAHO), ORYX Initiative Performance Measures: www.jcaho.org/pms
[4]National Diabetes Quality Improvement Alliance (NDQIA): www.nationaldiabetesalliance.org

Brief Description of Performance Measure & Source and Reporting Instructions	CPT Code(s)	Short Code Descriptor
Community-Acquired Bacterial Pneumonia (CAP), cont'd		
Percentage of community-acquired bacterial pneumonia patients ≥ 18 years of age with a chest x-ray performed **Reporting Instructions:** For patients with appropriate exclusion criteria, report 3006F with modifier 1P, 2P, or 3P		
Composite Code: Community-Acquired Bacterial Pneumonia Assessment— See individual measures listed below for (includes all of the following components): Co-morbid conditions assessed (1026F) Vital signs recorded (2010F) Mental status assessed (2014F) Hydration status assessed (2018F)	**0012F**	Cap bacterial assess
Assessment of Comorbid Conditions[1]—Whether or not patient was assessed for comorbid conditions **Numerator:** All patients assessed for history of comorbid conditions **Denominator:** All patients with the diagnosis of community-acquired bacterial pneumonia **Percentage** of patients ≥ 18 years of age with community-acquired bacterial pneumonia who were assessed for comorbid conditions	**1026F**	Co-morbid condition assess
Vital Signs[1]—Whether or not patient had vital signs recorded **Numerator:** All patients with vital signs recorded **Denominator:** All patients with the diagnosis of community-acquired bacterial pneumonia **Percentage** of community-acquired bacterial pneumonia patients ≥ 18 years of age with vital signs recorded	**2010F**	Vital signs recorded
Assessment of Oxygen Saturation[1]—Whether or not patient had oxygen saturation assessed **Numerator:** All patients with oxygen saturation assessed **Denominator:** All patients with the diagnosis of community-acquired bacterial pneumonia **Exclusion Criteria:** Documentation of medical reason(s) for not assessing oxygen saturation; documentation of patient reason(s) for not assessing oxygen saturation (eg, economic, social, religious, other patient reasons); documentation of system reason(s) for not assessing oxygen saturation (eg, oxygen saturation equipment not available) **Percentage** of patients ≥ 18 years of age with community-acquired bacterial pneumonia with oxygen saturation assessed **Reporting Instructions:** For patients with appropriate exclusion criteria, report 3028F with modifier 1P, 2P, or 3P	**3028F**	O_2 saturation doc rev
Assessment of Mental Status[1]—Whether or not patient had mental status assessed **Numerator:** All patients with mental status assessed **Denominator:** All patients with the diagnosis of community-acquired bacterial pneumonia **Percentage** of community-acquired bacterial pneumonia patients age ≥ 18 years of age with mental status assessed	**2014F**	Mental status assess
Assessment of Hydration Status[1]—Whether or not the patient had hydration status assessed **Numerator:** All patients with hydration status assessed **Denominator:** All patients with the diagnosis of community-acquired bacterial pneumonia **Percentage** of community-acquired bacterial pneumonia patients age ≥ 18 years of age with hydration status assessed	**2018F**	Hydration status assessed

[1]Physician Consortium for Performance Improvement: www.physicianconsortium.org
[2]National Committee on Quality Assurance (NCQA): Health Employer Data Information Set (HEDIS®): www.ncqa.org
[3]Joint Commission on Accreditation of Healthcare Organizations (JCAHO), ORYX Initiative Performance Measures: www.jcaho.org/pms
[4]National Diabetes Quality Improvement Alliance (NDQIA): www.nationaldiabetesalliance.org

Brief Description of Performance Measure & Source and Reporting Instructions	CPT Code(s)	Short Code Descriptor
Community-Acquired Bacterial Pneumonia (CAP), cont'd		
Level of Care Rationale[1]—Whether or not an assessment was made to determine the level of care **Numerator:** All patients with documented rationale for level of care **Denominator:** All patients with the diagnosis of community-acquired bacterial pneumonia **Percentage** of community-acquired bacterial pneumonia patients ≥ 18 years of age who had a documented rationale for level of care based on severity of illness and safety of home care	6005F	Care level rationale doc
Empiric Antibiotic[1]—Whether or not patient was prescribed an appropriate empiric antibiotic **Numerator:** All patients with an appropriate empiric antibiotic prescribed **Denominator:** All patients with the diagnosis of community-acquired bacterial pneumonia **Denominator Exclusion:** Documentation of medical reason(s) for not prescribing an antibiotic (eg, allergy, drug interaction, contraindication, other medical reasons); documentation of patient reasons(s) for not prescribing an antibiotic (eg, economic, social, religious, other patient reasons); documentation of system reasons(s) for not prescribing an antibiotic **Percentage** of community-acquired bacterial pneumonia patients ≥ 18 years of age who were prescribed an appropriate empiric antibiotic **Reporting Instructions:** For patients with appropriate exclusion criteria, report 4045F with modifier 1P, 2P, or 3P	4045F	Empiric antibiotic RX (See measure developer's Web site for definition of appropriate antibiotic)
Smoking Assessment[1]—Whether or not patient was queried about smoking **Numerator:** All patients who were queried about smoking **Denominator:** All patients with the diagnosis of community-acquired bacterial pneumonia **Percentage** of patients with community-acquired bacterial pneumonia who were queried about smoking **Reporting Instructions:** When reporting 1000F, it is required to report 1034F, and/or 1035F, or 1036F	1000F 1034F 1035F 1036F	Tobacco use assessed Current tobacco smoker Smokeless tobacco user Tobacco non-user
Smoking Cessation Intervention[1]—Whether or not patient received a smoking cessation intervention **Numerator:** All patients who received a smoking cessation intervention **Denominator:** All patients with the diagnosis with community-acquired bacterial pneumonia identified as smokers **Percentage** of patients ≥ 18 years of age with community-acquired bacterial pneumonia who received a smoking cessation intervention **Reporting Instructions:** Report 1034F for each cigarette smoker. Report either 1034F, 1035F, or 1036F for each patient. If patient is a smoker and received cessation intervention, report 4000F or 4001F, or both. Report 4000F or 4001F only if 1034F has been reported	4000F 4001F **Denominator Codes:** 1034F 1035F 1036F	Tobacco use txmnt counseling Tobacco use txmnt pharmacol Current tobacco smoker Smokeless tobacco user Tobacco non-user
Assessment of Influenza Immunization Status[1,2]—Whether or not patient was assessed for influenza immunization status **Numerator:** All patients who were assessed for influenza immunization status **Denominator:** All patients with the diagnosis of community-acquired bacterial pneumonia **Denominator Exclusion:** Documentation of medical, patient or system reason that immunization was not indicated **Percentage** of patients age ≥ 18 years of age with community-acquired bacterial pneumonia who were assessed for influenza immunization status **Reporting Instructions:** Use 1030F if documentation shows that influenza vaccine was administered. For patients with appropriate occlusion criteria, report 1030F with modifier 1P, 2P, or 3P	1030F	Influenza immunization status assessed

[1]Physician Consortium for Performance Improvement: www.physicianconsortium.org
[2]National Committee on Quality Assurance (NCQA): Health Employer Data Information Set (HEDIS®): www.ncqa.org
[3]Joint Commission on Accreditation of Healthcare Organizations (JCAHO), ORYX Initiative Performance Measures: www.jcaho.org/pms
[4]National Diabetes Quality Improvement Alliance (NDQIA): www.nationaldiabetesalliance.org

Brief Description of Performance Measure & Source and Reporting Instructions	CPT Code(s)	Short Code Descriptor
Community-Acquired Bacterial Pneumonia (CAP), cont'd		
Assessment of Pneumococcus Immunization Status[1,2]—Whether or not patient was assessed for pneumococcus immunization status **Numerator:** All patients who were assessed for pneumococcus immunization status **Denominator:** All patients with the diagnosis of community-acquired bacterial pneumonia **Denominator exclusion:** Documentation that immunization was not indicated; documentation of medical, patient, or system reason that immunization was not indicated **Percentage** of patients ≥ 18 years of age with community-acquired bacterial pneumonia who were assessed for pneumococcus immunization status **Reporting Instructions:** Use 1022F if documentation shows that pneumococcus vaccine was administered. For patient with appropriate exclusion criteria report 1022F with modifier 1P, 2P, or 3P	1022F	Pneumo imm status assess
Coronary Artery Disease (CAD)		
Smoking Cessation Evaluation[1]—Whether or not patient with CAD was queried one or more times about cigarette smoking **Numerator:** Patients who were queried one or more times about cigarette smoking **Denominator:** All patients with CAD **Percentage** of patients who were queried one or more times about cigarette smoking **Reporting Instructions:** When reporting 1000F, it is required to report 1034F, and/or 1035F, or 1036F	1000F 1034F 1035F 1036F	Tobacco use assessed Current tobacco smoker Smokeless tobacco user Tobacco non-user
Smoking Cessation Intervention[1]—Whether or not patient identified as a cigarette smoker received intervention for smoking cessation **Numerator:** Patients who were received smoking cessation intervention **Denominator:** All patients with CAD identified as cigarette smokers **Percentage** of patients identified as cigarette smokers who received intervention for smoking cessation **Reporting Instructions:** Report 1034F for each cigarette smoker. Report either 1034F, 1035F, or 1036F for each patient. If patient is a smoker and received cessation intervention, report 4000F or 4001F, or both. Report 4000F or 4001F only if 1034F has been reported	4000F 4001F **Denominator Codes:** 1034F 1035F 1036F	Tobacco use txmnt counseling Tobacco use txmnt pharmacol Current tobacco smoker Smokeless tobacco user Tobacco non-user
Symptom & Activity Assessment[1]—Whether or not patient's level of activity and anginal symptoms were evaluated during office visit **Numerator:** Patients evaluated for both level of activity and anginal symptoms during one or more office visits **Denominator:** All patients with CAD **Percentage** of patients who were evaluated for both level of activity and anginal symptoms during one or more office visits	1002F	Assess anginal symptom/level
Blood Pressure Measurement[1]—Most recent systolic and diastolic blood pressure measurement **Numerator:** Patients who had a blood pressure measurement during the last office visit **Denominator:** All patients with CAD **Percentage** of patients who had a blood pressure measurement during the last office visit	2000F	Blood pressure measured
Lipid Profile[1]—Whether or not a lipid profile was obtained **Numerator:** Patients who received at least one lipid profile (or ALL component tests) **Denominator:** All patients with CAD **Percentage** of patients who received at least one lipid profile (or ALL component tests)	3011F	Lipid panel doc rev

[1]Physician Consortium for Performance Improvement: www.physicianconsortium.org
[2]National Committee on Quality Assurance (NCQA): Health Employer Data Information Set (HEDIS®): www.ncqa.org
[3]Joint Commission on Accreditation of Healthcare Organizations (JCAHO), ORYX Initiative Performance Measures: www.jcaho.org/pms
[4]National Diabetes Quality Improvement Alliance (NDQIA): www.nationaldiabetesalliance.org

Brief Description of Performance Measure & Source and Reporting Instructions	CPT Code(s)	Short Code Descriptor
Coronary Artery Disease (CAD), cont'd		
Drug Therapy for Lowering LDL-Cholesterol[1]—Whether or not patient was prescribed lipid-lowering therapy **Numerator:** Patients who were prescribed lipid-lowering therapy **Denominator:** All patients with CAD **Denominator Exclusion(s):** Documentation of medical, patient, or system reason(s) for not prescribing lipid-lowering therapy **Percentage** of patients who were prescribed a lipid-lowering therapy (based on current ACC/AHA guidelines) **Reporting Instructions:** For patients with appropriate exclusion criteria, report code 4002F with modifier 1P, 2P, or 3P	4002F	Statin therapy RX
Beta-blocker Therapy—Prior Myocardial Infarction (MI)[1]—Whether or not CAD patient with prior MI at any time was prescribed beta-blocker therapy **Numerator:** Patients who were prescribed beta-blocker therapy **Denominator:** All patients with CAD who also have a prior MI at any time **Denominator Exclusion(s):** Documentation of medical, patient or system reason(s) for not prescribing beta-blocker therapy **Percentage** of CAD patients who also have prior MI at any time who were prescribed beta-blocker therapy **Reporting Instructions:** For patients with appropriate exclusion criteria, report code 4006F with modifier 1P, 2P, or 3P	4006F	Beta-blocker therapy RX
Angiotensin Converting Enzyme (ACE) Inhibitor or Angiotensin Receptor Blocker (ARB) Therapy[1]—Whether or not CAD patient with diabetes and/or left ventricular systolic dysfunction (LVSD) was prescribed ACE inhibitor or ARB therapy **Numerator:** Patients who were prescribed ACE inhibitor or ARB therapy **Denominator:** All CAD patients aged ≥ 18 years of age with diabetes and/or left ventricular ejection fraction (LVEF) < 40% or moderately or severely depressed left ventricular systolic function **Exclusion Criteria:** Documentation of medical reason for not prescribing ACE or ARB therapy (eg contraindication); documentation of patient reason(s) for not prescribing ACE or ARB therapy (eg economic, social or religious); documentation of system reason for not prescribing ACE or ARB therapy **Percentage** of CAD patients who also have diabetes and/or left ventricular systolic dysfunction (LVSD) who were prescribed ACE inhibitor or ARB therapy **Reporting Instructions:** Report either 3021F or 3022F or corresponding ICD-9 diagnosis code for diabetes for each CAD patient. For patient with appropriate exclusion criteria, report 4009F with modifier 1P, 2P, or 3P	4009F **Denominator Codes:** 3021F 3022F	ACE/ARB inhibitor therapy RX Lvef mod/sever deprs syst Lvef ≥40% systolic
Antiplatelet Therapy[1]—Whether or not patient was prescribed antiplatelet therapy **Numerator:** Patients who were prescribed antiplatelet therapy **Denominator:** All patients with CAD **Denominator Exclusion(s):** Documentation of medical reason(s) for not prescribing antiplatelet therapy; documentation of patient reason(s) for not prescribing antiplatelet therapy; documentation of system reason(s) for not prescribing antiplatelet therapy **Percentage** of patients who were prescribed antiplatelet therapy **Reporting Instructions:** For patients with appropriate exclusion criteria, report code 4011F with modifier 1P, 2P, or 3P	4011F	Oral antiplatelet therapy RX

[1]Physician Consortium for Performance Improvement: www.physicianconsortium.org
[2]National Committee on Quality Assurance (NCQA): Health Employer Data Information Set (HEDIS®): www.ncqa.org
[3]Joint Commission on Accreditation of Healthcare Organizations (JCAHO), ORYX Initiative Performance Measures: www.jcaho.org/pms
[4]National Diabetes Quality Improvement Alliance (NDQIA): www.nationaldiabetesalliance.org

Brief Description of Performance Measure & Source and Reporting Instructions	CPT Code(s)	Short Code Descriptor
Diabetes (DM)		
A1c Management[4]—Whether or not patient received one or more A1c test(s) **Numerator:** Patients who received one or more A1c test(s) **Denominator:** Patients with diagnosed diabetes 18-75 years of age **Percentage** of patients with diagnosed diabetes aged 18-75 years with one or more A1c test(s) **Reporting Instructions:** In order to meet this measure, the date of test when it was performed and the corresponding result are required. For this reason, report one of the two Category II codes listed and use the date of service as the date of the test, not the date of the reporting of the Category II code. The measure may also be met by reporting the Category I code, 83036 Hemoglobin; by copper sulfate method, non-automated, glycated, when performed	3046F 3047F **Category I Codes:** 83036	Hemoglobin A1C level > 9.0% Hemoglobin A1C level ≤ 9.0% Glycosylated hemoglobin test
A1c Management[4]—Whether or not patient's most recent A1c level > 9.0% (poor control) **Numerator:** Patients with most recent A1c level > 9.0% (poor control) **Denominator:** Patients diagnosed with diabetes 18-75 years of age **Percentage** of patients with most recent A1c level > 9.0% (poor control) **Reporting Instructions:** In order to meet this measure, the date of test when it was performed and the corresponding result are required. For this reason, report one of the two Category II codes listed and use the date of service as the date of the test, not the date of the reporting of the Category II code	3046F 3047F	Hemoglobin A1C level > 9.0% Hemoglobin A1C level ≤ 9.0%
Lipid Management[4]—Whether or not patient received at least one LDL-C test **Numerator:** Patients who received at least one LDL-C test **Denominator:** Patients diagnosed with diabetes 18-75 years of age **Percentage** of patients diagnosed with diabetes aged 18-75 years with at least one LDL-C test **Reporting Instructions:** In order to meet this measure, the date of test when it was performed and the corresponding result are required. For this reason, report one of the three Category II codes listed and use the date of service as the date of the test, not the date of the reporting of the Category II code. The measure may also be met by reporting the listed lipid test Category I codes, when performed	3048F 3049F 3050F **Category I Codes:** 80061 82465 83700 83701 83704 83721	LDL-C <100 MG/DL LDL-C 100-129 MG/DL LDL-C ≥ 130 MG/DL Lipid panel Assay, bld/serum cholesterol Lipopro bld, electrophoretic Lipoprotein bld, by hr fraction Lipoprotein bld, by nmr Assay of blood lipoprotein
Lipid Management[4]—Whether or not patient's most recent LDL-C < 130 mg/dL **Numerator:** Patients with most recent LDL-C < 130 mg/dL **Denominator:** Patients diagnosed with diabetes aged 18-75 years **Percentage** of patients diagnosed with diabetes aged 18-75 years with most recent LDL-C < 130 mg/dL **Reporting Instructions:** In order to meet this measure, the date of test when it was performed and the corresponding result are required. For this reason, report one of the three Category II codes listed and use the date of service as the date of the test, not the date of the reporting of the Category II code	3048F 3049F 3050F	LDL-C <100 MG/DL LDL-C 100-129 MG/DL LDL-C ≥ 130 MG/DL 130 mg/dL

[1]Physician Consortium for Performance Improvement: www.physicianconsortium.org
[2]National Committee on Quality Assurance (NCQA): Health Employer Data Information Set (HEDIS®): www.ncqa.org
[3]Joint Commission on Accreditation of Healthcare Organizations (JCAHO), ORYX Initiative Performance Measures: www.jcaho.org/pms
[4]National Diabetes Quality Improvement Alliance (NDQIA): www.nationaldiabetesalliance.org

Brief Description of Performance Measure & Source and Reporting Instructions	CPT Code(s)	Short Code Descriptor
Diabetes (DM), cont'd		
Lipid Management[4]—Whether or not patient's most recent LDL-C < 100 mg/dL **Numerator:** Patients whose most recent LDL-C is < 100 mg/dL **Denominator:** Patients diagnosed with diabetes 18-75 years of age **Percentage** of patients diagnosed with diabetes 18-75 years of age whose most recent LDL-C < 100 mg/dL **Reporting Instructions:** In order to meet this measure, the date of test when it was performed and the corresponding result are required. For this reason, report one of the three Category II codes listed and use the date of service as the date of the test, not the date of the reporting of the Category II code	3048F 3049F 3050F	LDL-C <100 MG/DL LDL-C 100-129 MG/DL LDL-C ≥ 130 MG/DL
Urine Protein Screening[4]—Whether or not a patient received at least one test for microalbumin during the measurement year **or** had evidence of medical attention for existing nephropathy **or** has documentation of microalbuminuria or albuminuria **or** is on an angiotensin converting enzyme (ACE) inhibitor or angiotensin receptor blocker (ARB) **Numerator:** Patients with at least one test for microalbumin during the measurement year; or who had evidence of medical attention for existing nephropathy or documentation of microalbuminuria or albuminuria or are on an ACE inhibitor or ARB therapy **Denominator:** Patients diagnosed with diabetes 18-75 years of age **Percentage** of patients diagnosed with diabetes 18-75 years of age with at least one test for microalbumin during the measurement year; or who had evidence of medical attention for existing nephropathy or documentation of microalbuminuria or albuminuria or are on an ACE inhibitor or ARB therapy **Reporting Instructions:** Report any one of the codes listed using the following: 1. Codes 3060F, 3061F, and 3062F may be used to indicate that a patient received at least one test for microalbuminuria 2. Code 3066F may be used if there is evidence of nephropathy **or** if there was a patient visit to a nephrologist 3. Code 3062F may be used to indicate that a patient had documentation of microalbuminuria or albuminuria 4. Code 4009F may be used if patient is on an ACE inhibitor or ARB therapy 5. Any CPT Category I code and corresponding result, when performed, and reported with any of the following ICD-9-CM diagnosis or procedure codes found in specifications: ICD-9-CM codes: 39.27, 39.42, 39.43, 39.53, 39.93-39.95, 54.98, 55.4-55.6, 250.4, 403, 404, 405.01, 405.11, 405.91, 581.81, 582.9, 583.81, 584-586, 588, 753.0, 753.1, 791.0; V codes: V42.0, V45.1, V56 6. CPT Category I codes for microalbumin measurement or quantitative timed urine albumin measurement and corresponding result as follows: 82042, 82043, 82044, 83518, 84156 or (84160, 84165, 84166) with code 81050	3060F 3061F 3062F 3066F 4009F **Category I Codes:** 82042, 82043, 82044, 83518, 84156, 84160, 84165, 84166, 81050, 90920, 90921, 90924, 90925, 90935, 90937, 90945, 90947, 90989, 90993, 90999	Pos microalbuminuria rev Neg microalbuminuria rev Pos macroalbuminuria rev Nephropathy doc tx ACE/ARB inhibitor therapy RX
Eye Examination[4]—Whether or not patient received a dilated eye exam or seven standard field stereoscopic photos with interpretation by an ophthalmologist or optometrist or imaging validated to match diagnosis from these photos during the reporting year or during the prior year if the patient is at low risk* for retinopathy **Numerator:** Patients who received a dilated eye exam or seven standard field stereoscopic photos with interpretation by an ophthalmologist or optometrist or imaging validated to match diagnosis from these photos during the reporting year, or during the prior year, if patient is at low risk* for retinopathy *A patient is considered low risk if the following criterion is met: has no evidence of retinopathy on one of the accepted examinations in the prior year (continued)	2022F 2024F 2026F 3072F **Category I Codes:** 99201	Dil retina exam interp rev 7 field photo interp doc rev Eye image valid to dx rev OR Low risk for retinopathy Office/outpatient visit, new

[1]Physician Consortium for Performance Improvement: www.physicianconsortium.org

[2]National Committee on Quality Assurance (NCQA): Health Employer Data Information Set (HEDIS®): www.ncqa.org

[3]Joint Commission on Accreditation of Healthcare Organizations (JCAHO), ORYX Initiative Performance Measures: www.jcaho.org/pms

[4]National Diabetes Quality Improvement Alliance (NDQIA): www.nationaldiabetesalliance.org

Brief Description of Performance Measure & Source and Reporting Instructions	CPT Code(s)	Short Code Descriptor
Diabetes (DM), cont'd		
Denominator: Patients with diagnosed diabetes 18-75 years of age; Low risk patient (defined as a patient who had no evidence of retinopathy in the prior year) must have had an evaluation in the prior year **Percentage** of patients who received a dilated eye exam or seven standard field stereoscopic photos with interpretation by an ophthalmologist or optometrist or imaging validated to match diagnosis from these photos during the reporting year **Reporting Instructions:** Only one of these codes should be reported	99212 99241 92002 92004 92012 92014 92225 92226	Office/outpatient visit Office consultation Eye exam, new patient Eye exam, new patient Eye exam, established pat Eye exam & treatment Special eye exam, initial Special eye exam, subsequent
Foot Examination[4]—Whether or not patient received at least one foot exam, defined in any manner **Numerator:** Patients who received at least one foot exam, defined in any manner **Denominator:** Patients diagnosed with diabetes 18-75 years of age **Denominator Exclusions:** Patients with bilateral foot/leg amputation **Percentage** of patients diagnosed with diabetes 18-75 years of age receiving at least one foot exam, defined in any manner **Reporting Instructions:** Report 2028F with modifier 1P for patients with bilateral foot/leg amputation	2028F	Foot exam performed
Blood Pressure Management[4]—Whether or not patient's most recent blood pressure is < 140/80 mm Hg **Numerator:** Patients in whose most recent blood pressure < 140/80 mm Hg **Denominator:** Patients diagnosed with diabetes 18-75 years of age **Percentage** of patients diagnosed with diabetes 18-75 years of age with most recent blood pressure < 140/80 mm Hg **Reporting Instructions:** Two codes must be reported here. For the systolic blood pressure value, report one of the two systolic codes; for the diastolic blood pressure value, report one of the three diastolic codes	**Systolic Codes:** **3076F** **3077F** **Diastolic Codes:** **3078F** **3079F** **3080F**	Syst BP < 140 MM HG Syst BP ≥ 140 MM HG6 it Diast BP < 80 MM HG Diast BP 80-89 MM HG Diast BP ≥ 90 MM HG
Smoking Cessation[4]—Whether or not patient's smoking status was ascertained and documented **Numerator:** Patients whose smoking status was ascertained and documented **Denominator:** Patients diagnosed with diabetes 18-75 years of age **Percentage** of patients diagnosed with diabetes 18-75 years of age whose smoking status was ascertained and documented **Reporting Instructions:** Report 1034F for each cigarette smoker. Report either 1034F, 1035F, or 1036F for each patient. If patient is a smoker and received cessation intervention, report 4000F or 4001F, or both. Report 4000F or 4001F only if 1034F has been reported	**4000F** **4001F** **Denominator Codes:** **1034F** **1035F** **1036F**	Tobacco use txmnt counseling Tobacco use txmnt pharmacol Current tobacco smoker Smokeless tobacco user Tobacco non-user
Heart Failure (HF)		
Composite Code: Heart Failure Assessment[1]—See individual measures listed below for the following: Level of activity assessed (1003F) Clinical symptoms of volume overload (excess) assessed (1004F) Blood pressure measured (2000F) Weight recorded (2001F) Clinical signs of volume overload (excess) assessed (2002F)	0001F	Heart failure composite

[1]Physician Consortium for Performance Improvement: www.physicianconsortium.org
[2]National Committee on Quality Assurance (NCQA): Health Employer Data Information Set (HEDIS®): www.ncqa.org
[3]Joint Commission on Accreditation of Healthcare Organizations (JCAHO), ORYX Initiative Performance Measures: www.jcaho.org/pms
[4]National Diabetes Quality Improvement Alliance (NDQIA): www.nationaldiabetesalliance.org

Brief Description of Performance Measure & Source and Reporting Instructions	CPT Code(s)	Short Code Descriptor
Heart Failure (HF), cont'd		
Assessment of Activity Level[1]—Number of visits with assessment of activity level per number of visits **Numerator:** Patient visits with assessment of current level of activity OR documentation of standardized scale OR completion of assessment tool (May include use of New York Heart Association Functional Classification of Congestive Heart Failure; Kansas City Cardiomyopathy Questionnaire; Minnesota™ Living with Heart Failure Questionnaire; or Guyatt's Chronic Heart Failure Questionnaire) **Denominator:** All patient visits for patients aged ≥ 18 years with heart failure **Percentage** of patient visits with assessment of activity level	1003F	Level of activity assessed
Assessment of Clinical Symptoms of Volume Overload (Excess)[1]—Number of patient visits with assessment of clinical symptoms of volume overload (excess) per number of visits **Numerator:** Patient visits with assessment of clinical *symptoms* of volume overload (excess) Assessment for absence or presence of symptoms of volume overload must include dyspnea, orthopnea, or documentation of standardized scale or completion of assessment tool (may include New York Heart Association Functional Classification of Congestive Heart Failure; Kansas City Cardiomyopathy Questionnaire; Minnesota™ Living with Heart Failure Questionnaire; or Guyatt's Chronic Heart Failure Questionnaire) **Denominator:** All patient visits for patients aged ≥ 18 years with heart failure **Percentage** of patient visits with assessment of clinical symptoms of volume overload (excess)	1004F	Clin symp vol ovrld assessed
Blood Pressure Measurement[1]—Number of visits with blood pressure measurement recorded per number of visits **Numerator:** Patient visits with blood pressure measurement recorded **Denominator:** All patient visits for patients aged ≥ 18 years with HF **Percentage** of patient visits with a blood pressure measurement recorded	2000F	Blood pressure measure
Weight Measurement[1]—Number of visits with weight measurement recorded per number of visits **Numerator:** Patient visits with weight measurement recorded **Denominator:** All patient visits for patients aged ≥ 18 years with heart failure **Percentage** of patient visits with weight measurement recorded	2001F	Weight record
Assessment of Clinical Signs of Volume Overload (Excess)[1]—Number of visits with assessment of clinical *signs* of volume overload (excess) per number of visits **Numerator:** Patient visits with assessment of clinical *signs* of volume overload (excess) Assessment for presence or absence of signs of volume overload must include: peripheral edema OR; Rales OR; Hepatomegaly OR; Ascites OR; Assessment of jugular venous pressure OR; S3 or S4 gallop **Denominator:** All patient visits for patients aged ≥ 18 years with heart failure **Percentage** of patient visits with assessment of clinical signs of volume overload (excess)	2002F	Clin sign vol ovrld assess
Left Ventricular Function (LVF) Assessment[1]—Whether or not patient has quantitative or qualitative results of LVF assessment recorded **Numerator:** Patients with quantitative or qualitative results of LVF assessment recorded **Denominator:** All patients aged ≥ 18 years with heart failure **Percentage** of patients with quantitative or qualitative results of LVF assessment recorded	3020F	Lvf assess
Patient Education[1]—Whether or not patient education was provided **Numerator:** Patients provided with patient education at at one or more visit(s) Patient education should include one or more of the following: weight monitoring; diet (sodium restriction); symptom management; physical activity; smoking cessation; <div align="right">(continued)</div>	4003F	Pt ed write/oral, pts w/hf

[1]Physician Consortium for Performance Improvement: www.physicianconsortium.org
[2]National Committee on Quality Assurance (NCQA): Health Employer Data Information Set (HEDIS®): www.ncqa.org
[3]Joint Commission on Accreditation of Healthcare Organizations (JCAHO), ORYX Initiative Performance Measures: www.jcaho.org/pms
[4]National Diabetes Quality Improvement Alliance (NDQIA): www.nationaldiabetesalliance.org

Brief Description of Performance Measure & Source and Reporting Instructions	CPT Code(s)	Short Code Descriptor
Heart Failure (HF), cont'd		
medication instruction; minimizing or avoiding use of NSAIDs; referral for visiting nurse; referral for specific educational or management programs; or prognosis/end-of-life issues **Denominator:** All patients aged ≥ 18 years with heart failure and with one or more visit(s) **Denominator Inclusion(s):** Patients with one or more visit(s) **Percentage** of heart failure patients who were provided with patient education on disease management and health behavior changes during one or more visit(s)		
Beta-Blocker Therapy[1]—Whether or not HF patient with LVSD was prescribed beta-blocker therapy **Numerator:** Patients who were prescribed beta-blocker therapy **Denominator:** All heart failure patients ≥ 18 years of age with left ventricular ejection fraction (LVEF) <40% or with moderately or severely depressed left ventricular systolic function **Denominator Inclusion(s):** Patients with heart failure and left ventricular systolic dysfunction (LVSD) (LVEF <40% or with moderately or severely depressed left ventricular systolic function) **Denominator Exclusion(s):** Documentation of medical reason(s) for not prescribing beta-blocker therapy (eg, contraindication); documentation of patient reason(s) for not prescribing beta-blocker therapy (eg, economic, social and/or religious); documentation of system reason(s) for not prescribing beta-blocker therapy **Percentage** of heart failure patients with LVSD who were prescribed beta-blocker therapy **Reporting Instructions:** Report either 3021F or 3022F for each heart failure patient. For patient with appropriate exclusion criteria, report 4006F with modifier 1P, 2P, or 3P	**4006F** **Denominator Codes:** **3021F** **3022F**	Beta-blocker therapy RX LVEF mod/sever deprs syst LVEF ≥40% systolic
Angiotensin Converting Enzyme (ACE) Inhibitor or Angiotensin Receptor Blocker (ARB) Therapy for Left Ventricular Systolic Dysfunction (LVSD)[1]—Whether or not heart failure patients who also have LVSD were prescribed ACE inhibitor or ARB therapy **Numerator:** Patients who were prescribed ACE inhibitor or ARB therapy **Denominator Inclusion:** All heart failure patients aged ≥ 18 years with left ventricular ejection fraction (LVEF <40% or with moderately or severely depressed left ventricular systolic function) **Denominator Exclusion(s):** Documentation of medical reason(s) for not prescribing ACE inhibitor or ARB therapy; documentation of patient reasons for not prescribing ACE inhibitor or ARB therapy (economic, social or religious); documentation of system reasons for not prescribing ACE inhibitor or ARB therapy **Percentage** of heart failure patients who also have LVSD and who were prescribed ACE or ARB inhibitor **Reporting Instructions:** Report either 3021F or 3022F for each heart failure patient. For patients with appropriate exclusion criteria, report 4009F with modifier 1P, 2P, or 3P	**4009F** **Denominator Codes:** **3021F** **3022F**	ACE/ARB inhibitor therapy RX LVEF mod/sever deprs syst LVEF ≥40% systolic
Warfarin Therapy for Patients With Atrial Fibrillation[1]—Whether or not heart failure patient who also has paroxysmal or chronic atrial fibrillation was prescribed warfarin therapy **Numerator:** Patients who were prescribed warfarin therapy **Denominator:** All heart failure patients aged ≥ 18 years with paroxysmal or chronic atrial fibrillation **Denominator Inclusion:** Patients with heart failure and paroxysmal or chronic atrial fibrillation (continued)	**4012F**	Warfarin therapy RX

[1]Physician Consortium for Performance Improvement: www.physicianconsortium.org
[2]National Committee on Quality Assurance (NCQA): Health Employer Data Information Set (HEDIS®): www.ncqa.org
[3]Joint Commission on Accreditation of Healthcare Organizations (JCAHO), ORYX Initiative Performance Measures: www.jcaho.org/pms
[4]National Diabetes Quality Improvement Alliance (NDQIA): www.nationaldiabetesalliance.org

Brief Description of Performance Measure & Source and Reporting Instructions	CPT Code(s)	Short Code Descriptor
Heart Failure (HF), cont'd		
Denominator Exclusion(s): Documentation of medical reasons(s) for not prescribing warfarin therapy (eg, allergy to warfarin, risk of bleeding or bleeding disorder, compliance, etc); documentation of patient reason(s) (eg, economic, social, and/or religious) for not prescribing warfarin therapy, document of system reason **Percentage** of heart failure patients who also have paroxysmal or chronic atrial fibrillation who were prescribed warfarin therapy **Reporting Instructions:** For patients with appropriate exclusion criteria, report 4012F with modifier 1P, 2P, or 3P		
Heart Failure Discharge Instructions[3] **Numerator:** Heart failure patients in the denominator with documentation that they or their caregivers were given written discharge instructions or other educational material addressing all of the following: activity level, diet, discharge medications, follow-up appointment, weight monitoring, what to do if symptoms worsen **Denominator:** Heart failure patients discharged home **Exclusion(s):** Patients less than 18 years of age **Percentage** of hospitalized heart failure patients in the denominator who received written discharge instructions	4014F	Written discharge instr prvd
Hypertension (HTN)		
Blood Pressure Measurement[1]—Number of visits with blood pressure measurement recorded per number of visits **Numerator:** Patient visits with blood pressure measurement recorded **Denominator:** All patient visits for patients aged ≥ 18 years with hypertension **Percentage** of patient visits with blood pressure recorded for patients aged ≥ 18 years	2000F	Blood pressure measure
Plan of Care[1]—Number of visits with documented plan of care for hypertension per number of visits during which either systolic blood pressure ≥140 mm Hg or diastolic blood pressure ≥ 90 mm Hg **Numerator:** Patient visits with documented plan of care for hypertension Plan of care should include one or more of the following: Recheck blood pressure at specified future date, initiate or alter pharmacologic therapy, initiate or alter non-pharmacologic therapy **Denominator:** All patient visits during which patients ≥18 years of age diagnosed with hypertension have either systolic blood pressure ≥140 mm Hg or diastolic blood pressure ≥ 90 mm Hg **Percentage** of patient visits during which either systolic blood pressure ≥ 140 mm Hg or diastolic blood pressure ≥ 90 mm Hg, with documented plan of care for hypertension **Reporting Instructions:** For this measure to be met, three codes must be reported: one code for systolic blood pressure, one code for diastolic blood pressure, and the code for hypertension plan of care (4050F). If no documentation of plan of care, or patient does not have elevated blood pressure at the visit, report only two codes for corresponding systolic and diastolic blood pressure values	4050F **Denominator Codes:** **Systolic Codes:** 3076F 3077F **Diastolic Codes:** 3078F 3079F 3080F	Ht care plan doc Syst BP ≥ 140 MM HG Syst BP ≥ 140 MM HG Diast BP < 80 MM HG Diast BP 80-89 MM HG Diast BP ≥ 90 MM HG
Osteoarthritis (Adult) (OA)		
Composite Code: Osteoarthritis Assessment—See individual measures listed below for: Osteoarthritis symptoms and functional status assessed (1006F) Use of anti-inflammatory or over-the-counter (OTC) analgesic medications assessed (1007F) Initial examination of the involved joint(s) (includes visual inspection, palpation, range of motion) (2004F)	0005F	Osteoarthritis composite

[1]Physician Consortium for Performance Improvement: www.physicianconsortium.org
[2]National Committee on Quality Assurance (NCQA): Health Employer Data Information Set (HEDIS®): www.ncqa.org
[3]Joint Commission on Accreditation of Healthcare Organizations (JCAHO), ORYX Initiative Performance Measures: www.jcaho.org/pms
[4]National Diabetes Quality Improvement Alliance (NDQIA): www.nationaldiabetesalliance.org

Brief Description of Performance Measure & Source and Reporting Instructions	CPT Code(s)	Short Code Descriptor
Osteoarthritis (Adult) (OA), cont'd		
Symptom and Functional Assessment[1]—Patient visits with assessment for function and pain per number of visits during the reporting year **Numerator:** Patient visits with assessment for level of function and pain documented during the reporting year **Denominator:** All visits for patients aged ≥ 21 years of age with osteoarthritis **Percentage** of visits for patients ≥ 21 years of age with osteoarthritis who were assessed for function and pain during the reporting year **Reporting Instructions:** Use when osteoarthritis is addressed during the patient encounter	1006F	Osteoarthritis assess
Assessment for Use of Anti-inflammatory or Analgesic OTC Medications[1]—Patient visits with assessment for use of anti-inflammatory or analgesic OTC medications per number of visits during the reporting year **Numerator:** Patient visits with assessment for use of anti-inflammatory or analgesic OTC medications documented during the reporting year **Denominator:** All visits for patients aged ≥ 21 years of age with osteoarthritis **Percentage** of visits for patients ≥ 21 years of age with osteoarthritis with assessment for use of anti-inflammantory or analgesic over-the-counter (OTC) medications during the reporting year **Reporting Instructions:** Use when osteoarthritis is addressed during the patient encounter	1007F	Use of anti-inflam/anlgsc OTC assess
Non-steroidal Anti-inflammatory Drug (NSAID) Risk Assessment[1]—Whether or not patient on prescribed or OTC NSAIDs was assessed for GI/renal risk factors during the reporting year **Numerator:** Patients who were assessed for *all* of the following GI and Renal risk factors during the reporting year: • GI bleed • History of peptic ulcer disease (PUD) • Concomitant use of glucocorticoids or anticoagulants • Smoking • Significant alcohol use • Age > 65 years • Renal disease (Cr > 2.0 mg/dl) • Hypertension • Heart failure • Concomitant use of diuretic or angiotensin-converting enzyme (ACE) inhibitor **Denominator:** All patients ≥ 21 years of age with osteoarthritis on a prescribed or OTC NSAID **Percentage** of patients ≥ 21 years of age with osteoarthritis on prescribed or OTC NSAIDs who were assessed for gastrointestinal and renal risk factors during the reporting year	1008F	GI/renal risk assess
Physical Examination of the Involved Joint[1]—Whether or not a physical examination of the involved joint was performed during the initial visit during the reporting year **Numerator:** Patients for whom a physical examination of the involved joint was performed during the initial visit during the reporting year **Denominator:** All patients ≥ 21 years of age with osteoarthritis **Percentage** of patients ≥ 21 years of age with osteoarthritis for whom a physical examination of the involved joint was performed during the initial visit during the reporting year **Reporting Instructions:** Use only for initial osteoarthritis visit or for visits for new joint involvement	2004F	Initial exam involved joints

[1]Physician Consortium for Performance Improvement: www.physicianconsortium.org
[2]National Committee on Quality Assurance (NCQA): Health Employer Data Information Set (HEDIS®): www.ncqa.org
[3]Joint Commission on Accreditation of Healthcare Organizations (JCAHO), ORYX Initiative Performance Measures: www.jcaho.org/pms
[4]National Diabetes Quality Improvement Alliance (NDQIA): www.nationaldiabetesalliance.org

Brief Description of Performance Measure & Source and Reporting Instructions	CPT Code(s)	Short Code Descriptor
Osteoarthritis (Adult) (OA), cont'd		
Anti-inflammatory/Analgesic Therapy[1]—Patient visits during which an anti-inflammatory agent or analgesic was considered/Number of visits during the reporting year **Numerator:** Patient visits during which an anti-inflammatory agent or analgesic was considered during the reporting year **Denominator:** All patient visits for patients aged ≥ 21 years of age with osteoarthritis **Numerator Inclusion(s):** Documentation that an anti-inflammatory agent or analgesic was prescribed; Documentation of medical reason(s) for not prescribing an anti-inflammatory agent or analgesic (eg, allergy, drug interaction, contraindication); documentation of patient reasons(s) for not prescribing an anti-inflammatory agent or analgesic (eg, economic, social, religious) **Percentage** of visits for patients aged ≥ 21 years of age with osteoarthritis during which an anti-inflammatory agent or analgesic was considered during the reporting year **Reporting Instructions:** Report 4016F alone or with modifier (1P if medical reason for not prescribing an anti-inflammatory or analgesic was documented or 2P modifier if patient reason for not prescribing an anti-inflammatory or analgesic was documented.) For this measure, the modifiers do not act as denominator exclusions, but rather demonstate that therapy was considered and are included in the numerator when calculating the measure	**4016F**	Anti-inflm/anlgsc agent RX
Gastrointestinal Prophylaxis[1]—Patient visits during which GI prophylaxis was considered/Number of visits during the reporting year **Numerator:** Patient visits during which GI prophylaxis was considered during the reporting year **Denominator:** All visits for patients aged ≥ 21 years of age with osteoarthritis on a prescribed or OTC NSAID **Numerator Inclusion(s):** Documentation that GI prophylaxis was prescribed; documentation of medical reason(s) for not prescribing GI prophylaxis (eg, allergy, drug interaction, contraindication); documentation of patient reason(s) for not prescribing GI prophylaxis (eg, economic, social, or religious) **Percentage** of visits for patients ≥ 21 years of age with osteoarthritis during which GI prophylaxis was considered during the reporting year **Reporting Instructions:** Report 4017F alone or with modifier (1P if medical reason for not prescribing GI prophylaxis was documented or 2P modifier if patient reason for not prescribing GI prophylaxis was documented). For this measure, the modifiers do not act as denominator exclusions, but rather demonstrate that therapy was considered and are included in the numerator when calculating the measure	**4017F**	GI prophylaxis for NSAID RX
Therapeutic Exercise for the Involved Joint[1]—Patient visits during which therapeutic exercise for the hip or knee was considered/Number of visits during the reporting year **Numerator:** Patient visits during which therapeutic exercise for the knee or hip was considered during the reporting year **Denominator:** All patient visits for patients ≥ 21 years of age with osteoarthritis of the hip or knee **Numerator Inclusion(s):** Documentation of medical reason(s) for not instructing therapeutic exercise or prescribing physical therapy for the hip or knee; documentation of patient reason(s) for not instructing therapeutic exercise or prescribing physical therapy for the hip or knee (eg, economic, social, religious); documentation that therapeutic exercise for the hip or knee was instructed; documentation that physical therapy for the hip or knee was prescribed (continued)	**4018F**	Therapy exercise joint RX

[1]Physician Consortium for Performance Improvement: www.physicianconsortium.org
[2]National Committee on Quality Assurance (NCQA): Health Employer Data Information Set (HEDIS®): www.ncqa.org
[3]Joint Commission on Accreditation of Healthcare Organizations (JCAHO), ORYX Initiative Performance Measures: www.jcaho.org/pms
[4]National Diabetes Quality Improvement Alliance (NDQIA): www.nationaldiabetesalliance.org

Brief Description of Performance Measure & Source and Reporting Instructions	CPT Code(s)	Short Code Descriptor
Osteoarthritis (Adult) (OA), cont'd		
Percentage of visits for patients ≥ 21 years of age with osteoarthritis of the hip or knee during which therapeutic exercise for the hip or knee (therapeutic exercise instructed or physical therapy prescribed) was considered during the reporting year **Reporting Instructions:** Report 4018F alone or or with modifier (1P if medical reason for not instructing therapeutic exercise or prescribing physical therapy was documented; 2P if patient reason for not instructing therapeutic exercise or prescribing physical therapy was documented.) For this measure, the modifiers do not act as denominator exclusions, but rather demonstate that therapy was considered and are included in the numerator when calculating the measure.		
Prenatal-Postpartum Care (Prenatal)		
Timeliness of Prenatal Care[2] **Numerator:** Number of women who received a prenatal care visit as a member of the managed care organization (MCO) in the first trimester or within 42 days of enrollment in the MCO **Denominator:** Women who had live births between November 6th of the year prior to the measurement year and November 5th of the measurement year, who were continuously enrolled at least 43 days prior to delivery through 56 days after delivery **Percentage** of patients in the denominator who received prenatal care	0500F	Initial prenatal care visit
Prenatal Flow Sheet[1]—Whether or not patient has a prenatal flow sheet in use by the date of the first physician visit **Numerator:** Number of patients with a flow sheet in use by the date of the first physician visit, which contains at a minimum: blood pressure, weight, urine protein, uterine size, fetal heart tones, and estimated date of delivery **Denominator:** Pregnant women seen for prenatal care **Exclusion(s):** Patients seen for consultation only, not for continuing care **Percentage** of patients in the denominator with a prenatal flow sheet in use by the first physician visit	0501F	Prenatal flow sheet
Frequency of Ongoing Prenatal Care[2] **Numerator:** Number of women in the denominator who had an unduplicated count of less than 21%, 21%-40%, 41%-60%, 61%-80%, or greater than or equal to 81% of the expected number of prenatal care visits, adjusted for the month of pregnancy at time of enrollment and gestational age **Denominator:** Women who had live births during the measurement year **Exclusion(s):** MCOs must exclude members for whom a prenatal visit is not indicated **Percentage** of patients in the denominator with expected number of prenatal visits	0502F	Subsequent prenatal care
Postpartum Care[2] **Numerator:** Number of women in the denominator who had a postpartum visit on or between 21 days and 56 days after delivery **Denominator:** Women who had live births between November 6th of the year prior to the measurement year and November 5th of the measurement year, who were continuously enrolled at least 43 days prior to delivery through 56 days after delivery **Percentage** of patients in the denominator who had a postpartum visit between 21 and 56 days after delivery	0503F	Postpartum care visit
Preventive Care & Screening (PV)		
Adult Influenza Immunization[1]—Whether or not patient received an influenza immunization **Numerator:** Patients who received an influenza immunization	4037F 90656	Influenza imm order/admin Flu vaccine no preserv 3 & >
(continued)		

[1]Physician Consortium for Performance Improvement: www.physicianconsortium.org

[2]National Committee on Quality Assurance (NCQA): Health Employer Data Information Set (HEDIS®): www.ncqa.org

[3]Joint Commission on Accreditation of Healthcare Organizations (JCAHO), ORYX Initiative Performance Measures: www.jcaho.org/pms

[4]National Diabetes Quality Improvement Alliance (NDQIA): www.nationaldiabetesalliance.org

Brief Description of Performance Measure & Source and Reporting Instructions	CPT Code(s)	Short Code Descriptor
Preventive Care & Screening (PV), cont'd		
Denominator: All patients greater than or equal to 50 years of age **Exclusion Criteria:** Documentation of medical reason(s) for not providing immunization; documentation of patient reason(s) for declining immunization; documentation of system reason(s) for declining immunization **Percentage** of patients who received an influenza immunization **Reporting Instructions:** For patients with appropriate exclusion criteria use 4037F with modifier 1P, 2P, or 3P. Use 4037F with modifier 1P if previously immunized for current season	**90658** **90660**	Flu vaccine age 3 & over, im Flu vaccine, nasal
Adult Colorectal Cancer Screening[1]—Whether or not patient was screened for colorectal cancer during the one-year measurement period **Numerator:** Patients with any of the recommended colorectal cancer screening test(s) performed (fecal occult blood testing annually; flexible sigmoidoscopy every five years; annual fecal occult blood testing plus flexible sigmoidoscopy every five years; double contrast barium enema every five years; colonoscopy every ten years) **Denominator:** All patients aged greater than or equal to 50 years of age **Denominator Exclusion:** Documentation of medical reason(s) for not providing colorectal cancer screening; documentation of patient reason(s) for not providing colorectal cancer screening; documentation of system reason(s) for not providing colorectal cancer screening **Percentage** of patients screened for colorectal cancer **Reporting Instructions:** For patients with appropriate exclusion criteria, report 3017F with modifier 1P, 2P, or 3P	**3017F**	Colorectal ca screen doc rev
Screening Mammography[1]—Whether or not female patient had a mammogram performed during the two-year measurement period **Numerator:** Female patients who had a mammogram performed **Denominator:** All female patients aged 50-69 years **Exclusion criteria:** Documentation of medical reason(s) for not performing screening mammography; documentation of patient reason(s) for declining screening mammography; documentation of system reason(s) for declining screening mammography **Percentage** of female patients who had a mammogram performed during the two-year measurement period **Reporting Instructions:** For patients with appropriate exclusion criteria use 3014F with modifier 1P, 2P, or 3P	**3014F**	Screen mammo doc rev
Tobacco Use[1]—Whether or not patient was queried about tobacco use one or more times **Numerator:** Patients who were queried about tobacco use one or more times **Denominator:** All patients aged ≥ 18 years at the beginning of the two-year measurement period **Percentage** of patients queried about tobacco use one or more times during the two-year measurement period **Reporting Instructions:** When reporting 1000F, it is required to report 1034F, and/or 1035F, or 1036F	**1000F** **1034F** **1035F** **1036F**	Tobacco use assessed Current tobacco smoker Smokeless tobacco user Tobacco non-user
Tobacco Use Intervention[1]—Whether or not patient identified as a tobacco user received cessation intervention **Numerator:** Patients identified as tobacco users who received cessation intervention **Denominator:** All patients ≥ 18 years at the beginning of the two-year measurement period identified as tobacco users **Percentage** of patients identified as tobacco users who received cessation intervention during the two-year measurement period **Reporting Instructions:** Report 1034F, 1035F, or 1036F for each patient. If patient is a tobacco user (1034F or 1035F) and received cessation intervention, report 4000F or 4001F or both	**4000F** **4001F** **Denominator Codes:** **1034F** **1035F** **1036F**	Tobacco use txmnt counseling Tobacco use txmnt pharmacol Current tobacco smoker Smokeless tobacco user Tobacco non-user

[1]Physician Consortium for Performance Improvement: www.physicianconsortium.org
[2]National Committee on Quality Assurance (NCQA): Health Employer Data Information Set (HEDIS®): www.ncqa.org
[3]Joint Commission on Accreditation of Healthcare Organizations (JCAHO), ORYX Initiative Performance Measures: www.jcaho.org/pms
[4]National Diabetes Quality Improvement Alliance (NDQIA): www.nationaldiabetesalliance.org

Appendix I

Genetic Testing Code Modifiers

This listing of modifiers is intended for reporting with molecular laboratory procedures related to genetic testing. Genetic testing modifiers should be used in conjunction with CPT and HCPCS codes to provide diagnostic granularity of service to enable providers to submit complete and precise genetic testing information without altering test descriptors. These two-character modifiers are categorized by mutation. The first (numeric) character indicates the disease category and the second (alpha) character denotes gene type. Introductory guidelines in the molecular diagnostic and molecular cytogenetic code sections of the CPT codebook provide further guidance in interpretation and application of genetic testing modifiers.

Neoplasia (Solid Tumor, Excluding Sarcoma and Lymphoma)

0A BRCA1 (hereditary breast/ovarian cancer)

0B BRCA2 (hereditary breast cancer)

0C Neurofibromin (neurofibromatosis, type 1)

0D Merlin (neurofibromatosis, type 2)

0E c-RET (multiple endocrine neoplasia, types 2A/B, familial medullary thyroid carcinoma)

0F VHL (Von Hippel Lindau disease, renal carcinoma)

0G SDHD (hereditary paraganglioma)

0H SDHB (hereditary paraganglioma)

0I ERRB2, commonly called Her-2/neu

0J MLH1 (HNPCC, mismatch repair genes)

0K MSH2, MSH6, or PMS2 (HNPCC, mismatch repair genes)

0L APC (hereditary polyposis coli)

0M Rb (retinoblastoma)

0N TP53, commonly called p53

0O PTEN (Cowden's syndrome)

0P KIT, also called CD117 (gastrointestinal stromal tumor)

0Z Solid tumor gene, not otherwise specified

Neoplasia (Sarcoma)

1A WT1 or WT2 (Wilm's tumor)

1B PAX3, PAX7, or FOXO1A (alveolar rhabdomyosarcoma)

1C FLI1, ERG, ETV1, or EWSR1 (Ewing's sarcoma, desmoplastic round cell)

1D DDIT3 or FUS (myxoid liposarcoma)

1E NR4A3, RBF56, or TCF12 (myxoid chondrosarcoma)

1F SSX1, SSX2, or SYT (synovial sarcoma)

1G MYCN (neuroblastoma)

1H COL1A1 or PDGFB (dermatofibrosarcoma protruberans)

1I TFE3 or ASPSCR1 (alveolar soft parts sarcoma)

1J JAZF1 or JJAZ1 (endometrial stromal sarcoma)

1Z Sarcoma gene, not otherwise specified

Neoplasia (Lymphoid/Hematopoietic)

2A RUNX1 or CBFA2T1, commonly called AML1 or ETO, genes associated with t(8;21) AML1—also ETO (acute myelogenous leukemia)

2B BCR or ABL1, genes associated with t(9;22) (chronic myelogenous or acute leukemia) BCR—also ABL (chronic myeloid, acute lymphoid leukemia)

2C PBX1 or TCF3, genes associated with t(1;19) (acute lymphoblastic leukemia) CGF1

2D CBFB or MYH11, genes associated with inv 16 (acute myelogenous leukemia) CBF beta (leukemia)

2E MLL (acute leukemia)

2F PML or RARA, genes associated with t(15;17) (acute promyelocytic leukemia) PML/RAR alpha (promyelocytic leukemia)

2G ETV6, commonly called TEL, gene associated with t(12;21) (acute leukemia) TEL (Leukemia)

2H BCL2 (B cell lymphoma, follicle center cell origin) bcl-2 (Lymphoma)

2I CCND1, commonly called BCL1, cyclin D1 (Mantle cell lymphoma, myeloma) bcl-1 (lymphoma)

2J MYC (Burkitt lymphoma) c-myc (lymphoma)

2K IgH (lymphoma/leukemia)

2L IGK (lymphoma/leukemia)

2M TRB, T cell receptor beta (lymphoma/leukemia)

2N TRG, T cell receptor gamma (lymphoma/leukemia)

2O SIL or TAL1 (T cell leukemia)

2T BCL6 (B cell lymphoma)

2Q API1 or MALT1 (MALT lymphoma)

2R NPM or ALK, genes associated with t(2;5) (anaplastic large cell lymphoma)

2S FLT3 (Acute myelogenous leukemia)

2Z Lymphoid/hematopoietic neoplasia, not otherwise specified

Non-Neoplastic Hematology/Coagulation

3A F5, commonly called Factor V (Leiden, others) (hypercoagulable state)

3B FACC (Fanconi anemia)

3C FACD (Fanconi anemia)

3D HBB, beta globin (thalassemia, sickle cell anemia, other hemoglobinopathies)

3E HBA, commonly called alpha globin (thalassemia)

3F MTHFR (elevated homocystinemia)

3G F2, commonly called prothrombin (20210, others) (hypercoagulable state) prothrombin (factor II, 20210A) (hypercoagulable state)

3H F8, commonly called factor VIII (hemophilia A/VWF)

3I F9, commonly called factor IX (hemophilia B)

3K F13, commonly called factor XIII (bleeding or hypercoagulable state) beta globin

3Z Non-neoplastic hematology/coagulation, not otherwise specified

Histocompatiblity/Blood Typing/ Identity/Microsatellite

4A HLA-A

4B HLA-B

4C HLA-C

4D HLA-D

4E HLA-DR

4F HLA-DQ

4G HLA-DP

4H Kell

4I Fingerprint for engraftment (post allogeneic progenitor cell transplant)

4J Fingerprint for donor allelotype (allogeneic transplant)

4K Fingerprint for recipient allelotype (allogeneic transplant)

4L Fingerprint for leukocyte chimerism (allogeneic solid organ transplant)

4M Fingerprint for maternal versus fetal origin

4N Microsatellite instability

4O Microsatellite loss (loss of heterozygosity)

4Z Histocompatiblity/blood typing, not otherwise specified

Neurologic, Non-Neoplastic

5A ASPA, commonly called Aspartoacylase A (Canavan disease)

5B FMR-1 (fragile X, FRAXA, syndrome)

5C FRDA, commonly called Frataxin (Freidreich ataxia)

5D HD, commonly called Huntington (Huntington's disease)

5E GABRA5, NIPA1, UBE3A, or ANCR GABRA (Prader Willi-Angelman syndrome)

5F GJB2, commonly called Connexin-26 (hereditary hearing loss) Connexin-32 (GJB2) (hereditary deafness)

5G GJB1, commonly called Connexin-32 (X-linked Charcot-Marie-Tooth disease)

5H SNRPN (Prader Willi-Angelman syndrome)

5I SCA1, commonly called Ataxin-1 (spinocerebellar ataxia, type 1)

5J SCA2, commonly called Ataxin-2 (spinocerebellar ataxia, type 2)

5K MJD, commonly called Ataxin-3 (spinocerebellar ataxia, type 3, Machado-Joseph disease)

5L CACNA1A (spinocerebellar ataxia, type 6)

5M ATXN7 Ataxin-7 (spinocerebellar ataxia, type 7)

5N PMP-22 (Charcot-Marie-Tooth disease, type 1A)

5O MECP2 (Rett syndrome)

5Z Neurologic, non-neoplastic, not otherwise specified

Muscular, Non-Neoplastic

6A DMD, commonly called dystrophin (Duchenne/Becker muscular dystrophy)

6B DMPK (myotonic dystrophy, type 1)

6C ZNF-9 (myotonic dystrophy, type 2)

6D SMN1/SMN2 (autosomal recessive spinal muscular atrophy)

6E MTTK, commonly called tRNAlys (myotonic epilepsy, MERRF)

6F MTTL1, commonly called tRNAleu (mitochondrial encephalomyopathy, MELAS)

6Z Muscular, not otherwise specified

Metabolic, Other

7A APOE, commonly called apolipoprotein E (cardiovascular disease or Alzheimer's disease)

7B NPC1 or NPC2, commonly called sphingomyelin phosphodiesterase (Nieman-Pick disease)

7C GBA, commonly called acid beta glucosidase (Gaucher disease)

7D HFE (hemochromatosis)

7E HEXA, commonly called hexosaminidase A (Tay-Sachs disease)

7F ACADM (medium chain acyl CoA dehydrogenase deficiency)

7Z Metabolic, other, not otherwise specified

Metabolic, Transport

8A CFTR (cystic fibrosis)

8B PRSS1 (hereditary pancreatitis)

8C Long QT syndrome, KCN (Jervell and Lange-Nielsen syndromes, types 1, 2, 5, and 6) and SCN (Brugada syndrome, SIDS and type 3)

8Z Metabolic, transport, not otherwise specified

Metabolic-Pharmacogenetics

9A TPMT, commonly called (thiopurine methyltransferase) (patients on antimetabolite therapy)

9B CYP2 genes, commonly called cytochrome p450 (drug metabolism)

9C ABCB1, commonly called MDR1 or p-glycoprotein (drug transport)

9D NAT2 (drug metabolism)

9L Metabolic-pharmacogenetics, not otherwise specified

Dysmorphology

9M FGFR1 (Pfeiffer and Kallman syndromes)

9N FGFR2 (Crouzon, Jackson-Weiss, Apert, Saethre-Chotzen syndromes)

9O FGFR3 (achondroplasia, hypochondroplasia, thanatophoric dysplasia, types I and II, Crouzon syndrome with acanthosis nigricans, Muencke syndromes)

9P TWIST (Saethre-Chotzen syndrome)

9Q DGCR, commonly called CATCH-22 (DiGeorge and 22q11 deletion syndromes)

9Z Dysmorphology, not otherwise specified

Appendix J

Electrodiagnostic Medicine Listing of Sensory, Motor, and Mixed Nerves

This summary assigns each sensory, motor, and mixed nerve with its appropriate nerve conduction study code in order to enhance accurate reporting of codes 95900, 95903, and 95904. Each nerve constitutes one unit of service.

Motor Nerves Assigned to Codes 95900 and 95903

I. Upper extremity, cervical plexus, and brachial plexus motor nerves
  A. Axillary motor nerve to the deltoid
  B. Long thoracic motor nerve to the serratus anterior
  C. Median nerve
    1. Median motor nerve to the abductor pollicis brevis
    2. Median motor nerve, anterior interosseous branch, to the flexor pollicis longus
    3. Median motor nerve, anterior interosseous branch, to the pronator quadratus
    4. Median motor nerve to the first lumbrical
    5. Median motor nerve to the second lumbrical
  D. Musculocutaneous motor nerve to the biceps brachii
  E. Radial nerve
    1. Radial motor nerve to the extensor carpi ulnaris
    2. Radial motor nerve to the extensor digitorum communis
    3. Radial motor nerve to the extensor indicis proprius
    4. Radial motor nerve to the brachioradialis
  F. Suprascapular nerve
    1. Suprascapular motor nerve to the supraspinatus
    2. Suprascapular motor nerve to the infraspinatus
  G. Thoracodorsal motor nerve to the latissimus dorsi
  H. Ulnar nerve
    1. Ulnar motor nerve to the abductor digiti minimi
    2. Ulnar motor nerve to the palmar interosseous
    3. Ulnar motor nerve to the first dorsal interosseous
    4. Ulnar motor nerve to the flexor carpi ulnaris
  I. Other
II. Lower extremity motor nerves
  A. Femoral motor nerve to the quadriceps
    1. Femoral motor nerve to vastus medialis
    2. Femoral motor nerve to vastus lateralis
    3. Femoral motor nerve to vastus intermedialis
    4. Femoral motor nerve to rectus femoris
  B. Ilioinguinal motor nerve
  C. Peroneal (fibular) nerve
    1. Peroneal motor nerve to the extensor digitorum brevis
    2. Peroneal motor nerve to the peroneus brevis
    3. Peroneal motor nerve to the peroneus longus
    4. Peroneal motor nerve to the tibialis anterior
  D. Plantar motor nerve
  E. Sciatic nerve
  F. Tibial nerve
    1. Tibial motor nerve, inferior calcaneal branch, to the abductor digiti minimi
    2. Tibial motor nerve, medial plantar branch, to the abductor hallucis
    3. Tibial motor nerve, lateral plantar branch, to the flexor digiti minimi brevis
  G. Other

III. Cranial nerves and trunk
    A. Cranial nerve VII (facial motor nerve)
        1. Facial nerve to the frontalis
        2. Facial nerve to the nasalis
        3. Facial nerve to the orbicularis oculi
        4. Facial nerve to the orbicularis oris
    B. Cranial nerve XI (spinal accessory motor nerve)
    C. Cranial nerve XII (hypoglossal motor nerve)
    D. Intercostal motor nerve
    E. Phrenic motor nerve to the diaphragm
    F. Recurrent laryngeal nerve
    G. Other
IV. Nerve Roots
    A. Cervical nerve root stimulation
        1. Cervical level 5 (CT)
        2. Cervical level 6 (C6)
        3. Cervical level 7 (C7)
        4. Cervical level 8 (C8)
    B. Thoracic nerve root stimulation
        1. Thoracic level 1 (T1)
        2. Thoracic level 2 (T2)
        3. Thoracic level 3 (T3)
        4. Thoracic level 4 (T4)
        5. Thoracic level 5 (T5)
        6. Thoracic level 6 (T6)
        7. Thoracic level 7 (T7)
        8. Thoracic level 8 (T8)
        9. Thoracic level 9 (T9)
      10. Thoracic level 10 (T10)
      11. Thoracic level 11 (T11)
      12. Thoracic level 12 (T12)
    C. Lumbar nerve root stimulation
        1. Lumbar level 1 (L1)
        2. Lumbar level 2 (L2)
        3. Lumbar level 3 (L3)
        4. Lumbar level 4 (L4)
        5. Lumbar level 5 (L5)
    D. Sacral nerve root stimulation
        1. Sacral level 1 (S1)
        2. Sacral level 2 (S2)
        3. Sacral level 3 (S3)
        4. Sacral level 4 (S4)

Sensory and Mixed Nerves Assigned to Code 95904

  I Upper extremity sensory and mixed nerves
    A. Lateral antebrachial cutaneous sensory nerve
    B. Medial antebrachial cutaneous sensory nerve
    C. Medial brachial cutaneous sensory nerve
    D. Median nerve
        1. Median sensory nerve to the first digit
        2. Median sensory nerve to the second digit
        3. Median sensory nerve to the third digit
        4. Median sensory nerve to the fourth digit
        5. Median palmar cutaneous sensory nerve
        6. Median palmar mixed nerve
    E. Posterior antebrachial cutaneous sensory nerve

    F. Radial sensory nerve
       1. Radial sensory nerve to the base of the thumb
       2. Radial sensory nerve to digit 1
    G. Ulnar nerve
       1. Ulnar dorsal cutaneous sensory nerve
       2. Ulnar sensory nerve to the fourth digit
       3. Ulnar sensory nerve to the fifth digit
       4. Ulnar palmar mixed nerve
    H. Intercostal sensory nerve
    I. Other

II. Lower extremity sensory and mixed nerves
    A. Lateral femoral cutaneous sensory nerve
    B. Medial calcaneal sensory nerve
    C. Medial femoral cutaneous sensory nerve
    D. Peroneal nerve
       1. Deep peroneal sensory nerve
       2. Superficial peroneal sensory nerve, medial dorsal cutaneous branch
       3. Superficial peroneal sensory nerve, intermediate dorsal cutaneous branch
    E. Posterior femoral cutaneous sensory nerve
    F. Saphenous nerve
       1. Saphenous sensory nerve (distal technique)
       2. Saphenous sensory nerve (proximal technique)
    G. Sural nerve
       1. Sural sensory nerve, lateral dorsal cutaneous branch
       2. Sural sensory nerve
    H. Tibial sensory nerve (digital nerve to toe 1)
    I. Tibial sensory nerve (medial plantar nerve)
    J. Tibial sensory nerve (lateral plantar nerve)
    K. Other

III. Head and trunk sensory nerves
    A. Dorsal nerve of the penis
    B. Greater auricular nerve
    C. Ophthalmic branch of the trigeminal nerve
    D. Pudendal sensory nerve
    E. Suprascapular sensory nerves
    F. Other

The following table provides a reasonable maximum number of studies performed per diagnostic category necessary for a physician to arrive at a diagnosis in 90% of patients with that final diagnosis. The numbers in each column represent the number of studies recommended. The appropriate number of studies to be performed is based upon the physician's discretion.

Indication	Type of Study/Maximum Number of Studies				
		Nerve Conduction Studies (95900, 95903, 95904)		Other EMG Studies (95934, 95936, 95937)	
	Needle EMG (95860-95864 95867-95870)	Motor NCS With and/or Without F wave	Sensory NCS	H-Reflex	Neuromuscular Junction Testing (Repetitive Stimulation)
Carpal Tunnel (Unilateral)	1	3	4	—	—
Carpal Tunnel (Bilateral)	2	4	6	—	—
Radiculopathy	2	3	2	2	—
Mononeuropathy	1	3	3	2	—
Polyneuropathy/ Mononeuropathy Multiplex	3	4	4	2	—
Myopathy	2	2	2	—	2
Motor Neuronopathy (eg, ALS)	4	4	2	—	2
Plexopathy	2	4	6	2	—
Neuromuscular Junction	2	2	2	—	3
Tarsal Tunnel Syndrome (Unilateral)	1	4	4	—	—
Tarsal Tunnel Syndrome (Bilateral)	2	5	6	—	—
Weakness, Fatigue, Cramps, or Twitching (Focal)	2	3	4	—	2
Weakness, Fatigue, Cramps, or Twitching (General)	4	4	4	—	2
Pain, Numbness, or Tingling (Unilateral)	1	3	4	2	—
Pain, Numbness, or Tingling (Bilateral)	2	4	6	2	—

Notes

⊙=Moderate sedation ✚=Add-on code ✗=FDA approval pending

Appendix K

Product Pending FDA Approval

Some vaccine products have been assigned a CPT Category I code in anticipation of future approval from the Food and Drug Administration (FDA). Following is the vaccine product code pending FDA approval status that is identified in the CPT codebook with the (✒) symbol. Upon revision of the approval status by the FDA, notation of this revision will be provided via the AMA CPT "Category I Vaccine Codes" Internet listing (www.ama-assn.org/ama/pub/category/10902.html) and in subsequent publications of the CPT codebook.

90698

Appendix L

Vascular Families

Assignment of branches to first, second, and third order in this table makes the assumption that the starting point is catheterization of the aorta. This categorization would not be accurate, for instance, if a femoral or carotid artery were catheterized directly in an antegrade direction. Arteries highlighted in bold are those more commonly reported during arteriographic procedures.

First Order	**Second Order Branch**	**Third Order Branch**	**Beyond Third Order Branches**
	R. common carotid	**R. internal carotid**	R. ophthalmic / R. p. communicating / R. middle cerebral / R. a. cerebral
		R. external carotid	R. superior thyroid / R. ascending pharyngeal / R. facial / R. lingual / R. occipital / R. p. auricular / R. superficial temporal / R. internal maxillary / R. middle meningeal
Innominate		**R. vertebral** — Basilar	
		R. internal thoracic (internal mammary)	
		R. thyrocervical trunk	R. inferior thyroid / R. suprascapular / R. transverse cervical
		R. costocervical trunk	R. highest intercostal / R. deep cervicall
	R. subclavian & axillary	R. lateral thoracic / R. thoracoacromial / R. humeral circumflex (A/P)	
		R. subscapular — R. circumflex scapular	
		R. brachial	
		R. deep brachial	R. ulnar / R. radial / R. interosseous / R. deep palmar arch / R. superficial palmar arch / R. metacarpals and digitals
L. common carotid	**L. internal carotid**	L. ophthalmic / L. p. communicating / L. middle cerebral / L. a. cerebral	
	L. external carotid	L. superior thyroid / L. ascending pharyngeal / L. facial / L. lingual / L. occipital / L. p. auricular / L. superficial temporal	
		L. internal maxillary — L. middle meningeal	

R = right, L = left, A = anterior, P = posterior

First Order	Second Order Branch	Third Order Branch	Beyond Third Order Branches

L. subclavian & axillary

L. vertebral
L. internal thoracic (internal mammary)

L. thyrocervical trunk
- L. inferior thyroid
- L. suprascapular
- L. transverse cervical

L. costocervical trunk
- L. highest intercostal
- L. deep cervical

L. lateral thoracic
L. thoracoacromial
L. humeral circumflex (A/P)
L. subscapular ——— L. circumflex scapular
L. brachial

L. deep brachial
- L. ulnar
- L. radial
- L. interosseous
  - L. deep palmar arch
  - L. superficial palmar arch
  - L. metacarpals and digitals

Intercostals

Bronchials

Recurrent esophageal

Inferior phrenic ——— Superior suprarenal

Celiac trunk

L. gastric ——— Esophageal branch

Splenic
- Dorsal pancreatic ——— Inferior transverse pancreatic
- Great pancreatic
- Caudal pancreatic
- Gastroepiploic
- Short gastrics

Common hepatic
- Gastroduodenal
  - P. superior pancreaticoduodenal
  - A. superior pancreaticoduodenal
- Proper Hepatic
  - L. hepatic
  - R. hepatic
  - Cystic
  - Gastroepiploic
  - Supraduodenal
  - Intermediate hepatic

Middle suprarenal

Superior mesenteric

Middle colic

Inferior pancreaticoduodenal
- P. inferior pancreaticoduodenal
- A. inferior pancreaticoduodenal

Jejunal
Ileocolic
Appendicular
P. cecal
A. cecal
Marginal
R. colic

R = right, L = left, A = anterior, P = posterior

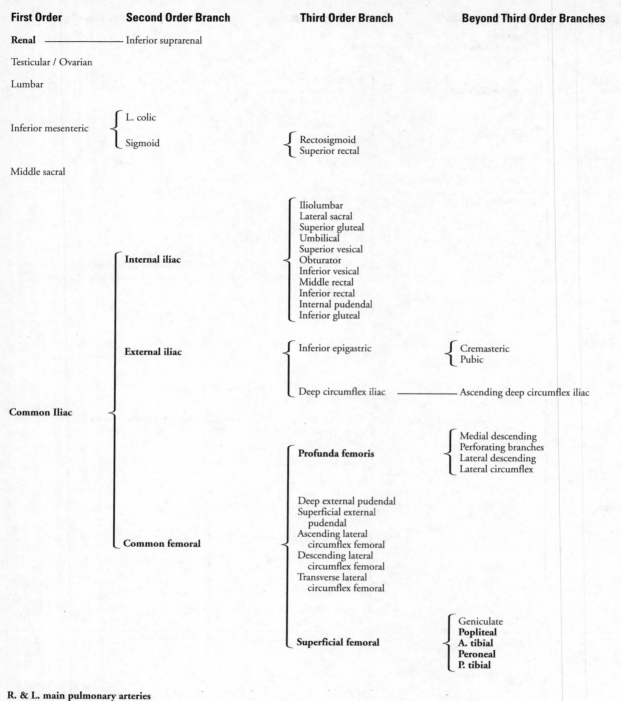

First Order	Second Order Branch	Third Order Branch	Beyond Third Order Branches
Renal ———————— Inferior suprarenal			
Testicular / Ovarian			
Lumbar			
Inferior mesenteric	L. colic		
	Sigmoid	Rectosigmoid	
		Superior rectal	
Middle sacral			

Internal iliac:
- Iliolumbar
- Lateral sacral
- Superior gluteal
- Umbilical
- Superior vesical
- Obturator
- Inferior vesical
- Middle rectal
- Inferior rectal
- Internal pudendal
- Inferior gluteal

External iliac:
- Inferior epigastric — Cremasteric, Pubic
- Deep circumflex iliac ——— Ascending deep circumflex iliac

Common Iliac

Common femoral:
- **Profunda femoris** — Medial descending, Perforating branches, Lateral descending, Lateral circumflex
- Deep external pudendal
- Superficial external pudendal
- Ascending lateral circumflex femoral
- Descending lateral circumflex femoral
- Transverse lateral circumflex femoral
- **Superficial femoral** — Geniculate, **Popliteal**, **A. tibial**, **Peroneal**, **P. tibial**

R. & L. main pulmonary arteries
(venous selective)

Reference: Kadir S. *Atlas of Normal and Variant Angiographic Anatomy.* Philadephia, Pa: WB Saunders Co; 1991.
R = right, L = left, A = anterior, P = posterior

Appendix M

Crosswalk to Deleted CPT Codes

This listing is a summary of the deleted *CPT 2006* codes and descriptors that have been crosswalked to *CPT 2007* codes.

Deleted CPT 2006 Code	CPT 2007 Code	CPT 2006 Code Descriptor
15000	15002, 15004	Surgical preparation or creation of recipient site by excision of open wounds, burn eschar, or scar (including subcutaneous tissues), or incisional release of scar contracture; first 100 sq cm or one percent of body area of infants and children
+15001	+15003, 15005	Surgical preparation or creation of recipient site by excision of open wounds, burn eschar, or scar (including subcutaneous tissues), or incisional release of scar contracture; each additional 100 sq cm or each additional one percent of body area of infants and children (List separately in addition to code for primary procedure)
15831	15830, 15847, 17999	Excision, excessive skin and subcutaneous tissue (includes lipectomy); abdomen (abdominoplasty)
17304	17311	Chemosurgery (Mohs micrographic technique), including removal of all gross tumor, surgical excision of tissue specimens, mapping, color coding of specimens, microscopic examination of specimens by the surgeon, and complete histopathologic preparation including the first routine stain (eg, hematoxylin and eosin, toluidine blue); first stage, fresh tissue technique, up to 5 specimens
17305	17312, 17314	Chemosurgery (Mohs micrographic technique), including removal of all gross tumor, surgical excision of tissue specimens, mapping, color coding of specimens, microscopic examination of specimens by the surgeon, and complete histopathologic preparation including the first routine stain (eg, hematoxylin and eosin, toluidine blue); second stage, fixed or fresh tissue, up to 5 specimens
17306	17312, 17314	Chemosurgery (Mohs micrographic technique), including removal of all gross tumor, surgical excision of tissue specimens, mapping, color coding of specimens, microscopic examination of specimens by the surgeon, and complete histopathologic preparation including the first routine stain (eg, hematoxylin and eosin, toluidine blue); third stage, fixed or fresh tissue, up to 5 specimens
17307	17312, 17314	Chemosurgery (Mohs micrographic technique), including removal of all gross tumor, surgical excision of tissue specimens, mapping, color coding of specimens, microscopic examination of specimens by the surgeon, and complete histopathologic preparation including the first routine stain (eg, hematoxylin and eosin, toluidine blue); additional stage(s), up to 5 specimens, each stage
+17310	+17315	Chemosurgery (Mohs micrographic technique), including removal of all gross tumor, surgical excision of tissue specimens, mapping, color coding of specimens, microscopic examination of specimens by the surgeon, and complete histopathologic preparation including the first routine stain (eg, hematoxylin and eosin, toluidine blue); each additional specimen, after the first 5 specimens, fixed or fresh tissue, any stage (List separately in addition to code for primary procedure)
19140	19300	Mastectomy for gynecomastia
19160	19301	Mastectomy, partial (eg, lumpectomy, tylectomy, quadrantectomy, segmentectomy);
19162	19302	Mastectomy, partial (eg, lumpectomy, tylectomy, quadrantectomy, segmentectomy); with axillary lymphadenectomy
19180	19303	Mastectomy, simple, complete
19182	19304	Mastectomy, subcutaneous
19200	19305	Mastectomy, radical, including pectoral muscles, axillary lymph nodes
19220	19306	Mastectomy, radical, including pectoral muscles, axillary and internal mammary lymph nodes (Urban type operation)

Deleted CPT 2006 Code	CPT 2007 Code	CPT 2006 Code Descriptor
19240	19307	Mastectomy, modified radical, including axillary lymph nodes, with or without pectoralis minor muscle, but excluding pectoralis major muscle
25611	25606	Percutaneous skeletal fixation of distal radial fracture (eg, Colles or Smith type) or epiphyseal separation, with or without fracture of ulnar styloid, requiring manipulation, with or without external fixation
25620	25607-25609	Open treatment of distal radial fracture (eg, Colles or Smith type) or epiphyseal separation, with or without fracture of ulnar styloid, with or without internal or external fixation
26504	26390	Reconstruction of tendon pulley, each tendon; with tendon prosthesis (separate procedure)
27315	27325	Neurectomy, hamstring muscle
27320	27326	Neurectomy, popliteal (gastrocnemius)
28030	28055	Neurectomy, intrinsic musculature of foot
33253	33254-33256	Operative incisions and reconstruction of atria for treatment of atrial fibrillation or atrial flutter (eg, maze procedure)
35381	35302-35306	Thromboendarterectomy, with or without patch graft; femoral and/or popliteal, and/or tibioperoneal
35507	35506	Bypass graft, with vein; subclavian-carotid
35541	35537, 35538	Bypass graft, with vein; aortoiliac or bi-iliac
35546	35539, 35540	Bypass graft, with vein; aortofemoral or bifemoral
35641	35637, 35638	Bypass graft, with other than vein; aortoiliac or bi-iliac
44152	44799	Colectomy, total, abdominal, without proctectomy; with rectal mucosectomy, ileoanal anastomosis, with or without loop ileostomy
44153	44799	Colectomy, total, abdominal, without proctectomy; with rectal mucosectomy, ileoanal anastomosis, creation of ileal reservoir (S or J), with or without loop ileostomy
47716	47719	Anastomosis, choledochal cyst, without excision
48005	48105	Resection or debridement of pancreas and peripancreatic tissue for acute necrotizing pancreatitis
48180	48548	Pancreaticojejunostomy, side-to-side anastomosis (Puestow-type operation)
49085	49402	Removal of peritoneal foreign body from peritoneal cavity
54152	54150	Circumcision, using clamp or other device; except newborn
54820	54865	Exploration of epididymis, with or without biopsy
55859	55875	Transperineal placement of needles or catheters into prostate for interstitial radioelement application, with or without cystoscopy
56720	56442	Hymenotomy, simple incision
57820	57558	Dilation and curettage of cervical stump
67350	67346	Biopsy of extraocular muscle
+75998	+77001	Fluoroscopic guidance for central venous access device placement, replacement (catheter only or complete), or removal (includes fluoroscopic guidance for vascular access and catheter manipulation, any necessary contrast injections through access site or catheter with related venography radiologic supervision and interpretation, and radiographic documentation of final catheter position) (List separately in addition to code for primary procedure)
76003	77002	Fluoroscopic guidance for needle placement (eg, biopsy, aspiration, injection, localization device)
76005	77003	Fluoroscopic guidance and localization of needle or catheter tip for spine or paraspinous diagnostic or therapeutic injection procedures (epidural, transforaminal epidural, subarachnoid, paravertebral facet joint, paravertebral facet joint nerve or sacroiliac joint), including neurolytic agent destruction
76006	77071	Manual application of stress performed by physician for joint radiography, including contralateral joint if indicated

Deleted CPT 2006 Code	CPT 2007 Code	CPT 2006 Code Descriptor
76012	72291	Radiological supervision and interpretation, percutaneous vertebroplasty or vertebral augmentation including cavity creation, per vertebral body; under fluoroscopic guidance
76013	72292	Radiological supervision and interpretation, percutaneous vertebroplasty or vertebral augmentation including cavity creation, per vertebral body; under CT guidance
76020	77072	Bone age studies
76040	77073	Bone length studies (orthoroentgenogram, scanogram)
76061	77074	Radiologic examination, osseous survey; limited (eg, for metastases)
76062	77075	Radiologic examination, osseous survey; complete (axial and appendicular skeleton)
76065	77076	Radiologic examination, osseous survey, infant
76066	77077	Joint survey, single view, two or more joints (specify)
76070	77078	Computed tomography, bone mineral density study, one or more sites; axial skeleton (eg, hips, pelvis, spine)
76071	77079	Computed tomography, bone mineral density study, one or more sites; appendicular skeleton (peripheral) (eg, radius, wrist, heel)
76075	77080	Dual energy X-ray absorptiometry (DXA), bone density study, one or more sites; axial skeleton (eg, hips, pelvis, spine)
76076	77081	Dual energy X-ray absorptiometry (DXA), bone density study, one or more sites; appendicular skeleton (peripheral) (eg, radius, wrist, heel)
76077	77082	Dual energy X-ray absorptiometry (DXA), bone density study, one or more sites; vertebral fracture assessment
76078	77083	Radiographic absorptiometry (eg, photodensitometry, radiogrammetry), one or more sites
+76082	+77051	Computer-aided detection (computer algorithm analysis of digital image data for lesion detection) with further physician review for interpretation, with or without digitization of film radiographic images; diagnostic mammography (List separately in addition to code for primary procedure)
+76083	+77052	Computer-aided detection (computer algorithm analysis of digital image data for lesion detection) with further physician review for interpretation, with or without digitization of film radiographic images; screening mammography (List separately in addition to code for primary procedure)
76086	77053	Mammary ductogram or galactogram, single duct, radiological supervision and interpretation
76088	77054	Mammary ductogram or galactogram, multiple ducts, radiological supervision and interpretation
76090	77055	Mammography; unilateral
76091	77056	Mammography; bilateral
76092	77057	Screening mammography, bilateral (two view film study of each breast)
76093	77058	Magnetic resonance imaging, breast, without and/or with contrast material(s); unilateral
76094	77059	Magnetic resonance imaging, breast, without and/or with contrast material(s); bilateral
76095	77031	Stereotactic localization guidance for breast biopsy or needle placement (eg, for wire localization or for injection), each lesion, radiological supervision and interpretation
76096	77032	Mammographic guidance for needle placement, breast (eg, for wire localization or for injection), each lesion, radiological supervision and interpretation
76355	77011	Computed tomography guidance for stereotactic localization
76360	77012	Computed tomography guidance for needle placement (eg, biopsy, aspiration, injection, localization device), radiological supervision and interpretation
76362	77013	Computed tomography guidance for, and monitoring of, parenchymal tissue ablation
76370	77014	Computed tomography guidance for placement of radiation therapy fields
76393	77021	Magnetic resonance guidance for needle placement (eg, for biopsy, needle aspiration, injection, or placement of localization device) radiological supervision and interpretation

Deleted CPT 2006 Code	CPT 2007 Code	CPT 2006 Code Descriptor
76394	77022	Magnetic resonance guidance for, and monitoring of, parenchymal tissue ablation
76400	77084	Magnetic resonance (eg, proton) imaging, bone marrow blood supply
76778	76775, 76776	Ultrasound, transplanted kidney, B-scan and/or real time with image documentation, with or without duplex Doppler study
76986	76998	Ultrasonic guidance, intraoperative
78704	78707-78709	Kidney imaging; with function study (ie, imaging renogram)
78715	78701-78709	Kidney vascular flow only
78760	78761	Testicular imaging
92573	92700	Lombard test
94656	94002, 94004	Ventilation assist and management, initiation of pressure or volume preset ventilators for assisted or controlled breathing; first day
94657	94003, 94004	Ventilation assist and management, initiation of pressure or volume preset ventilators for assisted or controlled breathing; subsequent days
0018T	0160T, 0161T	Delivery of high power, focal magnetic pulses for direct stimulation to cortical neurons
0044T	96904	Whole body integumentary photography, at request of a physician, for monitoring of high-risk patients; with dysplastic nevus syndrome or familial melanoma
0045T	96904	Whole body integumentary photography, at request of a physician, for monitoring of high-risk patients; with history of dysplastic nevi or personal history of melanoma
0082T	77371-77373	Stereotactic body radiation therapy, treatment delivery, one or more treatment areas, per day
0083T	77371-77373	Stereotactic body radiation therapy, treatment management, per day
0091T	22857	Total disc arthroplasty (artificial disc), anterior approach, including diskectomy to prepare interspace (other than for decompression); single interspace, lumbar
0094T	22865	Removal of total disc arthroplasty, anterior approach; single interspace, lumbar
0097T	22862	Removal of total disc arthroplasty, anterior approach; single interspace, lumbar
0120T	19105	Ablation, cryosurgical, of fibroadenoma, including ultrasound guidance, each fibroadenoma

Index

Instructions for the Use of the CPT Index

Main Terms

The index is organized by main terms. Each main term can stand alone, or be followed by up to three modifying terms. There are four primary classes of main entries:

1. Procedure or service.
   For example: Endoscopy; Anastomosis; Splint

2. Organ or other anatomic site.
   For example: Tibia; Colon; Salivary Gland

3. Condition.
   For example: Abscess; Entropion; Tetralogy of Fallot

4. Synonyms, Eponyms and Abbreviations.
   For example: EEG; Bricker Operation; Clagett Procedure

Modifying Terms

A main term may be followed by a series of up to three indented terms that modify the main term. When modifying terms appear, one should review the list, as these subterms do have an effect on the selection of the appropriate code for the procedure.

Code Ranges

Whenever more than one code applies to a given index entry, a code range is listed. If several non-sequential codes apply, they will be separated by a comma. For example:

Esophagus
    Reconstruction 43300, 43310, 43313

If two or more sequential codes apply, they will be separated by a hyphen. For example:

Debridement
    Burns 01951-01953, 16010-16030

Conventions

As a space saving convention, certain words infer some meaning. This convention is primarily used when a procedure or service is listed as a subterm. For example:

Knee
    Incision (of)

In this example, the word in parentheses (of) does not appear in the index, but it is inferred. As another example:

Pancreas
    Anesthesia (for procedures on)

In this example, as there is no such entity as pancreas anesthesia, the words in parentheses are inferred. That is, anesthesia for procedures on the pancreas.

The alphabetic index is NOT a substitute for the main text of *CPT*. Even if only one code appears, the user must refer to the main text to ensure that the code selection is accurate.

A

A Vitamin
See Vitamin, A

A-II
See Angiotensin II

Abbe-Estlander Procedure
See Reconstruction; Repair, Cleft Lip

Abdomen
Abdominal Wall
  Removal
    Mesh 11008
    Prosthesis 11008
  Repair
    Hernia 49491-49496, 49501, 49507,
               49521, 49590
  Tumor
    Excision 22900
  Unlisted Services and Procedures 22999
Abscess
  Incision and Drainage 49020, 49040
    Open 49040
    Percutaneous 49021
Angiography 74175, 75635
Artery
  Ligation 37617
Biopsy 49000
Bypass Graft 35907
Cannula/Catheter
  Removal 49422
Celiotomy
  for Staging 49220
CT Scan 74150-74175, 75635
Cyst
  Destruction/Excision 49200-49201
Drainage
  Fluid 49080-49081
Ectopic Pregnancy 59130
Endometrioma
  Destruction/Excision 49200-49201
Exploration 49000-49002
  Blood Vessel 35840
  Staging 58960
Incision 49000
  Staging 58960
Incision and Drainage
  Pancreatitis 48000
Infraumbilical Panniculectomy 15830
Injection
  Air 49400
  Contrast Material 49400
Insertion
  Catheter 49419-49421, 49324
  Venous Shunt 49425
Intraperitoneal
  Catheter Exit Site 49436
  Catheter Insertion 49324, 49435
  Catheter Removal 49422
  Catheter Revision 49325
Shunt
  Ligation 49428
  Removal 49429

Laparotomy
  Staging 49220
Magnetic Resonance Imaging
(MRI) 74181-74183
Needle Biopsy
  Mass 49180
Peritoneocentesis 49080-49081
Radical Resection 51597
Repair
  Blood Vessel 35221
    with Other Graft 35281
    with Vein Graft 35251
  Hernia 49491-49525, 49560-49587
  Suture 49900
Revision
  Venous Shunt 49426
Suture 49900
Tumor
  Destruction/Excision 49200-49201
Ultrasound 76700-76705
Unlisted Services and Procedures 49999
Wound Exploration
  Penetrating 20102
X-Ray 74000-74022

Abdominal Aorta
See Aorta, Abdominal

Abdominal Aortic Aneurysm
See Aorta, Abdominal, Aneurysm

Abdominal Deliveries
See Cesarean Delivery

Abdominal Hysterectomy
See Hysterectomy, Abdominal

Abdominal Lymphangiogram
See Lymphangiography, Abdomen

Abdominal Paracentesis
See Abdomen, Drainage

Abdominal Radiographies
See Abdomen, X-Ray

Abdominal Wall
Debridement
  Infected 11005-11006
Reconstruction 49905
Removal
  Mesh 11008
  Prosthesis 11008
Surgery 22999
Tumor
  Excision 22900

Abdominohysterectomy
See Hysterectomy, Abdominal

Abdominopelvic Amputation
See Amputation, Interpelviabdominal

Abdominoplasty
See Panniculectomy
Excision 15847

Ablation
Anal
  Polyp 46615
  Tumor 46615

Bone
  Tumor 20982
Colon
  Tumor 45339
Cryosurgical
  Renal Mass 50250
  Renal Tumor
    Percutaneous 0135T
CT Scan Guidance 77013
Endometrial 58353-58356, 58563
Endometrium
  Ultrasound Guidance 58356
Heart
  Arrhythmogenic Focus 93650-93652
    See Cardiology; Diagnostic, Intracardiac
      Pacing and Mapping
Liver
  Tumor
    Laparoscopic 47370-47371
    Open 47380-47382
Lung
  Tumor
    Radiofrequency 32998
Magnetic Resonance Guidance 77022
Parenchymal Tissue
  CT Scan Guidance 77013
Prostate 55873
Pulmonary Tumor 32998
Radiofrequency 32998
Renal Cyst 50541
Renal Mass 50542
  Radiofrequency 50592
Renal Tumor
  Cryotherapy
    Percutaneous 0135T
Turbinate Mucosa 30801-30802
Ultrasound
  Guidance 76940
  Uterine Tumor 0071T-0072T
Uterine Tumor
  Ultrasound, Focused 0071T-0072T
Vein
  Endovenous 36475-36479

Abortion
See Obstetrical Care
Incomplete 59812
Induced
  by Dilation and Curettage 59840
  by Dilation and Evacuation 59841
  by Saline 59850-59851
  by Vaginal Suppositories 59855-59856
  with Hysterectomy 59100, 59852, 59857
Missed
  First Trimester 59820
  Second Trimester 59821
Septic 59830
Spontaneous 59812
Therapeutic
  by Saline 59850
    with Dilation and Curettage 59851
    with Hysterectomy 59852

Abrasion
Skin
  Chemical Peel 15788-15793
  Dermabrasion 15780-15783
  Lesion 15786-15787

Abscess

Abdomen .49040-49041
　Incision and Drainage
　　Open 49040
　　Percutaneous 49021
Anal
　Incision and Drainage 46045-46050
Ankle 27603
Appendix
　Incision and Drainage 44900
　　Open 44900
　　Percutaneous 44901
Arm, Lower 25028
　Excision 25145
　Incision and Drainage 25035
Arm, Upper
　Incision and Drainage 23930-23935
Auditory Canal, External 69020
Bartholin's Gland
　Incision and Drainage 56420
Bladder
　Incision and Drainage 51080
Brain
　Drainage 61150-61151
　Excision 61514, 61522
　Incision and Drainage 61320-61321
Breast
　Incision and Drainage 19020
Carpals
　Incision, Deep 25035
Clavicle
　Sequestrectomy 23170
Drainage
　with X-Ray 75989
Ear, External
　Complicated 69005
　Simple 69000
Elbow
　Incision and Drainage 23930-23935
Epididymis
　Incision and Drainage 54700
Excision
　Olecranon Process 24138
　Radius 24136
　Ulna 24138
Eyelid
　Incision and Drainage 67700
Facial Bones
　Excision 21026
Finger 26010-26011
　Incision and Drainage 26034
Foot
　Incision 28005
Gums
　Incision and Drainage 41800
Hand
　Incision and Drainage 26034
Hematoma
　Incision and Drainage 27603
Hip
　Incision and Drainage 26990-26992
Humeral Head 23174
Humerus
　Excision 24134
　Incision and Drainage 23935
Kidney
　Incision and Drainage 50020

　　Open 50020
　　Percutaneous 50021
Leg, Lower
　Incision and Drainage 27603
Liver 47010
　Drainage
　　Open 47010
　　Injection 47015
　　Repair 47300
Localization
　Nuclear Medicine 78806-78807
Lung
　Percutaneous Drainage 32200-32201
Lymph Node
　Incision and Drainage 38300-38305
Lymphocele Drainage 49062
Mandible
　Excision 21025
Mouth
　Incision and Drainage 40800-40801,
　　　　　　　　　　41005-41009, 41015-41018
Nasal Septum
　Incision and Drainage 30020
Neck
　Incision and Drainage 21501-21502
Ovarian
　Incision and Drainage 58820-58822
　　Abdominal Approach 58822
　　Vaginal Approach 58820
Ovary
　Drainage
　　Percutaneous 58823
Palate
　Incision and Drainage 42000
Paraurethral Gland
　Incision and Drainage 53060
Parotid Gland Drainage 42300-42305
Pelvic
　Drainage
　　Percutaneous 58823
Pelvis
　Incision and Drainage . .26990-26992, 45000
Pericolic
　Drainage
　　Percutaneous 58823
Perineum
　Incision and Drainage 56405
Perirenal or Renal
　Drainage 50020-50021
　　Percutaneous 50021
Peritoneum
　Incision and Drainage
　　Open 49020
　　Percutaneous 49021
Prostate
　Incision and Drainage 55720-55725
　Transurethral Drainage 52700
Radius
　Incision, Deep 25035
Rectum
　Incision and Drainage 45005-45020,
　　　　　　　　　　　　　　　　46040, 46060
Retroperitoneal 49060-49061
　Drainage
　　Open 49060
　　Percutaneous 49061

Salivary Gland
　Drainage 42300-42320
Scapula
　Sequestrectomy 23172
Scrotum
　Incision and Drainage 54700, 55100
Shoulder
　Drainage 23030
Skene's Gland
　Incision and Drainage 53060
Skin
　Incision and Drainage 10060-10061
　Puncture Aspiration 10160
Soft Tissue
　Incision 20000-20005
Spine
　Incision and Drainage 22010-22015
Subdiaphragmatic 49040-49041
Sublingual Gland
　Drainage 42310-42320
Submaxillary Gland
　Drainage 42310-42320
Subphrenic 49040-49041
Testis
　Incision and Drainage 54700
Thoracostomy 32020
Thorax
　Incision and Drainage 21501-21502
Throat
　Incision and Drainage 42700-42725
Tongue
　Incision and Drainage 41000-41006
Tonsil
　Incision and Drainage 42700
Ulna
　Incision, Deep 25035
Urethra
　Incision and Drainage 53040
Uvula
　Incision and Drainage 42000
Vagina
　Incision and Drainage 57010
Vulva
　Incision and Drainage 56405
Wrist
　Excision 25145
　Incision and Drainage 25028, 25035
X-Ray 76080

Abscess, Nasal
See Nose, Abscess

Abscess, Parotid Gland
See Parotid Gland, Abscess

Absorptiometry
Dual Energy
　Body Composition 0028T
　Bone
　　Appendicular 77081
　　Axial Skeleton 77080
　　Vertebral 77082
Dual Photon
　Bone 78351
Radiographic
　Photodensity .77083
Single Photon
　Bone 78350

Absorption Spectrophotometry, Atomic
See Atomic Absorption Spectroscopy

Accessory Nerve, Spinal
See Nerves, Spinal Accessory

Accessory, Toes
See Polydactyly, Toes

ACE
See Angiotensin Converting Enzyme (ACE), Performance Measures

Acetabuloplasty 27120-27122

Acetabulum
Fracture
    Closed Treatment 27220-27222
    Open Treatment 27226-27228
    with Manipulation 27222
    without Manipulation 27220
Reconstruction 27120
    with Resection, Femoral Head 27122
Tumor
    Excision 27076

Acetaldehyde
Blood 82000

Acetaminophen
Urine 82003

Acetic Anhydrides 84600

Acetone
Blood or Urine 82009-82010

Acetone Body 82009-82010

Acetylcholinesterase
Blood or Urine 82013

AcG
See Clotting Factor

Achilles Tendon
Incision 27605-27606
Lengthening 27612
Repair 27650-27654

Achillotomy
See Tenotomy, Achilles Tendon

Acid
Gastric......................82926-82928

Acid Diethylamide, Lysergic
See Lysergic Acid Diethylamide

Acid Fast Bacilli (AFB)
Culture 87116

Acid Fast Bacillus Culture
See Culture, Acid Fast Bacilli

Acid Fast Stain 88312

Acid Perfusion Test
Esophagus 91012, 91030

Acid Phosphatase 84060-84066

Acid Probes, Nucleic
See Nucleic Acid Probe

Acid Reflux Test
Esophagus 91034-91038

Acid, Adenylic
See Adenosine Monophosphate (AMP)

Acid, Aminolevulinic
See Aminolevulinic Acid (ALA)

Acid, Ascorbic
See Ascorbic Acid

Acid, Deoxyribonucleic
See Deoxyribonucleic Acid

Acid, Folic
See Folic Acid

Acid, Glycocholic
See Cholylglycine

Acid, Lactic
See Lactic Acid

Acid, N-Acetylneuraminic
See Sialic Acid

Acid, Phenylethylbarbituric
See Phenobarbital

Acid, Uric
See Uric Acid

Acidity/Alkalinity
See pH

Acids, Amino
See Amino Acids

Acids, Bile
See Bile Acids

Acids, Fatty
See Fatty Acid

Acids, Guanylic
See Guanosine Monophosphate

Acids, N-Acetylneuraminic
See Sialic Acid

Acne Surgery
Incision and Drainage
    Abscess 10060-10061
    Comedones 10040
    Cyst 10040
    Milia, Multiple 10040
    Pustules 10040

Acne Treatment
Abrasion 15786-15787
Chemical Peel 15788-15793
Cryotherapy 17340
Dermabrasion 15780-15783
Exfoliation
    Chemical 17360

Acoustic Evoked Brain Stem Potential
See Evoked Potential, Auditory Brainstem

Acoustic Neuroma
See Brain, Tumor, Excision; Brainstem; Mesencephalon; Skull Base Surgery

Acoustic Recording
Heart Sounds
    with Computer Analysis 0068T-0070T

Acromioclavicular Joint
Arthrocentesis 20605
Arthrotomy 23044
    with Biopsy 23101
Dislocation 23540-23552
    Open Treatment 23550-23552
X-Ray 73050

Acromion
Excision
    Shoulder 23130

Acromionectomy
Partial 23130

Acromioplasty 23415-23420
Partial 23130

ACTH
See Adrenocorticotropic Hormone (ACTH)

ACTH Releasing Factor
See Corticotropic Releasing Hormone (CRH)

Actigraphy
Sleep Study 0089T

Actinomyces
Antibody 86602

Actinomycosis 86000

Actinomycotic Infection
See Actinomycosis

Actinotherapy 0168T, 96900
See Dermatology

Activated Factor X
See Thrombokinase

Activated Partial Thromboplastin Time
See Thromboplastin, Partial, Time

Activation, Lymphocyte
See Blastogenesis

Activities of Daily Living
See Physical Medicine/Therapy/Occupational Therapy

Activity, Glomerular Procoagulant
See Thromboplastin

Acupuncture
with Electrical Stimulation 97813-97814
without Electrical Stimulation 97810-97811

Acute Poliomyelitis
See Polio

Acylcarnitines 82016-82017

Adamantinoma, Pituitary
See Craniopharyngioma

Addam Operation
See Dupuytren's Contracture

Adductor Tenotomy of Hip
See Tenotomy, Hip, Adductor

Adenoidectomy 42820-42821,
42830-42836

Adenoids
Excision 42830-42836
   with Tonsils 42820-42821
Unlisted Services and Procedures .... .42999

Adenoma
Pancreas
   Excision .... .48120
Thyroid Gland Excision .... .60200

Adenosine 3'5' Monophosphate
See Cyclic AMP

Adenosine Diphosphate
Blood .... .82030

Adenosine Monophosphate (AMP)
Blood .... .82030

Adenovirus
Antibody .... .86603
Antigen Detection
   Enzyme Immunoassay .... .87301
   Immunofluorescense .... .87260

Adenovirus Vaccine
See Vaccines

Adenylic Acid
See Adenosine Monophosphate (AMP)

ADH
See Antidiuretic Hormone

Adhesions
Epidural .... .0027T, 62263-62264
Eye
   Corneovitreal .... .65880
   Incision
      Anterior Segment 65860-65870
      Posterior Segment .... .65875
Intermarginal
   Construction .... .67880
      Transposition of Tarsal Plate .... .67882
Intestinal
   Enterolysis .... .44005
   Laparoscopic .... .44180
Intracranial
   Lysis .... .62161
Intrauterine
   Lysis .... .58559
Labial
   Lysis .... .56441
Lungs
   Lysis .... .32124
Pelvic
   Lysis .... .58660, 58662, 58740
Penile
   Lysis
      Post-circumcision .... .54162
Preputial
   Lysis .... .54450
Urethral
   Lysis .... .53500

Adipectomy
See Lipectomy

ADL
See Activities of Daily Living

Administration
Immunization
   Each Additional Vaccine/Toxoid ..... .90472,
90474
      with Counseling .... .90466, 90468
   One Vaccine/Toxoid .... .90471, 90473
      with Counseling .... .90465, 90467

ADP
See Adenosine Diphosphate

ADP Phosphocreatine Phosphotransferase
See CPK

Adrenal Cortex Hormone
See Corticosteroids

Adrenal Gland
Biopsy 60540-60545
Excision
   Laparoscopy .... .60650
   Retroperitoneal Tumor .... .60545
Exploration 60540-60545
Nuclear Medicine
   Imaging .... .78075

Adrenal Medulla
See Medulla

Adrenalectomy .... .60540
Anesthesia .... .00866
Laparoscopic .... .50545

Adrenalin
See Catecholamines
Blood .... .82383
Urine .... .82384

Adrenaline-Noradrenaline
Testing 82382-82384

Adrenocorticotropic Hormone
(ACTH) .. .80400-80406, 80412, 80418, 82024
Blood or Urine .... .82024
Stimulation Panel 80400-80406

Adrenogenital Syndrome .56805, 57335

Adult T Cell Leukemia Lymphoma Virus I
See HTLV I

Advanced Life Support
See Emergency Department Services
Physician Direction .... .99288

Advancement
Genioglossus .... .21199
Tendon
   Foot .... .28238

Advancement Flap
See Skin, Adjacent Tissue Transfer

Aerosol Inhalation
See Pulmonology, Therapeutic
Pentamidine .... .94642

AFB
See Acid Fast Bacilli (AFB)

Afferent Nerve
See Sensory Nerve

AFP
See Alpha-Fetoprotein

After Hours Medical Services .... .99050

Agents, Anticoagulant
See Clotting Inhibitors

Agglutinin
Cold 86156-86157
Febrile .... .86000

Aggregation
Platelet .... .85576

AHG
See Clotting Factor

AICD (Pacing Cardioverter-Defibrillator)
See Defibrillator, Heart; Pacemaker, Heart

Aid, Hearing
See Hearing Aid

AIDS Antibodies
See Antibody, HIV

AIDS Virus
See HIV-1

Akin Operation
See Bunion Repair

ALA
See Aminolevulinic Acid (ALA)

Alanine 2 Oxoglutarate Aminotransferase
See Transaminase, Glutamic Pyruvic

Alanine Amino (ALT) .... .84460

Alanine Transaminase
See Transaminase, Glutamic Pyruvic

Albarran Test
See Water Load Test

Albumin
Ischemia modified .... .82045
Serum .... .82040
Urine 82042-82044

Alcohol
Breath .... .82075
Ethyl
   Blood .... .82055
   Urine .... .82055
Ethylene Glycol .... .82693

Alcohol Dehydrogenase
See Antidiuretic Hormone

Antiprothrombin Antibody ..... .0030T

Antistreptococcal Antibody ... .86215

Antistreptokinase Titer .... .86590

Antistreptolysin O 86060-86063

Antithrombin III 85300-85301

Antithrombin VI
See Fibrin Degradation Products

Antitoxin Assay .... .87230

Antiviral Antibody
See Viral Antibodies

Antrostomy
Sinus
    Maxillary 31256-31267

Antrotomy
Sinus
    Maxillary 31020-31032
Transmastoid .... .69501

Antrum of Highmore
See Sinus, Maxillary

Antrum Puncture
Sinus
    Maxillary .... .31000
    Sphenoid .... .31002

Anus
See Hemorrhoids; Rectum
Ablation .... .46615
Abscess
    Incision and Drainage 46045-46050
Biofeedback .... .90911
Biopsy
    Endoscopy .... .46606
Crypt
    Excision 46210-46211
Dilation
    Endoscopy .... .46604
Endoscopy
    Biopsy .... .46606
    Dilation .... .46604
    Exploration .... .46600
    Hemorrhage .... .46614
    Removal
        Foreign Body .... .46608
        Polyp .... .46610, 46612
        Tumor .... .46610, 46612
Excision
    Tag .... .46220, 46230
Exploration
    Endoscopy .... .46600
    Surgical .... .45990
Fissure
    Destruction 46940-46942
    Excision .... .46200
Fistula
    Excision 46270-46285
    Repair .... .0170T, 46706
Hemorrhage
    Endoscopic Control .... .46614
Hemorrhoids
    Clot Excision .... .46320
    Destruction 46934-46936

Excision 46250-46262
Injection .... .46500
Ligation .... .46221, 46945-46946
Stapling .... .46947
Suture 46945-46946
Imperforated
    Repair 46715-46742
Incision
    Septum .... .46070
Lesion
    Destruction 46900-46917, 46924
    Excision .... .45108, 46922
Manometry .... .91122
Placement
    Seton .... .46020
Reconstruction .... .46742
    Congenital Absence 46730-46740
    Sphincter 46750-46751, 46760-46762
    with Graft .... .46753
    with Implant .... .46762
Removal
    Foreign Body .... .46608
    Seton .... .46030
    Suture .... .46754
    Wire .... .46754
Repair
    Anovaginal Fistula 46715-46716
    Cloacal Anomaly .... .46748
    Fistula .... .0170T, 46706
    Stricture 46700-46705
Sphincter
    Chemodenervation .... .46505
    Electromyography 51784-51785
    Needle .... .51785
Unlisted Services and Procedures .... .46999

Aorta
Abdominal
    Aneurysm ...... .0078T, 0079T, 0080T, 0081T,
                    34800-34805, 34825-34832,
                    35081-35103, 75952-75953
    Thromboendarterectomy .... .35331
Anastomosis
    to Pulmonary Artery .... .33606
Angiogram
    Radiologic Injection .... .93544
        See Cardiac Catheterization, Injection
Angioplasty .... .35452
Aortography 75600-75630
Balloon .... .33967, 33970
Catheterization
    Catheter .... .36200
    Intracatheter/Needle .... .36160
Circulation Assist .... .33967, 33970
Conduit to Heart .... .33404
Excision
    Coarctation 33840-33851
Insertion
    Balloon Device .... .33967
    Graft 33330-33335
    Intracatheter/Needle .... .36160
Removal
    Balloon Assist Device .... .33968, 33971
Repair 33320-33322, 33802-33803
    Coarctation 33840-33851
    Graft 33860-33877
Hypoplastic or Interrupted Aortic Arch
    with Cardiopulmonary Bypass ...... .33853
    without Cardiopulmonary Bypass ... .33852

Sinus of Valsalva 33702-33720
Suspension .... .33800
Suture 33320-33322
Thoracic
    Repair 75956-75959
        Endovascular 33880-33891
Valve
    Incision .... .33415
    Repair 33400-33403
        Left Ventricle .... .33414
        Supravalvular Stenosis .... .33417
    Replacement 33405-33413
X-Ray with Contrast 75600-75630

Aorta-Pulmonary ART Transposition
See Transposition, Great Arteries

Aortic Sinus
See Sinus of Valsalva

Aortic Stenosis
Repair .... .33415
    Supravalvular .... .33417

Aortic Valve
See Heart, Aortic Valve

Aortic Valve Replacement
See Replacement, Aortic Valve

Aortocoronary Bypass
See Coronary Artery Bypass Graft (CABG)

Aortocoronary Bypass for Heart Revascularization
See Artery, Coronary, Bypass

Aortography 75600-75605,
                           75630, 93544
See Angiography
Serial .... .75625
with Iliofemoral Artery .... .75630

Aortoiliac
Embolectomy 34151-34201
Thrombectomy 34151-34201

Aortopexy .... .33800

Aortoplasty
Supravalvular Stenosis .... .33417

AP
See Voiding Pressure Studies

Apert-Gallais Syndrome
See Adrenogenital Syndrome

Aphasia Testing .... .96105
See Neurology, Diagnostic

Apheresis
Therapeutic 36511-36516

Apical-Aortic Conduit .... .33404

Apicectomy
with Mastoidectomy .... .69605
    Petrous .... .69530

Apoaminotransferase, Aspartate
See Transaminase, Glutamic Oxaloacetic

Arteriovenous Fistula

Cannulization
- Vein 36815

Repair
- Abdomen 35182
  - Acquired or Traumatic 35189
- Head 35180
  - Acquired or Traumatic 35188
- Lower Extremity 35184
  - Acquired or Traumatic 35190
- Neck 35180
  - Acquired or Traumatic 35188
- Thorax 35182
  - Acquired or Traumatic 35189
- Upper Extremity 35184
  - Acquired or Traumatic 35190

Revision
- Hemodialysis Graft or Fistula
  - with Thrombectomy 36833
  - without Thrombectomy 36832

Thrombectomy
- Dialysis Graft
  - without Revision 36831
- Graft 36870

Arteriovenous Malformation

Cranial
- Repair 61680-61692, 61705-61708

Spinal
- Excision 63250-63252
- Injection 62294
- Repair 63250-63252

Arteriovenous Shunt

Angiography 75790
Catheterization 36145

Artery

Abdomen
- Angiography 75726
- Catheterization 36245-36248
- Ligation 37617

Adrenal
- Angiography 75731-75733

Anastomosis
- Cranial 61711

Angioplasty 75962-75968

Aorta
- Angioplasty 35452
- Atherectomy 35481, 35491

Aortobi-iliac
- Bypass Graft 35538, 35638

Aortobifemoral
- Bypass Graft 35540

Aortofemoral
- Bypass Graft 35539

Aortoiliac
- Bypass Graft 35537, 35637
- Embolectomy 34151-34201
- Thrombectomy 34151-34201

Aortoiliofemoral 35363

Arm
- Angiography 75710-75716
- Harvest of Artery for Coronary Artery
- Bypass Graft 35600

Atherectomy
- Open 35480-35485
- Percutaneous 35490-35495

Axillary
- Aneurysm 35011-35013
- Angioplasty 35458
- Bypass Graft 35516-35522, 35533, 35616-35623, 35650, 35654
- Embolectomy 34101
- Thrombectomy 34101
- Thromboendarterectomy 35321

Basilar
- Aneurysm 61698, 61702

Biopsy
- Transcatheter 75970

Brachial
- Aneurysm 35011-35013
- Angiography 75658
- Bypass Graft 35510, 35512, 35522-35525
- Catheterization 36120
- Embolectomy 34101
- Exploration 24495
- Exposure 34834
- Thrombectomy 34101
- Thromboendarterectomy 35321

Brachiocephalic
- Angioplasty 35458
- Atherectomy 35484, 35494
- Catheterization 36215-36218

Bypass Graft
- with Composite Graft 35681-35683

Cannulization
- for Extra Corporeal Circulation 36823
- to Vein 36810-36815

Carotid
- Aneurysm 35001-35002, 61697-61705
  - Vascular Malformation or Carotid
  - Cavernous Fistula 61710
- Angiography 75660-75680
- Bypass Graft ...33891, 35501-35510, 35526, 35601-35606, 35626, 35642
- Catheterization 36100
- Decompression ..61590-61591, 61595-61596
- Embolectomy 34001
- Exploration 35701
- Ligation 37600-37606, 61611-61612
- Thrombectomy 34001
- Thromboendarterectomy 35301, 35390
- Transection 61611-61612
- Transposition 33889

Carotid, Common
- Intima-Media Thickness (IMT) Study ..0126T

Celiac
- Aneurysm 35121-35122
- Bypass Graft 35531, 35631
- Embolectomy 34151
- Thrombectomy 34151
- Thromboendarterectomy 35341

Chest
- Ligation 37616

Coronary
- Angiography 93556
- Atherectomy 92995-92996
- Bypass 33517-33519
  - Arterial 33533-33536
- Bypass Venous Graft 33510-33516
- Graft 33503-33505
- Ligation 33502
- Repair 33500-33507
- Thrombectomy
  - Percutaneous 92973

Digital
- Sympathectomy 64820

Ethmoidal
- Ligation 30915

Extra Corporeal Circulation
- for Regional Chemotherapy
- of Extremity 36823

Extracranial
- Vascular Studies
  - Non-Invasive, Physiologic 93875

Extremities
- Vascular Studies 93922-93923

Extremity
- Bypass Graft Revision 35879-35884
- Catheterization 36140
- Ligation 37618

Femoral
- Aneurysm 35141-35142
- Angioplasty 35456
- Atherectomy 35483, 35493
- Bypass Graft ...35521, 35533, 35551-35558, 35566, 35621, 35646-35647, 35651-35661, 35666, 35700
- Bypass Graft Revision 35883-35884
- Bypass In-Situ 35583-35585
- Embolectomy 34201
- Exploration 35721
- Exposure 34812-34813
- Thrombectomy 34201
- Thromboendarterectomy ...35371-35372

Great Vessel
- Repair 33770-33781

Head
- Angiography 75650

Hepatic
- Aneurysm 35121-35122

Iliac
- Aneurysm 35131-35132, 75954
- Angioplasty 35454
- Atherectomy 35482, 35492
- Bypass Graft 35563, 35663
- Embolectomy 34151-34201
- Exposure 34820, 34833
- Graft 34900
- Occulsion Device 34808
- Thrombectomy 34151-34201
- Thromboendarterectomy 35351, 35361-35363

Iliofemoral
- Bypass Graft 35548-35549, 35565, 35665
- Thromboendarterectomy 35355, 35363
- X-Ray with Contrast 75630

Innominate
- Aneurysm 35021-35022
- Embolectomy 34001-34101
- Thrombectomy 34001-34101
- Thromboendarterectomy 35311

Leg
- Angiography 75710-75716
- Catheterization 36245-36248

Mammary
- Angiography 75756

Maxillary
- Ligation 30920

Mesenteric
- Aneurysm 35121-35122
- Bypass Graft 35531, 35631
- Embolectomy 34151

Artery Catheterization, Pulmonary

See Catheterization, Pulmonary Artery

Arthrectomy

Arthrocentesis

Arthrodeses

See Arthrodesis

Arthrodesis

Destruction
   Calculi (Stone) 43265
Dilation
   Endoscopy 43271, 47555-47556
Drainage
   Transhepatic 75980
Endoscopy
   Biopsy 47553
   Destruction
     Calculi (Stone) 43265
     Tumor 43272
   Dilation 43271, 47555-47556
   Exploration 47552
   Intraoperative 47550
   Removal
     Calculi (Stone) 43264, 47554
     Foreign Body 43269
     Stent 43269
   Specimen Collection 43260
   Sphincter Pressure 43263
   Sphincterotomy 43262
   Tube Placement 43267-43268
Exploration
   Atresia 47700
   Endoscopy 47552
Incision
   Sphincter 43262, 47460
Incision and Drainage 47420-47425
Insertion
   Catheter 47510, 47525, 75982
     Revision 47530
   Stent 47511, 47801
Nuclear Medicine
   Imaging 78223
Reconstruction
   Anastomosis 47800
Removal
   Calculi (Stone) 43264, 47420-47425
     Percutaneous 47630
   Foreign Body 43269
   Stent 43269
Repair 47701
   Cyst 47719
   Gastrointestinal Tract 47785
   with Intestines 47760, 47780
Tube Placement
   Nasobiliary 43267
   Stent 43268
Tumor
   Destruction 43271
   Excision 47711-47712
Unlisted Services and Procedures 47999
X-Ray
   Guide Dilation 74360
   with Contrast 74300-74320
     Calculus Removal 74327
     Guide Catheter 74328, 74330

Bile Duct, Common, Cystic Dilatation
See Cyst, Choledochal

Bilirubin
Blood 82247-82248
Feces 82252
Total
   Direct 82247-82248
   Transcutaneous 88400

Billroth I or II
See Gastrectomy, Partial

Bilobectomy 32482

Bimone
See Testosterone

Binding Globulin, Testosterone-Estradiol
See Globulin, Sex Hormone Binding

Binet Test 96101-96103

Binet-Simon Test 96101-96103

Binocular Microscopy 92504

Biofeedback
See Training, Biofeedback
Anorectal 90911
Psychiatric Treatment 90875-90876

Biofeedback Training
See Training, Biofeedback

Bioimpedance
Breast 0060T
Thorax 93701

Biological Skin Grafts
See Allograft, Skin

Biometry
Eye 76516-76519, 92136

Biopsies, Needle
See Needle Biopsy

Biopsy
See Brush Biopsy; Needle Biopsy
Abdomen 49000
Adrenal Gland 60540-60545
Anal
   Endoscopy 46606
Ankle 27613-27614, 27620
Arm, Lower 25065-25066
Arm, Upper 24065-24066
Artery
   Temporal 37609
Auditory Canal, External 69105
Back/Flank 21920-21925
Bile Duct
   Endoscopy 47553
Bladder 52354
   Cystourethroscope 52204
   Cystourethroscopy 52224, 52250
Blood Vessel
   Transcatheter 75970
Bone .20220-20245
Bone Marrow 38221
Brain 61140
   Stereotactic 61750-61751
Brainstem 61575-61576
Breast 19100-19103
   Stereotactic Localization 77031
Bronchi
   Catheterization 31717
   Endoscopic 31625-31629, 31632-31633
Brush
   Bronchi .31717
   Renal Pelvis 52007

Ureter 52007
   with Cystourethroscopy 52204
Carpometacarpal Joint
   Synovium 26100
Cervix 57454-57455, 57460, 57500, 57520
Chorionic Villus 59015
Colon 44025, 44100
   Endoscopy 44389, 45380, 45391-45392
   Multiple
     with Colostomy, Cecostomy 44322
Colon-Sigmoid
   Endoscopy 45305, 45331
Conjunctiva 68100
Cornea 65410
Duodenum 44010
Ear
   External .69100
Elbow 24065-24066, 24101
   Synovium 24100
Embryo Blastomere 89290-89291
Endometrium 58100-58110, 58558
Epididymis 54800, 54865
Esophagus
   Endoscopy 43202
Eye Muscle 67346
Eyelid 67810
Forearm
   Soft Tissue 25065-25066
Gallbladder
   Endoscopy 43261
Gastrointestinal, Upper
   Endoscopy 43239
Hand Joint
   Synovium 26100
Heart 93505
Hip 27040-27041
   Joint 27052
Hypopharynx 42802
Ileum
   Endoscopy 44382
Interphalangeal Joint
   Finger 26110
   Toe 28054
Intertarsal Joint
   Toe 28050
Intestines, Small 44020, 44100
   Endoscopy 44361, 44377
Kidney 50200-50205
   Endoscopic 50555-50557,
                50574-50576, 52354
Knee 27323-27324
   Synovium 27330
Knee Joint
   Synovium 27330
Lacrimal Gland 68510
Lacrimal Sac 68525
Larynx
   Endoscopy 31510, 31576
Leg
   Lower 27613-27614
   Upper 27323-27324
Lip 40490
Liver 47000-47001, 47100
Lung
   Needle 32405
   Thoracotomy 32095-32100

Urethrocystography 74450-74455
Urethrotomy 52270-52276
Urinary Incontinence Procedures
   Laparoscopy 51990-51992
   Pulsed Magnetic Neuromodulation . . .0029T
X-Ray 74430
   with Contrast 74450-74455

Bladder Voiding Pressure Studies 51795

Blalock-Hanlon Procedure 33735-33737
See Septostomy, Atrial

Blalock-Taussig Procedure
See Shunt, Great Vessel

Blast Cells
See Stem Cell

Blast Transformation
See Blastogenesis

Blastocyst Implantation
See Implantation

Blastocyst Transfer
See Embryo Transfer

Blastogenesis 86353

Blastomyces
Antibody 86612

Blastomycosis, European
See Cryptococcus

Bleeding
See Hemorrhage
Anal
  See Anus, Hemorrhage
Disorder
  See Coagulopathy
Time 85002
Tube
  Passage and Placement 91100
Uterine
  See Hemorrhage, Uterus
Vaginal
  See Hemorrhage, Vaginal

Blepharoplasty 15820-15823
See Canthoplasty
Anesthesia 00103

Blepharoptosis
Repair 67901-67909
  Frontalis Muscle Technique 67901
   with Fascial Sling 67902
  Superior Rectus Technique with
  Fascial Sling 67906
  Tarso Levator Resection/Advancement
   External Approach 67904
   Internal Approach 67903

Blepharorrhaphy
See Tarsorrhaphy

Blepharospasm
Chemodenervation 64612

Blepharotomy 67700

Blister
See Bulla

Blom-Singer Prosthesis 31611

Blood
See Blood Cell Count, Complete Blood Count
Bleeding Time 85002
Collection, for Autotransfusion
  Intraoperative 86891
  Preoperative 86890
Feces 82270, 82272
  by Hemoglobin Immunoassay 82274
Gastric Contents 82273
Hemoglobin Concentration 85046
Nuclear Medicine
  Flow Imaging 78445
  Red Cell 78140
  Red Cell Survival 78130-78135
Osmolality 83930
Other Source .82273
Plasma
  Exchange 36514-36516
Platelet
  Aggregation 85576
  Automated Count 85049
  Count 85008
  Manual Count 85032
Stem Cell
  Count 86367
  Donor Search 38204
  Harvesting 38205-38206
  Transplantation 38240-38242
   Cell Concentration 38215
   Cryopreservation 38207, 88240
   Plasma Depletion 38214
   Platelet Depletion 38213
   Red Blood Cell Depletion 38212
   T-cell Depletion 38210
   Thawing 38208-38209, 88241
   Tumor Cell Depletion 38211
   Washing .38209
Transfusion 36430
  Exchange .36455
  Newborn .36450
  Fetal 36460
  Push
   Infant 36440
Unlisted Services and Procedures 85999
Urine 83491
Viscosity 85810

Blood Banking
Frozen Blood Preparation 86930-86932
Frozen Plasma Preparation 86927
Physician Services 86077-86079

Blood Cell
CD4 and CD8
  Including Ratio 86360
Enzyme Activity 82657
Exchange 36511-36513
Sedimentation Rate
  Automated 85652
  Manual 85651

Blood Cell Count
Automated 85049
B-Cells 86355

Blood Smear 85007-85008
Differential WBC Count 85004-85007, 85009
Hematocrit 85014
Hemoglobin 85018
Hemogram
  Added Indices 85025-85027
  Automated 85025-85027
  Manual 85032
Microhematocrit 85013
Natural Killer (NK) Cells 86357
Red Blood Cells 85032-85041
Reticulocyte 85044-85046
Stem Cells 86367
T-Cells .86359-86361
White Blood Cells 85032, 85048, 89055

Blood Cell Count, Red
See Red Blood Cell (RBC), Count

Blood Cell Count, White
See White Blood Cell, Count

Blood Cell, Red
See Red Blood Cell (RBC)

Blood Cell, White
See Leukocyte

Blood Clot
Assay 85396
Clot Lysis Time 85175
Clot Retraction 85170
Clotting Factor 85250-85293
Clotting Factor Test 85210-85244
Clotting Inhibitors . . .85300-85302, 85305, 85307
Coagulation Time 85345-85348

Blood Coagulation
Defect
  See Coagulopathy
Disorders
  See Clot
Factor
  See Clotting Factor
Factor I
  See Fibrinogen
Factor II
  See Prothrombin
Factor III
  See Thromboplastin
Factor IV
  See Calcium
Factor VII
  See Proconvertin
Factor VIII
  See Clotting Factor
Factor IX
  See Christmas Factor
Factor X
  See Stuart-Prower Factor
Factor X, Activated
  See Thrombokinase
Factor XI
  See Plasma Thromboplastin, Antecedent
Factor XIII
  See Fibrin Stabilizing Factor
Test
  See Coagulation

Boil

See Furuncle

Boil, Vulva

See Abscess, Vulva

Bone

See Specific Bone
Ablation
    Tumor 20982
Biopsy 20220-20245
Carpal
    See Carpal Bone
Cheek
    See Cheekbone
CT Scan
    Density Study 77078-77079
Cyst
    Drainage 20615
    Injection 20615
Dual Energy X-Ray
Absorptiometry 77080-77081
Excision
    Epyphyseal Bar 20150
    Facial Bones 21026
    Mandible 21025
Facial
    See Facial Bone
Fixation
    Caliper 20660
    Cranial Tong 20660
    Halo 20661-20663, 21100
    Interdental 21110
    Multiplane 20692
    Pin/Wire 20650
    Skeletal
        Humeral Epicondyle
            Percutaneous 24566
    Stereotactic Frame 20660
    Uniplane 20690
Hyoid
    See Hyoid Bone
Insertion
    Needle 36680
    Osseointegrated Implant
        for External Speech Processor/Cochlear
        Stimulator 69714-69718
Metatarsal
    See Metatarsal Bone
Nasal
    See Nasal Bone
Navicular
    See Navicular
Nuclear Medicine
    Density Study 78350-78351
    Imaging 78300-78320
    SPECT 78320
    Unlisted Services and Procedures 78399
Protein 83937
Removal
    Fixation Device 20670-20680
Replacement
    Osseointegrated Implant
        for External Speech Processor/Cochlear
        Stimulator 69717-69718
Scan
    See Bone, Nuclear Medicine; Nuclear
    Medicine Imaging

Semilunar
    See Lunate
Sesamoid
    See Sesamoid Bone
Spur
    See Exostosis
Tarsal
    See Ankle Bone
Temporal
    See Temporal Bone
X-Ray
    Age Study 77072
    Dual Energy Absorptiometry ...77080-77081
    Length Study 77073
    Osseous Survey 77074-77077

Bone 4-Carboxyglutamic Protein

See Osteocalcin

Bone Conduction Hearing Device, Electromagnetic

Implantation/Replacement 69710
Removal/Repair 69711

Bone Density Study

Appendicular Skeleton 77079, 77081
Axial Skeleton 77078, 77080
Ultrasound 76977
Vertebral Fracture Assessment 77082

Bone Graft

Augmentation
    Mandibular Body 21127
Femur 27170
Fracture
    Orbit 21408
Harvesting 20900-20902
Malar Area 21210
Mandible 21215
Mandibular Ramus 21194
Maxilla 21210
Microvascular Anastomosis
    Fibula 20955
    Other 20962
Nasal Area 21210
Nasomaxillary Complex Fracture 21348
Open Treatment
    Craniofacial Separation 21436
Osteocutaneous Flap 20969-20973
Reconstruction
    Mandibular Rami 21194
    Midface 21145-21160
Skull 61316
    Excision 62148
Spine Surgery
    Allograft
        Morselized 20930
        Structural 20931
    Autograft
        Local 20936
        Morselized 20937
        Structural 20938
Vascular Pedicle 25430

Bone Healing

Electrical Stimulation
    Invasive 20975
    Noninvasive 20974
Ultrasound Stimulation 20979

Bone Infection

See Osteomyelitis

Bone Marrow

Aspiration 38220
Harvesting 38230
Magnetic Resonance Imaging (MRI) 77084
Needle Biopsy 38221
Nuclear Medicine
    Imaging 78102-78104
Smear 85097
T-Cell Transplantation 38240-38242
Trocar Biopsy 38221

Bone Plate

Mandible 21244

Bone Wedge Reversal

Osteotomy 21122

Bordetella

Antibody 86615
Antigen Detection
    Direct Fluorescence 87265

Borrelia

Antibody 86618-86619

Borrelia burgdorferi ab

See Antibody, Lyme Disease

Borreliosis, Lyme

See Lyme Disease

Borthen Operation

See Iridotasis

Bost Fusion

See Arthrodesis, Wrist

Bosworth Operation

See Acromioclavicular Joint, Dislocation;
Arthrodesis, Vertebrae; Fasciotomy,

Bottle Type Procedure 55060

Botulinum Toxin

See Chemodenervation

Boutonniere Deformity 26426-26428

Bowel

See Intestine

Bowleg Repair 27455-27457

Boyce Operation

See Nephrotomy

Boyd Hip Disarticulation

See Amputation, Leg, Upper; Radical Resection;
Replantation

Brace

See Cast
for Leg Cast 29358

Brachial Arteries

See Artery, Brachial

Cardiomyotomy
See Esophagomyotomy

Cardioplasty 43320

Cardiopulmonary Bypass 33926
See Heart; Lung, Transplantation

Cardiopulmonary Resuscitation 92950

Cardiotomy 33310-33315

Cardiovascular Stress Test
See Exercise Stress Tests

Cardioversion 92960-92961

Care
Custodial
   See Nursing Facility Services
Intensive
   See Intensive Care
Neonatal Intensive
   See Intensive Care, Neonatal
Self
   See Self Care

Care Plan Oversight Services
See Physician Services

Carneous Mole
See Abortion

Carnitine 82379

Carotene 82380

Caroticum, Glomus
See Carotid Body

Carotid Artery
Aneurysm Repair
   Vascular Malformation or Carotid-Cavernous
   Fistula 61710
Excision 60605
Ligation 37600-37606
Stent, Transcatheter Placement 0075T-0076T
Transection
   with Skull Base Surgery 61609

Carotid Body
Lesion
   Carotid Artery 60605
   Excision 60600

Carpal Bone
See Wrist
Arthroplasty
   with Implant 25443
Cyst
   Excision 25130-25136
Dislocation
   Closed Treatment 25690
   Open Treatment 25695
Excision 25210-25215
   Partial 25145
Fracture
   Closed Treatment 25622, 25630
   Open Treatment 25628, 25645
   with Manipulation 25624, 25635
   without Manipulation 25630

Incision and Drainage 26034
Insertion
   Vascular Pedicle 25430
Osteoplasty 25394
Repair 25431-25440
Sequestrectomy 25145
Tumor
   Excision 25130-25136

Carpal Tunnel
Injection
   Therapeutic 20526

Carpal Tunnel Syndrome
Decompression 64721

Carpals
Incision and Drainage 25035

Carpectomy 25210-25215

Carpometacarpal Joint
Arthrodesis
   Hand 26843-26844
   Thumb 26841-26842
Arthrotomy 26070
Biopsy
   Synovium 26100
Dislocation
   Closed Treatment 26670
     with Manipulation 26675-26676
   Open Treatment 26685-26686
Exploration 26070
Fusion
   Hand 26843-26844
   Thumb 26841-26842
Removal
   Foreign Body 26070
Repair 25447
Synovectomy 26130

Cartilage Graft
Ear to Face 21235
Harvesting 20910-20912
Rib to Face 21230

Cartilage, Arytenoid
See Arytenoid

Cartilage, Ear
See Ear Cartilage

Cartilaginous Exostoses
See Exostosis

Case Management Services
Anticoagulant Management 99363-99364
Team Conferences 99361-99373
Telephone Calls 99361-99373

Cast
See Brace; Splint
Body
   Risser Jacket 29010-29015
Body Cast
   Halo 29000
   Turnbuckle Jacket 29020-29025
   Upper Body and Head 29040
   Upper Body and Legs 29046

   Upper Body and One Leg 29044
   Upper Body Only 29035
Clubfoot 29450
Cylinder 29365
Finger 29086
Hand 29085
Hip 29305-29325
Leg
   Rigid Total Contact 29445
Long Arm 29065
Long Leg 29345-29355, 29365, 29450
Long Leg Brace 29358
Patellar Tendon Bearing (PTB) 29435
Removal 29700-29715
Repair 29720
Short Arm 29075
Short Leg 29405-29435, 29450
Shoulder 29049-29058
Walking 29355, 29425
   Revision 29440
Wedging 29740-29750
Windowing 29730
Wrist 29085

Casting
Unlisted Services and Procedures 29799

Castration
See Orchiectomy

Castration, Female
See Oophorectomy

CAT Scan
See CT Scan

Cataract
Excision 66830
Incision 66820-66821
   Laser 66821
   Stab Incision 66820
Removal/Extraction
   Extracapsular 66982, 66984
   Intracapsular 66983

Catecholamines 80424, 82382-82384
Blood 82383
Urine 82382

Cathepsin-D 82387

Catheter
See Cannulization; Venipuncture
Aspiration
   Nasotracheal 31720
   Tracheobronchial 31725
Bladder 51701-51703
   Irrigation 51700
Breast Cytology 0046T, 0047T
Declotting 36550
Exchange
   Intravascular 37209, 75900
   Peritoneal 49423
Intracatheter
   Irrigation 99507
   Obstruction Clearance 36596
Pericatheter
   Obstruction
     Clearance 36595

Cell, Mother
See Stem Cell

Cell-Stimulating Hormone, Interstitial
See Luteinizing Hormone (LH)

Cellobiase
See Beta Glucosidase

Cellular Inclusion
See Inclusion Bodies

Central Shunt 33764

Central Venous Catheter Placement
Insertion
 Central 36555-36558
 Peripheral 36568-36569
Repair 36575
Replacement 36580-36585
Repositioning 36597

Central Venous Catheter Removal 36589

Cephalic Version
of Fetus
 External 59412

Cephalocele
See Encephalocele

Cephalogram, Orthodontic
See Orthodontic Cephalogram

Cerclage
Cervix 57700
 Abdominal 59325
 Removal Under Anesthesia 59871
 Vaginal 59320

Cerebellopontine Angle Tumor
See Brain, Tumor, Excision; Brainstem; Mesencephalon; Skull Base Surgery

Cerebral Cortex Decortication
See Decortication

Cerebral Death
See Brain Death

Cerebral Hernia
See Encephalocele

Cerebral Perfusion Analysis ...0042T

Cerebral Thermography
See Thermogram, Cephalic

Cerebral Ventriculographies
See Ventriculography

Cerebral Vessels
Angioplasty 61630
Dilation
 Intracranial Vasospasm 61640-61642
Occlusion 61623
Placement
 Stent 61635

Cerebrose
See Galactose

Cerebrospinal Fluid 86325
Nuclear Imaging 78630-78650

Cerebrospinal Fluid Leak 63744
Brain
 Repair 61618-61619, 62100
Nasal/Sinus Endoscopy
 Repair 31290-31291
Spinal Cord
 Repair 63707-63709

Cerebrospinal Fluid Shunt 63740, 63746
Creation 62180-62192, 62200-62223
Irrigation 62194
Removal 62256-62258
Replacement 62160, 62194, 62225-62230
Reprogramming 62252

Ceruloplasmin 82390

Cerumen
Removal 69210

Cervical Cap 57170

Cervical Lymphadenectomy 38720-38724

Cervical Mucus Penetration Test 89330

Cervical Plexus
Injection
 Anesthetic 64413

Cervical Pregnancy 59140

Cervical Puncture 61050-61055

Cervical Smears 88141, 88155, 88164-88167, 88174-88175
See Cytopathology

Cervical Spine
See Vertebra, Cervical

Cervical Sympathectomy
See Sympathectomy, Cervical

Cervicectomy 57530

Cervicography 0003T

Cervicoplasty 15819

Cervicothoracic Ganglia
See Stellate Ganglion

Cervix
See Cytopathology
Amputation
 Total 57530
Biopsy 57500, 57520
 Colposcopy 57454-57455, 57460
Cauterization 57522
 Cryocautery 57511
 Electro or Thermal 57510
 Laser Ablation 57513
Cerclage 57700
 Abdominal 59325
 Removal Under Anesthesia 59871
 Vaginal 59320

Cervicography 0003T
Colposcopy 57452-57461
Conization 57461, 57520-57522
Curettage
 Endocervical 57454, 57456, 57505
Dilation
 Canal 57800
 Stump 57558
Dilation and Curettage 57558
Ectopic Pregnancy 59140
Excision
 Radical 57531
 Stump
  Abdominal Approach 57540-57545
  Vaginal Approach 57550-57556
 Total 57530
Exploration
 Endoscopy 57452
Insertion
 Dilation 59200
 Laminaria 59200
 Prostaglandin 59200
 Sensor, Fetal Oximetry 0021T
Repair
 Cerclage 57700
 Abdominal 59325
 Suture 57720
 Vaginal 59320
Unlisted Services and Procedures 58999

Cesarean Delivery
Antepartum Care 59610, 59618
Delivery
 after Attempted Vaginal Delivery 59618
  Delivery Only 59620
  Postpartum Care 59622
  Routine Care 59610, 59618
Delivery Only 59514
Postpartum Care 59515
Routine Care 59510
Tubal Ligation at Time of 58611
with Hysterectomy 59525

CGMP
See Cyclic GMP

Chalazion
Excision 67805
 Multiple
  Different Lids 67805
  Same Lid 67801
 Single 67800
 Under Anesthesia 67808

Challenge Tests
Bronchial Ingestion 95070-95075

Chambers Procedure 28300

Change
Catheter
 Bile Duct 75984
Fetal Position
 by Manipulation 59412
Tube or Stent
 Endoscopic
  Bile or Pancreatic Duct 43269

Change of, Dressing
See Dressings, Change

Cholangiostomy
See Hepaticostomy

Cholangiotomy
See Hepaticostomy

Cholecalciferol
See Vitamin, D-3

Cholecystectomy 47562-47564,
                                                            47600-47620
Any Method 47562-47564
    with Cholangiography . .47563, 47605, 47620
    with Exploration Common
    Duct .... .47564, 47610

Cholecystenterostomy .... .47570,
                                                            47720-47741

Cholecystography 74290-74291

Cholecystotomy .... .47480, 48001
Percutaneous .... .47490

Choledochoplasty
See Bile Duct, Repair

Choledochoscopy .... .47550

Choledochostomy 47420-47425

Choledochotomy 47420-47425

Choledochus, Cyst
See Cyst, Choledochal

Cholera Vaccine
Injectable .... .90725

Cholesterol
Measurement .... .83721
Serum .... .82465
Testing 83718-83719

Choline Esterase I
See Acetylcholinesterase

Choline Esterase II
See Cholinesterase

Cholinesterase
Blood 82480-82482

Cholylglycine
Blood .... .82240

Chondroitin Sulfate .... .82485

Chondromalacia Patella
Repair .... .27418

Chondropathia Patellae
See Chondromalacia Patella

Chondrosteoma
See Exostosis

Chopart Procedure 28800-28805
See Amputation, Foot; Radical Resection;
Replantation

Chordotomies
See Cordotomy

Chorioangioma
See Lesion, Skin

Choriogonadotropin
See Chorionic Gonadotropin

Choriomeningitides, Lymphocytic
See Lymphocytic Choriomeningitis

Chorionic Gonadotropin ...... .80414,
                                                            84702-84703
Stimulation 80414-80415

Chorionic Growth Hormone
See Lactogen, Human Placental

Chorionic Tumor
See Hydatidiform Mole

Chorionic Villi
See Biopsy, Chorionic Villus

Chorionic Villus
Biopsy .... .59015

Choroid
Destruction
    Lesion .... .0016T, 67220-67225

Choroid Plexus
Excision .... .61544

Christmas Factor .... .85250

Chromaffinoma, Medullary
See Pheochromocytoma

Chromatin, Sex
See Barr Bodies

Chromatography
Column/Mass Spectrometry 82541-82544
Gas Liquid or HPLC .... .82486, 82491-82492
Paper 82487-82488
Thin-Layer .... .82489

Chromium .... .82495

Chromogenic Substrate Assay .85130

Chromosome Analysis
See Amniocentesis
Added Study 88280-88289
Amniotic Fluid 88267-88269
    Culture .... .88235
Biopsy Culture
    Tissue .... .88233
Bone Marrow Culture .... .88237
Chorionic Villus .... .88267
    5 Cells .... .88261
    15-20 Cells .... .88262
    20-25 Cells .... .88264
    45 Cells .... .88263
    Culture .... .88235
for Breakage Syndromes 88245-88249
Fragile-X .... .88248
Lymphocyte Culture .... .88230
Pregnancy Associated Plasma Protein-A . . .84163
Skin Culture
    Tissue .... .88233

Tissue Culture .... .88239
Unlisted Services and Procedures .... .88299

Chromotubation .... .58350
Oviduct .... .58350

Chronic Erection
See Priapism

Chronic Interstitial Cystitides
See Cystitis, Interstitial

Ciliary Body
Cyst
    Destruction
        Cryotherapy .... .66720
        Cyclodialysis .... .66740
        Cyclophotocoagulation 66710-66711
        Diathermy .... .66700
        Nonexcisional .... .66770
Destruction
    Cyclophotocoagulation 66710-66711
    Endoscopic .... .66711
Lesion
    Destruction .... .66770
Repair .... .66680

Cimino Type Procedure .... .36821

Cinefluorographies
See Cineradiography

Cineplasty
Arm, Lower or Upper .... .24940

Cineradiography
Esophagus .... .74230
Pharynx .... .70371, 74230
Speech Evaluation .... .70371
Swallowing Evaluation .... .74230
Unlisted Services and Procedures . .76120-76125

Circulation Assist
Aortic .... .33967, 33970
Balloon .... .33967, 33970
External 33960-33961

Circulation, Extracorporeal
See Extracorporeal Circulation

Circulatory Assist
See Circulation Assist

Circumcision
Repair .... .54163
Surgical Excision .... .54161
    Newborn .... .54160
with Clamp or Other Device .... .54152
    Newborn .... .54150

Cisternal Puncture 61050-61055

Cisternography .... .70015
Nuclear .... .78630

Citrate
Blood or Urine .... .82507

Clagett Procedure
See Chest Wall, Repair, Closure

Factor XI
  See Plasma Thromboplastin, Antecedent
Factor XII
  See Hageman Factor
Factor XIII
  See Fibrin Stabilizing Factor

Coagulation Time 85345-85348

Coagulation, Blood
See Blood Clot

Coagulation, Light
See Photocoagulation

Coagulin
See Thromboplastin

Coagulopathy .... .85390
Assay .... .85130

Cocaine
Blood or Urine .... .82520
Screen .... .82486

Coccidioides
Antibody .... .86635

Coccidioidin Test
See Streptokinase, Antibody

Coccidioidomycosis
Skin Test .... .86490

Coccygeal Spine Fracture
See Coccyx, Fracture

Coccygectomy 15920-15922, 27080

Coccyx
Excision .... .27080
Fracture
    Closed Treatment .... .27200
    Open Treatment .... .27202
Tumor
    Excision .... .49215
X-Ray .... .72220

Cochlear Device
Insertion .... .69930
Programming 92601-92604

Codeine
Alkaloid Screening .... .82101

Codeine Screen .... .82486

Cofactor Protein S
See Protein S

Coffey Operation
See Uterus, Repair, Suspension

Cognitive Function Tests .... .96116
See Neurology, Diagnostic

Cognitive Skills
Development .... .97532
See Physical Medicine/Therapy/Occupational
Therapy

Cold Agglutinin 86156-86157

Cold Pack Treatment .... .97010

Cold Preservation
See Cryopreservation

Cold Therapies
See Cryotherapy

Colectomy
Partial .... .44140
    Laparoscopic .... .44213
    with Anastomosis .... .44140
      Laparoscopic .... .44204, 44207-44208
    with Coloproctostomy 44145-44146
    with Colostomy 44141-44144
      Laparoscopic .... .44206, 44208
    with Ileocolostomy
      Laparoscopic .... .44205
    with Ileostomy .... .44144
    with Ileum Removal .... .44160
    with Transcanal Approach .... .44147
Total
    Laparoscopic 44210-44212
      with Proctectomy and
      Ileostomy 44210-44212
      without Proctectomy .... .44210
    Open
      with Complete Proctectomy ...... .45121
      with Ileostomy 44150-44151
      with Proctectomy 44155-44158

Collagen Cross Links .... .82523

Collagen Injection 11950-11954

Collar Bone
See Clavicle

Collateral Ligament
Ankle
    Repair 27695-27698
Interphalangeal Joint .... .26545
Knee Joint
    Repair .... .27409
Knee Repair .... .27405
Metacarpophalangeal Joint 26540-26542
Repair
    Ankle 27695-27698

Collection and Processing
Allogenic Blood
    Harvesting of Stem Cells .... .38205
Autologous Blood
    Harvesting of Stem Cells .... .38206
    Intraoperative .... .86891
    Preoperative .... .86890
Specimen
    Capillary Blood .... .36416
    Venous Blood .... .36415, 36540
Washings
    Esophagus .... .91000
    Stomach .... .91055

Colles Fracture 25600-25605

Colles Fracture Reversed
See Smith Fracture

Collins Syndrome, Treacher
See Treacher-Collins Syndrome

Collis Procedure
See Gastroplasty with Esophagogastric
Fundoplasty

Colon
See Colon-Sigmoid
Biopsy .... .44025, 44100, 44322
    Endoscopic ..... .44389, 45380, 45391-45392
Colostomy
    Revision 44340-44346
Colotomy .... .44322
    Colostomy .... .44320
CT Scan
    Colonography .... .0066T, 0067T
    Virtual Colonoscopy .... .0066T, 0067T
Destruction
    Lesion .... .44393, 45383
    Tumor .... .44393, 45383
Endoscopy
    Biopsy .... .44389, 45380, 45391-45392
    Destruction
      Lesion .... .44393
      Tumor .... .44393, 45383
    Dilation .... .45386
    Exploration .... .44388, 45378, 45381, 45386
    Hemorrhage .... .44391, 45382
    Injection, Submucosal .... .45381
    Placement
      Stent .... .45387
    Removal
      Foreign Body .... .44390, 45379
      Polyp .... .44392, 45384-45385
      Tumor 45384-45385
    Specimen Collection .... .45380
    Ultrasound 45391-45392
    via Colotomy .... .45355
    via Stoma 44388-44397
    Virtual .... .0066T, 0067T
Excision
    Partial 44140-44147, 44160
      Laparoscopic 44204-44208
    Total 44150-44158
      Laparoscopic 44210-44212
Exploration .... .44025
    Endoscopy ..... .44388, 45378, 45381, 45386
Hemorrhage
    Endoscopic Control .... .44391, 45382
Hernia .... .44050
Incision
    Creation
      Stoma 44320-44322
    Exploration .... .44025
    Revision
      Stoma 44340-44346
Lavage
    Intraoperative .... .44701
Lesion
    Destruction .... .45383
    Excision 44110-44111
Lysis
    Adhesions .... .44005
Obstruction 44025-44050
Reconstruction
    Bladder from .... .50810
Removal
    Foreign Body .... .44025, 44390, 45379
    Polyp .... .44392

Common Sensory Nerve
Repair/Suture 64834

Common Truncus
See Truncus Arteriosus

Communication Device
Non-Speech-Generating 92605-92606
Speech-Generating 92606-92609

Community/Work Reintegration
Training 97537
   See Physical Medicine/Therapy/Occupational
   Therapy

Compatibility Test
Blood 86920, 86923

Complement
Antigen 86160
Fixation Test 86171
Functional Activity 86161
Hemolytic
   Total 86162
Total 86162

**Complete Blood Count
(CBC)** 85025-85027
See Blood Cell Count

Complete Colectomy
See Colectomy, Total

Complete Pneumonectomy
See Pneumonectomy, Completion

**Complete Transposition of Great
Vessels**
See Transposition, Great Arteries

Complex, Factor IX
See Christmas Factor

Complex, Vitamin B
See B Complex Vitamins

Component Removal, Blood
See Apheresis

Composite Graft 15760-15770,
                                      35681-35683

Compound B
See Corticosterone

Compound F
See Cortisol

Compression, Nerve, Median
See Carpal Tunnel Syndrome

**Computed Tomographic
Scintigraphy**
See Emission Computerized Tomography

Computed Tomography (CT)
See CT Scan; Specific Anatomic Site

Computer Analysis
Acoustic Recording
   Heart Sounds
      with Computer Analysis 0068T-0069T,
                                      0070T

Computer Assisted Navigation
Orthopedic Surgery 0054T, 0055T, 0056T

Computer Data Analysis 99090

Computer-aided Detection
Chest X-Ray 0152T
Mammography 77051-77052
   Magnetic Resonance Imaging (MRI) . . .0159T

**Computer-Assisted Psychological
Testing** 96103

**Computerized Emission
Tomography**
See Emission Computerized Tomography

Concentration of Specimen 87015

Concentration, Hydrogen-Ion
See pH

Concentration, Minimum Inhibitory
See Minimum Inhibitory Concentration

Concentric Procedure 28296

Concha Bullosa Resection
with Nasal/Sinus Endoscopy 31240

Conchae Nasale
See Nasal Turbinate

Conduction, Nerve
See Nerve Conduction

Conduit, Ileal
See Ileal Conduit

Condyle
Humerus
   Fracture
      Closed Treatment 24576-24577
      Open Treatment 24579
      Percutaneous 24582
Metatarsal
   Excision 28288
Phalanges
   Toe
      Excision 28126

Condyle, Mandibular
See Mandibular Condyle

Condylectomy
Temporomandibular Joint 21050
with Skull Base Surgery 61596-61597

Condyloma
Destruction 54050-54065

Conference
Medical
   with Interdisciplinary Team 99361-99373

Confirmation
Drug 80102

**Congenital Arteriovenous
Malformation**
See Arteriovenous Malformation

Congenital Elevation of Scapula
See Sprengel's Deformity

Congenital Heart Septum Defect
See Septal Defect

Congenital Kidney Abnormality
Nephrolithotomy 50070
Pyeloplasty 50405
Pyelotomy 50135

Congenital Laryngocele
See Laryngocele

Congenital Vascular Anomaly
See Vascular Malformation

Conisation
See Cervix, Conization

Conization
Cervix 57461, 57520-57522

Conjoint Psychotherapy 90847
See Psychiatric Treatment, Family

Conjunctiva
Biopsy 68100
Cyst
   Incision and Drainage 68020
Fistulize for Drainage
   with Tube 68750
   without Tube .68745
Graft 65782
   Harvesting 68371
Harvesting 68371
Incision 0124T
Insertion Stent .68750
Lesion
   Destruction 68135
   Excision 68110-68130
      Over 1 cm .68115
      with Adjacent Sclera 68130
Reconstruction 68320-68335
   Symblepharon
      with Graft .68335
   with Flap
      Bridge or Partial 68360
      Total 68362
Repair
   Symblepharon
      Division 68340
      with Graft .68335
      without Graft 68330
   Wound
      Direct Closure 65270
      Mobilization and Rearrangement . . .65272-
                                            65273
Unlisted Services and Procedures 68399

**Conjunctivo-Tarso-Muller
Resection** 67908

Conjunctivocystorhinostomy
See Conjunctivorhinostomy

Conjunctivodacryocystostomy
See Conjunctivorhinostomy

**Coronary Artery Bypass Graft
(CABG)** 33503-33505, 33510-33516
Arterial 33533-33536
Arterial Graft 33548
Arterial-Venous 33517-33523
Harvest
   Upper Extremity Artery 35600
Reoperation 33530
Venous 33510-33516

Coronary Endarterectomy 33572

Coroner's Exam 88045

Coronoidectomy
Temporomandibular Joint 21070

Corpectomy 63101-63103

Corpora Cavernosa
Corpus Spongiosum Shunt 54430
Glans Penis Fistulization 54435
Injection 54235
Irrigation
   Priapism 54220
Saphenous Vein Shunt 54420
X-Ray with Contrast 74445

**Corpora Cavernosa, Plastic
Induration**
See Peyronie Disease

Corpora Cavernosography 74445

Corpus Callosum
Transection 61541

Corpus Vertebrae (Vertebrale)
See Vertebral Body

Correction of Cleft Palate
See Cleft Palate, Repair

Correction of Lid Retraction
See Repair, Eyelid, Retraction

**Correction of Malrotation of
Duodenum**
See Ladd Procedure

Correction of Syndactyly
See Syndactyly, Repair

**Correction of Ureteropelvic
Junction**
See Pyeloplasty

Cortex Decortication, Cerebral
See Decortication

Cortical Mapping
Transection
   by Electric Stimulation 95961-95962

Corticoids
See Corticosteroids

Corticoliberin
See Corticotropic Releasing Hormone (CRH)

Corticosteroid Binding Globulin
See Transcortin

Corticosteroid Binding Protein
See Transcortin

Corticosteroids
Blood 83491
Urine 83491

Corticosterone
Blood or Urine 82528

**Corticotropic Releasing Hormone
(CRH)** 80412

Cortisol 80400-80406, 80418-80420,
80436, 82530
Stimulation 80412
Total 82533

Cortisol Binding Globulin 84449

Costectomy
See Resection, Ribs

Costen Syndrome
See Temporomandibular Joint (TMJ)

Costotransversectomy 21610

Cothromboplastin
See Proconvertin

Cotte Operation 58400-58410
See Repair, Uterus, Suspension; Revision

Cotton Procedure
Bohler Procedure 28405

Counseling
See Preventive Medicine

**Counseling and/or Risk Factor
Reduction InterventionPreventive
Medicine, Individual Counseling**
See Preventive Medicine, Counseling and/or Risk
Factor Reduction Intervention, Individual
Counseling

Count
Blood Cell
   See Blood Cell Count
Blood Platelet
   See Blood, Platelet, Count
Cell
   See Cell Count
Complete Blood
   See Complete Blood Count (CBC)
Erythrocyte
   See Red Blood Cell (RBC), Count
Leukocyte
   See White Blood Cell, Count
Reticulocyte
   See Reticulocyte, Count

**Counterimmuno-
electrophoresis** 86185

Counters, Cell
See Cell Count

Countershock, Electric
See Cardioversion

Coventry Tibial Wedge Osteotomy
See Osteotomy, Tibia

Cowper's Gland
Excision 53250

Coxa
See Hip

Coxiella Burnetii
Antibody 86638

Coxsackie
Antibody 86658

CPAP
See Continuous Positive Airway Pressure

CPK
Blood 82550-82552

**CPR (Cardiopulmonary
Resuscitation)** 92950

Cranial Bone
Halo
   Thin Skull Osteology 20664
Reconstruction
   Extracranial 21181-21184
Tumor
   Excision 61563-61564

Cranial Halo 20661

Cranial Nerve
Avulsion 64732-64760, 64771
Cranial Nerve II
   See Optic Nerve
Cranial Nerve V
   See Trigeminal Nerve
Cranial Nerve VII
   See Facial Nerve
Cranial Nerve X
   See Vagus Nerve
Cranial Nerve XI
   See Accessory Nerve
Cranial Nerve XII
   See Hypoglossal Nerve
Decompression 61458, 64716
Implantation
   Electrode 64553, 64573
Incision 64732-64752, 64760, 65771
Injection
   Anesthetic 64400-64408, 64412
   Neurolytic 64600-64610
Insertion
   Electrode 64553, 64573
Neuroplasty 64716
Release 64716
Repair
   Suture, with or without Graft . . .64864-64865
Section 61460
Transection 64732-64760, 64771
Transposition 64716

Cranial Tongs
Application/Removal 20660
Removal 20665

Retinal Detachment
 Prophylaxis 67141
 Repair 67101
Trichiasis
 Correction 67825

Cryptectomy 46210-46211

Cryptococcus
Antibody 86641
Antigen Detection
 Enzyme Immunoassay 87327

Cryptococcus Neoformans
Antigen Detection
 Enzyme Immunoassay 87327

Cryptorchism
See Testis, Undescended

Cryptosporidium
Antigen Detection
 Direct Fluorescence 87272
 Enzyme Immunoassay 87328

Crystal Identification
Any Body Fluid 89060
Tissue 89060

CSF
See Cerebrospinal Fluid Leak

CT Angiography
Coronary Arteries 0146T, 0148T
 Coronary Calcium Evaluation ...0147T, 0149T

CT Scan
3D Rendering 76376-76377
Bone
 Density Study 77078-77079
Drainage 75989
Follow-up Study 76380
Guidance
 Localization 77011
 Needle Placement 77012
 Parenchymal Tissue Ablation 77013
 Radiation Therapy 77014
 Vertebroplasty 72292
Unlisted Services and Procedures 76497
with Contrast 70460
 Abdomen 74160
 Arm 73201
 Brain 0042T, 70460
 Cerebral Blood Flow/Volume 0042T
 Ear 70481
 Face 70487
 Head 70460
 Leg 73701
 Maxilla 70487
 Neck 70491
 Orbit 70481
 Pelvis 72193
 Sella Turcica 70481
 Spine
  Cervical 72126
  Lumbar 72132
  Thoracic 72129
 Thorax 71260
without and with Contrast
 Abdomen 74170-74175, 75635

Arm 73202-73206
Brain 70470, 70496
Chest 71275
Ear 70482
Face 70488
Head 70470, 70496
Heart
 3D Rendering 0145T, 0146T, 0147T,
           0148T, 0149T, 0150T-0151T
 Coronary Calcium Evaluation .0147T, 0149T
 Functional Evaluation 0151T
 Morphology ...0145T, 0148T, 0149T, 0150T
Leg 73702-73706, 75635
Maxilla 70488
Neck 70492, 70498
Orbit 70482
Pelvis 72191, 72194
Sella Turcica 70482
Spine
 Cervical 72127
 Lumbar 72133
 Thoracic 72130
Thorax 71270-71275
without Contrast 70450
 Abdomen 74150
 Arm 73200
 Brain 70450
 Colon
  Colonography 0066T, 0067T
  Virtual Colonoscopy 0066T, 0067T
 Ear 70480
 Face 70486
 Head 70450
 Heart
  3D Rendering 0144T
  Coronary Calcium Evaluation 0144T
 Leg 73700
 Maxilla 70486
 Neck 70490
 Orbit 70480
 Pelvis 72192
 Sella Turcica 70480
 Spine
  Cervical 72125
  Lumbar 72131
  Thoracic 72128
 Thorax 71250

CT Scan, Radionuclide
See Emission Computerized Tomography

Cuff, Rotator
See Rotator Cuff

Culdocentesis
See Colpocentesis

Culture
Acid Fast Bacilli 87116
Amniotic Fluid
 Chromosome Analysis 88235
Bacteria
 Additional Methods 87077
 Aerobic 87040-87070
 Anaerobic 87073-87076
 Blood 87040
 Other 87070-87073
 Screening 87081

Stool 87045-87046
Urine 87086-87088
Bone Marrow
 Chromosome Analysis 88237
Chlamydia 87110
Chorionic Villus
 Chromosome Analysis 88235
Fertilized Oocytes
 for In Vitro Fertilization 89250
  Co-Culture of Embryo 89251
Fungus
 Blood 87103
 Hair 87101
 Identification 87106
 Nail 87101
 Other 87102
 Skin 87101
Lymphocyte
 Chromosome Analysis 88230
Mold 87107
Mycobacteria 87116-87118
Mycoplasma 87109
Oocyte/Embryo 89250
 Co-Culture of Oocyte/Embryo 89251
 Extended Culture 89272
Pathogen
 by Kit 87084
Skin
 Chromosome Analysis 88233
Tissue
 Toxin/Antitoxin 87230
 Virus 87252-87253
Tubercle Bacilli 87116
Typing 87140-87158
Unlisted Services and Procedures 87999
Yeast 87106

Curettage
See Dilation and Curettage
Cervix
 Endocervical 57454, 57456, 57505
Cornea 65435-65436
 Chelating Agent 65436
Hydatidiform Mole 59870
Postpartum 59160

Curettage and Dilatation
See Dilation and Curettage

Curettage, Uterus
See Uterus, Curettage

Curettement
Skin Lesion 11055-11057, 17004, 17110,
            17270, 17280

Curietherapy
See Brachytherapy

Custodial Care
See Domiciliary Services; Nursing Facility
Services

Cutaneolipectomy
See Lipectomy

**Cutaneous Electrostimulation,
Analgesic**
See Application, Neurostimulation

Cutaneous Tag
See Skin, Tags

Cutaneous Tissue
See Integumentary System

Cutaneous-Vesicostomy
See Vesicostomy, Cutaneous

CVS
See Biopsy, Chorionic Villus

Cyanacobalamin
See Cyanocobalamin

Cyanide
Blood 82600
Tissue 82600

Cyanocobalamin 82607-82608

Cyclic AMP 82030

Cyclic GMP 83008

Cyclic Somatostatin
See Somatostatin

Cyclocryotherapy
See Cryotherapy, Destruction, Ciliary Body

Cyclodialysis
Destruction
　Ciliary Body 66740

Cyclophotocoagulation
Destruction
　Ciliary Body 66710-66711

Cyclosporine
Assay 80158

Cyst
Abdomen
　Destruction/Excision 49200-49201
Ankle
　Capsule 27630
　Tendon Sheath 27630
Bartholin's Gland Excision 56740
　See Bartholin's Gland, Cyst
　Repair 56440
Bile Duct 47715
Bladder
　Excision 51500
Bone
　Drainage 20615
　Injection 20615
Brain
　Drainage .61150-61151, 61156, 62161-62162
　Excision 61516, 61524, 62162
Branchial Cleft
　Excision 42810-42815
Breast
　Incision and Drainage 19020
　Puncture Aspiration 19000-19001
Calcaneus 28100-28103
Carpal 25130-25136
Choledochal 47715, 47719
Ciliary Body
　Destruction 66770

Clavicle
　Excision 23140-23146
Conjunctiva 68020
Dermoid
　Nose
　　Excision 30124-30125
Drainage
　Contrast Injection 49424
　with X-Ray 76080
Excision
　Cheekbone 21030
　Clavicle 23140
　　with Allograft 23146
　　with Autograft 23145
　Femur 27355-27358
　Ganglion
　　See Ganglion
　Humerus
　　with Allograft 23156
　　with Autograft 23155
　Hydatid
　　See Echinococcosis
　Lymphatic
　　See Lymphocele
　Maxilla 21030
　Mediastinum 32662
　Olecranon Process
　　with Allograft 24126
　　with Autograft 24125
　Pericardial 32661
　Pilonidal 11770-11772
　Radius
　　with Allograft 24126
　　with Autograft 24125
　Scapula 23140
　　with Allograft 23146
　　with Autograft 23145
　Ulna
　　with Allograft 24126
　　with Autograft 24125
　Zygoma 21030
Facial Bones
　Excision 21030
Femur 27065-27067
Fibula 27635-27638
Ganglion
　Aspiration/Injection 20612
Gums
　Incision and Drainage 41800
Hip 27065-27067
Humerus
　Excision 23150-23156, 24110
　　with Allograft 24116
　　with Autograft 24115
Ileum 27065-27067
Incision and Drainage 10060-10061
　Pilonidal 10080-10081
Iris
　Destruction 66770
Kidney
　Ablation 50541
　Aspiration 50390
　Excision 50280-50290
　Injection 50390
　X-Ray 74470

Knee
　Baker's 27345
　Excision 27347
Leg, Lower
　Capsule 27630
　Tendon Sheath 27630
Liver 47010
　Drainage 47010
　Open 47010
　Repair 47300
Lung
　Incision and Drainage 32200
　Removal 32140
Lymph Node
　Axillary/Cervical
　　Excision 38550-38555
Mandible
　Excision 21040, 21046-21047
Maxilla
　Excision 21030, 21048-21049
Mediastinal
　Excision 39200
Metacarpal 26200-26205
Metatarsal 28104-28107
Mouth 41005-41009, 41015-41018
　Incision and Drainage 40800-40801
Mullerian Duct
　Excision 55680
Nose
　Excision 30124-30125
Olecranon 24120
Ovarian
　Excision 58925
　Incision and Drainage 58800-58805
Pancreas 48500
　Anastomosis 48520-48540
　Excision 48120
Pelvis
　Aspiration 50390
　Injection 50390
Pericardial
　Excision 33050
Phalanges
　Finger 26210-26215
　Toe 28108
Pilonidal
　Excision 11770-11772
　Incision and Drainage 10080-10081
Pubis 27065-27067
Radius 24120, 25120-25126
Rathke's Pouch
　See Craniopharyngioma
Removal
　Skin 10040
Retroperitoneal
　Destruction/Excision 49200-49201
Salivary Gland Creation
　Destruction/Excision
　Drainage 42409
　Excision 42408
Scapula
　Excision 23140-23146
Seminal Vesicle
　Excision 55680
Skin
　Puncture Aspiration 10160

Spinal Cord
    Aspiration 62268
    Incision and Drainage 63172-63173
Sublingual Gland Drainage 42409
    Excision 42408
Talus 28100-28103
Tarsal 28104-28107
Thyroglossal Duct
    Excision 60280-60281
    Incision and Drainage 60000
Thyroid Gland Aspiration 60001
    Excision 60200
    Injection 60001
Tibia 27635-27638
Tongue 41000-41006, 41015
Ulna 24120, 25120-25126
Urachal
    Bladder
      Excision 51500
Vaginal
    Excision 57135
Wrist 25130-25136
    Excision 25111-25112
Zygoma
    Excision 21030

Cyst Ovary
See Ovary, Cyst

Cystatins, Kininogen
See Kininogen

Cystectomy
Complete 51570
    with Bilateral Pelvic
      Lymphadenectomy 51575, 51585, 51595
    with Continent Diversion 51596
    with Ureteroileal Conduit 51590
    with Ureterosigmoidostomy 51580
Ovarian 58925
    Laparoscopic 58661
Partial
    Complicated 51555
    Reimplantation of Ureters 51565
    Simple 51550

Cystic Hygroma
See Hygroma

Cystine
Urine 82615

Cystitis
Interstitial 52260-52265

Cystography 74430
Injection 52281
    Radiologic 51600

Cystolithotomy 51050

Cystometrogram 51725-51726

Cystoplasty 51800

Cystorrhaphy 51860-51865

Cystoscopy 52000

Cystoscopy, with Biopsy
See Biopsy, Bladder, Cystourethroscopy

Cystostomy
Change Tube 51705-51710
Closure 51880
Home Visit 99505
with Fulguration 51020
with Insertion Radioactive Material 51020
with Urethrectomy
    Female 53210
    Male 53215

Cystotomy
Excision
    Bladder Diverticulum 51525
    Bladder Tumor 51530
    Repair of Ureterocele 51535
    Vesical Neck 51520
Repair Ureterocele 51535
with Calculus Basket Extraction 51065
with Destruction Intravesical Lesion 51030
with Drainage 51040
with Fulguration 51020
with Insertion
    Radioactive Material 51020
    Ureteral Catheter 51045
with Removal Calculus 51050, 51065

Cystourethrogram, Retrograde
See Urethrocystography, Retrograde

Cystourethropexy
See Vesicourethropexy

Cystourethroplasty 51800-51820

Cystourethroscopy 52000, 52351,
        52601, 52647-52648, 53500
Biopsy 52204, 52354
    Brush 52007
Calibration and/or Dilation Urethral Stricture or
Stenosis 52281
Catheterization
    Ejaculatory Duct 52010
    Ureteral 52005
Destruction
    Lesion 52400
Dilation
    Bladder 52260-52265
    Intra-Renal Stricture 52343, 52346
    Ureter 52341-52342, 52344-52345
    Urethra 52281
Evacuation
    Clot 52001
Female Urethral Syndrome 52285
Incision
    Ejaculatory Duct 52402
Injection of Implant Material 52327
Insertion
    Indwelling Ureteral Stent 50947, 52332
    Radioactive Substance 52250
    Ureteral Guide Wire 52334
    Urethral Stent 52282
Lithotripsy 52353
Manipulation of Ureteral Calculus 52330
Meatotomy
    Ureteral 52290-52305
Removal
    Calculus .52310-52315, 52320-52325, 52352
    Foreign Body 52310-52315
    Urethral Stent 52310-52315

Resection
    Ejaculatory Duct 52402
    External Sphincter 52277
    Tumor 52355
Urethral Syndrome 52285
Vasectomy
    Transurethral 52402
Vasotomy
    Transurethral 52402
with Direct Vision Internal Urethrotomy ..52276
with Ejaculatory Duct Catheterization 52010
with Fulguration 52214, 52354
    Lesion 52224
    Tumor 52234-52240
with Internal Urethrotomy
    Female 52270
    Male 52275
with Steroid Injection 52283
with Ureteral Catheterization 52005
with Ureteral Meatotomy 52290-52305

Cytochrome Reductase, Lactic
See Lactic Dehydrogenase

Cytogenetic Study
Molecular
    DNA Probe 88271-88275, 88291, 88365
Unlisted Services and Procedures 88299

Cytomegalovirus
Antibody 86644-86645
Antigen Detection
    Direct Fluorescence 87271
    Enzyme Immunoassay 87332
    Nucleic Acid 87495-87497

Cytometries, Flow
See Flow Cytometry

Cytopathology
Cervical or Vaginal
    Requiring Interpretation by Physician ..88141
    Thin Layer Prep ..88142-88143, 88174-88175
Concentration Technique 88108
    See Saccomonno Technique
Evaluation 88172
Fluids, Washings, Brushings 88104-88108
Forensic 88125
Other Source 88160-88162
Selective Cellular Enhancement Technique .88112
Smears
    Cervical or Vaginal 88141-88167,
        88174-88175
Unlisted Services and Procedures 88199

Cytoscopy
See Bladder, Endoscopy

Cytosol Aminopeptidase
See Leucine Aminopeptidase

Cytotoxic Screen
Lymphocyte 86805-86806
Percent Reactive Antibody (PRA) ...86807-86808
Serum Antibodies 86807-86808

D

D & C Yellow No. 7
See Fluorescein

D 2, Vitamin
See Calciferol

D and C
See Dilation and Curettage

D and E
See Dilation and Evacuation

D Galactose
See Galactose

D Glucose
See Glucose

D Vitamin
See Vitamin, D

D-Xylose Absorption Test ..... .84620

Dacryoadenectomy
Partial .... .68505
Total .... .68500

Dacryocystectomy .... .68520

Dacryocystogram
See Dacryocystography

Dacryocystography .... .68850, 70170
Nuclear Imaging .... .78660

Dacryocystorhinostomy .... .68720
Total
    with Nasal/Sinus Endoscopy .... .31239

Dacryocystostomies
See Dacryocystotomy

Dacryocystotomy .... .68420

Daily Living Activities
See Activities of Daily Living

Damus-Kaye-Stansel Procedure
See Anastomosis, Pulmonary

Dana Operation
See Rhizotomy

Dandy Operation
See Ventriculocisternostomy

Dark Adaptation Examination . .92284

Dark Field Examination . . .87164-87166

Darkroom Test
See Glaucoma, Provocative Test

Darrach Procedure
See Excision, Ulna, Partial

Day Test
See Blood, Feces

de Quervain's Disease
Treatment .... .25000

Death, Brain
See Brain Death

Debridement
Brain .... .62010
Burns 01951-01953, 16020-16030
Mastoid Cavity
    Complex .... .69222
    Simple .... .69220
Metatarsophalangeal Joint .... .28289
Muscle
    Infected 11004-11006
Nails 11720-11721
Nose
    Endoscopic .... .31237
Pancreatic Tissue .... .48105
Skin
    Eczematous 11000-11001
    Full Thickness .... .11041
    Infected 11000-11006
    Partial Thickness .... .11040
    Subcutaneous Tissue 11042-11044
      Infected 11004-11006
    with Open Fracture and/or
    Dislocation 11010-11012
Sternum .... .21627
Wound
    Non-Selective .... .97602
    Selective 97597-97598

Debulking Procedure
Ovary/Pelvis 58952-58958

Decompression
See Section
Arm, Lower .... .24495, 25020-25025
Auditory Canal, Internal .... .69960
Brainstem 61575-61576
Cauda Equina ..... .63011, 63017, 63047-63048,
              63056-63057, 63087-63091
Cranial Nerve .... .61458
Esophagogastric Varices .... .37181
Facial Nerve .... .61590
    Intratemporal
      Lateral to Geniculate Ganglion .... .69720,
                           69740
      Medial to Geniculate Ganglion .... .69725,
                           69745
    Total .... .69955
Finger .... .26035
Gasserian Ganglion
    Sensory Root .... .61450
Hand 26035-26037
Intestines
    Small .... .44021
Jejunostomy
    Laparoscopic .... .44186
Leg
    Fasciotomy 27600-27602
Nerve 64702-64727
    Root 63020-63048, 63055-63103
Nucleus of Disk
    Lumbar .... .62287
Optic Nerve .... .67570
Orbit .... .61330
    Removal of Bone .... .67414, 67445

Skull 61322-61323, 61340-61345
Spinal Cord 63001-63017, 63045-63103
    Cauda Equina .... .63005
Tarsal Tunnel Release .... .28035
Volvulus .... .45321, 45337
with Nasal/Sinus Endoscopy
    Optic Nerve .... .31294
    Orbit Wall 31292-31293
Wrist 25020-25025

Decortication
Lung
    Endoscopic 32651-32652
    Partial .... .32225
    Total .... .32220
    with Parietal Pleurectomy .... .32320

Decubiti
See Pressure Ulcer (Decubitus)

Decubitus Ulcers
See Debridement; Pressure Ulcer (Decubitus);
Skin Graft and Flap

Deetjeen's Body
See Blood, Platelet

Defect, Coagulation
See Coagulopathy

Defect, Heart Septal
See Septal Defect

Defect, Septal Closure, Atrial
See Heart, Repair, Atrial Septum

Deferens, Ductus
See Vas Deferens

Defibrillation
See Cardioversion

Defibrillator, Heart
See Pacemaker, Heart
Evaluation and Testing 93640-93642,
                           93741-93744
Insertion Single/Dual Chamber
    Electrodes 33216-33217,
                     33224-33225, 33249
    Pulse Generator .... .33240
Removal Single/Dual Chamber
    Electrodes 33243-33244
    Pulse Generator .... .33241
Repair 33218-33220
Repositioning Single/Dual Chamber
    Electrodes .... .33215, 33226
Revise Pocket Chest .... .33223
Wearable Device 93741-93742, 93745

Deformity, Boutonniere
See Boutonniere Deformity

Deformity, Sprengel's
See Sprengel's Deformity

Degenerative, Articular Cartilage,
Patella
See Chondromalacia Patella

Degradation Products, Fibrin
See Fibrin Degradation Products

Dislocation, Radiocarpal Joint
See Radiocarpal Joint, Dislocation

Disorder
Blood Coagulation
  See Coagulopathy
Penis
  See Penis
Retinal
  See Retina

Displacement Therapy
Nose 30210

Dissection
Hygroma, Cystic
  Axillary/Cervical 38550-38555
Lymph Nodes 38542

Dissection, Neck, Radical
See Radical Neck Dissection

Distention
See Dilation

Diverticula, Meckel's
See Diverticulum, Meckel's

Diverticulectomy 44800
Esophagus 43130-43135

Diverticulectomy, Meckel's
See Meckel's Diverticulum, Excision

Diverticulum
Bladder
  See Bladder, Diverticulum
Meckel's
  Excision 44800
Repair
  Urethra 53400-53405

Division
Muscle
  Foot 28250
Plantar Fascia
  Foot 28250

Division, Isthmus, Horseshoe Kidney
See Symphysiotomy, Horseshoe Kidney

Division, Scalenus Anticus Muscle
See Muscle Division, Scalenus Anticus

Dl-Amphetamine
See Amphetamine

DMO
See Dimethadione

DNA
Antibody 86225-86226

DNA Endonuclease
See DNAse

DNA Probe
See Cytogenetics Studies; Nucleic Acid Probe

DNAse
Antibody 86215

Domiciliary Services
See Nursing Facility Services
Assisted Living 99339-99340
Discharge Services 99315-99316
Established Patient 99334-99337
New Patient 99324-99328

Donor Procedures
Conjunctival Graft 68371
Heart Excision 33940
Heart/Lung Excision 33930
Liver Segment 47140-47142
Stem Cells
  Donor Search 38204

Dopamine
See Catecholamines
Blood 82383-82384
Urine 82382, 82384

Doppler Echocardiography 76827-
  76828, 93307-93308, 93320-93350
Extracranial 93875
Intracardiac 93662
Transesophageal 93318
Transthoracic 93303-93317

Doppler Scan
Arterial Studies
  Extremities 93922-93924
  Fetal
    Middle Cerebral Artery 76821
    Umbilical Artery 76820
  Extremities 93965
  Intracranial Arteries 93886-93893

Dorsal Vertebra
See Vertebra, Thoracic

Dose Plan
See Dosimetry

Dosimetry
Radiation Therapy 77300, 77331
  Brachytherapy 77326-77328
  Intensity Modulation 77301
  Teletherapy 77305-77321

Double-Stranded DNA
See Deoxyribonucleic Acid

Doxepin
Assay 80166

DPH
See Phenytoin

Drainage
See Excision; Incision; Incision and Drainage; Paracentesis
Abdomen
  Abdomen Fluid 49080-49081
Abscess
  Appendix 44900-44901
    Percutaneous 44901
  Brain 61150-61151
  Eyelid 67700
  Liver 47010-47011
  Ovary
    Percutaneous 58823

Pelvic
  Percutaneous 58823
Pericolic
  Percutaneous 58823
Perirenal or Renal 50020-50021
  Percutaneous 50021
Prostate 52700
Retroperitoneal 49060-49061
  Percutaneous 49061
Subdiaphragmatic or
Subphrenic 49040-49041
  Percutaneous 49040-49041
with X-Ray 75989
Amniotic Fluid
  Diagnostic Aspiration 59000
  Therapeutic Aspiration 59001
Bile Duct
  Transhepatic 75980
Brain Fluid 61070
Bursa 20600-20610
Cerebrospinal Fluid 61000-61020, 61050,
  61070, 62272
Cervical Fluid 61050
Cisternal Fluid 61050
Cyst
  Bone 20615
  Brain 61150-61151, 62161-62162
  Breast 19000-19001
  Ganglion 20612
  Liver 47010-47011
    Percutaneous 47011
  Salivary Gland 42409
  Sublingual Gland 42409
Extraperitoneal Lymphocele
  Laparoscopic 49323
  Open 49062
Eye
  Paracentesis
    with Aqueous Aspiration 65800
    with Aqueous-Release 65805
  with Removal
    Blood 65815
    Discission of Anterior Hyaloid
    Membrane 65810
    Vitreous 65810
Fetal Fluid 59074
Ganglion Cyst 20612
Hematoma
  Brain 61154-61156
  Vagina 57022-57023
Hematoma, Subungual 11740
Joint 20600-20610
Liver
  Abscess or Cyst 47010-47011
  Percutaneous 47011
Lymphocele
  Endoscopic 49323
Onychia 10060-10061
Orbit 67405, 67440
Pancreas
  See Anastomosis, Pancreas to Intestines
  Pseudocyst 48510-48511
    Percutaneous 48511
Paronychia 10060-10061
Pericardial Sac 32659
Pericardium
  See Aspiration, Pericardium

E

Electrocautery 17000-17286
See Destruction

Electrochemistry
See Electrolysis

Electroconvulsive Therapy 90870

Electrocorticogram
Intraoperative 95829

Electrode, Depth
See Depth Electrode
Electrode Array Intracranial 61850-61868,
61885-61886
Peripheral Nerve 64553-64581
Retinal 0100T
Spinal 63650-63655

Electrodesiccation 17000-17286
Lesion
Penis 54055

Electroejaculation 55870

**Electroencephalography
(EEG)** 95816
Brain Death 95824
Coma 95822
Digital Analysis 95957
Electrode Placement 95830
Intraoperative 95955
Monitoring ...95812-95813, 95950-95953, 95956
with Drug Activation 95954
with Physical Activation 95954
with WADA Activation 95958
Sleep 95822, 95827
Standard 95819

Electrogastrography 91132-91133

Electrogram, Atrial
Esophageal Recording 93615-93616

Electrolysis 17380

Electromyographs
See Electromyography, Needle

Electromyography
Anorectal with Biofeedback 90911
Fine Wire
Dynamic 96004
Needle
Extremities 95861-95864
Extremity 95860
Face and Neck Muscles 95867-95868
Guidance
for Chemodenervation 95874
Hemidiaphragm 95866
Larynx 95865
Ocular 92265
Other than Thoracic Paraspinal 95870
Single Fiber Electrode 95872
Thoracic Paraspinal Muscles 95869
Sphincter Muscles
Anus 51784-51785
Needle 51785
Urethra 51784-51785
Needle 51785
Surface
Dynamic 96002-96004

Electron Microscopy 88348-88349

Electronic Analysis
Drug Infusion Pump 62367-62368
Implantable Loop Recorder System 93727
Neurostimulator Pulse Generator 0162T,
95970-95979
Pacing Cardioverter-Defibrillator ...93741-93744

Electrophoresis
Counterimmuno- 86185
Immuno- 86320-86327
Immunofixation 86334-86335
Protein 84165-84166
Unlisted Services and Procedures 82664

**Electrophysiology
Procedure** 93600-93660

Electroretinogram
See Electroretinography

Electroretinography 92275

**Electrostimulation, Analgesic
Cutaneous**
See Application, Neurostimulation

Electrosurgery
Trichiasis
Correction 67825

Electroversion, Cardiac
See Cardioversion

Elevation, Scapula, Congenital
See Sprengel's Deformity

Elliot Operation
See Excision, Lesion, Sclera

Eloesser Procedure
See Thoracostomy, Empyema

Eloesser Thoracoplasty
See Thoracoplasty

Embolectomy
Aortoiliac Artery 34151-34201
Axillary Artery 34101
Brachial Artery 34101
Carotid Artery 34001
Celiac Artery 34151
Femoral 34201
Iliac 34151-34201
Innominate Artery 34001-34101
Mesentery Artery 34151
Peroneal Artery 34203
Popliteal Artery 34203
Pulmonary Artery 33910-33916
Radial Artery 34111
Renal Artery 34151
Subclavian Artery 34001-34101
Tibial Artery 34203
Ulnar Artery 34111

Embolization
Leiomyomata 37210

Embryo
Biopsy 89290-89291
Cryopreservation 89258

Cryopreserved
Preparation
Thawing 89352
Culture 89250
with Co-Culture Oocyte 89251
Hatching
Assisted
Microtechnique 89253
Preparation
for Transfer 89255
Storage 89342

Embryo Implantation
See Implantation

Embryo Transfer
In Vitro Fertilization 58974-58976
Intrafallopian Transfer 58976
Intrauterine Transfer 58974

Embryo/Fetus Monitoring
See Monitoring, Fetal

Embryonated Eggs
Inoculation 87250

**Emergency Department
Services** 99281-99288
See Critical Care; Emergency Department
Services
Anesthesia 99140
Physician Direction of Advanced
Life Support 99288

Emesis Induction 99175

EMG
See Electromyography, Needle

EMI Scan
See CT Scan

**Emission Computerized
Tomography** 78607

**Emission-Computed Tomography,
Single-Photon**
See SPECT

Emmet Operation
See Vagina, Repair, Obstetric

Empyema
Closure
Chest Wall 32810
Thoracostomy 32020-32036

Empyema, Lung
See Abscess, Thorax

Empyemectomy 32540

Encephalitis
Antibody 86651-86654

Encephalitis Virus Vaccine 90735

Encephalocele
Repair 62120
Craniotomy 62121

Encephalon
See Brain

End-Expiratory Pressure, Positive
See Pressure Breathing, Positive

End-Stage Renal Disease
Services 90918-90925

Endarterectomy
Coronary Artery .33572
Pulmonary 33916

Endemic Flea-Borne Typhus
See Murine Typhus

Endobronchial Challenge Tests
See Bronchial Challenge Test

Endocavitary Fulguration
See Electrocautery

Endocrine System
Unlisted Services and Procedures . .60699, 78099

Endocrine, Pancreas
See Islet Cell

Endolymphatic Sac
Exploration
    with Shunt 69806
    without Shunt .69805

Endometrial Ablation 58353
Curettage 58356
Exploration
    via Hysteroscopy 58563

Endometrioma
Abdomen
    Destruction/Excision 49200-49201
Retroperitoneal
    Destruction/Excision 49200-49201

Endometriosis, Adhesive
See Adhesions, Intrauterine

Endometrium
Ablation 58356
Biopsy 58100-58110, 58558

Endonuclease, DNA
See DNAse

Endoscopic Retrograde
Cannulation of Pancreatic Duct
(ERCP)
See Cholangiopancreatography

Endoscopies, Pleural
See Thoracoscopy

Endoscopy
See Arthroscopy; Thoracoscopy
Adrenal Gland
    Biopsy 60650
    Excision 60650
Anus
    Biopsy 46606
    Dilation 46604
    Exploration 46600
    Hemorrhage 46614
    Removal
        Foreign Body 46608
        Polyp 46610, 46612
        Tumor 46610, 46612

Atria
    Surgical 33265-33266
Bile Duct
    Biopsy 47553
    Destruction
        Calculi (Stone) 43265
        Tumor 43272
    Dilation 43271, 47555-47556
    Exploration 47552
    Intraoperative .47550
    Percutaneous 47552-47555
    Removal
        Calculi (Stone) 43264, 47554
        Foreign Body 43269
        Stent 43269
    Specimen Collection 43260
    Sphincter Pressure 43263
    Sphincterotomy 43262
    Tube Placement 43267-43268
Bladder 52000
    Biopsy 52204, 52354
    Catheterization 52005, 52010
    Destruction 52354
        Lesion 52400
    Evacuation
        Clot 52001
    Excision
        Tumor 52355
    Exploration 52351
    Lithotripsy 52353
    Removal
        Calculus .52352
        Urethral Stent 52282
Bladder Neck
    Injection of Implant Material 51715
Brain
    Shunt
        Creation .62201
Bronchi
    Aspiration 31645-31646
    Biopsy 31625-31629, 31632-31633
    Destruction
        Lesion 31641
        Tumor 31641
    Dilation 31630-31631, 31636-31638
    Exploration 31622
    Injection 31656
    Lesion
        Destruction 31641
    Needle Biopsy 31629, 31633
    Placement
        Stent 31631, 31636-31637
    Revision
        Stent 31638
    Specimen Collection 31623-31624
    Stenosis 31641
    Tumor
        Destruction 31641
    Ultrasound 31620
Cervix
    Biopsy 57454-57455, 57460
    Curettage 57454, 57456
    Exploration 57452
    Loop Electrode Biopsy 57460
    Loop Electrode Conization 57461
Chest Cavity
    Exploration 32601-32606
    Surgical 32650-32665

Colon
    Biopsy 44389, 45380, 45392
    Destruction
        Lesion 44393, 45383
        Tumor 44393, 45383
    Exploration 45378
    Hemorrhage 44391, 45382
    Injection 45381
    Placement
        Stent 45387
    Removal
        Foreign Body 44390, 45379
        Polyp 44392, 45384-45385
        Tumor 44392, 45384-45385
    Specimen Collection 45380
    Ultrasound 45391-45392
    via Colotomy 45355
    via Stoma 44388-44393, 44397
    Virtual 0066T, 0067T
Colon-Sigmoid
    Ablation
        Polyp 45339
        Tumor 45339
    Biopsy 45331
    Dilation 45340
    Exploration 45330, 45335
    Hemorrhage .45334
    Needle Biopsy 45342
    Placement
        Stent 45327, 45345
    Removal
        Foreign Body 45332
        Polyp 45333, 45338
        Tumor 45333, 45338
    Specimen Collection 45331
    Ultrasound 45341-45342
    Volvulus 45337
Esophagus
    Biopsy 43202
    Dilation 43220-43226
    Exploration 43200
    Hemorrhage .43227
    Injection 43201, 43204
    Insertion Stent 43219
    Needle Biopsy 43232
    Removal
        Foreign Body 43215
        Polyp 43216-43217, 43228
        Tumor 43216, 43228
    Ultrasound 43231-43232
    Vein Ligation .43205
Eye 66990
Foot
    Plantar Fasciotomy 29893
Gastrointestinal
    Upper
        Biopsy 43239
        Catheterization 43241
        Destruction of Lesion 43258
        Dilation 43245, 43248-43249
        Drainage of Pseudocyst 43240
        Exploration 43234-43235
        Foreign Body 43247
        Gastric Bypass 43644-43645
        Gastroenterostomy 43644-43645
        Hemorrhage 43255
        Inject Varices 43243
        Injection 0133T, 43236

Needle Biopsy 43238, 43242
Removal 43247, 43250-43251
Roux-En-Y 43644
Stent Placement 43256
Suturing 0008T
Thermal Radiation 43257
Tube Placement 43246
Ultrasound . . .43237-43242, 43259, 76975
Vein Ligation 43244
Heart
Atria .33265-33266
Ileum
via Stoma 44383
Intestines, Small
Biopsy 44361, 44377
Destruction
Lesion 44369
Tumor 44369
Diagnostic .44376
Exploration 44360
Hemorrhage 44366, 44378
Insertion
Stent 44370, 44379
Tube 44379
Pelvic Pouch 44385-44386
Removal
Foreign Body 44363
Lesion 44365
Polyp 44364-44365
Tube Placement 44372
Tube Revision 44373
via Stoma 44380-44383
Tumor 44364-44365
Intracranial 62160-62165
Kidney
Biopsy 50555, 50574-50576, 52354
Catheterization 50553, 50572
Destruction 50557, 50576, 52354
Dilation of Ureter 50553
Excision
Tumor 52355
Exploration 52351
Lithotripsy 52353
Removal
Calculus 50561, 50580, 52352
Foreign Body 50561, 50580
via Incision 50562-50580
via Stoma 50551-50561
Larynx
Biopsy 31510, 31535-31536
Direct 31515-31571
Exploration 31505, 31520-31526, 31575
Fiberoptic 31575-31579
Indirect 31505-31513
Operative 31530-31561
Removal
Foreign Body 31530-31531
Lesion 31511, 31545-31546
See Endoscopic
Lysis
Device 0027T
Mediastinoscopy
Biopsy 39400
Exploration 39400
Nose
Diagnostic 31231-31235
Surgical 31237-31294
Unlisted Services and Procedures 31299

Pancreatic Duct
Destruction
Calculi (Stone) 43265
Tumor 43272
Dilation 43271
Removal
Calculi (Stone) 43264
Foreign Body 43269
Stent 43269
Specimen Collection 43260
Sphincter Pressure 43263
Sphincterotomy 43262
Tube Placement 43267-43268
Pelvis
Aspiration .49322
Destruction of Lesion 58662
Lysis of Adhesions 58660
Oviduct Surgery 58670-58671
Removal of Adnexal Structures 58661
Peritoneum
Biopsy 47561
Drainage
Lymphocele 49323, 54690
Radiologic 47560
Rectum
Biopsy 45305
Destruction
Tumor 45320
Dilation 45303
Exploration 45300
Hemorrhage 45317
Removal
Foreign Body 45307
Polyp 45308-45315
Tumor 45308-45315
Volvulus 45321
Spleen
Removal 38120
Testis
Removal 54690
Trachea
Dilation 31630-31631, 31636-31638
via Tracheostomy 31615
Ureter
Biopsy . . .50955-50957, 50974-50976, 52354
Catheterize 50953, 50972
Destruction 50957, 50976, 52354
Excision
Tumor 52355
Exploration 52351
Injection of Implant Material 52327
Lithotripsy 52353
Manipulation of Ureteral Calculus 52330
Placement
Stent 50947
Removal
Calculus 50961, 50980, 52352
Foreign Body 50961, 50980
Resection .52355
via Incision 50970-50980
via Stoma 50951-50961
Ureteral
Biopsy 52007
Catheterization 52005
Urethra 52000
Biopsy 52204, 52354
Catheterization 52010

Destruction .52354
Lesion 52400
Evacuation
Clot 52001
Excision
Tumor 52355
Exploration 52351
Incision
Ejaculatory Duct 52402
Injection of Implant Material 51715
Lithotripsy 52353
Removal
Calculus .52352
Resection
Ejaculatory Duct 52402
Vasectomy 52402
Vasotomy .52402
Uterus
Anesthesia 00952
Hysteroscopy
Diagnostic 58555
with Division/Resection Intrauterine
Septum .58560
with Lysis of Intrauterine
Adhesions 58559
Placement
Fallopian Tube 58565
Removal
Endometrial 58563
Impacted Foreign Body 58562
Leiomyomata 58561
Surgical with Biopsy 58558
Vagina
Anesthesia 00950
Biopsy 57454
Exploration 57452
Vascular
Surgical 33508, 37500-37501
Virtual
Colon 0066T, 0067T

Endosteal Implant
Reconstruction
Mandible 21248-21249
Maxilla 21248-21249

Endothelioma, Dural
See Meningioma

Endotracheal Intubation
See Insertion, Endotracheal Tube

Endotracheal Tube
Intubation 31500

Endovascular Repair 0078T, 0079T,
0080T, 0081T, 33880-33891,
34800-34805, 34812-34826, 34833-34900
Angiography 75952-75959

Endovascular Therapy
Ablation
Vein 36475-36479
Occlusion 61623

Enema
Home Visit for Fecal Impaction 99511
Intussusception 74283
Therapeutic
for Intussusception 74283

Energies, Electromagnetic
See Irradiation

ENT
See Ear, Nose, and Throat; Otorhinolaryngology,
Diagnostic
Therapeutic
 See Otorhinolaryngology

Entamoeba Histolytica
Antigen Detection
 Enzyme Immunoassay 87336-87337

Enterectomy 44120-44121,
    44126-44128, 44137, 44202
Donor 44132-44133
with Enterostomy 44125

Enterocele
Repair 57556
 Hysterectomy
  with Colpectomy 58280

Enterocystoplasty 51960
Camey 50825

Enteroenterostomy
See Anastomosis, Intestines

Enterolysis 44005
Laparoscopic 44180

Enteropancreatostomy
See Anastomosis, Pancreas to Intestines

Enterorrhaphy 44602-44603, 44615

Enterostomy 44300
Closure 44625-44626
with Enterectomy
 Intestine, Small 44125

Enterotomy 44615

Enterovirus
Antibody 86658

Entropion
Repair 67921-67924
 Excision Tarsal Wedge 67923
 Suture 67921
 Thermocauterization 67922

Enucleation
Eye
 with Implant 65103
  Muscles Attached 65105
 without Implant 65101
Pleural 32540

Enucleation, Cyst, Ovarian
See Cystectomy, Ovarian

Environmental Intervention
for Psychiatric Patients 90882

Enzyme Activity 82657
Radioactive Substrate 82658

Enzyme, Angiotensin Converting
See Angiotensin Converting Enzyme (ACE)

Enzyme, Angiotensin-Forming
See Renin

EOG
See Electro-oculography

Eosinocyte
See Eosinophils

Eosinophils
Nasal Smear 89190

Epiandrosterone 82666

Epicondylitides, Lateral Humeral
See Tennis Elbow

Epicondylitis, Radiohumeral
See Tennis Elbow

Epidemic Parotitis
See Mumps

Epididymectomy
Bilateral 54861
Unilateral 54860

Epididymis
Abscess
 Incision and Drainage 54700
Anastomosis
 to Vas Deferens
  Bilateral 54901
  Unilateral 54900
Biopsy 54800, 54865
Epididymography 74440
Excision
 Bilateral 54861
 Unilateral 54860
Exploration
 Biopsy 54865
Hematoma
 Incision and Drainage 54700
Lesion
 Excision
  Local 54830
  Spermatocele 54840
Needle Biopsy 54800
Spermatocele
 Excision 54840
Unlisted Services and Procedures ...55899
X-Ray with Contrast 74440

Epididymograms 55300

Epididymography 74440

Epididymoplasty
See Repair, Epididymis

Epididymovasostomy
Bilateral 54901
Unilateral 54900

Epidural
Electrode
 Insertion 61531
 Removal 61535
Injection 62281-62282, 62310-62319,
     64479-64484
Lysis 0027T, 62263-62264

Epidural Anesthesia
See Anesthesia, Epidural

Epidurography 72275

Epigastric
Hernia Repair 49572

Epiglottidectomy 31420

Epiglottis
Excision 31420

Epikeratoplasty 65767

Epilation
See Removal, Hair

Epinephrine
See Catecholamines
Blood 82383-82384
Urine 82384

Epiphyseal Arrest
Femur 20150, 27185, 27475, 27479-27485, 27742
Fibula 20150, 27477-27485, 27730-27742
Radius 20150, 25450-25455
Tibia ..20150, 27477-27485, 27730, 27734-27742
Ulna 20150, 25450-25455

Epiphyseal Separation
Radius
 Closed Treatment 25600
 Open Treatment 25607-25609

Epiphysiodesis
See Epiphyseal Arrest

Epiphysis
See Bone; Specific Bone

Epiploectomy 49255

Episiotomy 59300

Epispadias
Penis
 Reconstruction 54385
Repair 54380-54390
 with Exstrophy of Bladder 54390
 with Incontinence 54380-54390

Epistaxis 30901-30906
with Nasal/Sinus Endoscopy 31238

EPO
See Erythropoietin

Epstein-Barr Virus
Antibody 86663-86665

Equina, Cauda
See Cauda Equina

ERCP
See Bile Duct; Cholangiopancreatography;
Pancreatic Duct

ERG
See Electroretinography

Ergocalciferol
See Calciferol

Ergocalciferols
See Calciferol

Exploration, Larynx by Incision
See Laryngotomy, Diagnostic

Exploratory Laparotomy
See Abdomen, Exploration

Expression
Lesion

Exteriorization, Small Intestine
See Enterostomy

External Auditory Canal
See Auditory Canal

External Cephalic Version   .59412

External Ear
See Ear, External

External Extoses
See Exostosis

External Fixation

Extirpation, Lacrimal Sac
See Dacryocystectomy

Extracorporeal Circulation   .33960-33961
for Regional Chemotherapy

Extracorporeal Dialyses
See Hemodialysis

Extracorporeal Membrane Oxygenation

Extracorporeal Photochemotherapies
See Photopheresis

Extracorporeal Shock Wave Therapy
See Lithotripsy

Extracranial

Extraction
Lens

Extraction, Cataract
See Cataract, Excision

Extradural Anesthesia
See Anesthesia, Epidural

Extradural Injection
See Epidural, Injection

Extraocular Muscle
See Eye Muscles

Extrauterine Pregnancy
See Ectopic Pregnancy

Extravasation Blood
See Hemorrhage

Extremity
Lower
Upper

Eye
See Ciliary Body; Cornea; Iris; Lens; Retina;
Sclera; Vitreous

Paracentesis
    with Aqueous Aspiration 65800
    with Aqueous Release 65805
    with Discission of Anterior Hyaloid
    Membrane 65810
    with Removal
      Blood 65815
      Vitreous 65810
Radial Keratotomy 65771
Reconstruction
  Graft
    Conjunctiva 65782
    Stem Cell 65781
  Transplantation
    Amniotic Membrane 65780
Removal
  Blood Clot 65930
  Bone 65112
  Foreign Body
    Conjunctival Embedded 65210
    Conjunctival Superficial 65205
    Corneal with Slit Lamp 65222
    Corneal without Slit Lamp 65220
    Intraocular 65235-65265
  Implant 65175
    Anterior Segment 65920
    Muscles, Not Attached 65103
    Posterior Segment 67120-67121
Repair
  Conjunctiva
    by Mobilization and Rearrangement with
    Hospitalization 65273
    by Mobilization and Rearrangement
    without Hospitalization 65272
    Direct Closure 65270
  Cornea
    Nonperforating 65275
    Perforating 65280-65285
    Muscles 65290
  Sclera
    Anterior Segment 66250
    with Graft 66225
    with Tissue Glue 65286
    without Graft 66220
    Trabeculae 65855
  Wound
    by Mobilization and
    Rearrangement 65272-65273
    Direct Closure 65270
Shunt, Aqueous
  to Extraocular Reservoir 66180
Ultrasound 76510-76514
  Biometry 76516-76519
  Foreign Body 76529
Unlisted Services and Procedures
  Anterior Segment 66999
  Posterior Segment 67299
with Muscle or Myocutaneous Flap 65114
  Muscles Attached 65105
  Ocular Contents
    with Implant 65093
    without Implant 65091
  Orbital Contents 65110
    without Implant 65101
X-Ray 70030

Eye Allergy Test 95060
See Allergy Tests

Eye Evisceration
See Evisceration, Ocular Contents

Eye Exam
Established Patient 92012-92014
New Patient 92002-92004
Radiologic 70030
with Anesthesia 92018-92019

Eye Exercises
Training 92065

Eye Muscles
Biopsy 67346
Repair
  Strabismus
    Adjustable Sutures 67335
    Exploration and/or Repair Detached
    Extraocular Muscle 67340
    on Patient with Previous Surgery ...67331
    One Vertical Muscle 67314
    Posterior Fixation Suture 67334
    Recession or Resection 67311-67312
    Release of Scar Tissue without Detaching
    Extraocular Muscle 67343
    Two or More Vertical Muscles 67316
    with Scarring Extraocular Muscles ..67332
    with Superior Oblique Muscle 67318
Transposition 67320
Unlisted Services and Procedures 67399

Eye Prosthesis
See Prosthesis

Eye Socket
See Orbit; Orbital Contents; Orbital Floor;
Periorbital Region

Eyebrow
Repair
  Ptosis 67900

Eyeglasses
See Spectacle Services

Eyelashes
Repair Trichiasis
  Epilation
    by Forceps Only 67820
    by Other than Forceps 67825
  Incision of Lid Margin 67830
    with Free Mucous Membrane Graft .67835

Eyelid
Abscess
  Incision and Drainage 67700
Biopsy 67810
Blepharoplasty 15820-15823
Chalazion
  Excision 67805
    Multiple 67801-67805
    Single 67800
    with Anesthesia 67808
Closure by Suture 67875

Incision
  Canthus 67715
  Sutures 67710
Injection
  Subconjunctival 68200
Lesion
  Destruction 67850
  Excision
    Multiple 67801-67805
    Single 67800
    with Anesthesia 67808
    without Closure 67840
Reconstruction
  Canthus 67950
  Total 67973-67975
  Total Eyelid
    Lower 67973-67975
    Second Stage 67975
    Upper 67974
  Transfer of Tarsoconjunctival Flap from
  Opposing Eyelid 67971
Removal
  Foreign Body 67938
Repair 21280-21282
  Blepharoptosis
    Conjunctivo-Tarso-Muller's
    Muscle-Levator Resection 67908
    Frontalis Muscle Technique ..67901-67904
    Reduction Overcorrection of Ptosis ..67909
    Superior Rectus Technique with Fascial
    Sling 67906
  Ectropion
    Blepharoplasty 67914
    Suture 67914
  Entropion
    Excision Tarsal Wedge 67923
    Extensive 67924
    Suture 67921
    Thermocauterization 67922
  Excisional 67961
    over One-Fourth of Lid Margin 67966
  Lagophthalmos 67912
  Lashes
    Epilation, by Forceps Only 67820
    Epilation, by Other than Forceps 67825
    Lid Margin 67830-67835
  Wound
    Full Thickness 67935
    Partial Thickness 67930
Repair with Graft
  Retraction 67911
Skin Graft
  Full Thickness 67961
  Split 67961
Suture 67880
  with Transposition of Tarsal Plate 67882
Tissue Transfer, Adjacent 67961
Unlisted Services and Procedures 67999

Eyelid Ptoses
See Blepharoptosis

F

Face
CT Scan 70486-70488
Lesion
    Destruction 17000-17004, 17280-17286
Magnetic Resonance Imaging
(MRI) 70540-70543
Tumor Resection 21015

Face Lift 15824-15828

Facial Asymmetries
See Hemifacial Microsomia

Facial Bone
See Mandible; Maxilla
Tumor
    Excision 21034

Facial Bones
Abscess
    Excision 21026
Reconstruction
    Secondary 21275
Repair 21208-21209
Tumor
    Excision 21029-21030
    Resection
      Radical 21015
X-Ray 70140-70150

Facial Nerve
Anastomosis
    to Hypoglossal 64868
    to Phrenic Nerve 64870
    to Spinal Accessory 64866
Avulsion 64742
Decompression 61590, 61596
    Intratemporal
      Lateral to Geniculate
      Ganglion 69720, 69740
      Medial to Geniculate
      Ganglion 69725, 69745
    Total 69955
Function Study 92516
Incision 64742
Injection
    Anesthetic 64402
Mobilization 61590
Repair
    Lateral to Geniculate Ganglion 69740
    Medial to Geniculate Ganglion 69745
Repair/Suture
    with or without Graft 64864-64865
Suture
    Lateral to Geniculate Ganglion 69740
    Medial to Geniculate Ganglion 69745
Transection 64742

Facial Nerve Paralysis
Graft 15840-15845
Repair 15840-15845

Facial Prosthesis
Impression 21088

Facial Rhytidectomy
See Face Lift

Factor, ACTH-Releasing
See Corticotropic Releasing Hormone (CRH)

Factor, Antinuclear
See Antinuclear Antibodies (ANA)

Factor, Blood Coagulation
See Clotting Factor
Factor I
    See Fibrinogen
Factor II
    See Prothrombin
Factor III
    See Thromboplastin
Factor IV
    See Calcium
Factor VII
    See Proconvertin
Factor VIII
    See Clotting Factor
Factor IX
    See Christmas Factor
Factor X
    See Stuart-Prower Factor
Factor X, Activated
    See Thrombokinase
Factor Xa Inhibitor
    See Antithrombin III
Factor XI
    See Plasma Thromboplastin, Antecedent
Factor XII
    See Hageman Factor
Factor XIII
    See Fibrin Stabilizing Factor

Factor, Fitzgerald
See Fitzgerald Factor

Factor, Fletcher
See Fletcher Factor

Factor, Hyperglycemic-Glycogenolytic
See Glucagon

Factor Inhibitor Test 85335

Factor, Intrinsic
See Intrinsic Factor

Factor, Rheumatoid
See Rheumatoid Factor

Factor, Sulfation
See Somatomedin

Fallopian Tube
Anastomosis........................58750
Catheterization 58345, 74742
Destruction
    Endoscopy 58670

Ectopic Pregnancy 59121
    with Salpingectomy and/or
    Oophorectomy 59120
Excision 58700-58720
Ligation 58600-58611
Lysis
    Adhesions 58740
Occlusion 58615
    Endoscopy 58671
Placement
    Implant for Occlusion 58565
Repair 58752
    Anastomosis 58750
    Create Stoma 58770
Tumor
    Resection 58950, 58952-58958
Unlisted Services and Procedures 58999
X-Ray 74742

Fallopian Tube Pregnancy
See Ectopic Pregnancy, Tubal

Fallot, Tetralogy of
See Tetralogy of Fallot

Family Psychotherapy
See Psychotherapy, Family

Fanconi Anemia
Chromosome Analysis 88248

Farnsworth-Munsell Color Test
See Color Vision Examination

Farr Test
See Gammaglobulin, Blood

Fasanella-Servat Procedure ...67908

Fascia Graft 15840

Fascia Lata Graft
Harvesting 20920-20922

Fascial Defect
Repair 50728

Fascial Graft
Free
    Microvascular Anastomosis 15758
Open Treatment
    Sternoclavicular Dislocation 23532

Fasciectomy
Foot 28060
    Radical 28060-28062
Palm 26121-26125

Fasciocutaneous Flaps ...15731-15738

Fasciotomy
Arm, Lower 24495, 25020-25025
Elbow 24350-24356
Foot 28008
Hand Decompression 26037
Hip 27025
Knee 27305, 27496-27499

Fruit Sugar
See Fructose

FSF 85290-85291

FSH
See Follicle Stimulating Hormone (FSH)

FSP
See Fibrin Degradation Products

FT-4 84439

Fulguration
See Destruction
Bladder 51020
Cystourethroscopy with 52214
    Lesion 52224
    Tumor 52234-52240
Ureter 50957, 50976
Ureterocele
    Ectopic 52301
    Orthotopic 52300

Fulguration, Endocavitary
See Electrocautery

Full Thickness Graft 15200-15261

Function Test, Lung
See Pulmonology, Diagnostic

Function Test, Vestibular
See Vestibular Function Tests

Function, Study, Nasal
See Nasal Function Study

Functional Ability
See Activities of Daily Living

Fundoplasty
Esophagogastric 43324-43325
    Laparoscopic 43280
    with Gastroplasty 43326

Fundoplication
See Fundoplasty, Esophagogastric

Fungus
Antibody 86671
Culture
    Blood 87103
    Hair 87101
    Identification 87106
    Nail 87101
    Other 87102
    Skin 87101
Tissue Exam 87220

Funnel Chest
See Pectus Excavatum

Furuncle
Incision and Drainage 10060-10061

Furuncle, Vulva
See Abscess, Vulva

Fusion
See Arthrodesis
Pleural Cavity 32005
Thumb
    in Opposition 26820

Fusion, Epiphyseal-Diaphyseal
See Epiphyseal Arrest

Fusion, Joint
See Arthrodesis

Fusion, Joint, Ankle
See Ankle, Arthrodesis

Fusion, Joint, Interphalangeal, Finger
See Arthrodesis, Finger Joint, Interphalangeal

G

Gago Procedure
See Repair, Tricuspid Valve; Revision

Gait Training 97116
See Physical Medicine/Therapy/Occupational Therapy

Galactogram 77053-77054
Injection 19030

Galactokinase
Blood 82759

Galactose
Blood 82760
Urine 82760

Galactose-1-Phosphate
Uridyl Transferase 82775-82776

Gall Bladder
See Gallbladder

Gallbladder
See Bile Duct
Anastomosis
    with Intestines 47720-47741
Excision 47562-47564, 47600-47620
Exploration 47480
Incision 47490
Incision and Drainage 47480
Nuclear Medicine
    Imaging 78223
Removal
    Calculi (Stone) 47480
Repair
    with Gastroenterostomy 47741
    with Intestines 47720-47740
Unlisted Services and Procedures 47999
X-Ray with Contrast 74290-74291

Galvanocautery
See Electrocautery

Galvanoionization
See Iontophoresis

Gamete Intrafallopian Transfer (GIFT) 58976

Gamete Transfer
In Vitro Fertilization 58976

Gamma Camera Imaging
See Nuclear Medicine

Gamma Glutamyl Transferase 82977

Gamma Seminoprotein
See Antigen, Prostate Specific

Gammacorten
See Dexamethasone

Gammaglobulin
Blood 82784-82787

Gamulin Rh
See Immune Globulins, Rho (D)

Ganglia, Trigeminal
See Gasserian Ganglion

Ganglion
See Gasserian Ganglion
Cyst
    Aspiration/Injection 20612
    Drainage 20612
    Wrist
        Excision 25111-25112
Injection
    Anesthetic 64505, 64510

Ganglion Cervicothoracicum
See Stellate Ganglion

Ganglion Pterygopalatinum
See Sphenopalatine Ganglion

Ganglion, Gasser's
See Gasserian Ganglion

Gardner Operation
See Meningocele Repair

Gardnerella Vaginalis Detection 87510-87512

Gasser Ganglion
See Gasserian Ganglion

Gasserian Ganglion
Sensory Root
    Decompression 61450
    Section 61450
Stereotactic 61790

Gastrectomy
Partial 43631-43635, 43845
    with Gastrojejunostomy 43632
Total 43621-43622
    with Esophagoenterostomy 43620
with Gastroduodenostomy 43631

Gastric Acid 82926-82928

Gastric Analysis Test 91052

Gastric Electrodes
Implantation
    Laparoscopic
        Neurostimulator 43647
        Stimulation 0155T
    Open
        Neurostimulator 43881
        Stimulation 0157T

Gentamicin .... .80170
Assay .... .80170

Gentamycin Level
See Gentamicin

Gentiobiase
See Beta Glucosidase

Genus: Human Cytomegalovirus Group
See Cytomegalovirus

GERD
See Gastroesophageal Reflux Test

German Measles
See Rubella

Gestational Trophoblastic Tumor
See Hydatidiform Mole

GGT
See Gamma Glutamyl Transferase

GI Tract
See Gastrointestinal Tract

Giardia
Antigen Detection
　Enzyme Immunoassay .... .87329
　Immunofluorescence .... .87269

Giardia Lamblia
Antibody .... .86674

Gibbons Stent .... .52332

GIF
See Somatostatin

GIFT
See Gamete Intrafallopian Transfer

Gill Operation .... .63012

Gillies Approach
Fracture
　Zygomatic Arch .... .21356

Gingiva
See Gums

Gingiva, Abcess
See Abscess
Fracture
　See Abscess, Gums; Gums
　Zygomatic Arch
　　See Abscess, Gums; Gums, Abscess

Gingivectomy .... .41820

Gingivoplasty .... .41872

Girdlestone Laminectomy
See Laminectomy

Girdlestone Procedure
See Acetabulum, Reconstruction

Gla Protein (Bone)
See Osteocalcin

Gland
See Specific Gland

Gland, Adrenal
See Adrenal Gland

Gland, Bartholin's
See Bartholin's Gland

Gland, Bulbourethral
See Bulbourethral Gland

Gland, Lacrimal
See Lacrimal Gland

Gland, Mammary
See Breast

Gland, Parathyroid
See Parathyroid Gland

Gland, Parotid
See Parotid Gland

Gland, Pituitary
See Pituitary Gland

Gland, Salivary
See Salivary Glands

Gland, Sublingual
See Sublingual Gland

Gland, Sweat
See Sweat Glands

Gland, Thymus
See Thymus Gland

Gland, Thyroid
See Thyroid Gland

Glasses
See Spectacle Services

Glaucoma
Cryotherapy .... .66720
Cyclophotocoagulation 66710-66711
Diathermy .... .66700
Fistulization of Sclera .... .66150
Provocative Test .... .92140

Glaucoma Drainage Implant
See Aqueous Shunt

Glenn Procedure 33766-33767

Glenohumeral Joint
Arthrotomy .... .23040
　with Biopsy .... .23100
　with Synovectomy .... .23105
Exploration .... .23107
Removal
　Foreign or Loose Body .... .23107

Glenoid Fossa
Reconstruction .... .21255

GLN
See Glutamine

Globulin
Antihuman 86880-86886
Immune 90281-90399
Sex Hormone Binding .... .84270

Globulin, Corticosteroid-Binding
See Transcortin

Globulin, Rh Immune
See Immune Globulins, Rho (D)

Globulin, Thyroxine-Binding
See Thyroxine Binding Globulin

Glomerular Procoagulant Activity
See Thromboplastin

Glomus Caroticum
See Carotid Body

Glossectomies
See Excision, Tongue

Glossopexy
See Tongue, Fixation

Glossorrhaphy
See Suture, Tongue

Glucagon .... .82943
Tolerance Panel 80422-80424
Tolerance Test .... .82946

Glucose 80422-80424, 80430-80435,
　　　　　　　　　　　　　　95250-95251
Blood Test 82947-82950, 82962
Body Fluid .... .82945
Interstitial Fluid
　Continuous Monitoring 95250-95251
Tolerance Test 82951-82952
　with Tolbutamide .... .82953

Glucose Phosphate Isomerase
See Phosphohexose Isomerase

Glucose Phosphate Isomerase Measurement
See Phosphohexose Isomerase

Glucose-6-Phosphate
Dehydrogenase 82955-82960

Glucosidase .... .82963

Glucuronide Androstanediol ... .82154

Glue
Cornea Wound .... .65286
Sclera Wound .... .65286

Glukagon
See Glucagon

Glutamate Dehydrogenase
Blood .... .82965

Glutamate Pyruvate Transaminase
See Transaminase, Glutamic Pyruvic

Glutamic Alanine Transaminase
See Transaminase, Glutamic Pyruvic

Glutamic Aspartic Transaminase
See Transaminase, Glutamic Oxaloacetic

Glutamic Dehydrogenase
See Glutamate Dehydrogenase

Glutamine .... .82975

Glutamyltransferase, Gamma .. .82977

Glutathione .... .82978

Groin Area
Repair
　　Hernia 49550-49557

Group Health Education . .98961-98962,
　　　　　　　　　　　　　　　　　　　99078

Grouping, Blood
See Blood Typing

Growth Factors, Insulin-Like
See Somatomedin

Growth Hormone 83003
Human 80418, 80428-80430, 86277

**Growth Hormone Release
Inhibiting Factor**
See Somatostatin

GTT
See Hydatidiform Mole

Guaiac Test
See Blood, Feces

Guanosine Monophosphate 83008

Guanosine Monophosphate, Cyclic
See Cyclic GMP

Guanylic Acids
See Guanosine Monophosphate

Guard Stain 88313

Gullet
See Esophagus

Gums
Abscess
　　Incision and Drainage 41800
Alveolus
　　Excision 41830
Cyst
　　Incision and Drainage 41800
Excision
　　Gingiva 41820
　　Operculum 41821
Graft
　　Mucosa 41870
Hematoma
　　Incision and Drainage 41800
Lesion
　　Destruction 41850
　　Excision 41822-41828
Mucosa
　　Excision 41828
Reconstruction
　　Alveolus 41874
　　Gingiva 41872
Removal
　　Foreign Body 41805
Tumor
　　Excision 41825-41827
Unlisted Services and Procedures 41899

Gunning-Lieben Test
See Acetone, Blood or Urine

Guthrie Test 84030

H

H Flu
See Hemophilus Influenza

H-Reflex Study 95934-95936

**HAA (Hepatitis Associated
Antigen)**
See Hepatitis Antigen, B Surface

HAAb
See Antibody, Hepatitis

Haemoglobin F
See Fetal Hemoglobin

Haemorrhage
See Hemorrhage

Haemorrhage Rectum
See Hemorrhage, Rectum

Hageman Factor 85280

HAI Test
See Hemagglutination Inhibition Test

Hair
Electrolysis 17380
KOH Examination 87220
Microscopic Evaluation 96902
Transplant
　　Punch Graft 15775-15776
　　Strip Graft 15220-15221

Hair Removal
See Removal, Hair

Hallux
See Great Toe

Halo
Body Cast 29000
Cranial 20661
　　for Thin Skull Osteology 20664
Femur 20663
Maxillofacial 21100
Pelvic 20662
Removal 20665

Haloperidol
Assay 80173

Halsted Mastectomy
See Mastectomy, Radical

Halsted Repair
See Hernia, Repair, Inguinal

Ham Test
See Hemolysins

Hammertoe Repair 28285-28286

Hamster Penetration Test 89329

Hand
See Carpometacarpal Joint; Intercarpal Joint

Amputation
　　at Metacarpal 25927
　　at Wrist 25920
　　　　Revision 25922
　　Revision 25924, 25929-25931
Arthrodesis
　　Carpometacarpal Joint 26843-26844
　　Intercarpal Joint 25820-25825
Bone
　　Incision and Drainage 26034
Cast 29085
Decompression 26035-26037
Fracture
　　Metacarpal 26600
Insertion
　　Tendon Graft 26392
Magnetic Resonance Imaging
(MRI) 73218-73223
Reconstruction
　　Tendon Pulley 26500-26502
Removal
　　Implantation 26320
　　Tube/Rod 26390-26392, 26416
Repair
　　Blood Vessel 35207
　　Cleft Hand 26580
　　Muscle 26591-26593
　　Tendon
　　　　Extensor 26410-26416, 26426-26428,
　　　　　　　　　　　　　　　　26433-26437
　　　　Flexor 26350-26358, 26440
　　　　Profundus 26370-26373
Replantation 20808
Strapping 29280
Tendon
　　Excision 26390
　　Extensor 26415
Tenotomy 26450, 26460
Tumor
　　Excision 26115-26117
Unlisted Services and Procedures 26989
X-Ray 73120-73130

Hand Abscess
See Abscess, Hand

Hand Phalange
See Finger, Bone

Hand(s) Dupuytrens Contracture(s)
See Dupuytren's Contracture

Handling
Device 99002
Radioelement 77790
Specimen 99000-99001

Hanganutziu Deicher Antibodies
See Antibody, Heterophile

Haptoglobin 83010-83012

Hard Palate
See Palate

Harelip Operation
See Cleft Lip, Repair

Harii Procedure 25430

Hexadecadrol
See Dexamethasone

Hexosephosphate Isomerase
See Phosphohexose Isomerase

Heyman Procedure 27179, 28264

Hg Factor
See Glucagon

HGB
See Hemoglobin, Concentration

HGH
See Growth Hormone, Human

HHV-4
See Epstein-Barr Virus

HIAA
See Hydroxyindolacetic Acid, Urine

Hib Vaccine
4 Dose Schedule
   HbOC 90645
   PRP-T 90648
PRP-D
   Booster 90646
PRP-OMP
   3 Dose Schedule 90647

Hibb Operation
See Spinal Cord; Spine, Fusion; Vertebra;
Vertebral Body; Vertebral Process

Hickmann Catheterization
See Cannulization; Catheterization, Venous,
Central Line; Venipuncture

Hidradenitis
See Sweat Gland
Excision 11450-11471
Suppurative
   Incision and Drainage 10060-10061

**High Altitude
Simulation Test** 94452-94453

High Density Lipoprotein
See Lipoprotein

High Molecular Weight Kininogen
See Fitzgerald Factor

Highly Selective Vagotomy
See Vagotomy, Highly Selective

Highmore Antrum
See Sinus/Sinuses, Maxillary

Hill Procedure 43324
Laparoscopic 43280

Hinton Positive
See RPR

Hip
See Femur; Pelvis
Abscess
   Incision and Drainage 26990
Arthrocentesis 20610
Arthrodesis 27284-27286

Arthrography 73525
Arthroplasty 27130-27132
Arthroscopy 29860-29863
Arthrotomy 27030-27033
Biopsy 27040-27041
Bone
   Drainage 26992
Bursa
   Incision and Drainage 26991
Capsulectomy
   with Release, Flexor Muscles 27036
Cast 29305-29325
Craterization 27070
Cyst
   Excision 27065-27067
Denervation 27035
Echography
   Infant 76885-76886
Endoprosthesis
  See Prosthesis, Hip
Excision 27070
Exploration 27033
Fasciotomy 27025
Fusion 27284-27286
Hematoma
   Incision and Drainage 26990
Injection
   Radiologic 27093-27096
Reconstruction
   Total Replacement 27130
Removal
   Cast 29710
   Foreign Body 27033, 27086-27087
     Arthroscopic 29861
   Loose Body
     Arthroscopic 29861
   Prosthesis 27090-27091
Repair
   Muscle Transfer 27100-27105, 27111
   Osteotomy 27146-27156
   Tendon 27097
Saucerization 27070
Stem Prostheses
  See Arthroplasty, Hip
Strapping 29520
Tenotomy
   Abductor Tendon 27006
   Adductor Tendon 27000-27003
   Iliopsoas 27005
Total Replacement 27130-27132
Tumor
   Excision 27047-27049, 27065-27067
   Radical 27075-27076
Ultrasound
   Infant 76885-76886
X-Ray 73500-73520, 73540
   Intraoperative 73530
   with Contrast 73525

Hip Joint
Arthroplasty 27132
   Revision 27134-27138
Arthrotomy 27052
Biopsy 27052
Capsulotomy
   with Release, Flexor Muscles 27036
Dislocation 27250-27252
   Congenital 27256-27259

   Open Treatment 27253-27254
   without Trauma 27265-27266
Manipulation 27275
Reconstruction
   Revision 27134-27138
Synovium
   Excision 27054
    Arthroscopic 29863
Total Replacement 27132

Hip Stem Prostheses
See Arthroplasty, Hip

Hippocampus
Excision 61566

Histamine 83088

Histamine Release Test 86343

Histochemistry 88318-88319

Histocompatibility Testing
See Tissue Typing

Histoplasma
Antibody 86698
Antigen 87385

Histoplasma capsulatum
Antigen Detection
   Enzyme Immunoassay 87385

Histoplasmin Test
See Histoplasmosis, Skin Test

Histoplasmoses
See Histoplasmosis

Histoplasmosis
Skin Test 86510

History and Physical
See Evaluation and Management, Office and/or
Other Outpatient Services
Pelvic Exam 57410

HIV
Antibody 86701-86703
   Confirmation Test 86689

HIV-1
Antigen Detection
   Enzyme Immunoassay 87390

HIV-2
Antigen Detection
   Enzyme Immunoassay 87391

HK3 Kallikrein
See Antigen, Prostate Specific

HLA Typing 86812-86817

HMRK
See Fitzgerald Factor

HMW Kininogen
See Fitzgerald Factor

Hoffman Apparatus 20690

Hofmeister Operation
See Gastrectomy, Total

Holotranscobalamin 0103T

Holten Test
See Creatinine, Urine, Clearance

Home Services
Activities of Daily Living 99509
Anticoagulant Management 99363-99364
Apnea Monitoring 94774-94777
Catheter Care 99507
Enema Administration 99511
Established Patient 99347-99350
Hemodialysis 99512
Home Infusion Procedures 99601-99602
Individual or Family Counseling 99510
Intramuscular Injections 99506
Mechanical Ventilation 99504
New Patient 99341-99345
Newborn Care 99502
Postnatal Assessment 99501
Prenatal Monitoring 99500
Respiratory Therapy 99503
Sleep Studies 95805-95811
Stoma Care 99505
Unlisted Services and Procedures 99600
Ventilation Assist 94005

Home Visit
See House Calls

Homocyst(e)ine 83090
Urine 82615

Homogenization, Tissue 87176

Homograft
Skin 15300-15336

Homologous Grafts
See Graft

Homologous Transplantation
See Homograft

Homovanillic Acid
Urine 83150

Hormone Assay
ACTH 82024
Aldosterone
    Blood or Urine 82088
Androstenedione
    Blood or Urine 82157
Androsterone
    Blood or Urine 82160
Angiotensin II 82163
Corticosterone 82528
Cortisol
    Total 82533
Dehydroepiandrosterone 82626
Dihydroelestosterone 82651
Dihydrotestosterone 82651
Epiandrosterone 82666
Estradiol 82670
Estriol 82677
Estrogen 82671-82672
Estrone 82679
Follicle Stimulating Hormone 83001
Growth Hormone 83003
Hydroxyprogesterone 83498-83499
Luteinizing Hormone 83002

Somatotropin 83003
Testosterone 84403
Vasopressin 84588

**Hormone Pellet
Implantation** 11980

Hormone, Adrenocorticotrophic
See Adrenocorticotropic Hormone (ACTH)

Hormone, Corticotropin-Releasing
See Corticotropic Releasing Hormone (CRH)

Hormone, Growth
See Growth Hormone

Hormone, Human Growth
See Growth Hormone, Human

**Hormone, Interstitial Cell-
Stimulating**
See Luteinizing Hormone (LH)

Hormone, Parathyroid
See Parathormone

Hormone, Pituitary Lactogenic
See Prolactin

Hormone, Placental Lactogen
See Lactogen, Human Placental

**Hormone, Somatotropin Release-
Inhibiting**
See Somatostatin

Hormone, Thyroid-Stimulating
See Thyroid Stimulating Hormone (TSH)

Hormone-Binding Globulin, Sex
See Globulin, Sex Hormone Binding

Hormones, Adrenal Cortex
See Corticosteroids

Hormones, Antidiuretic
See Antidiuretic Hormone

Hospital Discharge Services
See Discharge Services, Hospital

Hospital Services
Inpatient Services 99238-99239
    Discharge Services 99238-99239
    Initial Care
       New or Established Patient ..99221-99233
    Initial Hospital Care 99221-99223
    Newborn 99431-99433
    Prolonged Services 99356-99357
    Subsequent Hospital Care 99231-99233
Observation
    Discharge Services 99234-99236
    Initial Care 99218-99220
       New or Established Patient ..99218-99220
Same Day Admission
    Discharge Services 99234-99236
Subsequent Newborn Care 99433

Hot Pack Treatment 97010
See Physical Medicine and Rehabilitation

House Calls 99341-99350

Howard Test
See Cystourethroscopy, Catheterization, Ureter

HPL
See Lactogen, Human Placental

HTLV I
Antibody
    Confirmatory Test 86689
    Detection 86687

HTLV II
Antibody 86688

HTLV III
See HIV

HTLV III Antibodies
See Antibody, HIV

HTLV IV
See HIV-2

Hubbard Tank Therapy 97036
See Physical Medicine/Therapy/Occupational
Therapy

Hue Test 92283

Huggin Operation
See Orchiectomy, Simple

Huhner Test 89300, 89320

Human Chorionic Gonadotropin
See Chorionic Gonadotropin

**Human Chorionic
Somatomammotropin**
See Lactogen, Human Placental

Human Cytomegalovirus Group
See Cytomegalovirus

**Human Growth
Hormone (HGH)** 80418, 80428-80430

Human Herpes Virus 4
See Epstein-Barr Virus

Human Immunodeficiency Virus
See HIV

Human Immunodeficiency Virus 1
See HIV-1

Human Immunodeficiency Virus 2
See HIV-2

**Human Papillomavirus
Detection** 87620-87622

Human Placental Lactogen
See Lactogen, Human Placental

Human T Cell Leukemia Virus I
See HTLV I

**Human T Cell Leukemia Virus I
Antibodies**
See Antibody, HTLV I

Human T Cell Leukemia Virus II
See HTLV II

Hypopharynges
See Hypopharynx

Hypopharynx
Biopsy 42802

Hypophysectomy 61546-61548, 62165

Hypophysis
See Pituitary Gland

Hypopyrexia
See Hypothermia

Hypospadias
Repair 54300, 54352
   Complications 54340-54348
   First Stage 54304
      Proximal Penile or Penoscrotal 54332
   One Stage
      Meatal Advancement 54322
      Perineal 54336
   Urethroplasty
      Local Skin Flaps 54324
      Local Skin Flaps and Mobilization of
      Urethra 54326
      Local Skin Flaps, Skin Graft Patch
      and/or Island Flap 54328
   Urethroplasty for Second Stage .54308-54316
      Free Skin Graft 54316
   Urethroplasty for Third Stage 54318

Hypothermia 99185-99186

Hypoxia
Breathing Response 94450
High Altitude Simulation Test 94452-94453

Hysterectomy
Abdominal
   Radical 58210
   Resection of Ovarian Malignancy 58951,
                         58953-58956
   Supracervical .58180
   Total 58150, 58200, 58956
      with Colpo-Urethrocystopexy 58152
      with Omentectomy 58956
      with Partial Vaginectomy 58200
Cesarean
   after Cesarean Delivery 59525
   with Closure of Vesicouterine Fistula . .51925
Laparoscopic 58541-58544
   Radical 58548
Removal
   Lesion 59100
Supracervical
   Laparoscopic 58541-58544
Vaginal 58260-58270, 58290-58294, 58550-58554
   Laparoscopic .58550
   Radical 58285
   Removal Tubes/Ovaries 58262-58263,
            58291-58292, 58552, 58554
      Repair of Enterocele .58263, 58292, 58294
   with Colpectomy 58275-58280
   with Colpo-Urethrocystopexy . .58267, 58293

Hysterolysis
See Lysis, Adhesions, Uterus

Hysteroplasty 58540

Hysterorrhaphy 58520, 59350

Hysterosalpingography 74740
Catheterization 58345
Injection Procedure 58340

Hysterosalpingostomy
See Implantation, Tubouterine

Hysteroscopy
Ablation
   Endometrial .58563
Diagnostic 58555
Lysis
   Adhesions 58559
Placement
   Fallopian Tube Implants 58565
Removal
   Impacted Foreign Body 58562
   Leiomyomata 58561
Resection
   of Intrauterine Septum 58560
Surgical with Biopsy 58558
Unlisted Services and Procedures . .58578-58579

Hysterosonography
See Ultrasound; Sonohysterography

Hysterotomy 59100
See Ligation, Uterus
Induced Abortion
   with Amniotic Injections 59852
   with Vaginal Suppositories 59857

Hysterotrachelectomy
See Amputation, Cervix

I

I Antibodies, HTLV
See Antibody, HTLV-I

I, Angiotensin
See Angiotensin I

I, Coagulation Factor
See Fibrinogen

I, Heparin Co-Factor
See Antithrombin III

ICCE
See Extraction, Lens, Intracapsular

Ichthyosis, Sex Linked
See Syphilis Test

ICSH
See Luteinizing Hormone (LH)

Identification
Oocyte
   from Follicular Fluid 89254
Sperm
   from Aspiration 89257
   from Tissue .89264

IDH
See Isocitric Dehydrogenase, Blood

IG
See Immune Globulins

IgE 86003-86005

IgG 86001

II, Coagulation Factor
See Prothrombin

II, Cranial Nerve
See Optic Nerve

Ileal Conduit
Visualization 50690

Ileoscopy
via Stoma 44383

Ileostomy 44310, 45136
Continent (Kock Procedure) 44316
Laparoscopic 44186-44187
Non-Tube 44187
Revision 44312-44314

Iliac Arteries
See Artery, Iliac

Iliac Crest
Free Osteocutaneous Flap with Microvascular
Anastomosis 20970

Iliohypogastric Nerve
Injection
   Anesthetic 64425

Ilioinguinal Nerve
Injection
   Anesthetic 64425

Ilium
Craterization 27070
Cyst
   Excision 27065-27067
Excision 27070
Fracture
   Open Treatment 27215, 27218
Saucerization 27070
Tumor
   Excision 27065-27067

Ilizarov Procedure
Monticelli Type 20692
      See Application, Bone Fixation Device

IM Injection
See Injection, Intramuscular

Imaging
See Vascular Studies

Imaging, Gamma Camera
See Nuclear Medicine

Imaging, Magnetic Resonance
See Magnetic Resonance Imaging (MRI)

Imaging, Ultrasonic
See Echography

Bursa
  Ankle 27604
  Arm, Lower 25031
  Elbow 23931
  Foot 28001
  Hip 26991
  Knee 27301
  Leg, Lower 27604
  Leg, Upper 27301
  Palm 26025-26030
  Pelvis 26991
  Wrist 25031
Carbuncle
  Skin 10060-10061
Carpals 25035, 26034
Comedones
  Skin 10040
Cyst
  Conjunctiva 68020
  Gums 41800
  Liver
    Open 47010
    Percutaneous 47011
  Lung 32200
    Percutaneous 32201
  Mouth 40800-40801, 41005-41009,
                 41015-41018
  Ovarian 58800-58805
  Skin 10040, 10060-10061
    Pilonidal 10080-10081
    Puncture Aspiration 10160
  Spinal Cord 63172-63173
  Thyroid Gland 60000
  Tongue 41000-41006, 41015, 60000
Elbow
  Abscess 23935
  Arthrotomy 24000
Femur 27303
Fluid Collection
  Skin 10140
Foreign Body
  Skin 10120-10121
Furuncle 10060-10061
Gallbladder 47480
Hematoma
  Ankle 27603
  Arm, Lower 25028
  Arm, Upper 23930
  Brain 61312-61315
  Ear, External
    Complicated 69005
    Simple 69000
  Elbow 23930
  Epididymis 54700
  Gums 41800
  Hip 26990
  Knee 27301
  Leg, Lower 27603
  Leg, Upper 27301
  Mouth 40800-40801, 41005-41009,
                 41015-41018
  Nasal Septum 30020
  Neck 21501-21502
  Nose 30000-30020
  Pelvis 26990
  Scrotum 54700
  Skin 10140
    Puncture Aspiration 10160

Skull 61312-61315
Testis 54700
Thorax 21501-21502
Tongue 41000-41006, 41015
Vagina 57022-57023
Wrist 25028
Hepatic Duct 47400
Hip
  Bone 26992, 27030
Humerus
  Abscess 23935
Interphalangeal Joint
  Toe 28024
Intertarsal Joint 28020
Kidney 50040, 50125
Knee 27303, 27310
Lacrimal Gland 68400
Lacrimal Sac 68420
Liver
  Abscess or Cyst 47010-47011
    Percutaneous 47011
Mediastinum 39000-39010
Metatarsophalangeal Joint 28022
Milia, Multiple 10040
Onychia 10060-10061
Orbit 67405, 67440
Paronychia 10060-10061
Pelvic
  Bone 26992
Penis 54015
Pericardium 33025
Phalanges
  Finger 26034
Pilonidal Cyst 10080-10081
Pustules
  Skin 10040
Radius 25035
Seroma
  Skin 10140
Shoulder
  Abscess 23030
  Arthrotomy
    Acromioclavicular Joint 23044
    Sternoclavicular Joint 23044
  Bursa 23031
  Hematoma 23030
Shoulder Joint
  Arthrotomy
    Glenohumeral Joint 23040
Spine
  Abscess 22010-22015
Tarsometatarsal Joint 28020
Tendon Sheath
  Finger 26020
  Palm 26020
Thorax
  Deep 21510
Toe 28024
Ulna 25035
Ureter 50600
Vagina 57020
Wound Infection
  Skin 10180
Wrist 25028, 25040

Incisional Hernia Repair
See Hernia, Repair, Incisional

Inclusion Bodies

Fluid 88106
Smear 87207, 87210

Incomplete Abortion
See Abortion, Incomplete

**Indicator Dilution
Studies** 93561-93562

Induced Abortion
See Abortion

Induced Hyperthermia
See Thermotherapy

Induced Hypothermia
See Hypothermia

Induratio Penis Plastica
See Peyronie Disease

Infant, Newborn, Intensive Care
See Intensive Care, Neonatal

Infantile Paralysis
See Polio

Infection
Immunoassay 86317-86318
Rapid Test 86403-86406

Infection, Actinomyces
See Actinomycosis

Infection, Bone
See Osteomyelitis

Infection, Filarioidea
See Filariasis

Infection, Postoperative Wound
See Postoperative Wound Infection

Infection, Wound
See Wound, Infection

Infectious Agent
Antigen Detection
  Direct Fluorescence 87265-87272, 87276,
                 87278, 87280, 87285-87290
    Bordetella 87265
    Chlamydia Trachomatis 87270
    Cryptosporidium 87272
    Cytomegalovirus 87271
    Enterovirus 87267
    Giardia 87269
    Influenza A 87276
    Legionella Pneumophila 87278
    Respiratory Syncytial Virus ... 87280
    Treponema Pallidum 87285
    Varicella-Zoster 87290
  Enzyme Immunoassay
    Adenovirus 87301
    Aspergillus 87305
    Chlamydia Trachomatis 87320
    Clostridium Difficile 87324
    Cryptococcus Neoformans 87327
    Cryptosporidium 87328
    Cytomegalovirus 87332
    Entamoeba Histolytica Dispar Group .87336
    Entamoeba Histolytica Group ... 87337
    Escherichia Coli 0157 87335
    Giardia 87329

Helicobacter Pylori 87338-87339
Hepatitis B Surface Antigen
(HBsAg) 87340
Hepatitis B Surface Antigen (HBsAg)
Neutralization 87341
Hepatitis Be Antigen (HBeAg) 87350
Hepatitis, Delta Agent 87380
Histoplasma capsulatum 87385
HIV-1......................87390
HIV-2......................87391
Influenza A 87400
Influenza B 87400
Multiple Step Method 87301-87449,
87451

See specific agent
Not Otherwise Specified 87449, 87451
Respiratory Syncytial Virus 87420
Rotavirus 87425
Shiga-like Toxin 87427
Single Step Method 87450
Streptococcus, Group A 87430
Immunofluorescence ...87260, 87273-87275,
87277, 87279, 87281-87283, 87299-87300
Adenovirus 87260
Herpes Simplex 87273-87274
Influenza B 87275
Legionella Micdadei 87277
Not Otherwise Specified 87299
Parainfluenza Virus 87279
Pneumocystis Carinii 87281
Polyvalent 87300
Rubeola 87283
Concentration 87015
Detection
by Immunoassay
Chlamydia Trachomatis 87810
Clostridium Difficile 87803
Influenza 87804
Neisseria Gonorrheae 87850
Not Otherwise Specified 87899
Respiratory Syncytial Virus 87807
Streptococcus, Group A 87880
Streptococcus, Group B 87802
Trichomonas Vaginalis 87808
with Direct Optical
Observation 87802-87899
by Nucleic Acid
Bartonella Henselae 87470-87472
Bartonella Quintana 87470-87472
Borrelia Burgdorferi 87475-87477
Candida Species 87480-87482
Chlamydia Pneumoniae 87485-87487
Chlamydia Trachomatis 87490-87492
Cytomegalovirus 87495-87497
Enterovirus 87498
Gardnerella Vaginalis 87510-87512
Hepatitis B Virus 87515-87517
Hepatitis C 87520-87522
Hepatitis G 87525-87527
Herpes Simplex Virus 87528-87530
Herpes Virus-6 87531-87533
HIV-1 87534-87536
HIV-2 87537-87539
Legionella Pneumophila 87540-87542
Multiple Organisms 87800-87801
Mycobacteria
Avium-Intracellulare 87560-87562
Mycobacteria Species 87550-87552

Mycobacteria Tuberculosis ...87555-87557
Mycoplasma Pneumoniae ..87580-87582
Neisseria Gonorrheae 87590-87592
Not Otherwise Specified ...87797-87799
Papillomavirus, Human 87620-87622
Staphylococcus Aureus 87640-87641
Streptococcus, Group A 87650-87652
Streptococcus, Group B 87653
Trichomonas Vaginalis 87660
Urinalysis 0041T
Genotype Analysis
by Nucleic Acid
Hepatitis C Virus 87902
HIV-1 Protease/Reverse
Transcriptase 87901
Phenotype Analysis
by Nucleic Acid
HIV-1 Drug Resistance 87903-87904
Phenotype Prediction
by Genetic Database 87900

Infectious Mononucleosis Virus
See Epstein-Barr Virus

Inflammatory Process
Localization
Nuclear Medicine 78805-78807

Inflation
Ear, Middle
Eustachian Tube
with Catheterization 69400
without Catheterization 69401
Eustachian Tube
Myringotomy 69420
Anesthesia 69424

Influenza A
Antigen Detection
Direct Fluorescence 87276
Enzyme Immunoassay 87400

Influenza B
Antigen Detection
Enzyme Immunoassay 87400
Immunofluorescence 87275

Influenza Vaccine
See Vaccines

Influenza Virus
Antibody 86710
by Immunoassay
with Direct Optical Observation 87804

Infraorbital Nerve
Avulsion 64734
Incision 64734
Transection 64734

Infrared Light Treatment 97026
See Physical Medicine/Therapy/Occupational
Therapy

Infratentorial
Craniectomy 61520-61521

Infusion
Amnion
Transabdominal 59072

Cerebral
Intravenous
for Thrombolysis 37195
Intra-Arterial.........................90773
Unlisted 90779
Intraosseous 36680
Intravenous 90779
Diagnostic/Prophylactic/
Therapeutic 90760-90768
Radioelement 77750
Transcatheter Therapy 37201-37202

Infusion Pump
Electronic Analysis
Spinal Cord 62367-62368
Insertion
Intra-Arterial 36260
Intraarterial
Removal 36262
Revision 36261
Intravenous
Insertion 36563
Repair 36576
Replacement 36583
Maintenance 95990-95991, 96521-96522
See Chemotherapy, Pump Services
Spinal Cord 62361-62362
Ventricular Catheter 61215

Infusion Therapy 62350-62351,
62360-62362

See Injection, Chemotherapy
Arterial Catheterization 36640
Chemotherapy 96401-96542, 96545, 96549
Home Infusion Procedures 99601-99602
Intravenous 90760-90768
Pain 62360-62362, 62367-62368
Transcatheter Therapy 75896

Ingestion Challenge Test 95075
See Allergy Tests

Inguinal Hernia Repair
See Hernia, Repair, Inguinal

INH
See Drug Assay

Inhalation
Pentamidine 94642

Inhalation Provocation Tests
See Bronchial Challenge Test

Inhalation Treatment 94640,
94644-94645, 94664, 99503
See Pulmonology, Therapeutic

Inhibin A 86336

Inhibition Test, Hemagglutination
See Hemagglutination Inhibition Test

Inhibition, Fertilization
See Contraception

Inhibitor, Alpha 1-Protease
See Alpha-1 Antitrypsin

Inhibitor, Alpha 2-Plasmin
See Alpha-2 Antiplasmin

Inspiratory Positive Pressure Breathing

See Intermittent Positive Pressure Breathing (IPPB)

Instillation

Instillation, Bladder

See Bladder, Instillation

Instrumentation

See Application; Bone, Fixation; Spinal Instrumentation

Insufflation, Eustachian Tube

See Eustachian Tube, Inflation

Insulin

Insulin C-Peptide Measurement

See C-Peptide

Insulin Like Growth Factors

See Somatomedin

Insurance

Integumentary System

Integumentum Commune

See Integumentary System

Intelligence Test

Intensive Care

J

Jaboulay Operation
See Gastroduodenostomy

Jaboulay Operation Gastroduodenostomy
See Gastroduodenostomy

Jannetta Procedure
See Decompression, Cranial Nerve; Section

Japanese, River Fever
See Scrub Typhus

Jatene Type 33770-33781

Jaw Joint
See Facial Bones; Mandible; Maxilla

Jaws
Muscle Reduction 21295-21296
X-Ray
   for Orthodontics 70355

Jejunostomy
Catheterization 44015
Insertion
   Catheter 44015
Laparoscopic 44186-44187
Non-Tube 44187, 44310
with Pancreatic Drain 48001

Jejunum
Creation
   Stoma
   Laparoscopic 44186
Transfer
   with Microvascular Anastomosis
     Free 43496

Johannsen Procedure 53400

Johanson Operation
See Reconstruction, Urethra

Joint
See Specific Joint
Acromioclavicular
   See Acromioclavicular Joint
Arthrocentesis 20600-20610
Aspiration 20600-20610
Dislocation
   See Dislocation
Drainage 20600-20610
Finger
   See Intercarpal Joint
Fixation (Surgical)
   See Arthrodesis
Foot
   See Foot, Joint
Hip
   See Hip Joint
Injection 20600-20610
Intertarsal
   See Intertarsal Joint
Knee
   See Knee Joint
Ligament
   See Ligament
Metacarpophalangeal
   See Metacarpophalangeal Joint
Metatarsophalangeal
   See Metatarsophalangeal Joint
Nuclear Medicine
   Imaging 78300, 78315

Radiology
   Stress Views 77071
Sacroiliac
   See Sacroiliac Joint
Shoulder
   See Glenohumeral Joint
Sternoclavicular
   See Sternoclavicular Joint
Survey 77077
Temporomandibular
   See Temporomandibular Joint (TMJ)
   Dislocation Temporomandibular
     See Dislocation, Temporomandibular Joint
   Implant
     See Prosthesis, Temporomandibular Joint
Wrist
   See Radiocarpal Joint

Joint Syndrome, Temporomandibular
See Temporomandibular Joint (TMJ)

Jones and Cantarow Test
See Blood Urea Nitrogen; Urea Nitrogen, Clearance

Jones Procedure 28760

Joplin Procedure 28294

Jugal Bone
See Cheekbone

Jugular Vein
See Vein, Jugular

K

K-Wire Fixation
Tongue 41500

Kader Operation
See Incision, Stomach, Creation, Stoma; Incision and Drainage

Kala Azar Smear 87207

Kallidin I /Kallidin 9
See Bradykinin

Kallikrein HK3
See Antigen, Prostate Specific

Kallikreinogen
See Fletcher Factor

Kasai Procedure 47701

Kedani Fever
See Scrub Typhus

Keel
Insertion/Removal
   Laryngoplasty 31580

Keen Operation
See Laminectomy

Kelikian Procedure 28280

Keller Procedure 28292

Kelly Urethral Plication 57220

Keratectomy
Partial
   for Lesion 65400

Keratomileusis 65760

Keratophakia 65765

Keratoplasty
Lamellar 65710
Penetrating 65730
   in Aphakia 65750
   in Pseudophakia 65755

Keratoprosthesis 65770

Keratotomy
Radial 65771

Ketogenic Steroids 83582

Ketone Body
Acetone 82009-82010

Ketosteroids 83586-83593

Kidner Procedure 28238

Kidney
Abscess
   Incision and Drainage 50020
     Open 50020
     Percutaneous 50021
Anesthesia 00862
Biopsy 50200-50205
   Endoscopic 50555-50557, 52354
Catheterization
   Endoscopic 50572
Cyst
   Ablation 50541
   Aspiration 50390
   Excision 50280-50290
   Injection 50390
   X-Ray 74470
Destruction
   Calculus 50590
   Endoscopic 50557, 50576, 52354
Dilation 50395
Endoscopy
   Biopsy 50555, 50574-50576, 52354
   Catheterization 50553, 50572
   Destruction 50557, 50576, 52354
   Dilation
     Intra-Renal Stricture 52343, 52346
     Ureter 50553
   Excision
     Tumor 52355
   Exploration 52351
   Lithotripsy 52353
   Removal
     Calculus 50561, 50580, 52352
     Foreign Body 50561, 50580
   via Incision 50562-50580
   via Stoma 50551-50561
Excision
   Donor 50300-50320, 50547

L

Stomach
  Excision 43611
Testis
  Excision 54512
Toe
  Excision 28092
Tongue
  Excision 41110-41114
Uvula
  Destruction 42145
  Excision 42104-42107
Vagina
  Destruction 57061-57065
Vulva
  Destruction
    Extensive 56515
    Simple 56501
Wrist Tendon
  Excision 25110

Leu 2 Antigens
See CD8

Leucine Aminopeptidase 83670

**Leukemia Lymphoma Virus I
Antibodies, Human T Cell**
See Antibody, HTLV-I

**Leukemia Lymphoma Virus I,
Adult T Cell**
See HTLV I

**Leukemia Lymphoma Virus II
Antibodies, Human T Cell**
See Antibody, HTLV-II

**Leukemia Virus II, Hairy Cell
Associated, Human T Cell**
See HTLV II

Leukoagglutinins 86021

Leukocyte
See White Blood Cell
Alkaline Phosphatase 85540
Antibody 86021
Count 85032, 85048, 89055
Histamine Release Test 86343
Phagocytosis 86344
Transfusion 86950

Levarterenol
See Noradrenalin

Levator Muscle Repair
See Blepharoptosis, Repair

LeVeen Shunt
Insertion 49425
Patency Test 78291
Revision 49426

Levulose
See Fructose

LGV
See Lymphogranuloma Venereum

LH
See Luteinizing Hormone (LH)

LHR
See Leukocyte Histamine Release Test

Lid Suture
See Blepharoptosis, Repair

Lidocaine
Assay 80176

Lift, Face
See Face Lift

Ligament
See Specific Site
Collateral
  Repair
    Knee
      with Cruciate Ligament 27409
Dentate
  Section 63180-63182
Injection 20550
Release
  Coracoacromial 23415
  Transverse Carpal 29848
Repair
  Elbow 24343-24346
  Knee Joint 27405-27409

Ligation
Artery
  Abdomen 37617
  Carotid 37600-37606
  Chest 37616
  Coronary 33502
  Ethmoidal 30915
  Extremity 37618
  Fistula 37607
  Maxillary 30920
  Neck 37615
  Temporal 37609
Esophageal Varices 43204, 43400
Fallopian Tube
  Oviduct 58600-58611, 58670
Gastroesophageal 43405
Hemorrhoids 46945-46946
Oviducts 59100
Salivary Duct 42665
Shunt
  Aorta
    Pulmonary 33924
  Peritoneal
    Venous 49428
Thoracic Duct 38380
  Abdominal Approach 38382
  Thoracic Approach 38381
Vas Deferens 55450
Vein
  Clusters 37785
  Esophagus 43205, 43244, 43400
  Femoral 37650
  Gastric 43244
  Iliac 37660
  Jugular, Internal 37565
  Perforate 37760
  Saphenous 37700-37735, 37780
  Vena Cava 37620

Ligature Strangulation
Skin Tags 11200-11201

Light Coagulation
See Photocoagulation

Light Scattering Measurement
See Nephelometry

Light Therapy, UV
See Actinotherapy

Limb
See Extremity

**Limited Lymphadenectomy for
Staging**
See Lymphadenectomy, Limited, for Staging

Limited Neck Dissection
with Thyroidectomy 60252

Limited Resection Mastectomies
See Breast, Excision, Lesion

Lindholm Operation
See Tenoplasty

Lingual Bone
See Hyoid Bone

Lingual Frenectomy
See Excision, Tongue, Frenum

Lingual Nerve
Avulsion 64740
Incision 64740
Transection 64740

Lingual Tonsil
See Tonsils, Lingual

Linton Procedure 37760

Lip
Biopsy 40490
Excision 40500-40530
  Frenum 40819
Incision
  Frenum 40806
Reconstruction 40525-40527
Repair 40650-40654
  Cleft Lip 40700-40761
  Fistula 42260
Unlisted Services and Procedures 40799

Lip, Cleft
See Cleft Lip

Lipase 83690

Lipectomy
Excision 15830-15839
Suction Assisted 15876-15879

Lipectomy, Aspiration
See Liposuction

Lipids
Feces 82705-82710

Lipo-Lutin
See Progesterone

Lipolysis, Aspiration
See Liposuction

Lung

Ablation 32998
Abscess
  Incision and Drainage
    Open 32200
    Percutaneous 32200-32201
Aspiration 32420
Biopsy 32095-32100
Bullae
  Excision 32141
  Endoscopic 32655
Cyst
  Incision and Drainage
    Open 32200
    Removal 32140
Decortication
  Endoscopic 32651-32652
  Partial 32225
  Total 32220
  with Parietal Pleurectomy 32320
Empyema
  Excision 32540
Excision
  Bronchus Resection 32486
  Completion 32488
  Donor
    Heart-Lung 33930
    Lung 32850
  Emphysematous 32491
  Empyema 32540
  Lobe 32480-32482
  Segment 32484
  Total 32440-32445
  Tumor 32503-32504
  Wedge Resection 32500
  Endoscopic 32657
Foreign Body
  Removal 32151
Hemorrhage 32110
Lavage
  Bronchial 31624
  Total 32997
Lysis
  Adhesions 32124
Needle Biopsy 32405
Nuclear Medicine
  Imaging, Perfusion 78580-78585
  Imaging, Ventilation 78586-78594
  Unlisted Services and Procedures 78599
Pneumocentesis 32420
Pneumolysis 32940
Pneumothorax 32960
Puncture 32420
Removal
  Bronchoplasty 32501
  Completion Pneumonectomy 32488
  Extrapleural 32445
  Single Lobe 32480
  Single Segment 32484
  Sleeve Lobectomy 32486
  Sleeve Pneumonectomy 32442
  Total Pneumonectomy 32440-32445
  Two Lobes 32482
  Volume Reduction 32491
  Wedge Resection 32500
Repair
  Hernia 32800
Segmentectomy 32484

Tear
  Repair 32110
Thoracotomy
  Biopsy 32095-32100
  Cardiac Massage 32160
  for Post-Op Complications 32120
  Removal
    Bullae 32141
    Cyst 32140
    Intrapleural Foreign Body 32150
    Intrapulmonary Foreign Body 32151
  Repair 32110
  with Excision-Plication of Bullae 32141
  with Open Intrapleural
    Pneumonolysis 32124
Transplantation 32851-32854, 33935
  Allograft Preparation ..32855-32856, 33933
  Donor Pneumonectomy
    Heart-Lung 33930
    Lung 32850
Tumor
  Removal 32503-32504
Unlisted Services and Procedures 32999

Lung Function Tests
See Pulmonology, Diagnostic

Lung Volume Reduction
Emphysematous 32491

Lupus Anticoagulant Assay 85705

Lupus Band Test
See Immunofluorescent Study

Luteinizing Hormone (LH) 80418,
80426, 83002

Luteinizing Releasing Factor ...83727

Luteotropic Hormone
See Prolactin

Luteotropin
See Prolactin

Luteotropin, Placental
See Lactogen, Human Placental

Lyme Disease 86617-86618

Lyme Disease ab
See Antibody, Lyme Disease

Lyme Disease Vaccine
See Vaccination

Lymph Duct
Injection 38790

Lymph Nodes
Abscess
  Incision and Drainage 38300-38305
Biopsy 38500, 38510-38530, 38570
  Needle 38505
Dissection 38542
Excision 38500, 38510-38530
  Abdominal 38747
  Inguinofemoral 38760-38765
  Laparoscopic 38571-38572
  Limited, for Staging
    Para-Aortic 38562

    Pelvic 38562
    Retroperitoneal 38564
  Pelvic 38770
  Radical
    Axillary 38740-38745
    Cervical 38720-38724
    Suprahyoid 38720-38724
    Retroperitoneal Transabdominal 38780
    Thoracic 38746
Exploration 38542
Hygroma, Cystic
  Axillary/Cervical
    Excision 38550-38555
Nuclear Medicine
  Imaging 78195
Removal
  Abdominal 38747
  Inguinofemoral 38760-38765
  Pelvic 38770
  Retroperitoneal Transabdominal 38780
  Thoracic 38746

Lymph Vessels
Imaging
  Lymphangiography
    Abdomen 75805-75807
    Arm 75801-75803
    Leg 75801-75803
    Pelvis 75805-75807
  Nuclear Medicine 78195
Incision 38308

Lymphadenectomy
Abdominal 38747
Bilateral Inguinofemoral ..54130, 56632, 56637
Bilateral Pelvic 51575, 51585, 51595, 54135,
55845, 55865
  Total 38571-38572, 57531, 58210
Diaphragmatic Assessment 58960
Gastric 38747
Inguinofemoral 38760-38765
Inguinofemoral, Iliac and Pelvic 56640
Injection
  Sentinel Node 38792
Limited Para-Aortic, Resection of Ovarian
  Malignancy 58951, 58954
Limited Pelvic 55842, 55862, 58954
Limited, for Staging
  Para-Aortic 38562
  Pelvic 38562
  Retroperitoneal 38564
Mediastinal 21632
Para-Aortic 58958
Pelvic 58958
Peripancreatic 38747
Portal 38747
Radical
  Axillary 38740-38745
  Cervical 38720-38724
  Pelvic 54135, 55845, 58548
  Suprahyoid 38700
Regional 50230
Retroperitoneal Transabdominal 38780
Thoracic 38746
Unilateral Inguinofemoral 56631, 56634

Lymphadenitis
Incision and Drainage 38300-38305

Lymphadenopathy Associated Antibodies/Virus
See Antibody, HIV

Lymphangiogram
See Lymphangiography

Lymphangiography
Abdomen 75805-75807
Arm 75801-75803
Injection 38790
Leg 75801-75803
Pelvis 75805-75807

Lymphangioma, Cystic
See Hygroma; Lymph Nodes, Hygroma

Lymphangiotomy 38308

Lymphatic Channels
Incision 38308

Lymphatic Cyst
See Lymphocele

Lymphatic System
Unlisted Procedure 38999

Lymphatics
See Specific Procedure

Lymphoblast Transformation
See Blastogenesis

Lymphocele
Drainage
    Laparoscopic .49323
    Open 49062

Lymphocoele
See Lymphocele

Lymphocyte
Culture 86821-86822
Toxicity Assay 86805-86806
Transformation 86353

Lymphocyte, Thymus-Dependent
See T-Cells

Lymphocytes, CD4
See CD4

Lymphocytes, CD8
See CD8

Lymphocytic Choriomeningitis
Antibody 86727

Lymphocytotoxicity 86805-86806

Lymphogranuloma Venereum
Antibody 86729

Lymphoma Virus, Burkitt
See Epstein-Barr Virus

Lynch Procedure 31075

Lysergic Acid Diethylamide 80102-80103, 80299

Lysergide
See Lysergic Acid Diethylamide

Lysis
Adhesions
    Epidural 0027T, 62263-62264
    Fallopian Tube 58740
    Foreskin 54450
    Intestinal .44005
    Labial 56441
    Lung 32124
    Nose 30560
    Ovary 58740
    Oviduct 58740
    Penile
        Post-Circumcision 54162
    Ureter 50715-50725
    Urethra 53500
    Uterus 58559
Euglobulin 85360
Labial
    Adhesions 56441
Nose
    Intranasal Synechia 30560

Lysozyme .85549

M

MacEwen Operation
See Hernia, Repair, Inguinal

Machado Test
See Complement, Fixation Test

MacLean-De Wesselow Test
See Blood Urea Nitrogen; Urea Nitrogen, Clearance

Macrodactylia
Repair 26590

Madlener Operation
See Tubal Ligation

Magnesium 83735

Magnet Operation
See Ciliary Body; Cornea; Eye, Removal, Foreign Body; Iris; Lens; Retina; Sclera; Vitreous

Magnetic Resonance
Unlisted Services and Procedures 76498

Magnetic Resonance Angiography (MRA)
Abdomen 74185
Arm 73225
Chest 71555
Head 70544-70546
Leg 73725
Neck 70547-70549
Pelvis 72198
Spine 72159

Magnetic Resonance Imaging (MRI)
3D Rendering 76376-76377
Abdomen 74181-74183

Ankle 73721-73723
Arm 73218-73220, 73223
Bone Marrow Study 77084
Brain 70551-70555
    Intraoperative 70557-70559
Breast 77058-77059
    with Computer-aided Detection 0159T
Chest 71550-71552
Elbow 73221
Face 70540-70543
Finger Joint 73221
Foot 73718-73719
Foot Joints 73721-73723
Guidance
    Needle Placement 77021
    Parenchymal Tissue Ablation 77022
Hand 73218-73220, 73223
Heart 75552
    Complete Study 75554
    Flow Mapping 75556
    Limited Study 75555
    Morphology 75553
Joint
    Lower Extremity 73721-73723
    Upper Extremity 73221-73223
Knee 73721-73723
Leg 73718-73720
Neck 70540-70543
Orbit 70540-70543
Pelvis 72195-72197
Spectroscopy .76390
Spine
    Cervical 72141-72142, 72156-72158
    Lumbar 72148-72158
    Thoracic 72146-72147, 72156-72158
Temporomandibular Joint (TMJ) 70336
Toe 73721-73723
Unlisted 76498
Wrist 73221

Magnetic Resonance Spectroscopy 76390

Magnetic Stimulation
Transcranial 0160T, 0161T

Magnetoencephalography (MEG) 95965-95967

Magnuson Procedure 23450

MAGPI Operation 54322

MAGPI Procedure
See Hypospadias, Repair

Major Vestibular Gland
See Bartholin's Gland

Malar Area
Augmentation 21270
Bone Graft 21210
Fracture
    Open Treatment 21360-21366
    with Bone Graft 21366
    with Manipulation 21355
Reconstruction .21270

Malar Bone
See Cheekbone

McIndoe Procedure
See Vagina, Construction

McKissock Surgery
See Breast, Reduction

McVay Operation
See Hernia, Repair, Inguinal

Measles Uncomplicated
See Rubeola

Measles Vaccine
See Vaccines

Measles, German
See Rubella

Meat Fibers
Feces .... .89160

Meatoplasty .... .69310

Meatotomy 53020-53025
Cystourethroscopy .... .52281
Infant .... .53025
Prostate
   Laser Coagulation .... .52647
   Laser Vaporization .... .52648
Transurethral Electrosurgical Resection
   Prostate .... .52601
Ureter .... .52290
Ureteral
   Cystourethroscopy 52290-52305

Meckel's Diverticulum
Excision .... .44800
Unlisted Services and Procedures .... .44899

Median Nerve
Decompression .... .64721
Neuroplasty .... .64721
Release .... .64721
Repair/Suture
   Motor .... .64835
Transposition .... .64721

Median Nerve Compression
See Carpal Tunnel Syndrome

Mediastinal Cyst
See Cyst, Mediastinal; Mediastinum, Cyst

Mediastinoscopy .... .39400

Mediastinotomy
Cervical Approach .... .39000
Transthoracic Approach .... .39010

Mediastinum
See Chest; Thorax
Cyst
   Excision .... .32662, 39200
Endoscopy
   Biopsy .... .39400
   Exploration .... .39400
Exploration 39000-39010
Incision and Drainage 39000-39010
Needle Biopsy .... .32405
Removal
   Foreign Body 39000-39010

Tumor
   Excision .... .32662, 39220
Unlisted Procedures .... .39499

Medical Disability Evaluation
Services 99455-99456

Medical Genetics .... .96040
Genetic Counseling .... .96040

Medical Testimony .... .99075

Medicine, Preventive
See Preventive Medicine

Medicine, Pulmonary
See Pulmonology

Medulla
Tractotomy .... .61470

Medullary Tract
Incision .... .61470
Section .... .61470

Meibomian Cyst
See Chalazion

Membrane Oxygenation, Extracorporeal
See Extracorporeal Membrane Oxygenation

Membrane, Mucous
See Mucosa

Membrane, Tympanic
See Ear, Drum

Meninges
Tumor
   Excision .... .61512, 61519

Meningioma
Excision .... .61512, 61519
Tumor
   Excision .... .61512, 61519

Meningitis, Lymphocytic Benign
See Lymphocytic Choriomeningitis

Meningocele Repair 63700-63702

Meningococcal
See Vaccines

Meningococcal Vaccine
See Vaccines

Meningococcus
See Neisseria Meningitidis

Meningomyelocele
See Myelomeningocele

Meniscectomy
Knee Joint 27332-27333
Temporomandibular Joint .... .21060

Meniscus
Knee
   Excision 27332-27333
   Repair .... .27403
   Transplantation .... .29868

Mental Nerve
Avulsion .... .64736
Incision .... .64736
Transection .... .64736

Meprobamate .... .83805

Mercury .... .83015, 83825

Merskey Test
See Fibrin Degradation Products

Mesencephalic Tract
Incision .... .61480
Section .... .61480

Mesencephalon
Tractotomy .... .61480

Mesenteric Arteries
See Artery, Mesenteric

Mesentery
Lesion
   Excision .... .44820
Repair .... .44850
Suture .... .44850
Unlisted Services and Procedures ...... .44899

Mesh
Implantation
   Hernia .... .49568
Insertion
   Pelvic Floor .... .57267
Removal
   Abdominal Infected .... .11008

Metabisulfite Test
See Red Blood Cell (RBC), Sickling

Metabolite .... .82520

Metacarpal
Amputation .... .26910
Craterization .... .26230
Cyst
   Excision 26200-26205
Diaphysectomy .... .26230
Excision .... .26230
   Radical
     for Tumor 26250-26255
Fracture
   Closed Treatment .... .26605
     with Fixation .... .26607
   Open Treatment .... .26615
   Percutaneous Fixation .... .26608
   with Manipulation 26605-26607
   without Manipulation .... .26600
Ostectomy
   Radical
     for Tumor 26250-26255
Repair
   Lengthening .... .26568
   Nonunion .... .26546
   Osteotomy .... .26565
Saucerization .... .26230
Tumor
   Excision 26200-26205

Metacarpophalangeal Joint
Arthrodesis 26850-26852
Arthroplasty 26530-26531

Milia, Multiple
Removal 10040

Miller Procedure 28737

Miller-Abbott Intubation 44500, 74340

Minerva Cast 29035
Removal 29710

Minimum Inhibitory Concentration 87186

Minimum Lethal Concentration 87187

Minnesota Multiphasic Personality Inventory
See MMPI

Miscarriage
Incomplete Abortion 59812
Missed Abortion
    First Trimester 59820
    Second Trimester 59821
Septic Abortion .59830

Missed Abortion
See Abortion

Mitchell Procedure 28296

Mitogen Blastogenesis 86353

Mitral Valve
Incision .33420-33422
Repair 33420-33427
    Incision 33420-33422
Replacement 33430

Mitrofanoff Operation 50845
See Appendico-Vesicostomy

Miyagawanella
See Chlamydia

MLC
See Lymphocyte, Culture

MMPI .96101-96103
Computer-Assisted 96103

MMR Shots 90707
See Vaccines

Mobilization
Splenic Flexure 44139
    Laparoscopic 44213
Stapes 69650

Modified Radical Mastectomy
See Mastectomy, Modified Radical

Mohs Micrographic Surgery 17311-17315

Molar Pregnancy
See Hydatidiform Mole

Mold
Culture 87107

Mole, Carneous
See Abortion

Mole, Hydatid
See Hydatidiform Mole

Molecular Cytogenetics . .88271-88275
Interpretation and Report 88291

Molecular Diagnostics . . .83890-83914
Amplification 83898-83901
Cell Lysis 83907
Dot/Slot Production 83893
Enzymatic Digestion 83892
Extraction 83890-83891
Interpretation .83912
Molecular Isolation (Extraction) 83890
Mutation Identification 83904-83906
    Enzymatic Ligation 83914
Mutation Scanning 83903
Nucleic Acid Amplification . .83900-83901, 83908
Nucleic Acid Extraction 83907
Nucleic Acid Probe 83896
Nucleic Acid Transfer 83897
Polymerase Reaction Chain 83898
Reverse Transcription 83902
RNA Stabilization 83913
Separation 83894
Separation and Identification
    High Resolution Technique 83909

Molecular Oxygen Saturation
See Oxygen Saturation

Molecular Probes 88384-88386
Multiple
    Array-Based Evaluation 88384-88386

Molluscum Contagiosum
Destruction 17110-17111, 54050-54065

Molteno Procedure 66180

Monilia
See Candida

Monitoring
Blood Pressure, 24 Hour 93784-93790
Electrocardiogram 93224-93237
    See Electrocardiography
Electroencephalogram 95812-95813,
                   95950-95953, 95956
    with Drug Activation 95954
    with Physical Activation 95954
    with WADA Activation 95958
Fetal
    During Labor 59050-59051, 99500
        Interpretation Only 59051
Glucose
    Interstitial Fluid 95250-95251
Interstitial Fluid Pressure 20950
Pediatric Apnea 94774-94777
Seizure 61531, 61760

Monitoring, Sleep
See Polysomnography

Monoethylene Glycol
See Ethylene Glycol

Mononucleosis Virus, Infectious
See Epstein-Barr Virus

Monophosphate, Adenosine
See Adenosine Monophosphate (AMP)

Monophosphate, Adenosine Cyclic
See Cyclic AMP

Monophosphate, Guanosine
See Guanosine Monophosphate

Monophosphate, Guanosine Cyclic
See Cyclic GMP

Monospot Test
See Rapid Test for Infection

Monoxide, Carbon
See Carbon Monoxide

Monteggia Fracture 24620-24635

Monticelli Procedure
See Application, Bone Fixation Device

Morbilli
See Rubeola

Morphine Methyl Ether
See Codeine

Morphometric Analysis
Nerve 88356
Skeletal Muscle 88355
Tumor 88358-88361, 88367-88368

Morton's Neuroma
See Neuroma, Foot, Excision
Excision 28080

Moschcowitz Operation
See Repair, Hernia, Femoral; Revision

Mosenthal Test
See Urinalysis, Routine

Mother Cell
See Stem Cell

Motility Study
Duodenal 91022
Esophagus 91010-91012
    Imaging 78258
Sperm 89300

Motion Analysis
by Video and 3D Kinematics 96000, 96004
Computer-based 96000, 96004

Mouth
Abscess
    Incision and Drainage 40800-40801,
               41005-41009, 41015-41018
Biopsy .40808, 41108
Cyst
    Incision and Drainage 40800-40801,
               41005-41009, 41015-41018
Excision
    Frenum 40819
Hematoma
    Incision and Drainage 40800-40801,
               41005-41009, 41015-41018
Lesion
    Destruction 40820
    Excision 40810-40816, 41116

Sensitivity Studies 87190

Mycoplasma
Antibody 86738
Culture 87109
Detection 87580-87582

Mycota
See Fungus

Myectomy, Anorectal
See Myomectomy, Anorectal

Myelencephalon
See Medulla

Myelin Basic Protein
Cerebrospinal Fluid 83873

Myelography
Brain 70010
Spine
　　Cervical .72240
　　Lumbosacral 72265
　　Thoracic .72255
　　Total 72270

Myelomeningocele
Repair 63704-63706

Myelotomy 63170

Myocardial
Perfusion Imaging . . .78460-78465, 78478-78480
　　See Nuclear Medicine
Positron Emission Tomography (PET) 78459

Myocardial Imaging 78466-78469
Positron Emission Tomography
　　Perfusion Study 78491-78492
Repair
　　Postinfarction 33542

Myocutaneous Flaps 15731-15738, 15756

Myofascial Pain Dysfunction Syndrome
See Temporomandibular Joint (TMJ)

Myofibroma
See Leiomyomata

Myoglobin 83874

Myomectomy
Anorectal 45108
Uterus 58140-58146, 58545-58546

Myoplasty
See Muscle, Repair

Myotomy
Esophagus 43030
Hyoid 21685

Myringoplasty 69620

Myringostomy
See Myringotomy

Myringotomy 69420-69421

Myxoid Cyst
See Ganglion

N

N. Meningitidis
See Neisseria Meningitidis

Naffziger Operation
See Decompression, Orbit; Section

Nagel Test
See Color Vision Examination

Nail Bed
Reconstruction 11762
Repair 11760

Nail Fold
Excision
　　Wedge 11765

Nail Plate Separation
See Nails, Avulsion

Nails
Avulsion 11730-11732
Biopsy 11755
Debridement 11720-11721
Drainage 10060-10061
Evacuation
　　Hematoma, Subungual 11740
Excision 11750-11752
KOH Examination 87220
Removal 11730-11732, 11750-11752
Trimming 11719

Narcosynthesis
Diagnostic and Therapeutic 90865

Nasal Abscess
See Nose, Abscess

Nasal Area
Bone Graft 21210

Nasal Bleeding
See Epistaxis

Nasal Bone
Fracture
　　Closed Treatment 21310-21320
　　Open Treatment 21325-21335
　　with Manipulation 21315-21320
　　without Manipulation 21310
X-Ray 70160

Nasal Deformity
Repair 40700-40761

Nasal Function Study 92512

Nasal Polyp
See Nose, Polyp

Nasal Prosthesis
Impression 21087

Nasal Septum
Abscess
　　Incision and Drainage 30020

Fracture
　　Closed Treatment 21337
　　Open Treatment 21336
Hematoma
　　Incision and Drainage 30020
Repair 30630
Submucous Resection 30520

Nasal Sinuses
See Sinus/Sinuses

Nasal Smear
Eosinophils 89190

Nasal Turbinate
Fracture
　　Therapeutic 30930

Nasoethmoid Complex
Fracture
　　Open Treatment 21338-21339
　　Percutaneous Treatment 21340
Reconstruction 21182-21184

Nasogastric Tube
Placement 43752

Nasolacrimal Duct
Exploration 68810
　　with Anesthesia 68811
Insertion
　　Stent 68815
X-Ray
　　with Contrast 70170

Nasomaxillary
Fracture
　　Closed Treatment 21345
　　Open Treatment 21346-21348
　　with Bone Grafting 21348

Nasopharynges
See Nasopharynx

Nasopharyngoscopy 92511

Nasopharynx
See Pharynx
Biopsy 42804-42806
Hemorrhage 42970-42972
Unlisted Services and Procedures 42999

Natriuretic Peptide 83880

Natural Killer (NK) Cells
Count 86357

Natural Ostium
Sinus
　　Maxillary 31000
　　Sphenoid 31002

Navicular
Arthroplasty
　　with Implant 25443
Fracture
　　Closed Treatment 25622
　　Open Treatment 25628
　　with Manipulation 25624
Repair 25440

Tibial
  See Tibial Nerve
Ulnar
  See Ulnar Nerve
Vestibular
  See Vestibular Nerve

Nerve Conduction
Motor Nerve 95900-95903
Sensory Nerve or Mixed 95904

Nerve II, Cranial
See Optic Nerve

Nerve Root
See Cauda Equina; Spinal Cord
Decompression 63020-63048, 63055-63103
Incision 63185-63190
Section 63185-63190

Nerve Stimulation, Transcutaneous
See Application, Neurostimulation

Nerve Teasing 88362

Nerve V, Cranial
See Trigeminal Nerve

Nerve VII, Cranial
See Facial Nerve

Nerve X, Cranial
See Vagus Nerve

Nerve XI, Cranial
See Accessory Nerve

Nerve XII, Cranial
See Hypoglossal Nerve

Nerves
Anastomosis
  Facial to Hypoglossal 64868
  Facial to Phrenic 64870
  Facial to Spinal Accessory 64866
Avulsion 64732-64772
Biopsy 64795
Decompression 64702-64727
Destruction 64600-64681
  Laryngeal, Recurrent 31595
Foot
  Incision 28035
Graft 64885-64907
Implantation
  Electrode 64553-64581
  to Bone 64787
  to Muscle 64787
Incision 43640-43641, 64732-64772
Injection
  Anesthetic 01991-01992, 64400-64530
  Neurolytic Agent 64600-64681
Insertion
  Electrode 64553-64581
Lesion
  Excision 64774-64792
Neurofibroma
  Excision 64788-64792
Neurolemmoma
  Excision 64788-64792
Neurolytic
  Internal 64727

Neuroma
  Excision 64774-64786
Neuroplasty 64702-64721
Removal
  Electrode 64585
Repair
  Graft 64885-64911
  Microdissection 69990
  Suture 64831-64876
Spinal Accessory
  Incision 63191
  Section 63191
Suture 64831-64876
Sympathectomy
  Excision 64802-64818
Transection 43640-43641, 64732-64772
Transposition 64718-64721
Unlisted Services and Procedures 64999

Nervous System
Nuclear Medicine
  Unlisted Services and Procedures 78699

Nesidioblast
See Islet Cell

Neural Conduction
See Nerve Conduction

Neural Ganglion
See Ganglion

Neurectomy
Foot 28055
Gastrocnemius 27326
Hamstring Muscle 27325
Leg, Lower 27326
Leg, Upper 27325
Popliteal 27326
Tympanic 69676

Neuroendoscopy
Intracranial 62160-62165

Neurofibroma
Cutaneous Nerve
  Excision 64788
Extensive
  Excision 64792
Peripheral Nerve
  Excision 64790

Neurolemmoma
Cutaneous Nerve
  Excision 64788
Extensive
  Excision 64792
Peripheral Nerve
  Excision 64790

Neurologic System
See Nervous System

Neurology
Brain Cortex
Magnetic Stimulation 0160T-0161T
Brain Mapping 96020
Brain Surface Electrode
Stimulation 95961-95962

Central Motor
  Transcranial Motor
  Stimulation 95928-95929
Diagnostic
  Anal Sphincter 51785
  Autonomic Nervous Function
    Heart Rate Response 95921-95923
    Pseudomotor Response 95921-95923
    Sympathetic Function 95921-95923
Electrocorticogram
  Intraoperative 95829
Electroencephalogram (EEG) 95812-95827,
                                      95955
  Brain Death 95824
  Electrode Placement 95830
  Intraoperative 95955
  Monitoring 95812-95813, 95950-95953,
                                      95956
  Physical or Drug Activation 95954
  Sleep 95822, 95827
  Standard 95819
  WADA Activation 95958
Electroencephalography (EEG)
  Digital Analysis 95957
Electromyography
  Fine Wire
    Dynamic 96004
  Ischemic Limb Exercise Test 95875
  Needle 51785, 95860-95872
  Surface
    Dynamic 96002-96004
Higher Cerebral Function
  Aphasia Test 96105
  Cognitive Function Tests 96116
  Developmental Tests 96110-96111
  Neurobehavioral Status 96116
  Neuropsychological Testing 96118-96120
  Neuropsychological Testing, Computer-
    Assisted 96120
Magnetoencephalography
(MEG) 95965-95967
Motion Analysis
  by Video and 3D Kinematics ...96000, 96004
  Computer-based 96000, 96004
Muscle Testing
  Manual 95831-95834
Nerve Conduction
  Motor Nerve 95900-95903
  Sensory Nerve or Mixed 95904
Neurofunctional Testing 96020
Neuromuscular Junction Tests 95937
Neurophysiological Testing
  Intraoperative 95920
Neuropsychological Testing 96118-96120
  Computer-Assisted 96120
Plantar Pressure Measurements
  Dynamic 96001, 96004
Polysomnography 95808-95811
Range of Motion 95851-95852
Reflex
  Blink Reflex 95933
  H-Reflex 95933-95934
Sleep Study 95807-95810
Somatosensory Testing 95925-95927
Tensilon Test 95857

Obturator Nerve
Avulsion 64763-64766
Incision 64763-64766
Transection 64763-64766

Obturator Prosthesis 21076
Definitive 21080
Insertion
   Larynx 31527
Interim 21079

Occipital Nerve, Greater
Avulsion 64744
Incision 64744
Injection
   Anesthetic 64405
Transection 64744

Occlusion
Extracranial
   Intracranial 61623
Fallopian Tube
   Oviduct 58565, 58615
Penis
   Vein 37790
Umbilical Cord 59072

Occlusive Disease of Artery
See Repair, Artery; Revision

Occult Blood 82270-82272
by Hemoglobin Immunoassay 82274

Occupational Therapy
Evaluation 97003-97004

Ocular Implant
See Orbital Implant
Insertion
   in Scleral Shell 65130
   Muscles, Attached 65140
   Muscles, Not Attached 65135
Modification 65125
Reinsertion 65150
   with Foreign Material 65155
Removal 65175

Ocular Muscle
See Eye Muscles

Ocular Orbit
See Orbit

Ocular Photoscreening 0065T

Ocular Prostheses
See Prosthesis, Ocular

Oculomotor Muscle
See Eye Muscles

Oddi Sphincter
See Sphincter of Oddi

Odontoid Dislocation
Open Treatment/Reduction 22318
   with Grafting 22319

Odontoid Fracture
Open Treatment/Reduction 22318
   with Grafting 22319

Odontoid Process
Excision 22548

Oesophageal Neoplasm
See Tumor, Esophagus

Oesophageal Varices
See Esophageal Varices

Oesophagus
See Esophagus

Oestradiol
See Estradiol

Office and/or Other Outpatient Services
See History and Physical
Consultation
Established Patient 99211-99215
New Patient 99201-99205
Normal Newborn 99432
Office Visit
   Established Patient 99211-99215
   New Patient 99201-99205
Outpatient Visit
   Established Patient 99211-99215
   New Patient 99201-99205
   Prolonged Services 99354-99355

Office Medical Services
After Hours 99050
Emergency Care 99058
Extended Hours 99051

Office or Other Outpatient Consultations
See Consultation, Office and/or Other Outpatient

Olecranon
See Elbow; Humerus; Radius; Ulna
Bursa
   Arthrocentesis 20605
Cyst
   Excision 24125-24126
Tumor
   Cyst 24120
   Excision 24125-24126

Olecranon Process
Craterization 24147
Diaphysectomy 24147
Excision 24147
   Abscess 24138
Fracture
   See Elbow; Humerus; Radius
   Closed Treatment 24670-24675
   Open Treatment 24685
Osteomyelitis 24138, 24147
Saucerization 24147
Sequestrectomy 24138

Oligoclonal Immunoglobulins .83916

Omentectomy 49255, 58950-58958
Laparotomy 58960
Oophorectomy 58943
Resection Ovarian Malignancy 58950-58952
Resection Peritoneal Malignancy ...58950-58958
Resection Tubal Malignancy 58950-58958

Omentum
Excision 49255, 58950-58958
Flap 49904-49905
   Free
     with Microvascular Anastomosis ...49906
Omentopexy 49326
Unlisted Services and Procedures 49999

Omphalectomy 49250

Omphalocele
Repair 49600-49611

Omphalomesenteric Duct
Excision 44800

Omphalomesenteric Duct, Persistent
See Diverticulum, Meckel's

Oncoprotein
HER-2/neu 83950

One Stage Prothrombin Time ...85610-85611
See Prothrombin Time

Onychectomy
See Excision, Nails

Onychia
Drainage 10060-10061

Oocyte
Assisted Fertilization
   Microtechnique 89280-89281
Biopsy 89290-89291
Cryopreservation 0059T
Culture
   Extended 89272
   Less than 4 Days 89250
   with Co-Culture 89251
Identification
   Follicular Fluid 89254
Insemination 89268
Retrieval
   for In Vitro Fertilization 58970
Storage 89346
Thawing 89356

Oophorectomy .58262-58263, 58291-58292,
     58552, 58554, 58661, 58940-58943
Ectopic Pregnancy
   Laparoscopic Treatment 59120
   Surgical Treatment 59120

Oophorectomy, Partial
See Excision, Ovary, Partial

Oophorocystectomy
See Cystectomy, Ovarian

Open Biopsy, Adrenal Gland
See Adrenal Gland, Biopsy

Operating Microscope 69990

P

Gross Exam
   Level I 88300
Histochemistry 88318-88319
Immunocytochemistry 88342
Immunofluorescent Study 88346-88347
Morphometry
   Nerve 88356
   Skeletal Muscle 88355
   Tumor 88358-88361
Nerve Teasing 88362
Special Stain 88312-88314
Staining 88312-88314
Tissue Hybridization 88365
Unlisted Services and Procedures 88399,
    89240

Patterson's Test
See Blood Urea Nitrogen

Paul-Bunnell Test
See Antibody; Antibody Identification;
Microsomal Antibody

PBG
See Porphobilinogen

PCP
See Phencyclidine

PCR
See Polymerase Chain Reaction

Peans' Operation
See Amputation, Leg, Upper, at Hip; Radical
Resection; Replantation

Pectoral Cavity
See Chest Cavity

Pectus Carinatum
Reconstructive Repair 21740-21742
   with Thoracoscopy 21743

Pectus Excavatum
Reconstructive Repair 21740-21742
   with Thoracoscopy 21743

Pediatric Critical Care 99293-99294

Pediatric Intensive Care 99293

Pedicle Fixation
Insertion 22842-22844

Pedicle Flap
Formation 15570-15576
Island 15740
Neurovascular 15750
Transfer 15650

PEEP
See Pressure Breathing, Positive

Peet Operation
See Nerves, Sympathectomy, Excision

Pelvi-Ureteroplasty
See Pyeloplasty

Pelvic Adhesions
See Adhesions, Pelvic

Pelvic Exam 57410

Pelvic Exenteration 51597

Pelvic Fixation
Insertion 22848

Pelvic Lymphadenectomy 58210,
    58958

Pelvimetry 74710

Pelviolithotomy 50130

Pelvis
See Hip
Abscess
   Incision and Drainage 26990, 45000
Angiography 72191
Biopsy 27040-27041
Bone
   Drainage 26992
Brace Application 20662
Bursa
   Incision and Drainage 26991
CT Scan 72191-72194
Cyst
   Aspiration 50390
   Injection 50390
Destruction
   Lesion 58662
Endoscopy
   Destruction of Lesion 58662
   Lysis of Adhesions 58660
   Oviduct Surgery 58670-58671
Exclusion
   Small Intestine 44700
Exenteration 45126, 58240
Halo 20662
Hematoma
   Incision and Drainage 26990
Lysis
   Adhesions 58660
Magnetic Resonance Angiography 72198
Magnetic Resonance Imaging
(MRI) 72195-72197
Removal
   Foreign Body 27086-27087
Repair
   Osteotomy 27158
   Tendon 27098
Ring
   Dislocation 27193-27194, 27216-27218
   Fracture 27216-27218
   Closed Treatment 27193-27194
Tumor
   Excision 27047-27049
Ultrasound 76856-76857
Unlisted Services and Procedures for Hips and
Hip Joint 27299
X-Ray 72170-72190, 73540
   Manometry 74710

Pemberton Osteotomy of Pelvis
See Osteotomy, Pelvis

Penectomy
See Amputation, Penis

Penetrating Keratoplasties
See Keratoplasty, Penetrating

Penile Induration
See Peyronie Disease

Penile Prosthesis
Insertion
   Inflatable 54401-54405
   Noninflatable 54400
Removal
   Inflatable 54406, 54410-54417
   Semi-Rigid 54415-54417
Repair
   Inflatable 54408
Replacement
   Inflatable 54410-54411, 54416-54417
   Semi-Rigid 54416-54417

Penile Rigidity Test 54250

Penile Tumescence Test 54250

Penis
Amputation
   Partial 54120
   Radical 54130-54135
   Total 54125
Biopsy 54100-54105
Circumcision
   Repair 54163
   Surgical Excision
    Newborn 54150, 54160
Excision
   Partial 54120
   Prepuce 54150-54161, 54163
   Total 54125-54135
Frenulum
   Excision 54164
Incision
   Prepuce 54000-54001
Incision and Drainage 54015
Injection
   for Erection 54235
   Peyronie Disease 54200
    Surgical Exposure Plague 54205
   Vasoactive Drugs 54231
   X-Ray 54230
Insertion
   Prosthesis
    Inflatable 54401-54405
    Noninflatable 54400
Irrigation
   Priapism 54220
Lesion
   Destruction
    Cryosurgery 54056
    Electrodesiccation 54055
    Extensive 54065
    Laser Surgery 54057
    Simple 54050-54060
    Surgical Excision 54060
   Excision 54060
    Penile Plaque 54110-54112
Nocturnal Penile Tumescence Test 54250
Occlusion
   Vein 37790
Plaque
   Excision 54110-54112
Plethysmography 54240

Performance Test

Perfusion

Perfusion Pump

Perfusion, Intracranial Arterial

Pericardectomies

Pericardial Cyst

Pericardial Sac

Pericardial Window

Pericardial Window Technic

Pericardiectomy

Pericardiocentesis

Pericardiostomy

Pericardiotomy

Pericardium

Peridural Anesthesia

Peridural Injection

Perineal Prostatectomy

Perineoplasty

Perineorrhaphy

Perineum

Perionychia

Periorbital Region

Peripheral Artery Disease (PAD) Rehabilitation

Peripheral Nerve

Platysmal Flap 15825

PLC
See Lymphocyte, Culture; Tissue Typing

Pleoptic Training 92065

Plethysmography
See Vascular Studies
Extremities 93922-93923
    Veins 93965
Penis 54240
Total Body 93720-93722

Pleura
Biopsy 32095-32100, 32400-32402
Decortication 32320
Empyema
    Excision 32540
Excision 32310-32320
    Endoscopic 32656
Foreign Body
    Removal 32150-32151
Needle Biopsy 32400
Removal
    Foreign Body 32653
Repair 32215
Thoracotomy 32095-32100
Unlisted Services and Procedures 32999

Pleural Cavity
Aspiration 32000-32002
Catheterization 32019
Chemotherapy Administration 96440
    See Chemotherapy
Fusion 32005
Incision
    Empyema 32035-32036
    Pneumothorax 32020
Puncture and Drainage 32000-32002
Thoracostomy 32035-32036

Pleural Endoscopies
See Thoracoscopy

Pleural Scarification
for Repeat Pneumothorax 32215

Pleural Tap
See Thoracentesis

Pleurectomy
Anesthesia 00542
Parietal 32310-32320
    Endoscopic 32656

Pleuritis, Purulent
See Abscess, Thorax

Pleurocentesis
See Thoracentesis

Pleurodesis
Chemical 32005
Endoscopic 32650

Pleurosclerosis
See Pleurodesis

Pleurosclerosis, Chemical
See Pleurodesis, Chemical

Plexectomy, Choroid
See Choroid Plexus, Excision

Plexus
Brachialis
    See Brachial Plexus
Cervicalis
    See Cervical Plexus
Choroid
    See Choroid Plexus
Coeliacus
    See Celiac Plexus
Lumbalis
    See Lumbar Plexus

PLGN
See Plasminogen

Plication, Sphincter, Urinary Bladder
See Bladder, Repair, Neck

Pneumocentesis
Lung 32420

Pneumocisternogram
See Cisternography

Pneumococcal Vaccine
See Vaccines

Pneumocystis Carinii
Antigen Detection
    Immunofluorescence 87281

Pneumogastric Nerve
See Vagus Nerve

Pneumogram
Pediatric 94772

Pneumolysis 32940

Pneumonectomy 32440-32500
Completion 32488
Donor 32850, 33930
Sleeve 32442
Total 32440-32445

Pneumonology
See Pulmonology

Pneumonolysis 32940
Intrapleural 32652
Open Intrapleural 32124

Pneumonostomy 32200-32201

Pneumonotomy
See Incision, Lung

Pneumoperitoneum 49400

Pneumoplethysmography
Ocular 93875

Pneumothorax
Chemical Pleurodesis 32005
Pleural Scarification for Repeat 32215
Therapeutic
    Injection Intrapleural Air 32960
Thoracentesis with Tube Insertion 32002

Polio
Antibody 86658
Vaccine 90712-90713

Poliovirus Vaccine
See Vaccines

Pollicization
Digit 26550

Polya Gastrectomy
See Gastrectomy, Partial

Polydactylism
See Polydactyly; Supernumerary Digit

Polydactyly
Digit
    Reconstruction 26587
    Repair 26587
Toe 28344

Polymerase Chain Reaction 83898

Polyp
Antrochoanal
    Removal 31032
Esophagus
    Ablation 43228
Nose
    Excision
        Endoscopic 31237-31240
        Extensive 30115
        Simple 30110
Sphenoid Sinus
    Removal 31051
Urethra
    Excision 53260

Polypectomy
Nose
    Endoscopic 31237
Uterus 58558

Polypeptide, Vasoactive Intestinal
See Vasoactive Intestinal Peptide

Polysomnography 95808-95811

Polyuria Test
See Water Load Test

Pomeroy's Operation
See Tubal Ligation

Pooling
Blood Products 86965

Popliteal Arteries
See Artery, Popliteal

Popliteal Synovial Cyst
See Baker's Cyst

Poradenitistras
See Lymphogranuloma Venereum

PORP (Partial Ossicular Replacement Prosthesis) 69633, 69637

Porphobilinogen
Urine 84106-84110

Positive
  Continuous (CPAP) 94660

Pressure
  Blood
    See Blood Pressure
  Measurement of Sphincter of Oddi
    See Sphincter of Oddi, Pressure
    Measurement
  Sensor, Aneurysm
    Placement .0153T
    Study 0154T
  Ulcer (Decubitus)
    See Debridement; Skin Graft and Flap
    Excision 15920-15999
  Venous
    See Blood Pressure, Venous

Pretreatment
Red Blood Cell
  Antibody Identification 86970-86972
Serum
  Antibody Identification 86975-86978

Prevention & Control
See Prophylaxis

Preventive Medicine 99381-99397
See Immunization; Newborn Care, Normal; Office
and/or Other Outpatient Services; Performance
Measures, Prophylatic Treatment
Administration/Interpretation of Health Risk
Assessment 99420
Counseling and/or Risk Factor Reduction
Intervention 99401-99429
    Group Counseling 99411-99412
    Individual Counseling 99401-99404
Established Patient 99382-99397
New Patient 99381-99387
Newborn Care .99432
Respiratory Pattern Recording 94772
Unlisted Services and Procedures 99429

Priapism
Repair
  Fistulization 54435
  with Shunt 54420-54430

Primidone
Assay 80188

PRL
See Prolactin

Pro-Insulin C Peptide
See C-Peptide

Proalbumin
See Prealbumin

Probes, DNA
See Nucleic Acid Probe

Probes, Nucleic Acid
See Nucleic Acid Probe

Procainamide
Assay 80190-80192

Process
See Anatomic term (eg coracoid, odontoid)

Procidentia
Rectum
  Excision 45130-45135
  Repair 45900

Procoagulant Activity, Glomerular
See Thromboplastin

Proconvertin 85230

Proctectasis
See Dilation, Rectum

Proctectomy
Partial
  Open 45111, 45113-45116, 45123
Total 45110, 45112, 45119-45120
  Laparoscopic 45395-45397
  Open 45110, 45112, 45119-45120
    with Colon 45121
with Colectomy 44157-44158
with Colectomy/Ileostomy
  Laparoscopic 44212
  Open 44155

Proctocele
See Rectocele

Proctopexy
Laparoscopic 45400-45402
  with Sigmoid Resection 45402
Open 45540-45541
  with Sigmoid Excision 45550

Proctoplasty 45500-45505

Proctorrhaphy
See Rectum, Suture

Proctoscopies
See Anoscopy

Proctosigmoidoscopy
Ablation
  Polyp or Lesion 45320
Biopsy 45305
Destruction
  Tumor 45320
Dilation 45303
Exploration 45300
Hemorrhage Control 45317
Placement
  Stent 45327
Removal
  Foreign Body 45307
  Polyp 45308-45315
  Tumor 45315
Volvulus Repair 45321

Products, Gene
See Protein

Proetz Therapy
Nose 30210

Profibrinolysin
See Plasminogen

Progenitor Cell
See Stem Cell

Progesterone 84144

Progesterone Receptors 84234

Progestin Receptors
See Progesterone Receptors

Proinsulin .84206

Projective Test 96101-96103

Prokallikrein
See Fletcher Factor

Prokallikrein, Plasma
See Fletcher Factor

Prokinogenase
See Fletcher Factor

Prolactin 80418, 80440, 84146

Prolapse
See Procidentia

Prolapse, Rectal
See Procidentia, Rectum

Prolastin
See Alpha-1 Antitrypsin

Prolonged Services 99354-99357,
                                                          99360
without Direct Patient Contact 99358-99359

Prophylactic Treatment
See Preventive Medicine
Femoral Neck and Proximal Femur
  Nailing 27187
  Pinning 27187
  Wiring 27187
Femur 27495
  Nailing 27495
  Pinning 27495
  Wiring 27495
Humerus
  Pinning, Wiring 24498
Radius .25490, 25492
  Nailing 25490, 25492
  Pinning 25490, 25492
  Plating 25490, 25492
  Wiring 25490, 25492
Shoulder
  Clavicle 23490
  Humerus 23491
Tibia 27745
Ulna 25491-25492
  Nailing 25491-25492
  Pinning 25491-25492
  Plating 25491-25492
  Wiring 25491-25492

Prophylaxis
Retina
  Detachment
    Cryotherapy, Diathermy 67141
    Photocoagulation 67145

Prostaglandin 84150
Insertion 59200

Prostanoids
See Prostaglandin

Provitamin A
See Vitamin, A

Provocation Test
See Allergy Tests
for Glaucoma 92140

Provocation Tonography 92130

Prower Factor
See Stuart-Prower Factor

PSA
See Prostate Specific Antigen

Pseudocyst, Pancreas
See Pancreas, Pseudocyst

PSG
See Polysomnography

Psoriasis Treatment 96910-96922
See Dermatology; Photochemotherapy

Psychiatric Diagnosis
Evaluation of Records or Reports 90885
Interventional Evaluation
    Interactive 90802
Interview and Evaluation 90801-90802
Psychological Testing 96101-96103
    Computer-Assisted 96103
Unlisted Services and Procedures 90899

Psychiatric Treatment
See Psychotherapy
Biofeedback Training 90875-90876
Consultation with Family 90887
Drug Management 90862
Electroconvulsive Therapy 90870
Environmental Intervention 90882
Family 90846-90849, 99510
Group 90853-90857
Hypnotherapy 90880
Individual
    Insight-Oriented
        Home Visit 99510
        Hospital or Residential Care ..90816-90822
        Office or Outpatient 90804-90809
    Interactive
        Home Visit 99510
        Hospital or Residential Care ..90823-90829
        Office or Outpatient 90810-90815
Narcosynthesis Analysis 90865
Psychoanalysis 90845
Report Preparation 90889
Residential
    Facility Care 90816-90829
Unlisted Services and Procedures 90899

Psychoanalysis 90845

Psychophysiologic Feedback
See Biofeedback

Psychotherapy
Family 90846-90849, 99510
Group 90853-90857
    Insight-Oriented
        Hospital or Residential Care ..90816-90822
        Office or Outpatient 90804-90809

Interactive
    Hospital or Residential Care ..90823-90829
    Office or Outpatient 90810-90815

PTA 85270

PTA (Factor XI)
See Clotting Factor

PTC Factor 85250

PTCA
See Percutaneous Transluminal Angioplasty

Pteroylglutamic Acid
See Folic Acid

Pterygium
Excision 65420
    with Graft 65426

Pterygomaxillary Fossa
Incision 31040

Pterygopalatine Ganglion
See Sphenopalatine Ganglion

PTH
See Parathormone

Ptosis
See Blepharoptosis; Procidentia

PTT
See Thromboplastin, Partial, Time

Ptyalectasis
See Dilation, Salivary Duct

Pubic Symphysis 27282

Pubis
Craterization 27070
Cyst
    Excision 27065-27067
Excision 27070
Saucerization 27070
Tumor
    Excision 27065-27067

Pudendal Nerve
Avulsion 64761
Destruction 64630
Incision 64761
Injection
    Anesthetic 64430
    Neurolytic 64630
Transection 64761

Puestow Procedure 48548

Pulled Elbow
See Nursemaid Elbow

Pulmonary Artery
Banding 33690
Catheterization 36013-36015
Embolism......................33910-33916
    Excision 33910-33916
Percutaneous Transluminal
Angioplasty 92997-92998
Reimplantation 33788
Repair 33690, 33917-33920
    Reimplantation 33788

Shunt
    from Aorta 33755-33762, 33924
    from Vena Cava 33766-33767
    Subclavian 33750
Transection 33922

Pulmonary Function Test
See Pulmonology, Diagnostic

Pulmonary Haemorrhage
See Hemorrhage, Lung

Pulmonary Perfusion Imaging
Nuclear Medicine 78588

Pulmonary Valve
Incision 33470-33474
Repair 33470-33474
Replacement 33475

Pulmonary Vein
Repair
    Complete 33730
    Partial 33724
    Stenosis 33726
Stenosis
    Repair 33726

Pulmonology
Diagnostic
    Airway Closing Volume 94370
    Apnea Monitoring
        Pediatric 94774-94777
    Bronchodilation 94664
    Carbon Dioxide Response Curve ...94400
    Carbon Monoxide Diffusion Capacity ..94720
    Expired Gas Analysis
        CO 0043T
        CO_2 94770
        NO 95012
        O_2 and CO_2 94681
        O_2 Update, Direct 94680
        O_2 Uptake, Indirect 94690
        Quantitative 94250
        Spectroscopy 0064T
    Flow-Volume Loop 94375
    Function Study 78596
    Functional Residual Capacity 94240
    Hemoglobin O_2 Affinity 82820
    High Altitude Simulation
    Test (HAST) 94452-94453
    Hypoxia Response Curve 94450
    Inhalation Treatment 94640
    Maldistribution of Inspired Air 94350
    Maximum Breathing Capacity 94200
    Maximum Voluntary Ventilation 94200
    Membrane Compliance 94750
    Membrane Diffusion Capacity 94725
    Nitrogen Washout Curve 94350
    Oximetry
        Ear or Pulse 94760-94762
    Resistance to Airflow 94360
    Spectroscopy 0064T
    Spirometry 94010-94070
        Evaluation 94010-94070
        Patient Initiated with
        Bronchospasm 94014-94016
    Sputum Mobilization with
        Inhalants 94664
    Stress Test 94621

Radiation
See Irradiation

Radiation Physics
Consultation 77336-77370
Unlisted Services and Procedures 77399

Radiation Therapy 77280-77295
Consultation
   Radiation Physics 77336-77370
CT Guidance 77014
Dose Plan 77300, 77305-77331
   Brachytherapy 77326-77328
   Intensity Modulation 77301
   Teletherapy 77305-77321
Field Set-up 77280-77295
Planning 77261-77263, 77299
Special 77470
Stereotactic
   Body 77373
   Cerebral Lesions 77371-77372
   Guidance 77421
Treatment Delivery 77371-77373
   2 Areas 77407-77411
   3 or More Areas 77412-77416
   Beam Modulation 0073T
   High Energy Neutron Radiation .77422-77423
   Intensity Modulation 77418
   Proton Beam 77520-77525
   Single Area 77402-77406, 77422
   Stereotactic 77371-77373
    Body 77373
   Superficial 77401
   Weekly 77427
Treatment Device 77332-77334
Treatment Management
   1 or 2 Fractions Only 77431
   Stereotactic
    Body 77435
    Cerebral 77432
   Unlisted Services and Procedures 77499
   Weekly 77427

Radiation, X
See X-Ray

Radical Excision of Lymph Nodes
See Excision, Lymph Nodes, Radical

Radical Mastectomies, Modified
See Mastectomy, Modified Radical

Radical Neck Dissection
Laryngectomy 31365-31368
Pharyngolaryngectomy 31390-31395
with Auditory Canal Surgery 69155
with Thyroidectomy 60254
with Tongue Excision 41135, 41145, 41153-41155

Radical Resection
See Resection, Radical
Abdomen 51597
Acetabulum 27076
Ankle 27615
Arm, Lower 25077
Calcaneus 27647
Elbow
   Capsule, Soft Tissue, Bone
    with Contracture Release 24149
Face 21015

Fibula 27646
Finger 26117
Foot 28046
Forearm 25077
Hand 26115
Hip
   Soft Tissue 27049
   Tumor or Infection 27075-27076
Humerus 23220-23222
Innominate 27077
Ischial 27078-27079
Knee 27329
Leg
   Lower 27615
   Upper 27329
Metacarpal 26250-26255
Metatarsal 28173
Mouth
   with Tongue Excision 41150, 41155
Ovarian Tumor
   Bilateral Salpingo-Oophorectomy-
   Omentectomy 58950-58956
   with Radical Dissection for
   Debulking 58952-58954
   with Total Abdominal
   Hysterectomy 58951, 58953-58956
Pelvis
   Soft Tissue 27049
Peritoneal Tumor
   Bilateral Salpingo-Oophorectomy-
   Omentectomy 58952-58956
   with Radical Dissection for
   Debulking 58952-58954
Phalanges
   Finger 26260-26262
   Toe 28175
Radius 25170
Scalp 21015
Scapula 23210
Shoulder 23077
Sternum 21630-21632
Talus
   Tumor 27647
Tarsal 28171
Tibia 27645
Tonsil 42842-42845
Tumor
   Back/Flank 21935
   Femur 27365
   Knee 27329, 27365
   Leg, Upper 27329
   Neck 21557
   Thorax 21557
Ulna 25170
Wrist 25077

Radical Vaginal Hysterectomy
See Hysterectomy, Vaginal, Radical

Radical Vulvectomy
See Vulvectomy, Radical

Radio-Cobalt B12 Schilling Test
See Vitamin, B12, Absorption Study

Radioactive Colloid Therapy ...79300

Radioactive Substance
Insertion

Prostate 55860

Radiocarpal Joint
Arthrotomy 25040
Dislocation
   Closed Treatment 25660

Radiocinematographies
See Cineradiography

Radioelement
Application 77761-77778
   Surface 77789
   with Ultrasound 76965
Handling 77790
Infusion 77750

Radioelement Substance
Catheter Placement
   Breast 19296-19298
   Bronchus 31643
   Prostate 55875
Needle Placement
   Prostate 55875-55876

Radiography
See Radiology, Diagnostic; X-Ray

Radioimmunosorbent Test
See Gammaglobulin, Blood

Radioisotope Brachytherapy
See Brachytherapy

Radioisotope Scan
See Nuclear Medicine

Radiological Marker
Preoperative Placement
   Excision of Breast Lesion 19125-19126

Radiology
See Nuclear Medicine, Radiation Therapy, X-Ray,
Ultrasound
Diagnostic
   Unlisted Services and Procedures 76499
Stress Views 77071

Radionuclide CT Scan
See Emission Computerized Tomography

Radionuclide Imaging
See Nuclear Medicine

Radionuclide Therapy
See Radiopharmaceutical Therapy

Radionuclide Tomography, Single-Photon Emission-Computed
See SPECT

Radiopharmaceutical Therapy
Interstitial 79300
Intra-Arterial 79445
Intra-Articular 79440
Intracavitary 79200
Intravenous 79101, 79403
Oral 79005
Unlisted Services and Procedures 79999

Radiotherapeutic
See Radiation Therapy

Artificial Intervertebral Disc
　Cervical Interspace 0093T, 0095T
　Lumbar Interspace 22865, 0164T
Balloon
　Intra-Aortic .33974
Balloon Assist Device
　Intra-Aortic 33968, 33971
Blood Clot
　Eye 65930
Blood Component
　Apheresis 36511-36516
Breast
　Capsules 19371
　Implants 19328-19330
　Modified Radical 19307
　Partial 19300-19302
　Radical 19305-19306
　Simple, Complete 19303
　Subcutaneous 19304
Calcareous Deposits
　Subdeltoid .23000
Calculi (Stone)
　Bile Duct 43264, 47420-47425
　　Percutaneous 47554, 47630
　Bladder 51050, 52310-52318, 52352
　Gallbladder 47480
　Hepatic Duct 47400
　Kidney 50060-50081, 50130, 50561,
　　　　　　　　　　　　　　50580, 52352
　Pancreas 48020
　Pancreatic Duct 43264
　Salivary Gland 42330-42340
　Ureter 50610-50630, 50961, 50980,
　　　　　　　51060-51065, 52320-52330, 52352
　Urethra 52310-52315, 52352
Cardiac Event Recorder 33284
Cast 29700-29715
Cataract
　with Replacement
　　Extracapsular 66982, 66984
　　Intracapsular 66983
　　Not Associated with Concurrent 66983
Catheter
　Central Venous 36589
　Fractured .75961
　Peritoneum 49422
　Spinal Cord 62355
Cerclage
　Cervix 59871
Cerumen
　Auditory Canal, External 69210
Clot
　Pericardium 33020
　　Endoscopic 32658
Comedones 10040
Contraceptive Capsules 11976-11977
Cranial Tongs .20665
Cyst 10040
Dacryolith
　Lacrimal Duct 68530
　Lacrimal Gland 68530
Defibrillator
　Heart 33244
　　Pulse Generator Only 33241
　　via Thoracotomy 33243
Drug Delivery Implant 11982-11983
Ear Wax
　Auditory Canal, External 69210

Electrode
　Brain 61535, 61880
　Heart 33238
　Nerve 64585
　Spinal Cord 63660
　Stomach 0156T, 0158T, 43648, 43882
Embolus
　See Embolectomy
External Fixation System 20694
Eye
　Bone 67414, 67445
　Ocular Contents
　　with Implant 65093
　　without Implant 65091
　Orbital Contents Only 65110
　with Bone .65112
　with Implant
　　Muscles Attached 65105
　　Muscles, Not Attached 65103
　with Muscle or Myocutaneous Flap . . .65114
　without Implant 65101
Fallopian Tube
　Laparoscopy 58661
　　with Hysterectomy . .58542, 58544, 58548
Fat
　Lipectomy 15876-15879
Fecal Impaction
　Rectum 45915
Fibrin Deposit .32150
Fixation Device 20670-20680
Foreign Body 65205-65265
　Anal 46608
　Ankle Joint 27610, 27620
　Arm
　　Lower 25248
　　Upper 24200-24201
　Auditory Canal, External 69200
　　with Anesthesia 69205
　Bile Duct .43269
　Bladder 52310-52315
　Brain 61570, 62163
　Bronchi 31635
　Colon 44025, 44390, 45379
　Colon-Sigmoid 45332
　Conjunctival Embedded 65210
　Cornea
　　with Slit Lamp 65222
　　without Slit Lamp 65220
　Duodenum 44010
　Elbow 24000, 24101, 24200-24201
　Esophagus 43020, 43045, 43215, 74235
　External Eye 65205
　Eyelid 67938
　Finger 26075-26080
　Foot 28190-28193
　Gastrointestinal, Upper 43247
　Gum 41805
　Hand 26070
　Hip 27033, 27086-27087
　Hysteroscopy 58562
　Interphalangeal Joint
　　Toe 28024
　Intertarsal Joint 28020
　Intestines, Small 44020, 44363
　Intraocular 65235
　Kidney 50561, 50580
　Knee Joint 27310, 27331, 27372

Lacrimal Duct .68530
Lacrimal Gland 68530
Larynx 31511, 31530-31531, 31577
Leg, Upper 27372
Lung 32151
Mandible 41806
Mediastinum 39000-39010
Metatarsophalangeal Joint 28022
Mouth 40804-40805
Muscle 20520-20525
Nose 30300
　Anesthesia 30310
　Lateral Rhinotomy 30320
Orbit 61334, 67413, 67430
　with Bone Flap 67430
　without Bone Flap 67413
Pancreatic Duct 43269
Patella
　See Patellectomy
Pelvis 27086-27087
Penile Tissue 54115
Penis 54115
Pericardium .33020
　Endoscopic 32658
Peritoneum .49402
Pharynx 42809
Pleura 32150-32151
　Endoscopic 32653
Posterior Segment
　Magnetic Extraction 65260
　Nonmagnetic Extraction 65265
Rectum 45307, 45915
Scrotum 55120
Shoulder 23040-23044
　Complicated 23332
　Deep 23331
　Subcutaneous 23330
Skin
　with Debridement 11010-11012
Stomach 43500
Subcutaneous Tissue 10120-10121
　with Debridement 11010-11012
Tarsometatarsal Joint 28020
Tendon Sheath 20520-20525
Toe 28022
Ureter 50961, 50980
Urethra 52310-52315
Uterus 58562
Vagina 57415
Wrist 25040, 25101, 25248
Hair
　Electrolysis 17380
Halo 20665
Hearing Aid
　Bone Conduction 69711
Hematoma
　Brain 61312-61315
Implantation 20670-20680
　Ankle 27704
　Contraceptive Capsules 11976-11977
　Disc 22865
　Elbow 24160
　Eye 67120-67121
　Finger 26320
　Hand 26320
　Radius 24164
　Wrist 25449

Repair

See Revision
Abdomen 49900
    Hernia 49491-49525, 49565, 49570,
                      49582-49590
    Omphalocele 49600-49611
    Suture 49900
Abdominal Wall 15830, 15847
Anal
    Anomaly 46744-46748
    Fistula . . .0170T, 46288, 46706, 46715-46716
    Stricture 46700-46705
Anastomosis
    Cyst 47719
Aneurysm
    Aorta
        Abdominal 0078T-0081T
          Infrarenal 34800-34805, 34825-34832
          Imaging 75952-75953
          Thoracic 33877-33886
    Arteriovenous .36834
    Iliac Artery 75954
    Intracranial Artery 61697-61708
Ankle
    Ligament 27695-27698
    Tendon . . .27612, 27650-27654, 27680-27687
Aorta 33320-33322, 33802-33803
    Coarctation 33840-33851
    Graft 33860-33877
    Sinus of Valsalva 33702-33720
    Thoracic 75956-75959
        Endovascular 33880-33891
Aortic Arch
    with Cardiopulmonary Bypass 33853
    without Cardiopulmonary Bypass 33852
Aortic Valve 33400-33403
    Obstruction
        Outflow Tract 33414
    Septic Hypertrophy 33416
    Stenosis 33415
Arm
    Lower 25260-25263, 25270
        Fasciotomy 24495
        Secondary 25265, 25272-25274
        Tendon 25290
        Tendon Sheath 25275
        Muscle 24341
        Tendon 24332, 24341, 25280, 25295,
                      25310-25316
    Upper
        Muscle Revision 24330-24331
        Muscle Transfer 24301, 24320
        Tendon Lengthening 24305
        Tendon Revision 24320
        Tendon Transfer 24301
        Tenotomy 24310
Arteriovenous Aneurysm 36834
Arteriovenous Fistula
    Abdomen 35182
        Acquired or Traumatic 35189
    Head 35180
        Acquired or Traumatic 35188
    Lower Extremity 35184
        Acquired or Traumatic 35190
    Neck 35180
        Acquired or Traumatic 35188
    Thorax 35182
        Acquired or Traumatic 35189

    Upper Extremity 35184
        Acquired or Traumatic 35190
Arteriovenous Malformation
    Intracranial 61680-61692
    Intracranial Artery 61705-61708
    Spinal Artery 62294
    Spinal Cord 63250-63252
Artery
    Angioplasty 75962-75968
    Aorta 35452, 35472
    Axillary 35458
    Brachiocephalic 35458, 35475
    Bypass Graft 35501-35571, 35601-35683,
                  35691-35695, 35700
    Bypass In-Situ 35583-35587
    Bypass Venous Graft 33510-33516,
                      35510-35525
    Coronary 33507
    Femoral 35456, 35474
    Iliac 34900, 35454, 35473
    Occlusive Disease 35001, 35005-35021,
      35045-35081, 35091, 35102, 35111, 35121,
               35131, 35141, 35151
    Popliteal 35456, 35474
    Pulmonary 33690
    Renal 35450
    Renal or Visceral 35471
    Subclavian 35458
    Thromboendarterectomy 35301-35321,
                    35341-35390
    Tibioperoneal 35459, 35470
    Viscera 35450, 35471
Arytenoid Cartilage 31400
Atria
    Laparoscopic 33265-33266
    Open 33254-33256
Bile Duct 47701
    Cyst 47719
    with Intestines 47760, 47780-47785
    Wound 47900
Bladder
    Exstrophy 51940
    Fistula 44660-44661, 45800-45805,
                    51880-51925
    Neck 51845
    Resection 52500
    Wound 51860-51865
Blepharoptosis
    Frontalis Muscle Technique
        with Fascial Sling 67902
Blood Vessel
    Abdomen 35221
        with Other Graft 35281
        with Vein Graft 35251
    Chest 35211-35216
        with Other Graft 35271-35276
        with Vein Graft 35241-35246
    Finger 35207
    Graft Defect 35870
    Hand 35207
    Kidney 50100
    Lower Extremity 35226
        with Other Graft 35286
        with Vein Graft 35256
    Neck 35201
        with Other Graft 35261
        with Vein Graft 35231

    Upper Extremity 35206
        with Other Graft 35266
        with Vein Graft 35236
Body Cast 29720
Brain
    Wound 61571
Breast
    Suspension .19316
Bronchi
    Fistula 32815
Brow Pyrosis 67900
Bunion .28290-28299
Bypass Graft 35901-35907
    Fistula 35870
Calcaneus
    Osteotomy .28300
Cannula 36860-36861
Carpal 25440
Carpal Bone 25431
Cervix
    Cerclage 57700
        Abdominal 59320-59325
    Suture 57720
Chest Wall 32905
    Closure 32810
    Fistula 32906
Chin
    Augmentation 21120, 21123
    Osteotomy 21121-21123
Clavicle
    Osteotomy 23480-23485
Cleft Hand 26580
Cleft Lip 40525-40527, 40700-40761
    Nasal Deformity .40700-40701, 40720-40761
Cleft Palate
    See Cleft Palate Repair
Colon
    Fistula 44650-44661
    Hernia 44050
    Malrotation .44055
    Obstruction 44050
Cornea
    See Cornea, Repair
Coronary Chamber Fistula 33500-33501
Cyst
    Bartholin's Gland 56440
    Choledochal 47719
    Liver 47300
Diaphragm
    for Eventration 39545
    Hernia 39502-39541
    Laceration .39501
Ductus Arteriosus 33820-33824
Ear, Middle
    Oval Window Fistula 69666
    Round Window Fistula 69667
Elbow
    Fasciotomy 24350-24356
    Hemiepiphyseal Arrest 24470
    Ligament 24343-24346
    Muscle 24341
    Muscle Transfer 24301
    Tendon 24340-24342
        Each 24341
    Tendon Lengthening 24305
    Tendon Transfer 24301
    Tennis Elbow 24350-24356

Epigastric 49570
   Incarcerated 49572
Femoral 49550
   Incarcerated 49553
   Recurrent 49555
   Recurrent Incarcerated 49557
   Reducible Recurrent 49555
Incisional
   Incarcerated 49561
   Recurrent Incarcerated 49566
Inguinal 49491-49521
   Initial 49650
   Recurrent 49651
   Sliding 49525
Intestinal 44025-44050
Lumbar 49540
Lung 32800
Orchiopexy 54640
Reducible 49565, 49570
   Femoral .49550
   Incisional 49560
   Inguinal 49500, 49505
   Recurrent 49520
Sliding 49525
Spigelian .49590
Umbilical 49580, 49585
   Incarcerated 49582, 49587
   Reducible 49580
with Spermatic Cord 54640
Hip
   Muscle Transfer 27100-27105, 27111
   Osteotomy 27146-27156
   Tendon 27097
Humerus 24420-24430
   Osteotomy 24400-24410
   with Graft 24435
Ileostomy
   See Ileostomy, Repair
Interphalangeal Joint
   Volar Plate 26548
Intestine
  Large
   Ulcer 44605
   Wound 44605
Intestines
  Enterocele
   Abdominal Approach 57270
   Vaginal Approach 57268
  Large
   Closure Enterostomy 44620-44626
   Diverticula 44605
   Obstruction 44615
Intestines, Small
   Closure Enterostomy 44620-44626
   Diverticula 44602-44603
   Fistula 44640-44661
   Hernia 44050
   Malrotation 44055
   Obstruction 44025-44050
   Ulcer 44602-44603
   Wound 44602-44603
Introitus
   Vagina 56800
Iris, Ciliary Body 66680
Jejunum
  Free Transfer
   with Microvascular Anastomosis . . .43496

Kidney
   Fistula 50520-50526
   Horseshoe 50540
   Renal Pelvis 50400-50405
   Wound 50500
Knee
   Cartilage 27403
   Instability 27420
   Ligament 27405-27409
    Collateral 27405
    Collateral and Cruciate 27409
    Cruciate 27407-27409
   Meniscus 27403
   Tendon 27380-27381
Larynx
   Fracture .31584
  Reinnervation
   Neuromuscular Pedicle 31590
Leg
  Lower
   Fascia 27656
   Tendon 27658-27692
  Upper
   Muscle 27385-27386, 27400, 27430
   Tendon 27393-27400
Ligament
   See Ligament, Repair
Lip 40650-40654
   Cleft Lip 40700-40761
   Fistula 42260
Liver
   Abscess .47300
   Cyst 47300
   Wound 47350-47361
Lung
   Hernia 32800
   Pneumolysis 32940
   Tear 32110
Mastoidectomy
   Complete 69601
   Modified Radical 69602
   Radical .69603
   with Apicectomy 69605
   with Tympanoplasty 69604
Maxilla
   Osteotomy 21206
Mesentery 44850
Metacarpal
   Lengthening 26568
   Nonunion 26546
   Osteotomy 26565
Metacarpophalangeal Joint
   Capsulodesis 26516-26518
   Collateral Ligament 26540-26542
   Fusion 26516-26518
Metatarsal 28322
   Osteotomy 28306-28309
Microsurgery 69990
Mitral Valve 33420-33427
Mouth
   Laceration 40830-40831
   Vestibule of 40830-40845
Musculotendinous Cuff 23410-23412
Nail Bed .11760
Nasal Deformity
   Cleft Lip 40700-40761

Nasal Septum 30630
Navicular .25440
Neck Muscles
   Scalenus Anticus 21700-21705
   Sternocleidomastoid 21720-21725
Nerve 64876
   Graft 64885-64911
   Microrepair 69990
   Suture 64831-64876
Nose
   Adhesions 30560
   Fistula 30580-30600, 42260
   Rhinophyma 30120
   Septum 30540-30545, 30630
   Synechia 30560
   Vestibular Stenosis 30465
Omphalocele 49600-49611
Osteotomy
   Femoral Neck 27161
  Radius
   and Ulna 25365
  Ulna
   and Radius 25365
  Vertebra
   Additional Segment 22216, 22226
   Cervical 22210, 22220
   Lumbar 22214, 22224
   Thoracic 22212, 22222
Oviduct 58752
   Create Stoma 58770
Pacemaker
  Heart
   Electrode 33218-33220
Palate
   Laceration 42180-42182
   Vomer Flap 42235
Pancreas
   Cyst 48500
   Pseudocyst 48510-48511
    Percutaneous 48511
Paravaginal Defect 57284
Pectus Carinatum 21740-21742
   with Thoracoscopy 21743
Pectus Excavatum 21740-21742
   with Thoracoscopy 21743
Pelvic Floor
   Prosthetic Insertion 57267
Pelvis
   Osteotomy 27158
   Tendon .27098
Penis
   Fistulization 54435
   Injury 54440
   Priapism 54420-54435
   Shunt 54420-54430
Perineum .56810
Periorbital Region
   Osteotomy 21260-21263
Phalanx
  Finger
   Lengthening 26568
   Osteotomy 26567
   Nonunion 26546
  Toe
   Osteotomy 28310-28312
Pharynx
   with Esophagus 42953
Pleura 32215

Wrist 25260-25263, 25270, 25447
   Bone 25440
   Carpal Bone 25431
   Cartilage 25107
   Removal
     Implant 25449
   Secondary 25265, 25272-25274
   Tendon 25280-25316
   Tendon Sheath 25275
   Total Replacement 25446

Repeat Surgeries
See Reoperation

Replacement
Adjustable Gastric Band 43773
Aortic Valve 33405-33413
Arthroplasties, Hip
   See Arthroplasty, Hip
Artificial Heart
   Intracorporeal 0052T, 0053T
Cerebrospinal Fluid Shunt 62160, 62194,
                   62225-62230
Contact Lens
   See Contact Lens Services
Elbow
   Total 24363
Electrode
   Heart 33210-33211, 33216-33217
   Stomach 0155T, 0157T, 43647
Eye
   Drug Delivery System 67121
Gastrostomy Tube 43760
Hearing Aid
   Bone Conduction 69710
Hip 27130-27132
   Revision 27134-27138
Implant
   Bone
     for External Speech Processor/Cochlear
     Stimulator 69717-69718
Intervertebral Disc
   Cervical Interspace 0090T
   Lumbar Interspace 0163T, 22862
Knee
   Total 27447
Mitral Valve 33430
Nephrostomy Tube
   See Nephrostomy, Change Tube
Nerve 64726
Neurostimulator
   Pulse Generator/Receiver
     Intracranial .61885
     Peripheral Nerve 64590
     Spinal 63685
Ossicles
   with Prosthesis 69633, 69637
Ossicular Replacement
   See TORP (Total Ossicular Replacement
   Prosthesis)
Pacemaker 33206-33208
   Catheter 33210
   Electrode 33210-33211, 33216-33217
Pacing Cardioverter-Defibrillator
   Leads 33243-33244
   Pulse Generator Only 33241
Penile
   Prosthesis 54410-54411, 54416-54417

Prosthesis
   Skull 62143
   Urethral Sphincter 53448
Pulmonary Valve 33475
Pulse Generator
   Brain 61885
   Peripheral Nerve 64590
   Spinal Cord 63685
Receiver
   Brain 61885
   Peripheral Nerve 64590
   Spinal Cord 63685
Skin
   Acellular Dermal Matrix 15170-15176
Skull Plate 62143
Spinal Cord
   Reservoir 62360
Stent
   Ureteral 50382, 50387
Subcutaneous Port
   for Gastric Restrictive Procedure 43888
Tissue Expanders
   Skin 11970
Total Replacement
   See Hip, Total Replacement
Total Replacement Heart System
   Intracorporeal 0052T, 0053T
Tricuspid Valve .33465
Ureter
   with Intestines 50840
Venous Access Device 36582-36583, 36585
   Catheter 36578
Venous Catheter
   Central 36580-36581, 36584

Replantation
Arm, Upper 20802
Digit 20816-20822
Foot 20838
Forearm 20805
Hand 20808
Thumb 20824-20827

Report Preparation
Extended, Medical 99080
Psychiatric 90889

Reposition
Toe to Hand 26551-26556

Repositioning
Central Venous Catheter 36597
Electrode
   Heart 33215-33217, 33226
Gastrostomy Tube 43761
Heart
   Defibrillator
     Leads 33215-33216, 33226, 33249
Intraocular Lens 66825
Tricuspid Valve 33468

Reproductive Tissue
Cryopreserved
   Preparation
     Thawing 89354
   Storage 89344

Reprogramming
Shunt
   Brain 62252

Reptilase Test 85635

Reptilase Time
See Thrombin Time

Resection
Aortic Valve
   Stenosis 33415
Bladder Diverticulum 52305
Bladder Neck
   Transurethral 52500
Brain Lobe
   See Lobectomy, Brain
Chest Wall 19260-19272
Diaphragm 39560-39561
Endaural
   See Ear, Inner, Excision
Humeral Head .23195
Intestines, Small
   Laparoscopic 44202-44203
Lung 32503-32504
Mouth
   with Tongue Excision 41153
Myocardium
   Aneurysm 33542
   Septal Defect .33545
Nasal Septum Submucous
   See Nasal Septum, Submucous Resection
Nose
   Septum 30520
Ovary, Wedge
   See Overy, Wedge Resection
Palate 42120
Phalangeal Head
   Toe 28153
Prostate Transurethral
   See Prostatectomy, Transurethral
Radical
   Arm, Upper 24077
   Elbow 24077
     with Contracture Release 24149
   Foot 28046
   Humerus 24150-24151
   Radius 24152-24153
   Tumor
     Ankle 27615
     Calcaneus or Talus 27647
     Clavicle 23200
     Femur 27365
     Fibula 27646
     Humerus 23220
     Humerus with Autograft 23221
     Humerus with Prosthetic
      Replacement 23222
     Knee 27329, 27365
     Leg, Lower .27615
     Leg, Upper .27329
     Metatarsal .28173
     Phalanx, Toe 28175
     Scapula 23210
     Tarsal 28171
     Tibia 27645
Ribs 19260-19272, 32900
Synovial Membrane
   See Synovectomy
Temporal Bone .69535

Venous Access Device 36576-36578,
　　　　　　　　　　　　　36582-36583, 36585
Ventricle
　　Ventriculomyectomy 33416
　　Ventriculomyotomy 33416

Rh (D)
See Blood Typing

Rh Immune Globulin
See Immune Globulins, Rho (D)

Rheumatoid Factor 86430-86431

Rhinectomy
Partial 30150
Total 30160

Rhinomanometry 92512

Rhinopharynx
See Nasopharynx

Rhinophototherapy 0168T

Rhinophyma
Repair 30120

Rhinoplasty
Cleft Lip/Cleft Palate 30460-30462
Primary 30400-30420
Secondary 30430-30450

Rhinoscopy
See Endoscopy, Nose

Rhinotomy
Lateral 30118, 30320

Rhizotomy 63185-63190

Rho Variant Du 86905

Rhytidectomy 15824-15829

Rhytidoplasties
See Face Lift

Rib
Antibody 86756
Antigen Detection
　by Immunoassay
　　with Direct Optical Observation
　　Direct Fluorescense 87280
　　Enzyme Immunoassay 87420
Excision 21600-21616, 32900
Fracture
　　Closed Treatment 21800
　　External Fixation 21810
　　Open Treatment 21805
Graft
　　to Face 21230
Resection 19260-19272, 32900
X-Ray 71100-71111

Riboflavin 84252

**Richardson Operation
Hysterectomy**
See Hysterectomy, Abdominal, Total

Richardson Procedure 53460

Rickettsia
Antibody 86757

Ridell Operation
See Sinusotomy, Frontal

Ridge, Alveolar
See Alveolar Ridge

Right Atrioventricular Valve
See Tricuspid Valve

Right Heart Cardiac Catheterization
See Cardiac Catheterization, Right Heart

Ripstein Operation
See Proctopexy

Risk Factor Reduction Intervention
See Performance Measures, Preventive Medicine

Risser Jacket 29010-29015
Removal 29710

Rocky Mountain Spotted Fever 86000

Roentgen Rays
See X-Ray

Roentgenographic
See X-Ray

Roentgenography
See Radiology, Diagnostic

Ropes Test 83872

Rorschach Test 96101

Ross Procedure 33413

Rotation Flap
See Skin, Adjacent Tissue Transfer

Rotator Cuff
Repair 23410-23420

Rotavirus
Antibody 86759
Antigen Detection
　　Enzyme Immunoassay 87425

Rotavirus Vaccine 90680

Round Window
Repair Fistula 69667

Round Window Fistula
See Fistula, Round Window

Roux-En-Y Procedure 43621,
　　43633-43634, 43644, 43846, 47740-47741,
　　　　　　　　　47780-47785, 48540

RPR 86592-86593

RSV
See Immune Globulins; Respiratory Syncytial
Virus

RT3
See Triiodothyronine, Reverse

Rubbing Alcohol
See Isopropyl Alcohol

Rubella
Antibody 86762
Vaccine 90706

Rubella HI Test
See Hemagglutination Inhibition Test

Rubella/Mumps
See Vaccines

Rubeola
Antibody 86765
Antigen Detection
　　Immunofluorescence 87283

Rubeolla
See Rubeola

**Russell Viper Venom
Time** 85612-85613

S

Sac, Endolymphatic
See Endolymphatic Sac

Saccomanno Technique 88108

Sacral Nerve
Implantation
　　Electrode 64561, 64581
Insertion
　　Electrode 64561, 64581

Sacroiliac Joint
Arthrodesis 27280
Arthrotomy 27050
Biopsy 27050
Dislocation
　　Open Treatment 27218
Fusion 27280
Injection for Arthrography 27096
X-Ray 72200-72202, 73542

Sacrum
Tumor
　　Excision 49215
X-Ray 72220

Sahli Test
See Gastroenterology, Diagnostic, Stomach

Salicylate
Assay 80196

Saline-Solution Abortion
See Abortion, Induced, by Saline

Salivary Duct
Catheterization .42660
Dilation .42650-42660
Ligation 42665
Repair .42500-42505
　　Fistula 42600

Salivary Gland Virus
See Cytomegalovirus

Salivary Glands

Abscess
    Incision and Drainage 42310-42320
Biopsy 42405
Calculi (Stone)
    Excision 42330-42340
Cyst
    Drainage 42409
    Excision 42408
Injection
    X-Ray 42550
Needle Biopsy 42400
Nuclear Medicine
    Function Study 78232
    Imaging 78230-78231
Parotid
    Abscess 42300-42305
Unlisted Services and Procedures 42699
X-Ray 70380-70390
    with Contrast 70390

Salmonella

Antibody 86768

Salpingectomy 58262-58263,
    58291-58292, 58552, 58554, 58661, 58700
Ectopic Pregnancy
    Laparoscopic Treatment 59151
    Surgical Treatment 59120
Oophorectomy 58943

Salpingo-Oophorectomy . . .58720
Resection Ovarian Malignancy 58950-58958
Resection Peritoneal Malignancy . . .58950-58958
Resection Tubal Malignancy 58950-58958

Salpingohysterostomy
See Implantation, Tubouterine

Salpingolysis 58740

Salpingoneostomy 58673, 58770

Salpingoplasty
See Fallopian Tube, Repair

Salpingostomy 58673, 58770
Laparoscopic 58673

Salter Osteotomy of the Pelvis
See Osteotomy, Pelvis

Sampling
See Biopsy; Brush Biopsy; Needle Biopsy

Sang-Park Procedure 33735-33737

Sao Paulo Typhus
See Rocky Mountain Spotted Fever

Saucerization

Calcaneus 28120
Clavicle 23180
Femur 27070, 27360
Fibula 27360, 27641
Hip 27070
Humerus 23184, 24140
Ileum 27070
Metacarpal 26230
Metatarsal 28122
Olecranon Process 24147

Phalanges
    Finger 26235-26236
    Toe 28124
Pubis 27070
Radius .24145, 25151
Scapula 23182
Talus 28120
Tarsal 28122
Tibia 27360, 27640
Ulna 24147, 25150

Saundby Test
See Blood, Feces

Scabies
See Tissue, Examination for Ectoparasites

Scalenotomy
See Muscle Division, Scalenus Anticus

Scalenus Anticus
Division 21700-21705

Scaling
See Exfoliation

Scalp
Tumor Resection
    Radical 21015

Scalp Blood Sampling 59030

Scan
See Specific Site, Nuclear Medicine
Abdomen
    See Abdomen, CT Scan
CT
    See CT Scan
MRI
    See Magnetic Resonance Imaging
PET
    See Positron Emission Tomography
Radionuclide
    See Emission Computerized Tomography

Scanning, Radioisotope
See Nuclear Medicine

Scanogram .77073

Scaphoid
Fracture
    Closed Treatment 25622
    Open Treatment 25628
    with Manipulation 25624

Scapula
Craterization 23182
Cyst
    Excision 23140
    with Allograft 23146
    with Autograft 23145
Diaphysectomy .23182
Excision 23172, 23190
    Partial 23182
Fracture
    Closed Treatment
      with Manipulation 23575
      without Manipulation 23570
    Open Treatment 23585
Ostectomy 23190

Repair
    Fixation 23400
    Scapulopexy 23400
Saucerization 23182
Sequestrectomy 23172
Tumor
    Excision 23140, 23210
    with Allograft 23146
    with Autograft 23145
    Radical Resection 23210
X-Ray 73010

Scapulopexy 23400

Scarification
Pleural 32215

Scarification of Pleura
See Pleurodesis

Schanz Operation
See Femur, Osteotomy

Schauta Operation
See Hysterectomy, Vaginal, Radical

Schede Procedure 32905-32906

Scheie Procedure
See Iridectomy

Schilling Test 78270
See Vitamin B-12 Absorption Study

Schlatter Operation Total
Gastrectomy
See Excision, Stomach, Total

Schlicter Test 87197
See Bactericidal Titer, Serum

Schocket Procedure 66180
See Aqueous Shunt

Schonbein Test
See Blood, Feces

Schuchard Procedure
Osteotomy
    Maxilla 21206

Schwannoma, Acoustic
See Brain, Tumor, Excision

Sciatic Nerve
Decompression .64712
Injection
    Anesthetic 64445-64446
Lesion
    Excision 64786
Neuroma
    Excision 64786
Neuroplasty 64712
Release 64712
Repair/Suture 64858

Scintigraphy
See Nuclear Medicine
Computed Tomographic
    See Emission Computerized Tomography

Scissoring
Skin Tags 11200-11201

Sclera
Excision
    Sclerectomy with Punch or Scissors . . .66160
Fistulization
    for Glaucoma 0123T
    Iridencleisis or Iridotasis 66165
    Sclerectomy with Punch or Scissors with
    Iridectomy 66160
    Thermocauterization with Iridectomy . .66155
    Trabeculectomy ab Externo in Absence of
    Previous Surgery 66170
    Trephination with Iridectomy 66150
Incision
    Fistulization
        Iridencleisis or Iridotasis 66165
        Sclerectomy with Punch or Scissors with
        Iridectomy .66160
        Thermocauterization with Iridectomy 66155
        Trabeculectomy ab Externo in Absence of
        Previous Surgery 66170
        Trephination with Iridectomy 66150
Lesion
    Excision 66130
Repair
    Reinforcement
        with Graft 67255
        without Graft 67250
    Staphyloma
        with Graft 66225
        without Graft 66220
        with Glue 65286
    Wound
        Operative 66250
        Tissue Glue 65286

Scleral Buckling Operation
See Retina, Repair, Detachment

Scleral Ectasia
See Staphyloma, Sclera

Sclerectomy 66160

Sclerotherapy
Venous 36468-36471

Sclerotomy
See Incision, Sclera

Screening, Drug
See Drug Screen

Scribner Cannulization 36810

Scrotal Varices
See Varicocele

Scrotoplasty 55175-55180

Scrotum
Abscess
    Incision and Drainage 54700, 55100
Excision 55150
Exploration 55110
Hematoma
    Incision and Drainage 54700
Removal
    Foreign Body .55120
Repair 55175-55180
Ultrasound 76870
Unlisted Services and Procedures 55899

Scrub Typhus 86000

Second Look Surgery
See Reoperation

Section
See Decompression
Cesarean
    See Cesarean Delivery
Cranial Nerve 61460
    Spinal Access 63191
Dentate Ligament 63180-63182
Gasserian Ganglion
    Sensory Root 61450
Medullary Tract 61470
Mesencephalic Tract 61480
Nerve Root 63185-63190
Spinal Accessory Nerve 63191
Spinal Cord Tract 63194-63199
Tentorium Cerebelli 61440
Vestibular Nerve
    Transcranial Approach 69950
    Translabyrinthine Approach 69915

Sedation
Moderate 99143-99150
    with Independent Observation . .99143-99145

Seddon-Brookes Procedure . . .24320

Sedimentation Rate
Blood Cell
    Automated 85652
    Manual 85651

Segmentectomy
Breast .19301-19302
Lung 32484

Seidlitz Powder Test
See X-Ray, with Contrast

Selective Cellular Enhancement
Technique 88112

Selenium 84255

Self Care
See Physical Medicine/Therapy/Occupational
Therapy
Training 97535, 98960-98962, 99509

Sella Turcica
CT Scan .70480-70482
X-Ray 70240

Semen
See Sperm

Semen Analysis 89300-89321
Sperm Analysis
    Antibodies 89325
with Sperm Isolation 89260-89261

Semenogelase
See Antigen, Prostate Specific

Semicircular Canal
Incision
    Fenestration .69820
    Revised 69840

Semilunar
Bone
    See Lunate
Ganglion
    See Gasserian Ganglion

Seminal Vesicle
Cyst
    Excision 55680
Excision 55650
Incision .55600-55605
Mullerian Duct
    Excision 55680
Unlisted Services and Procedures 55899

Seminal Vesicles
Vesiculography .74440
X-Ray with Contrast 74440

Seminin
See Antigen, Prostate Specific

Semiquantitative 81005

Sengstaaken Tamponade
Esophagus 43460

Senning Procedure 33774-33777
See Repair, Great Arteries; Revision

Senning Type 33774-33777

Sensitivity Study
Antibiotic
    Agar 87181
    Disc 87184
    Enzyme Detection 87185
    Macrobroth 87188
    MIC 87186
    Microtiter 87186
    MLC 87187
    Mycobacteria 87190
Antiviral Drugs
    HIV-1
        Tissue Culture 87904

Sensor, Fetal Oximetry
Insertion
    Cervix 0021T
    Vagina 0021T

Sensor, Pressure
See also Sphincter of Oddi
Intravascular
    Complete Study 0154T
Placement
    Transcatheter
        Intravascular 0153T

Sensorimotor Exam 92060

Sensory Nerve
Common
    Repair/Suture 64834

Sentinel Node
Injection Procedure 38792

Separation
Craniofacial
    Closed Treatment 21431
    Open Treatment 21432-21436

Dislocation
　Open Treatment 23660
　with Greater Tuberosity Fracture
　　Closed Treatment 23665
　　Open Treatment 23670
　with Surgical or Anatomical Neck Fracture
　　Closed Treatment with Manipulation 23675
　　Open Treatment 23680
Excision
　Torn Cartilage 23101
Exploration 23040-23044
Incision and Drainage 23040-23044
Removal
　Foreign Body 23040-23044
X-Ray 73050

Shunt(s)

Aqueous
　to Extraocular Reservoir 66180
　　Revision 66185
Arteriovenous
　See Arteriovenous Shunt
Brain
　Creation 62180-62223
　Removal 62256-62258
　Replacement 62160, 62194,
　　　　　　　　　　　　62225-62230, 62258
　Reprogramming 62252
Cerebrospinal Fluid
　See Cerebrospinal Fluid Shunt
Creation
　Arteriovenous
　　Direct 36821
　　ECMO 36822
　　Thomas Shunt 36835
　　Transposition 36818-36820
　　with Bypass Graft 35686
　　with Graft 36825-36830
　Cerebrospinal Fluid 62200
　Thomas Shunt 36835
Fetal 59076
Great Vessel
　Aorta
　　Pulmonary 33924
　Aorta to Pulmonary Artery
　　Ascending 33755
　　Descending 33762
　　Central .33764
　　Subclavian Pulmonary Artery 33750
　　Vena Cava to Pulmonary Artery .33766-33768
Intra-Atrial 33735-33737
LeVeen
　See LeVeen Shunt
Nonvascular
　X-Ray 75809
Peritoneal
　Venous
　　Injection 49427
　　Ligation 49428
　　Removal 49429
　　X-Ray 75809
Pulmonary Artery
　See Pulmonary Artery, Shunt
Revision
　Arteriovenous 36832
Spinal Cord
　Creation 63740-63741
　Irrigation .63744

　　Removal .63746
　　Replacement 63744
Superior Mesenteric-Caval
　See Anastomosis, Caval to Mesenteric
Ureter to Colon 50815
Ventriculocisternal with Valve
　See Ventriculocisternostomy

Shuntogram .75809

Sialic Acid .84275

Sialodochoplasty 42500-42505

Sialogram
See Sialography

Sialography 70390

Sickling
Electrophoresis .83020

Siderocytes 85536

Siderophilin
See Transferrin

Sigmoid
See Colon-Sigmoid

Sigmoid Bladder
Cystectomy 51590

Sigmoidoscopy

Ablation
　Polyp 45339
　Tumor 45339
Biopsy 45331
Collection
　Specimen 45331
Exploration 45330, 45335
Hemorrhage Control 45334
Injection
　Submucosal 45335
Needle Biopsy .45342
Placement
　Stent 45345
Removal
　Foreign Body 45332
　Polyp 45333, 45338
　Tumor 45333, 45338
Repair
　Volvulus 45337
Ultrasound 45341-45342

Signal-Averaged
Electrocardiography
See Electrocardiogram

Silica 84285

Silicon Dioxide
See Silica

Silicone
Contouring Injections 11950-11954

Silver Operation
See Keller Procedure

Silver Procedure 28290

Simple Mastectomies
See Mastectomy

Single Photon Absorptiometry
See Absorptiometry, Single Photon

Single Photon Emission Computed
Tomography
See SPECT

Sinu, Sphenoid
See Sinus/Sinuses, Sphenoid

Sinus/Sinuses

Ethmoid
　Excision 31200-31205
　　with Nasal/Sinus Endoscopy .31254-31255
　Repair of Cerebrospinal Leak 31290
Ethmoidectomy
　Excision 31254
Frontal
　Destruction 31080-31085
　Exploration 31070-31075
　　with Nasal/Sinus Endoscopy 31276
　Fracture
　　Open Treatment 21343-21344
　Incision 31070-31087
Injection 20500
　Diagnostic .20501
Maxillary
　Antrostomy 31256-31267
　Excision 31225-31230
　Exploration 31020-31032
　　with Nasal/Sinus Endoscopy 31233
　Incision 31020-31032, 31256-31267
　Irrigation 31000
　Skull Base .61581
　Surgery 61581
Multiple
　Incision 31090
Paranasal
　Incision 31090
Pilonidal
　See Cyst, Pilonidal
Sinus of Valsalva
　Repair 33702-33722
Sinus Venosus
　Repair 33645
Sphenoid
　Biopsy 31050-31051
　Exploration 31050-31051
　　with Nasal/Sinus Endoscopy 31235
　Incision 31050-31051
　　with Nasal/Sinus Endoscopy .31287-31288
　Irrigation 31002
　Repair of Cerebrospinal Leak 31291
　Sinusotomy 31050-31051
　Skull Base Surgery 61580-61581
Unlisted Services and Procedures 31299
X-Ray .70210-70220

Sinusectomy, Ethmoid
See Sinus/Sinuses; Ethmoidectomy

Sinusoidal Rotational Testing
See Ear, Nose and Throat

Removal 63746
Replacement 63744
Stereotaxis
   Aspiration 63615
   Biopsy 63615
   Creation Lesion 63600
   Excision Lesion 63615
   Stimulation 63610
Syrinx
   Aspiration 62268
Tumor
   Excision 63275-63290

Spinal Cord Neoplasms
See Spinal Cord
Tumor
   See Spinal Cord, Tumor; Tumor
   Excision
      See Spinal Cord, Tumor; Tumor, Spinal
      Cord

Spinal Fluid
See Cerebrospinal Fluid

Spinal Fracture
See Fracture, Vertebra

Spinal Instrumentation
Anterior 22845-22847
   Removal 22855
Internal Fixation 22841
Pelvic Fixation 22848
Posterior Nonsegmental
   Harrington Rod Technique 22840
      Removal 22850
Posterior Segmental 22842-22844
   Removal 22852
Prosthetic Device 22851
Reinsertion of Spinal Fixation Device 22849

Spinal Manipulation
See Manipulation, Chiropractic

Spinal Nerve
Avulsion 64772
Transection 64772

Spinal Tap
See Cervical Puncture; Cisternal Puncture;
Subdural Tap; Ventricular Puncture
Drainage Fluid 62272
Lumbar 62270

Spine
See Intervertebral Disc; Spinal Cord; Vertebra;
Vertebral Body; Vertebral Process
Allograft
   Morselized 20930
   Structural 20931
Arthroplasty
   Cervical 0090T-0098T
   Lumbar 0163T-0165T, 22857-22865
Augmentation
   Lumbar Vertebra 22524-22525
   Thoracic Vertebra 22523, 22525
Autograft
   Local 20936
   Morselized 20937
   Structural 20938
Biopsy 20250-20251

CT Scan
   Cervical 72125-72127
   Lumbar 72131-72133
   Thoracic 72128-72130
Fixation 22842
Fusion
   Anterior 22808-22812
   Anterior Approach 22548-22585, 22812
   Exploration 22830
   Lateral Extracavitary 22532-22534
   Posterior Approach 22590-22802
Incision and Drainage
   Abscess 22010-22015
Insertion
   Instrumentation 22840-22848, 22851
Kyphectomy 22818-22819
Magnetic Resonance Angiography 72159
Magnetic Resonance Imaging
   Cervical 72141-72142, 72156-72158
   Lumbar 72148-72158
   Thoracic ...72146-72147, 72156-72158
Manipulation
   with Anesthesia 22505
Myelography
   Cervical 72240
   Lumbosacral 72265
   Thoracic 72255
   Total 72270
Reconstruction
   Dorsal Spine Elements 63295
Reinsertion
   Instrumentation 22849
Removal
   Instrumentation 22850, 22852-22855
Repair, Osteotomy
   Anterior 22220-22226
   Posterior 22210-22214
      Cervical Laminoplasty 63050-63051
      Posterolateral 22216
Ultrasound 76800
Unlisted Services and Procedures,
Surgery 22899
X-Ray 72020, 72090
   Absorptiometry 77080-77082
   Cervical 72040-72052
   Lumbosacral 72100-72120
   Standing 72069
   Thoracic 72070-72074
   Thoracolumbar 72080
   Total 72010
   with Contrast
      Cervical 72240
      Lumbosacral 72265
      Thoracic 72255
      Total 72270

Spine Chemotherapy
Administration 96450
   See Chemotherapy

Spirometry 94010-94070
See Pulmonology, Diagnostic
Patient Initiated 94014-94016

Splanchnicectomy
See Nerves, Sympathectomy, Excision

Spleen
Excision 38100-38102
   Laparoscopic 38120
Injection
   Radiologic 38200
Nuclear Medicine
   Imaging 78185, 78215-78216
Repair 38115

Splenectomy
Laparoscopic 38120
Partial 38101
Partial with Repair, Ruptured Spleen 38115
Total 38100
   En bloc 38102

Splenoplasty
See Repair, Spleen

Splenoportography 75810
Injection Procedures 38200

Splenorrhaphy 38115

Splint
See Casting; Strapping
Arm
   Long 29105
   Short 29125-29126
Finger 29130-29131
Foot 29590
Leg
   Long 29505
   Short 29515
Oral Surgical 21085
Ureteral
   See Ureteral Splinting

Split Grafts 15100-15101, 15120-15121

Split Renal Function Test
See Cystourethroscopy, Catheterization, Ureteral

Splitting
Blood Products 86985

Spontaneous Abortion
See Abortion

Sprengel's Deformity 23400

Spring Water Cyst
See Cyst, Pericardial

Spur, Bone
See Exostosis
Calcaneal
   See Heel Spur

Sputum Analysis 89220

SRIH
See Somatostatin

Ssabanejew-Frank Operation
See Incision, Stomach, Creation, Stoma; Incision
and Drainage

Stabilizing Factor, Fibrin
See Fibrin Stabilizing Factor

Stable Factor 85230

Radical Resection 21630-21632
Reconstruction 21740-21742, 21750
    with Thoracoscopy 21743
X-Ray 71120-71130

Steroid-Binding Protein, Sex
See Globulin, Sex Hormone Binding

Steroids
Anabolic
    See Androstenedione
Injection
    Urethral Stricture 52283
Ketogenic
    Urine 83582

STH (Somatotropic Hormone)
See Growth Hormone

Stimulating Antibody, Thyroid
See Immunoglobulin, Thyroid Stimulating

Stimulation
Electric
    See Electrical Stimulation
Lymphocyte
    See Blastogenesis
Spinal Cord
    Stereotaxis 63610
Transcutaneous Electric
    See Application, Neurostimulation

Stimulator, Long-Acting Thyroid
See Thyrotropin Releasing Hormone (TRH)

Stimulators, Cardiac
See Heart, Pacemaker

Stimulus Evoked Response 51792

Stoffel Operation
See Rhizotomy

Stoma
Creation
    Bladder 51980
    Kidney 50551-50561
    Stomach
        Neonatal 43831
        Temporary 43830-43831
    Ureter 50860
Ureter
    Endoscopy via 50951-50961

Stomach
Anastomosis
    with Duodenum 43810, 43850-43855
    with Jejunum . . .43820-43825, 43860-43865
Biopsy 43600-43605
Creation
    Stoma
        Temporary 43830-43831
    Temporary Stoma
        Laparoscopic 43653
Electrode
    Removal 0156T, 0158T, 43882
Electrogastrography 91132-91133
Excision
    Partial 43631-43635, 43845
    Total 43620-43622
Exploration 43500

Gastric Bypass 43644-43645, 43846
    Revision 43848
Gastric Restrictive Procedures 43770-43774,
                                43848, 43886-43888
Implantation
    Electrodes 0155T, 0157T, 43647, 43881
Incision 43830-43832
    Exploration 43500
    Pyloric Sphincter 43520
    Removal
        Foreign Body 43500
Intubation with Specimen Prep 91055
Laparoscopy 0155T-0156T, 43647-43648
Nuclear Medicine
    Blood Loss Study 78278
    Emptying Study 78264
    Imaging 78261
    Protein Loss Study 78282
    Reflux Study 78262
    Vitamin B-12 Absorption 78270-78272
Reconstruction
    for Obesity 43644-43645, 43842-43847
    Roux-En-Y 43644, 43846
Removal
    Foreign Body 43500
Repair 48547
    Fistula 43880
    Fundoplasty 43324-43325
        Laparoscopic 43280
    Laceration 43501-43502
    Stoma 43870
    Ulcer 43501
Replacement
    Electrodes 0155T, 0157T, 43647, 43881
Specimen Collection 89130-89141
Stimulation of Secretion 91052
Suture
    Fistula 43880
    for Obesity 43842-43843
    Stoma 43870
    Ulcer 43840
    Wound 43840
Tumor
    Excision 43610-43611
Ulcer
    Excision 43610
Unlisted Services and Procedures . .43659, 43999

Stomatoplasty
See Mouth, Repair

Stone, Kidney
See Calculus, Removal, Kidney

Stookey-Scarff Procedure
See Ventriculocisternostomy

Stool Blood
See Blood, Feces

Storage
Embryo 89342
Oocyte 89346
Reproductive Tissue 89344
Sperm 89343

Strabismus
Chemodenervation 67345
Repair
    Adjustable Sutures 67335

Extraocular Muscles 67340
One Horizontal Muscle 67311
One Vertical Muscle 67314
Posterior Fixation Suture
    Technique 67334-67335
Previous Surgery, Not Involving Extraocular
    Muscles 67331
Release Extensive Scar Tissue 67343
Superior Oblique Muscle 67318
Transposition 67320
Two Horizontal Muscles 67312
Two or More Vertical Muscles 67316

Strapping
See Cast; Splint
Ankle 29540
Back 29220
Chest 29200
Elbow 29260
Finger 29280
Foot 29540, 29590
Hand 29280
Hip 29520
Knee 29530
Shoulder 29240
Thorax 29200
Toes 29550
Unlisted Services and Procedures 29799
Unna Boot 29580
Wrist 29260

Strassman Procedure 58540

Strayer Procedure
Leg, Lower 27687

**Streptococcus pneumoniae
Vaccine**
See Vaccines

Streptococcus, Group A
Antigen Detection
    Enzyme Immunoassay 87430
    Nucleic Acid 87650-87652
Direct Optical Observation 87880

Streptococcus, Group B
by Immunoassay
    with Direct Optical Observation 87802

Streptokinase, Antibody 86590

Stress Tests
Cardiovascular 93015-93024
Multiple Gated Acquisition (MUGA) .78472-78473
Myocardial Perfusion Imaging 78460-78465
Pulmonary 94620-94621
    See Pulmonology, Diagnostic

Stricture
Repair
    Urethra 53400-53405
Urethra
    See Urethral Stenosis

Strictureplasty
Intestines 44615

Stroboscopy
Larynx 31579

Saucerization 28120
Tumor
  Excision 27647, 28100-28103

Tap
Cisternal
  See Cisternal Puncture
Lumbar Diagnostic
  See Spinal Tap

Tarsal
Fracture
  Percutaneous Fixation 28456

Tarsal Bone
See Ankle Bone

Tarsal Joint
See Foot
Arthrodesis 28730-28735, 28740
  with Advancement 28737
  with Lengthening 28737
Craterization 28122
Cyst
  Excision 28104-28107
Diaphysectomy 28122
Dislocation 28540-28545, 28555
  Percutaneous Fixation 28545-28546
Excision 28116, 28122
Fracture
  Open Treatment 28465
  with Manipulation 28455-28456
  without Manipulation 28450
Fusion 28730-28735, 28740
  with Advancement 28737
  with Lengthening 28737
Repair 28320
  Osteotomy 28304-28305
Saucerization 28122
Tumor
  Excision 28104-28107, 28171

Tarsal Strip Procedure 67917-67924

Tarsal Tunnel Release 28035

Tarsal Wedge Procedure .67916, 67923

Tarsometatarsal Joint
Arthrodesis 28730-28735, 28740
Arthrotomy 28020, 28050
Dislocation 28600-28605, 28615
  Percutaneous Fixation 28606
Exploration 28020
Fusion 28730-28735, 28740
Removal
  Foreign Body 28020
  Loose Body 28020
Synovial
  Biopsy 28050
  Excision 28070

Tarsorrhaphy 67875
Median 67880
Severing 67710
  with Transposition of Tarsal Plate 67882

Tattoo
Cornea 65600
Skin 11920-11922

TB Test
Antigen Response 86480
Skin Test 86580

TBG
See Thyroxine Binding Globulin

TBS
See Bethesda System

TCT
See Thrombin Time

Td Shots
See Tetanus Immunization; Vaccines

Team Conference
Case Management Services 99361-99373

Tear Duct
See Lacrimal Duct

Tear Gland
See Lacrimal Gland

Technique
Pericardial Window
  See Pericardiostomy
Projective
  See Projective Test

Teeth
X-Ray 70300-70320

Telangiectasia
Chromosome Analysis 88248
Injection 36468

Telangiectasia, Cerebello-Oculocutaneous
See Ataxia Telangiectasia

Telephone
Case Management Services 99361-99373
Pacemaker Analysis 93733, 93736
Transmission of ECG 93012

Teletherapy
Dose Plan 77305-77321

Temperature Gradient Studies 93740

Temporal Arteries
See Artery, Temporal

Temporal Bone
Electromagnetic Bone Conduction Hearing Device
  Implantation/Replacement 69710
  Removal/Repair 69711
Excision 69535
Resection 69535
Tumor
  Removal 69970
Unlisted Services and Procedures 69979

Temporal, Petrous
Excision
  Apex...........................69530

Temporomandibular Joint (TMJ)
Arthrocentesis 20605
Arthrography 70328-70332

Injection 21116
Arthroplasty 21240-21243
Arthroscopy
  Diagnostic 29800
  Surgical 29804
Arthrotomy 21010
Cartilage
  Excision 21060
Condylectomy 21050
Coronoidectomy 21070
Dislocation
  Closed Treatment 21480-21485
  Open Treatment 21490
Injection
  Radiologic 21116
Magnetic Resonance Imaging (MRI) 70336
Meniscectomy 21060
Prostheses
  See Prosthesis, Temporomandibular Joint
Reconstruction
  See Reconstruction, Temporomandibular Joint
X-Ray with Contrast 70328-70332

Tenago Procedure 53431

Tendinosuture
See Suture, Tendon

Tendon
Achilles
  See Achilles Tendon
Arm, Upper
  Revision 24320
Excision
  Finger 26180
  Forearm 25109
  Palm 26170
  Wrist 25109
Finger
  Excision 26180
Forearm
  Excision 25109
  Repair 25260-25274
Graft
  Harvesting 20924
Insertion
  Biceps Tendon 24342
Lengthening
  Ankle 27685-27686
  Arm, Upper 24305
  Elbow 24305
  Finger 26476, 26478
  Forearm 25280
  Hand 26476, 26478
  Leg, Lower 27685-27686
  Leg, Upper 27393-27395
  Toe 28240
  Wrist 25280
Palm
  Excision 26170
Release
  Arm, Lower 25295
  Arm, Upper 24332
  Wrist 25295
Shortening
  Ankle 27685-27686
  Finger 26477, 26479
  Hand 26477, 26479
  Leg, Lower 27685-27686

Surgery
   Video-Assisted
      See Thoracoscopy
Vertebra
   See Vertebra, Thoracic
Wall
   See Chest Wall

Thoracocentesis
See Thoracentesis

Thoracoplasty 32905
with Closure Bronchopleural Fistula 32906

Thoracoscopy
Diagnostic 32601-32606
   with Biopsy 32602, 32604, 32606
   without Biopsy 32601, 32603, 32605
Surgical 32650-32665
   with Control Traumatic Hemorrhage ...32654
   with Creation Pericardial Window 32659
   with Esophagomyotomy 32665
   with Excision Mediastinal Cyst, Tumor
   and/or Mass 32662
   with Excision Pericardial Cyst, Tumor
   and/or Mass 32661
   with Excision-Plication of Bullae 32655
   with Lobectomy 32663
   with Parietal Pleurectomy 32656
   with Partial Pulmonary Decortication ..32651
   with Pleurodesis 32650
   with Removal Intrapleural Foreign
   Body 32653
   with Removal of Clot/Foreign Body ...32658
   with Sternum Reconstruction 21743
   with Thoracic Sympathectomy 32664
   with Total Pericardiectomy 32660
   with Total Pulmonary Decortication ..32652
   with Wedge Resection of Lung 32657

Thoracostomy
Empyema 32035-32036
Tube, with/without Water Seal 32020

Thoracotomy
Cardiac Massage 32160
for Post-Op Complications 32120
Hemorrhage 32110
Removal
   Bullae 32141
   Cyst 32140
   Defibrillator 33243
   Electrodes 33238
   Foreign Body
      Intrapleural 32150
      Intrapulmonary 32151
   Pacemaker 33236-33237
      with Biopsy 32095-32100
      with Excision-Plication of Bullae ...32141
      with Lung Repair 32110
      with Open Intrapleural Pneumolysis .32124
Transmyocardial Laser Revascularization ..33140-
                                33141

Thorax
See Chest; Chest Cavity; Mediastinum
Angiography 71275
Bioimpedance 93701
Biopsy 21550
CT Scan 71250-71275

Incision
   Empyema 32035-32036
   Pneumothorax 32020
Incision and Drainage
   Abscess 21501-21502
   Deep 21510
   Hematoma 21501-21502
Strapping 29200
Tumor
   Excision 21555-21556
   Excision/Resection 21557
Unlisted Services and Procedures, Surgery .21899

Three Glass Test
See Urinalysis, Glass Test

Three-Day Measles
See Rubella

Throat
See Pharynx
Abscess
   Incision and Drainage 42700-42725
Biopsy 42800-42806
Hemorrhage 42960-42962
Reconstruction 42950
Removal
   Foreign Body 42809
Repair
   Pharyngoesophageal 42953
   Wound 42900
Suture
   Wound 42900
Unlisted Services and Procedures 42999

Thrombectomy
See Thromboendarterectomy
Aortoiliac Artery 34151-34201
Arteriovenous Fistula
   Graft 36870
Axillary Artery 34101
Axillary Vein 34490
Brachial Artery 34101
Bypass Graft
   Other than Hemodialysis Graft or
   Fistula 35875-35876
Carotid Artery 34001
Celiac Artery 34151
Dialysis Graft
   without Revision 36831
Femoral 34201
Femoropopliteal Vein 34421-34451
Iliac 34151-34201
Iliac Vein 34401-34451
Innominate Artery 34001-34101
Mesentery Artery 34151
Percutaneous
   Coronary Artery 92973
   Fluoroscopic Guidance 37184-37188
   Mechanical Arterial 37184-37186
   Mechanical Venous 37187-37188
Peroneal Artery 34203
Popliteal Artery 34203
Radial Artery 34111
Renal Artery 34151
Subclavian Artery 34001-34101
Subclavian Vein 34471-34490
Tibial Artery 34203
Ulnar Artery 34111

Vena Cava 34401-34451
Vena Caval 50230

Thrombin Inhibitor I
See Antithrombin III

Thrombin Time 85670-85675

Thrombocyte (Platelet)
See Blood, Platelet

Thrombocyte ab
See Antibody, Platelet

Thromboendarterectomy
See Thrombectomy
Aorta, Abdominal 35331
Aortoiliofemoral Artery 35363
Axillary Artery 35321
Brachial Artery 35321
Carotid Artery 35301, 35390
Celiac Artery 35341
Femoral Artery 35371-35372
Iliac Artery 35351, 35361-35363
Iliofemoral Artery 35355, 35363
Innominate Artery 35311
Mesenteric Artery 35341
Peroneal Artery 35305-35306
Popliteal Artery 35303
Renal Artery 35341
Subclavian Artery 35301, 35311
Superficial Femoral Artery 35302
Tibial Artery 35305-35306
Tibioperoneal Trunk Artery 35304
Vertebral Artery 35301

Thrombokinase 85260

Thrombolysin
See Plasmin

Thrombolysis
Catheter Exchange
   Intravascular 37209, 75900
Cerebral
   Intravenous Infusion 37195
Coronary Vessels 92975-92977
Cranial Vessels 37195

Thrombolysis Biopsy Intracranial
Arterial Perfusion 61624

Thrombolysis Intracranial 65205
See Ciliary Body; Cornea; Eye, Removal, Foreign
Body; Iris; Lens; Retina; Sclera; Vitreous

Thrombomodulin 85337

Thromboplastin
Inhibition 85705
Inhibition Test 85347
Partial Time 85730-85732

Thromboplastin Antecedent, Plasma
See Plasma Thromboplastin, Antecedent

Thromboplastinogen
See Clotting Factor

Thromboplastinogen B
See Christmas Factor

Thumb

See Phalanx
Amputation 26910-26952
Arthrodesis
    Carpometacarpal Joint 26841-26842
Dislocation
    with Fracture 26645-26650
      Open Treatment .... .26665
    with Manipulation .... .26641
Fracture
    with Dislocation 26645-26650
      Open Treatment .... .26665
Fusion
    in Opposition .... .26820
Reconstruction
    from Finger .... .26550
    Opponensplasty 26490-26496
Repair
    Muscle .... .26508
    Muscle Transfer .... .26494
    Tendon Transfer .... .26510
Replantation 20824-20827
Sesamoidectomy .... .26185
Unlisted Services and Procedures .... .26989

Thymectomy 60520-60521
Sternal Split/Transthoracic
Approach 60521-60522
Transcervical Approach .... .60520

Thymotaxin
See Beta-2-Microglobulin

Thymus Gland .... .60520
Excision 60520-60521

Thyramine
See Amphetamine

Thyrocalcitonin
See Calcitonin

Thyroglobulin .... .84432
Antibody .... .86800

Thyroglossal Duct
Cyst
    Excision 60280-60281

Thyroid Gland
Cyst
    Aspiration .... .60001
    Excision .... .60200
    Incision and Drainage .... .60000
    Injection .... .60001
Excision
    for Malignancy
      Limited Neck Dissection .... .60252
      Radical Neck Dissection .... .60254
    Partial 60210-60225
    Secondary .... .60260
    Total .... .60240, 60271
      Cervical Approach .... .60271
      Removal All Thyroid Tissue .... .60260
      Sternal Split/Transthoracic
      Approach .... .60270
      Transcervical Approach .... .60520
Metastatic Cancer
    Nuclear Imaging 78015-78018

Needle Biopsy .... .60100
Nuclear Medicine
    Imaging .... .78010
    Imaging for Metastases 78015-78018
    Imaging with Flow .... .78011
    Imaging with Uptake 78006-78007
    Metastases Uptake .... .78020
    Uptake 78000-78003
Tumor
    Excision .... .60200

Thyroid Hormone Binding
Ratio .... .84479

Thyroid Hormone Uptake ...... .84479

Thyroid Stimulating Hormone
(TSH) .... .80418, 80438-80440, 84443

Thyroid Stimulating Hormone
Receptor ab
See Thyrotropin Releasing Hormone (TRH)

Thyroid Stimulating Immune
Globulins .... .84445

Thyroid Stimulator, Long Acting
See Thyrotropin Releasing Hormone (TRH)

Thyroid Suppression Test
See Nuclear Medicine, Thyroid, Uptake

Thyroidectomy
Partial 60210-60225
Secondary .... .60260
Total .... .60240, 60271
    Cervical Approach .... .60271
    for Malignancy
      Limited Neck Dissection .... .60252
      Radical Neck Dissection .... .60254
    Removal All Thyroid Tissue .... .60260
    Sternal Split/Transthoracic Approach . .60270

Thyrolingual Cyst
See Cyst, Thyroglossal Duct

Thyrotomy .... .31300

Thyrotropin Receptor Ab
See Thyrotropin Releasing Hormone (TRH)

Thyrotropin Releasing Hormone
(TRH) 80438-80439

Thyroxine
Free .... .84439
Neonatal .... .84437
Total .... .84436
True .... .84436

Thyroxine Binding Globulin .... .84442

Tibia
See Ankle
Arthroscopy Surgical 29891-29892
Craterization .... .27360, 27640
Cyst
    Excision 27635-27638
Diaphysectomy .... .27360, 27640
Excision .... .27360, 27640
    Epiphyseal Bar .... .20150

Fracture
    Arthroscopic Treatment 29855-29856
      Plafond .... .29892
    Closed Treatment 27824-27825
    Distal 27824-27828
    Intercondylar 27538-27540
    Malleolus 27760-27766, 27808-27814
    Open Treatment 27535-27536,
                 27758-27759, 27826-27828
    Plateau 29855-29856
      Closed Treatment 27530-27536
    Shaft 27752-27759
    with Manipulation .... .27825
    without Manipulation .... .27824
Incision .... .27607
Osteoplasty
    Lengthening .... .27715
Prophylactic Treatment .... .27745
Reconstruction .... .27418
    at Knee 27440-27443, 27446
Repair 27720-27725
    Epiphysis 27477-27485, 27730-27742
    Osteochondritis Dissecans
      Arthroscopy .... .29892
    Osteotomy 27455-27457, 27705,
                   27709-27712
    Pseudoarthrosis .... .27727
Saucerization .... .27360, 27640
Tumor
    Excision 27635-27638, 27645
X-Ray .... .73590

Tibial
Arteries
    See Artery, Tibial
Nerve
    Repair/Suture
      Posterior .... .64840

Tibiofibular Joint
Arthrodesis .... .27871
Dislocation 27830-27832
Disruption
    Open Treatment .... .27829
Fusion .... .27871

TIG
See Immune Globulins, Tetanus

Time
Bleeding
    See Bleeding Time
Prothrombin
    See Prothrombin Time
Reptilase
    See Thrombin Time

Tinnitus
Assessment .... .92625

Tissue
Crystal Identification .... .89060
Culture
    Chromosome Analysis 88230-88239
    Homogenization .... .87176
    Non-neoplastic Disorder ...... .88230, 88237
    Skin Grafts 15100-15101, 15120-15121
      Harvesting .... .15040
    Solid Tumor .... .88239

Torus Mandibularis
Tumor Excision .... .21031

Total
Abdominal Hysterectomy
   See Hysterectomy, Abdominal, Total
Bilirubin Level
   See Bilirubin, Total
Catecholamines
   See Catecholamines, Urine
Cystectomy
   See Bladder, Excision, Total
Dacryoadenectomy
   See Dacryoadenectomy, Total
Elbow Replacement
   See Replacement, Elbow, Total
Esophagectomy
   See Esophagectomy, Total
Gastrectomy
   See Excision, Stomach, Total
Hemolytic Complement
   See Complement, Hemolytic, Total
Hip Arthroplasty
   See Hip, Total Replacement
Knee Arthroplasty
   See Prosthesis, Knee
Mastectomies
   See Mastectomy
Ostectomy of Patella
   See Patellectomy
Splenectomy
   See Splenectomy, Total

Touroff Operation .... .37615
See Ligation, Artery, Neck

Toxicology Screen 80100-80103

Toxin Assay .... .87230

Toxin, Botulinum
See Chemodenervation

Toxoplasma
Antibody 86777-86778

Trabeculectomies
See Trabeculoplasty

Trabeculectomy ab Externo
in Absence of Previous Surgery .... .66170
with Scarring Previous Surgery .... .66172

Trabeculoplasty
by Laser Surgery .... .65855

Trabeculotomy ab Externo
Eye .... .65850

Trachea
Aspiration .... .31720
   Catheter 31720-31725
Dilation 31630-31631, 31636-31638
Endoscopy
   via Tracheostomy .... .31615
Excision
   Stenosis 31780-31781
Fistula
   with Plastic Repair .... .31825
   without Plastic Repair .... .31820

Fracture
   Endoscopy .... .31630
Incision
   Emergency 31603-31605
   Planned 31600-31601
   with Flaps .... .31610
Introduction
   Needle Wire .... .31730
Puncture
   Aspiration and/or Injection .... .31612
Reconstruction
   Carina .... .31766
   Cervical .... .31750
   Fistula .... .31755
   Intrathoracic .... .31760
Repair
   Cervical .... .31750
   Fistula .... .31755
   Intrathoracic .... .31760
   Stoma 31613-31614
Revision
   Stoma
     Scars .... .31830
Scar
   Revision .... .31830
Stenosis
   Excision 31780-31781
   Repair 31780-31781
Stoma
   Repair
     with Plastic Repair .... .31825
     without Plastic Repair .... .31820
   Revision
     Scars .... .31830
Tumor
   Excision
     Cervical .... .31785
     Thoracic .... .31786
Unlisted Services and Procedures
   Bronchi .... .31899
Wound
   Suture
     Cervical .... .31800
     Intrathoracic .... .31805

Tracheal
Stent
   Placement .... .31631
Tubes
   See Endotracheal Tube

Trachelectomy .... .57530
Radical .... .57531

Tracheloplasty
See Cervicoplasty

Trachelorrhaphy .... .57720

Tracheo-Esophageal Fistula
See Fistula, Tracheoesophageal

Tracheobronchoscopy
through Tracheostomy .... .31615

Tracheoplasty
Cervical .... .31750
Intrathoracic .... .31760
Tracheopharyngeal Fistulization .... .31755

Tracheostoma
Revision 31613-31614

Tracheostomy
Emergency 31603-31605
Planned 31600-31601
Revision
   Scar .... .31830
Surgical Closure
   with Plastic Repair .... .31825
   without Plastic Repair .... .31820
Tracheobronchoscopy through .... .31615
with Flaps .... .31610

Tracheotomy
Tube Change .... .31502

Tracking Tests (Ocular) .... .92545
See Ear, Nose and Throat

Tract, Urinary
See Urinary Tract

Traction Therapy
See Physical Medicine/Therapy/Occupational
Therapy
Manual .... .97140
Mechanical .... .97012

Tractotomy
Medulla .... .61470
Mesencephalon .... .61480

Training
Activities of Daily Living .... .97535, 99509
Biofeedback 90901-90911
Cognitive Skills .... .97532
Community/Work Reintegration .... .97537
Home Management .... .97535, 99509
Orthoptic/Pleoptic .... .92065
Orthotics .... .97760
Prosthetics .... .97761
Self Care .... .97535, 98960-98962, 99509
Sensory Integration .... .97533
Walking (Physical Therapy) .... .97116
Wheelchair Management .... .97542

TRAM Flap
Breast Reconstruction 19367-19369

Trans-Scaphoperilunar
Fracture/Dislocation
   Closed Treatment .... .25680
   Open Treatment .... .25685

Transaminase
Glutamic Oxaloacetic .... .84450
Glutamic Pyruvic .... .84460

Transcatheter
Biopsy .... .37200
Closure
   Percutaneous
     Heart 93580-93581
   Transmyocardial
     Heart .... .0166T, 0167T
Embolization
   Percutaneous .... .37204
   Cranial 61624-61626

Peripheral Nerve
Major	64856
Vein Valve	34510

Transthoracic Echocardiography
See Echocardiography

Transthyretin
See Prealbumin

Transureteroureterostomy 50770

Transurethral Balloon Dilation
Prostatic Urethra 52510

Transurethral Fulguration
Postoperative Bleeding 52606

Transurethral Procedure
See Specific Procedure
Prostate
Incision	52450
Resection	52612-52614
Thermotherapy	53850-53853
Microwave	53850
Radiofrequency	53852

Trapezium
Arthroplasty
with Implant	25445

Travel, Unusual 99082

Treacher-Collins Syndrome
Midface Reconstruction 21150-21151

Treatment, Tocolytic
See Tocolysis

Trendelenburg Operation
See Varicose Vein, Removal, Secondary Varicosity

Trephine Procedure
Sinusotomy
Frontal	31070

Treponema Pallidum
Antibody
Confirmation Test	86781
Antigen Detection
Direct Fluorescence	87285

TRH
See Thyrotropin Releasing Hormone (TRH)

Triacylglycerol
See Triglycerides

Triacylglycerol Hydrolase
See Lipase

Tributyrinase
See Lipase

Trichiasis
Repair	67825
Epilation, by Forceps	67820
Epilation, by Other than Forceps	67825
Incision of Lid Margin	67830
with Free Mucous Membrane Graft	67835

Trichina
See Trichinella

Trichinella
Antibody	86784
Trichogram	96902

Trichomonas Vaginalis
Antigen Detection
Nucleic Acid	87660
by Immunoassay with Direct Optical Observation	87808

Trichrome Stain 88313

Tricuspid Valve
Excision	33460
Repair	33463-33465
Replacement	33465
Repositioning	33468

Tridymite
See Silica

Trigeminal Ganglia
See Gasserian Ganglion

Trigeminal Nerve
Destruction	64600-64610
Injection
Anesthetic	64400
Neurolytic	64600-64610

Trigeminal Tract
Stereotactic
Create Lesion	61791

Trigger Finger Repair 26055

Trigger Point
Injection
One or Two Muscles	20552
Two or More Muscles	20553

Triglyceridase
See Lipase

Triglyceride Lipase
See Lipase

Triglycerides 84478

Trigonocephaly 21175

Triiodothyronine
Free	84481
Reverse	84482
Total	84480
True	84480

Triolean Hydrolase
See Lipase

Trioxopurine
See Uric Acid

Tripcellim
See Trypsin

Trisegmentectomy 47122

Trocar Biopsy
Bone Marrow	38221

Trochanteric Femur Fracture
See Femur, Fracture, Trochanteric

Trophoblastic Tumor GTT
See Hydatidiform Mole

Troponin 84484
Qualitative	84512
Quantitative	84484

Truncal Vagotomies
See Vagotomy, Truncal

Truncus Arteriosus
Repair	33786

Truncus Brachiocephalicus
See Artery, Brachiocephalic

Trunk, Brachiocephalic
See Artery, Brachiocephalic

Trypanosomiases
See Trypanosomiasis

Trypanosomiasis 86171, 86280

Trypsin
Duodenum	84485
Feces	84488-84490

Trypsin Inhibitor, Alpha 1-Antitrypsin
See Alpha-1 Antitrypsin

Trypure
See Trypsin

Tsalicylate Intoxication
See Salicylate

TSH
See Thyroid Stimulating Hormone

TSI
See Thyroid Stimulating Immunoglobulin

Tsutsugamushi Disease
See Scrub Typhus

TT
See Thrombin Time

TT-3
See Triiodothyronine, True

TT-4
See Thyroxine, True

Tuba Auditoria (Auditiva)
See Eustachian Tube

Tubal Embryo Stage Transfer
See Embryo Transfer

Tubal Ligation 58600
Laparoscopic	58670
with Cesarean Delivery	58611

Tubal Occlusion
See Fallopian Tube, Occlusion; Occlusion
Create Lesion

Tubal Pregnancy 59121
with Salpingectomy and/or
Oophorectomy 59120

Tube Change
Tracheotomy 31502

Tube Placement
Endoscopic
   Bile Duct, Pancreatic Duct 43268
   Nasobiliary, Nasopancreatic
     for Drainage 43267
Gastrostomy Tube 43750
Nasogastric Tube 43752
Orogastric Tube .43752

Tube, Fallopian
See Fallopian Tube

Tubectomy
See Excision, Fallopian Tube

Tubed Pedicle Flap
Formation .15570-15576

Tubercle Bacilli
Culture 87116

Tubercleplasty
Tibia
   Anterior 27418

Tuberculin Test
See Skin, Tests, Tuberculosis

Tuberculosis
Antigen Response Test 86480
Culture 87116
Skin Test 86580

Tuberculosis Vaccine
(BCG) 90585-90586

Tubes
Endotracheal
   See Endotracheal Tube
Gastrostomy
   See Gastrostomy Tube

Tudor 'Rabbit Ear'
See Urethra, Repair

Tuffier Vaginal Hysterectomy
See Hysterectomy, Vaginal

Tumor
See Craniopharyngioma
Abdomen
   Destruction/Excision 49200-49201
Abdominal Wall
   Excision 22900
Acetabulum
   Excision 27076
Ankle 27615-27619
Arm, Lower 25075-25077
Arm, Upper
   Excision 24075-24077
Back/Flank
   Excision 21930
   Radical Resection 21935

Bile Duct
   Destruction .43272
   Extrahepatic .47711
   Intrahepatic .47712
Bladder 52234-52240
   Excision 51530, 52355
Bone
   Ablation 20982
Brain 61510
   Excision 61518, 61520-61521,
           61526-61530, 61545, 62164
Breast
   Excision 19120-19126
Bronchi
   Excision 31640
Calcaneus 28100-28103
   Excision 27647
Carpal .25130-25136
Cheekbone 21030, 21034
Chest Wall
   Excision 19260-19272
Clavicle
   Excision 23140, 23200
   with Allograft 23146
   with Autograft 23145
Coccyx 49215
Colon
   Destruction 44393, 45383
Cranial Bone
   Reconstruction 21181-21184
Destruction
   Chemosurgery 17311-17315
   Urethra 53220
Ear, Middle
   Extended 69554
   Transcanal 69550
   Transmastoid 69552
Elbow
   Excision 24075-24077
Esophagus
   Ablation 43228
Excision
   Femur 27355-27358
Facial Bone 21029-21030, 21034
Fallopian Tube
   Resection 58950, 58952-58958
Femoral 27355-27358
Femur .27065-27067
   Excision 27365
Fibroid
   See Leiomyomata
Fibula .27635-27638
   Excision 27646
Finger
   Excision 26115-26117
Foot 28043-28046
Forearm
   Radical Resection 25077
Gastrostomy
   See Lesion
Gums
   Excision 41825-41827
Hand
   Excision 26115-26117
Heart
   Excision 33120-33130
Hip 27047-27049, 27065-27067
   Excision 27075-27076

Humerus
   Excision 23150, 23220-23222, 24110
   with Allograft 23156, 24116
   with Autograft 23155, 24115
Ileum 27065-27067
Immunoassay for Antigen 86294, 86316
   CA 125 86304
   CA 15-3 86300
   CA 19-9 86301
Innominate
   Excision 27077
Intestines, Small
   Destruction .44369
Ischial
   Excision 27078-27079
Kidney
   Ablation
     Cryotherapy 0135T
     Radiofrequency 50592
   Excision 50562, 52355
Knee
   Excision 27327-27329, 27365
Lacrimal Gland
   Excision
     Frontal Approach 68540
     with Osteotomy 68550
Larynx
   Excision 31300
   Endoscopic 31540-31541, 31578
   Incision 31300
Leg, Lower 27615-27619
Leg, Upper
   Excision 27327-27329
Localization
   Nuclear Medicine 78800-78804
Mandible 21044-21047
Maxilla 21030, 21034, 21048-21049
Maxillary Torus Palatinus 21032
Mediastinal
   Excision 39220
Mediastinum 32662
Meningioma 61512
   Excision 61519
Metacarpal 26200-26205, 26250-26255
Metatarsal 28104-28107
   Excision 28173
Neck
   Excision 21555-21556
   Radical Resection 21557
Olecranon
   Excision 24120
Olecranon Process
   with Allograft
     Excision .24126
   with Autograft
     Excision .24125
Ovary
   Resection 58950-58958
Pancreatic Duct
   Destruction .43272
Parotid Gland
   Excision 42410-42426
Pelvis .27047-27049
Pericardial
   Endoscopic .32661
   Excision 33050
Peritoneum
   Resection 58950-58958

Phalanges
 Finger 26210-26215, 26260-26262
 Toe 28108
  Excision 28175
Pituitary Gland
 Excision 61546-61548, 62165
Positron Emission Tomography
(PET) 78811-78816
Pubis 27065-27067
Pulmonary
 Ablation 32998
Radiation Therapy 77295
Radius 25120-25126, 25170
 Excision 24120
 with Allograft
  Excision 24126
 with Autograft
  Excision 24125
Rectum
 Destruction ..... .45190, 45320, 46937-46938
 Excision 45160-45170
Resection
 Face 21015
 Scalp 21015
 with Cystourethroscopy 52355
Retroperitoneal
 Destruction/Excision 49200-49201
Sacrum 49215
Scapula
 Excision 23140, 23210
  with Allograft 23146
  with Autograft 23145
Shoulder
 Excision 23075-23077
Skull
 Excision 61500
Soft Tissue
 Elbow
  Excision 24075
 Finger
  Excision 26115
 Forearm
  Radical Resection 25077
 Hand
  Excision 26115
 Wrist
  Excision 25075
  Radical Resection 25077
Spinal Cord
 Excision 63275-63290
Stomach
 Excision 43610-43611
Talus 28100-28103
 Excision 27647
Tarsal 28104-28107
 Excision 28171
Temporal Bone
 Removal 69970
Testis
 Excision 54530-54535
Thorax
 Excision 21555-21556
 Radical Resection 21557
Thyroid
 Excision 60200
Tibia 27365, 27635-27638
 Excision 27645
Torus Mandibularis 21031

Trachea
 Excision
  Cervical 31785
  Thoracic 31786
Ulna 25120-25126, 25170
 Excision 24120
 with Allograft
  Excision 24126
 with Autograft
  Excision 24125
Ureter
 Excision 52355
Urethra 52234-52240, 53220
 Excision 52355
Uterus
 Excision 58140-58146
 Resection 58950-58958
Vagina
 Excision 57135
Vertebra
 Additional Segment
  Excision 22116
 Cervical
  Excision 22100
 Lumbar 22102
 Thoracic
  Excision 22101
Wrist 25075-25077, 25135-25136
 Radical Resection 25077

Tunica Vaginalis
Hydrocele
 Aspiration 55000
 Excision 55040-55041
 Repair 55060

Turbinate
Excision 30130-30140
Fracture
 Therapeutic 30930
Injection 30200
Submucous Resection
 Nose Excision 30140

Turbinate Mucosa
Cauterization 30801-30802

Turcica, Sella
See Sella Turcica

Turnbuckle Jacket 29020-29025
Removal 29715

TURP
See Prostatectomy, Transurethral

Tylectomy
See Breast, Excision, Lesion

Tylenol
Urine 82003

Tympanic Membrane
Create Stoma 69433-69436
Incision 69420-69421
Reconstruction 69620
Repair 69450, 69610

Tympanic Nerve
Excision 69676

Tympanolysis 69450

Tympanomastoidectomy
See Tympanoplasty

Tympanometry 92567
See Audiologic Function Tests

Tympanoplasty
See Myringoplasty
Radical or Complete 69645
 with Ossicular Chain Reconstruction ..69646
with Antrotomy or Mastoidotomy 69635
 with Ossicular Chain Reconstruction ..69636
  and Synthetic Prosthesis 69637
with Mastoidectomy 69641
 with Intact or Reconstructed Wall 69643
  and Ossicular Chain Reconstruction 69644
 with Ossicular Chain Reconstruction ..69642
without Mastoidectomy 69631
 with Ossicular Chain Reconstruction ..69632
  and Synthetic Prosthesis 69633

Tympanostomy 69433-69436

Tympanotomy
See Myringotomy

Typhoid Vaccine 90690-90693
AKD 90693
Oral 90690
Polysaccharide 90691

Typhus
Endemic
 See Murine Typhus
Mite-Borne
 See Scrub Typhus
Sao Paulo
 See Rocky Mountain Spotted Fever
Tropical
 See Scrub Typhus

Typing, Blood
See Blood Typing

Typing, HLA
See HLA Typing

Typing, Tissue
See Tissue Typing

Tyrosine 84510

Tzank Smear 88160-88161

U

Uchida Procedure
See Tubal Ligation

UDP Galactose Pyrophosphorylase
See Galactose-1-Phosphate, Uridyl Transferase

UFR
See Uroflowmetry

Ulcer

Anal
  See Anus, Fissure
Decubitus
  See Debridement; Pressure Ulcer (Decubitus);
  Skin Graft and Flap
Pinch Graft 15050
Pressure .15920-15999
Stomach
  Excision 43610

Ulcerative, Cystitis

See Cystitis, Interstitial

Ulna

See Arm, Lower; Elbow; Humerus; Radius
Arthrodesis
  Radioulnar Joint
    with Resection 25830
Arthroplasty
  with Implant .25442
Centralization or Wrist 25335
Craterization 24147, 25150-25151
Cyst
  Excision 24125-24126, 25120-25126
Diaphysectomy 24147, 25150-25151
Excision 24147
  Abscess 24138
  Complete 25240
  Epiphyseal Bar 20150
  Partial 25145-25151, 25240
Fracture
  Closed Treatment 25530-25535
  Olecranon 24670-24675
    Open Treatment 24685
  Open Treatment 25545
  Shaft 25530-25545
    Open Treatment 25574
  Styloid
    Closed Treatment 25650
    Open Treatment 25652
    Percutaneous Fixation 25651
  with Dislocation
    Closed Treatment 24620
    Open Treatment 24635
  with Manipulation 25535
  with Radius 25560-25565
    Open Treatment 25575
  without Manipulation 25530
Incision and Drainage 25035
Osteoplasty 25390-25393
Prophylactic Treatment 25491-25492
Reconstruction
  Radioulnar .25337
Repair
  Epiphyseal Arrest 25450-25455
  Malunion or Nonunion 25400, 25415
  Osteotomy 25360, 25370-25375
  and Radius 25365
  with Graft 25405, 25420-25426
Saucerization 24147, 25150-25151
Sequestrectomy 24138, 25145
Tumor
  Cyst 24120
  Excision . .24125-24126, 25120-25126, 25170

Ulnar Arteries

See Artery, Ulnar

Ulnar Nerve

Decompression 64718
Neuroplasty 64718-64719
Reconstruction 64718-64719
Release 64718-64719
Repair/Suture
  Motor 64836
Transposition 64718-64719

Ultrasonic

See Ultrasound

Ultrasonic Cardiography

See Echocardiography

Ultrasonic Procedure 52325

Ultrasonography

See Echography

Ultrasound

See Echocardiography; Echography
3D Rendering 76376-76377
Abdomen 76700-76705
Arm 76880
Artery
  Intracranial 93886-93893
  Middle Cerebral 76821
  Umbilical 76820
Bladder 51798
Bone Density Study 76977
Breast 76645
Bronchi
  Endoscopy 31620
Chest 76604
Colon
  Endoscopic 45391-45392
Colon-Sigmoid
  Endoscopic 45341-45342
Drainage
  Abscess 75989
Echoencephalography
  See Echoencephalography
Esophagus
  Endoscopy 43231-43232
Eye 76510-76513
  Arteries 93875
  Biometry 76516-76519
  Foreign Body 76529
  Pachymetry 76514
Fetus 76818-76828
Follow-Up 76970
for Physical Therapy 97035
Gastrointestinal 76975
Gastrointestinal, Upper
  Endoscopic 43237-43238, 43242, 43259
Guidance
  Amniocentesis 59001, 76946
  Amnioinfusion 59070
  Arteriovenous Fistulae 76936
  Chorionic Villus Sampling 76945
  Cryosurgery 55873
  Drainage
    Fetal Fluid 59074
  Endometrial Ablation 58356
  Fetal Cordocentesis 76941
  Fetal Transfusion 76941
  Heart Biopsy 76932
  Needle Biopsy 43232, 43238, 43242,
                  45342, 45392, 76942

Occlusion
  Umbilical Cord 59072
Ova Retrieval 76948
Pericardiocentesis 76930
Pseudoaneurysm 76936
Radiation Therapy 76950
Radioelement 76965
Shunt Placement
  Fetal .59076
Thoracentesis 76942
Tissue Ablation 76940
Vascular Access 76937
Head 76506, 76536
Heart
  Fetal .76825
Hips
  Infant 76885-76886
Hysterosonography 76831
Intraoperative 76998
Intravascular
  Intraoperative 37250-37251
Kidney 76770-76776
Leg 76880
Neck 76536
Non-Coronary
  Intravascular 75945-75946
Pelvis 76856-76857
Pregnant Uterus 76801-76817
Prostate .76873
Rectal 76872-76873
Retroperitoneal 76770-76775
Scrotum .76870
Sonohysterography 76831
Spine 76800
Stimulation to Aid Bone Healing 20979
Umbilical Artery 76820
Unlisted Services and Procedures 76999
Uterus
  Tumor Ablation 0071T-0072T
Vagina 76830

Ultraviolet Light Therapy

Dermatology
  Ultraviolet A 96912
  Ultraviolet B 96910
for Dermatology 96900
for Physical Medicine 97028
for Respiratory Medicine 0168T

Umbilectomy 49250

Umbilical

Artery Ultrasound 76820
Hernia
  See Omphalocele
Vein Catheterization
  See Catheterization, Umbilical Vein

Umbilical Cord

Occlusion .59072

Umbilicus

Excision 49250
Repair
  Hernia 49580-49587
  Omphalocele 49600-49611

Undescended Testicle

See Testis, Undescended

Unfertilized Egg
See Ova

Unguis
See Nails

Unilateral Simple Mastectomy
See Mastectomy

Unlisted Services and Procedures 99499, 99600
Abdomen 22999, 49329, 49999
Allergy/Immunology 95199
Anal 46999
Anesthesia 01999
Arm 25999
Arthroscopy 29999
Autopsy 88099
Bile Duct 47999
Bladder 51999
Brachytherapy 77799
Breast 19499
Bronchi 31899
Cardiac 33999
Cardiovascular Studies 93799
Casting 29799
Cervix 58999
Chemistry Procedure 84999
Chemotherapy 96549
Chest 32999
Coagulation 85999
Colon 44799
Conjunctiva Surgery 68399
Craniofacial 21299
CT Scan 76497
Cytogenetic Study 88299
Cytopathology 88199
Dermatology 96999
Dialysis 90999
Diaphragm 39599
Ear
    External 69399
    Inner 69949
    Middle 69799
Endocrine System 60699
Epididymis 55899
Esophagus 43289, 43499
Evaluation and Management Services ..99499
Eye Muscle 67399
Eye Surgery
    Anterior Segment 66999
    Posterior Segment 67299
Eyelid 67999
Fluoroscopy 76496
Forearm 25999
Gallbladder 47999
Gastroenterology Test 91299
Gum 41899
Hand 26989
Hemic System 38999
Hepatic Duct 47999
Hip Joint 27299
Home Services 99600
Hysteroscopy 58579
Immunization 90749
Immunology 86849
Infusion 90779
Injection 90779
Injection of Medication 90779

Intestine 44238, 44799
Kidney 49659
Lacrimal System 68899
Laparoscopy 38129, 38589, 43289, 43659,
    44238, 44979, 47379, 47579, 49329,
    49659, 50549, 50949, 54699, 55559,
    58578, 58679, 59898, 60659
Larynx 31599
Lip 40799
Liver 47379, 47399
Lungs 32999
Lymphatic System 38999
Magnetic Resonance 76498
Maxillofacial 21299
Maxillofacial Prosthetics 21089
Meckel's Diverticulum 44899
Mediastinum 39499
Mesentery Surgery 44899
Microbiology 87999
Mouth 40899, 41599
Musculoskeletal 25999, 26989
Musculoskeletal Surgery
    Abdominal Wall 22999
    Neck 21899
    Spine 22899
    Thorax 21899
Musculoskeletal System 20999
    Ankle 27899
    Arm, Upper 24999
    Elbow 24999
    Head 21499
    Knee 27599
    Leg, Lower 27899
    Leg, Upper 27599
Necropsy 88099
Nervous System Surgery 64999
Neurology/Neuromuscular Testing 95999
Nose 30999
Nuclear Medicine 78999
    Blood 78199
    Bone 78399
    Endocrine System 78099
    Genitourinary System 78799
    Heart 78499
    Hematopoietic System 78199
    Lymphatic System 78199
    Musculoskeletal System 78399
    Nervous System 78699
    Therapeutic 79999
Obstetrical Care 59898-59899
Omentum 49329, 49999
Ophthalmology 92499
Orbit 67599
Otorhinolaryngology 92700
Ovary 58679, 58999
Oviduct 58679, 58999
Palate 42299
Pancreas Surgery 48999
Pathology 89240
Pelvis 27299
Penis 55899
Peritoneum 49329, 49999
Pharynx 42999
Physical Therapy 97039, 97139, 97799
Pleura 32999
Pressure Ulcer 15999
Preventive Medicine 99429
Prostate 55899

Psychiatric 90899
Pulmonology 94799
Radiation Physics 77399
Radiation Therapy 77499
    Planning 77299
Radiology, Diagnostic 76499
Radionuclide Therapy 79999
Radiopharmaceutical Therapy 79999
Rectum 45499, 45999
Salivary Gland 42699
Scrotum 55899
Seminal Vesicle 55899
Shoulder Surgery 23929
Sinuses 31299
Skin 17999
Special Services and Reports 99199
Spine 22899
Stomach 43659, 43999
Strapping 29799
Surgical Pathology 88399
Temporal Bone 69979
Testis 54699, 55899
Throat 42999
Tongue 41599
Tonsil/Adenoid 42999
Toxoid 90749
Trachea 31899
Transfusion 86999
Ultrasound 76999
Ureter 50949
Urinary System 53899
Uterus 58578-58579, 58999
Uvula 42299
Vaccine 90749
Vagina 58999
Vas Deferens 55899
Vascular 37799
Vascular Endoscopy 37501
Vascular Injection 36299
Vascular Studies 93799
Wrist 25999

Unna Paste Boot 29580
Removal 29700

UPP
See Urethra Pressure Profile

Upper
Digestive System Endoscopy
    See Endoscopy, Gastrointestinal, Upper
Extremity
    See Arm, Upper; Elbow; Humerus
Gastrointestinal Bleeding
    See Gastrointestinal, Upper, Hemorrhage
Gastrointestinal Endoscopy, Biopsy
    See Biopsy
    Planning
        See Biopsy, Gastrointestinal, Upper
        Endoscopy; Endoscopy, Gastrointestinal
GI Tract
    See Gastrointestinal Tract, Upper

Urachal Cyst
See Cyst, Urachal

Urea Breath Test 78267-78268, 83014

Urea Nitrogen
See Blood Urea Nitrogen

Injection
Anesthetic 64408
Transection 43640-43641
Abdominal 64760
Selective 43652, 64755
Thoracic 64752
Truncal 43651

Valentine's Test
See Urinalysis, Glass Test

Valproic Acid
See Dipropylacetic Acid

Valproic Acid Measurement
See Dipropylacetic Acid

Valsalva Sinus
See Sinus of Valsalva

Valva Atrioventricularis Sinistra (Valva Mitralis)
See Mitral Valve

Valve
Aortic
See Heart, Aortic Valve
Bicuspid
See Mitral Valve
Mitral
See Mitral Valve
Pulmonary
See Pulmonary Valve
Tricuspid
See Tricuspid Valve

Valve Stenoses, Aortic
See Aortic Stenosis

Valvectomy
Tricuspid Valve 33460

Valvotomy
Mitral Valve .33420-33422
Pulmonary Valve 33470-33474
Reoperation 33530

Valvuloplasty
Aortic Valve 33400-33403
Femoral Vein 34501
Mitral Valve 33425-33427
Percutaneous Balloon
Aortic Valve .92986
Mitral Valve .92987
Pulmonary Valve 92990
Prosthetic Valve 33496
Reoperation 33530
Tricuspid Valve 33463-33465

Van Deen Test
See Blood, Feces

Van Den Bergh Test
See Bilirubin, Blood

Vancomycin
Assay 80202

Vanillylmandelic Acid
Urine 84585

Vanilmandelic Acid
See Vanillylmandelic Acid

Varicella (Chicken Pox)
See Vaccines

Varicella-Zoster
Antibody 86787
Antigen Detection
Direct Fluorescence 87290

Varices Esophageal
See Esophageal Varices

Varicocele
Spermatic Cord
Excision 55530-55540

Varicose Vein
Ablation .36475-36479
Removal .37765-37785
Secondary Varicosity 37785
with Tissue Excision 37735-37760

Vas Deferens
Anastomosis
to Epididymis 54900-54901
Excision 55250
Incision 55200
for X-Ray 55300
Ligation 55450
Repair
Suture 55400
Unlisted Services and Procedures 55899
Vasography 74440
X-Ray with Contrast 74440

Vascular Flow Check, Graft 15860

Vascular Injection
Unlisted Services and Procedures 36299

Vascular Lesion
Cranial
Excision 61600-61608, 61615-61616
Cutaneous
Destruction 17106-17108

Vascular Malformation
Cerebral
Repair 61710
Finger
Excision 26115
Hand
Excision 26115

Vascular Procedures
Angioscopy
Non-Coronary Vessels 35400
Brachytherapy
Intracoronary Artery 92974
Endoscopy
Surgical 37500
Harvest
Lower Extremity Vein 35572
Intravascular Ultrasound
Coronary Vessels 92978-92979
Non-Coronary Vessels 75945-75946
Stent
Intracoronary 92980-92981

Thrombolysis
Coronary Vessels 92975-92977
Cranial Vessels 37195

Vascular Rehabilitation
See Peripheral Artery Disease Rehabilitation (PAD)

Vascular Studies
See Doppler Scan, Duplex, Plethysmography
Angioscopy
Non-Coronary Vessels 35400
Aorta .93978-93979
Arterial Studies (Non-Invasive)
Extracranial 93875-93882
Extremities 93922-93924
Intracranial 93886-93890
Lower Extremity 93925-93926
Middle Cerebral Artery, Fetal 76821
Umbilical Artery, Fetal 76820
Artery Studies
Upper Extremity 93930-93931
Blood Pressure Monitoring,
24 Hour 93784-93790
Cardiac Catheterization
Imaging 93555-93556
Hemodialysis Access 93990
Kidney
Multiple Study
with Pharmacological Intervention . .78709
Single Study
with Pharmacological Intervention . .78708
Penile Vessels 93980-93981
Plethysmography
Total Body 93720-93722
Temperature Gradient 93740
Thermogram
Cephalic 93760
Peripheral .93762
Unlisted Services and Procedures 93799
Venous Studies
Extremity 93965-93971
Venous Pressure 93770
Visceral Studies 93975-93979

Vascular Surgery
Arm, Upper
Anesthesia 01770-01782
Elbow
Anesthesia 01770-01782
Endoscopy 37500
Unlisted Services and Procedures 37799

Vasectomy 55250
Laser Coagulation of Prostate 52647
Laser Vaporization 52648
Reversal
See Vasovasorrhaphy
Transurethral
Cystourethroscopic 52402
Transurethral Electrosurgical Resection of
Prostate 52601
Transurethral Resection of Prostate 52648

Vasoactive Drugs
Injection
Penis 54231

Vasoactive Intestinal Peptide 84586

Vasogram
See Vasography

Vasography 74440

Vasointestinal Peptide
See Vasoactive Intestinal Peptide

Vasopneumatic Device Therapy 97016
See Physical Medicine/Therapy/Occupational Therapy

Vasopressin 84588

Vasotomy 55200, 55300
Transurethral
  Cystourethroscopic 52402

Vasovasorrhaphy 55400

Vasovasostomy 55400

VATS
See Thoracoscopy

VDRL 86592-86593

Vein
Ablation
  Endovenous 36475-36479
Adrenal
  Venography 75840-75842
Anastomosis
  Caval to Mesenteric 37160
  Intrahepatic Portosystemic ...37182-37183
  Portocaval 37140
  Reniportal 37145
  Saphenopopliteal 34530
  Splenorenal 37180-37181
  to Vein 37140-37160, 37182-37183
Angioplasty 75978
  Transluminal 35460
Arm
  Harvest of Vein for Bypass Graft 35500
  Venography 75820-75822
Axillary
  Thrombectomy 34490
Biopsy
  Transcatheter 75970
Cannulization
  to Artery 36810-36815
  to Vein 36800
Catheterization
  Central Insertion 36555-36558
  Organ Blood 36500
  Peripheral Insertion 36568-36569
  Removal 36589
  Repair 36575
  Replacement 36578-36581, 36584
  Umbilical 36510
Division
  Saphenous 37718-37722
Endoscopic Harvest
  for Bypass Graft 33508
External Cannula
  Declotting 36860-36861

Extremity
  Non-Invasive Studies 93965-93971
Femoral
  Repair 34501
Femoropopliteal
  Thrombectomy 34421-34451
Guidance
  Fluoroscopic 77001
  Ultrasound 76937
Hepatic Portal
  Splenoportography 75810
  Venography 75885-75887
Iliac
  Thrombectomy 34401-34451
Injection
  Sclerosing Agent 36468-36471
Insertion
  IVC Filter 75940
Interrupt
  Femoral 37650
  Iliac 37660
  Vena Cava 37620
Jugular
  Venography 75860
Leg
  Harvest for Vascular Reconstruction ...35572
  Venography 75820-75822
Ligation
  Clusters 37785
  Esophagus 43205
  Jugular 37565
  Perforation 37760
  Saphenous 37700-37735, 37780
  Secondary 37785
Liver
  Venography 75889-75891
Neck
  Venography 75860
Nuclear Medicine
  Thrombosis Imaging 78456-78458
Orbit
  Venography 75880
Placement
  IVC Filter 75940
Portal
  Catheterization 36481
Pulmonary
  Repair 33730
Removal
  Clusters 37785
  Saphenous 37735, 37780
  Varicose 37765-37766
Renal
  Venography 75831-75833
Repair
  Aneurysm 36834
  Angioplasty 75978
  Graft 34520
Sampling
  Venography 75893
Sinus
  Venography 75870
Skull
  Venography 75870-75872
Spermatic
  Excision 55530-55540
  Ligation 55550

Splenic
  Splenoportography 75810
Stripping
  Saphenous 37718-37735
Subclavian
  Thrombectomy 34471-34490
Thrombectomy 37187-37188
  Other than Hemodialysis Graft or
  Fistula 35875-35876
Unlisted Services and Procedures 37799
Valve Transposition 34510
Varicose
  See Varicose Vein
Vena Cava
  Thrombectomy 34401-34451
  Venography 75825-75827

Velpeau Cast 29058

Vena Cava
Catheterization 36010
Reconstruction 34502
Resection with Reconstruction 37799

Vena Caval
Thrombectomy 50230

Venereal Disease Research Laboratory
See VDRL

Venesection
See Phlebotomy

Venipuncture
See Cannulation; Catheterization
Child/Adult
  Cutdown 36425
  Percutaneous 36410
Infant
  Cutdown 36420
  Percutaneous 36400-36406
Routine 36415

Venography
Adrenal 75840-75842
Arm 75820-75822
Epidural 75872
Hepatic Portal 75885-75887
Injection 36005
Jugular 75860
Leg 75820-75822
Liver 75889-75891
Neck 75860
Nuclear Medicine 78445, 78457-78458
Orbit 75880
Renal 75831-75833
Sagittal Sinus 75870
Vena Cava 75825-75827
Venous Sampling 75893

Venorrhaphy
See Suture, Vein

Venotomy
See Phlebotomy

Venous Access Device
Fluoroscopic Guidance 77001

VII, Cranial Nerve
See Facial Nerve

VIII, Coagulation Factor
See Clotting Factor

Villus, Chorionic
See Chorionic Villus

Villusectomy
See Synovectomy

VIP
See Vasoactive Intestinal Peptide

Viral Antibodies 86280

Viral Warts
See Warts

Virtual Colonoscopy
Diagnostic 0067T
Screening 0066T

Virus
AIDS
  See HIV-1
Burkitt Lymphoma
  See Epstein-Barr Virus
Human Immunodeficiency
  See HIV
Influenza
  See Influenza Virus
Respiratory Syncytial
  See Respiratory Syncytial Virus
Salivary Gland
  See Cytomegalovirus

Virus Identification
Immunofluorescence 87254

Virus Isolation 87250-87255

Visceral Larval Migrans 86280

Viscosities, Blood
See Blood, Viscosity

Visit, Home
See House Calls

Visual Acuity Screen 99172-99173

Visual Field Exam 92081-92083

Visual Function Screen ...0065T, 99172

Visual Reinforcement Audiometry 92579
See Audiologic Function Tests

Visualization
Ileal Conduit 50690

Vital Capacity Measurement ...94150

Vitamin 84591
A 84590
B Complex
  See B Complex Vitamins
B-1 84425
B-12 82607-82608
  Absorption Study 78270-78272
  Holotranscobalamin 0103T

B-2 84252
B-6 84207
B-6 Measurement
  See Pyridoxal Phosphate
BC
  See Folic Acid
C 82180
D 82307, 82652
D, 25-Hydroxy Measurement
  See Calcifediol
D-2
  See Calciferol
D-3 82306
E 84446
K 84597
K Dependent Bone Protein
  See Osteocalcin
K-Dependent Protein S
  See Protein S

Vitelline Duct
See Omphalomesenteric Duct

Vitrectomy
Anterior Approach
  Partial 67005
Pars Plana Approach 67036
Subtotal 67010
  with Endolaser Panretinal
  Photocoagulation 67040
with Epiretinal Membrane Stripping 67038
with Focal Endolaser Photocoagulation 67039
with Implantation or Replacement
  Drug Delivery System 67027

Vitreous
Aspiration 67015
Excision
  Pars Planta Approach 67036
  with Epiretinal Membrane Stripping ...67038
  with Focal Endolaser Photocoagulation 67039
Implantation
  Drug Delivery System 67027
Incision
  Strands 67030-67031
Injection
  Fluid Substitute 67025
  Pharmacologic Agent 67028
Removal
  Anterior Approach 67005
  Subtotal 67010
Replacement
  Drug Delivery System 67027
Strands
  Discission 67030
  Severing 67031
Subtotal 67010

VLDL
See Lipoprotein, Blood

VMA
See Vanillylmandelic Acid

Vocal Cords
Injection
  Endoscopy 31513
    Therapeutic 31570-31571

Voice Box
See Larynx

Voice Button 31611

Voiding Pressure Studies
Abdominal 51797
Bladder 51795

Volatiles 84600

Volhard's Test
See Water Load Test

Volkman Contracture 25315-25316

Volume Reduction
Blood Products 86960

Volume Reduction, Lung
See Lung Volume Reduction

Von Kraske Proctectomy
See Proctectomy, Partial

VP
See Voiding Pressure Studies

Vulva
Abscess
  Incision and Drainage 56405
Colposcopy 56820
  Biopsy 56821
Excision
  Complete 56625, 56633-56640
  Partial 56620, 56630-56632
  Radical 56630-56631, 56633-56640
    Complete 56633-56640
    Partial 56630-56632
  Simple
    Complete 56625
    Partial 56620
Lesion
  Destruction 56501-56515
Perineum
  Biopsy 56605-56606
  Incision and Drainage 56405
Repair
  Obstetric 59300

Vulvectomy
Complete 56625, 56633-56640
Partial 56620, 56630-56632
Radical 56630-56631, 56633-56640
  Complete
    with Bilateral Inguinofemoral
    Lymphadenectomy 56637
    with Inguinofemoral, Iliac, and Pelvic
    Lymphadenectomy 56640
    with Unilateral Inguinofemoral
    Lymphadenectomy 56634
  Partial
    with Bilateral Inguinofemoral
    Lymphadenectomy 56632
    with Unilateral Inguinofemoral
    Lymphadenectomy 56631
Simple
  Complete 56625
  Partial 56620

VZIG
See Immune Globulins, Varicella-Zoster

W

Wrist

See Arm, Lower; Carpal Bone
Abscess 25028
Arthrocentesis 20605
Arthrodesis 25800
   with Graft 25810
   with Sliding Graft 25805
Arthrography 73115
Arthroplasty 25332, 25443, 25447
   Revision 25449
   Total Replacement 25446
   with Implant 25441-25442, 25444-25445
Arthroscopy
   Diagnostic 29840
   Surgical 29843-29848
Arthrotomy 25040, 25100-25105
   for Repair 25107
Biopsy 25065-25066, 25100-25101
Bursa
   Excision 25115-25116
   Incision and Drainage 25031
Capsule
   Incision 25085
Cast 29085
Cyst 25130-25136
Decompression 25020-25025
Disarticulation 25920
   Reamputation 25924
   Revision 25922
Dislocation
   Closed Treatment 25660
   Intercarpal 25660
      Open Treatment 25670
   Open Treatment 25670, 25676
   Percutaneous Fixation 25671
   Radiocarpal 25660
      Open Treatment 25670
   Radioulnar
      Closed Treatment 25675
      Percutaneous Fixation 25671
   with Fracture
      Closed Treatment 25680
      Open Treatment 25685
   with Manipulation 25259, 25660, 25675
Excision
   Carpal 25210-25215
   Cartilage 25107
Exploration 25040, 25101
Fasciotomy 25020-25025
Fracture 25645
   Closed Treatment 25622, 25630
   Open Treatment 25628
   with Dislocation 25680-25685
   with Manipulation 25259, 25624, 25635
Ganglion Cyst
   Excision 25111-25112
Hematoma 25028
Incision 25040, 25100-25105
   Tendon Sheath 25000-25001
Injection
   Carpal Tunnel
      Therapeutic 20526
   X-Ray 25246
Joint
   See Radiocarpal Joint
Lesion, Tendon Sheath
   Excision 25110
Magnetic Resonance Imaging (MRI) 73221

Reconstruction
   Capsulectomy 25320
   Capsulorrhaphy 25320
   Carpal Bone 25394, 25430
   Realign 25335
Removal
   Foreign Body 25040, 25101, 25248
   Implant 25449
   Loose Body 25101
   Prosthesis 25250-25251
Repair 25447
   Bone 25440
   Carpal Bone 25431
   Muscle 25260, 25270
      Secondary 25263-25265, 25272-25274
   Tendon 25260, 25270, 25280-25316
      Secondary 25263-25265, 25272-25274
   Tendon Sheath 25275
Strapping 29260
Synovium
   Excision 25105, 25115-25119
Tendon
   Excision 25109
Tendon Sheath
   Excision 25115-25116
Tenodesis 25300-25301
Tenotomy 25290
Tumor 25130-25136
   Excision 25075-25077
Unlisted Services and Procedures 25999
X-Ray 73100-73110
   with Contrast 73115

X

X, Coagulation Factor
See Stuart-Prower Factor

X, Cranial Nerve
See Vagus Nerve

X-Linked Ichthyoses
See Syphilis Test

X-Ray
Abdomen 74000-74022
Abscess 76080
Acromioclavicular Joint 73050
Ankle 73600-73610
Arm, Lower 73090
Arm, Upper 73092
Artery
   Atherectomy 75992-75996
Auditory Meatus 70134
Bile Duct
   Guide Dilation 74360
Body Composition
   Dual Energy Absorptiometry 0028T
Body Section 76100
   Motion 76101-76102
Bone
   Age Study 77072
   Dual Energy Absorptiometry ...77080-77081
   Length Study 77073

   Osseous Survey 77074-77077
   Ultrasound 76977
Breast 77055-77057
   Localization Nodule 77032
   with Computer-aided Detection .77051-77052
Calcaneus 73650
Chest 71010-71035
   Complete (Four Views)
      with Fluoroscopy 71034
      Insert Pacemaker 71090
   Partial (Two Views)
      with Fluoroscopy 71023
      Stereo 71015
      with Fluoroscopy 71090
Clavicle 73000
Coccyx 72220
Consultation 76140
Duodenum 74260
Elbow 73070-73080
Esophagus 74220
Eye 70030
Facial Bones 70140-70150
Fallopian Tube 74742
Femur 73550
Fibula 73590
Finger 73140
Fistula 76080
Foot 73620-73630
Gastrointestinal Tract 74240-74245
   Guide Dilation 74360
   Guide Intubation 74340-74350
Hand 73120-73130
Head 70350
Heel 73650
Hip 73500-73520, 73540
   Intraoperative 73530
Humerus 73060
Intestines, Small 74245, 74249-74251
   Guide Intubation 74355
Intravascular Stent 75960
Jaws 70355
Joint
   Stress Views 77071
Knee 73560-73564, 73580
   Bilateral 73565
Larynx 70370
Leg 73592
Lumen Dilator 74360
Mandible 70100-70110
Mastoids 70120-70130
Nasal Bone 70160
Neck 70360
Nose to Rectum
   Foreign Body 76010
Orbit 70190-70200
Pelvis 72170-72190, 73540
   Manometry 74710
Peritoneum 74190
Pharynx 70370, 74210
Ribs 71100-71111
Sacroiliac Joint 72200-72202, 73542
Sacrum 72220
Salivary Gland 70380
Scapula 73010
Sella Turcica 70240
Shoulder 73020-73030, 73050
Sinus Tract 76080

X-Ray Tomography, Computed
See CT Scan

Xa, Coagulation Factor
See Thrombokinase

Xenoantibodies
See Antibody, Heterophile

Xenograft

Xenografts, Skin
See Heterograft, Skin

Xenotransplantation
See Heterograft

Xerography
See Xeroradiography

Xeroradiography

XI, Coagulation Factor
See Plasma Thromboplastin, Antecedent

XI, Cranial Nerve
See Accessory Nerve

XII, Coagulation Factor
See Hageman Factor

XII, Cranial Nerve
See Hypoglossal Nerve

XIII, Coagulation Factor
See Fibrin Stabilizing Factor

Xylose Absorption Test

Y

Yeast

Yellow Fever Vaccine

Yersinia

Z

Ziegler Procedure
Discission Secondary Membranous

Zinc

Zinc Manganese Leucine Aminopeptidase
See Leucine Aminopeptidase

Zygoma
See Cheekbone

Zygomatic Arch
Fracture

Notes

Notes

Time For a Practice Management Check-up?

The AMA offers a range of products to help your office run smooth and effectively

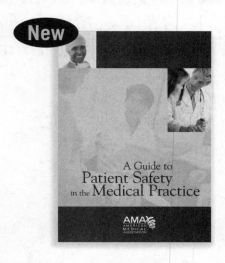

Maximizing Billing and Collections in the Medical Practice

Prevent undue financial losses in today's medical practice. Given the shrinking physician reimbursement environment, practices today need the tools and information necessary to maximize their billing and collections efforts; this book provides that and more. *Maximizing Billing and Collections in the Medical Practice* integrates the patient encounter with the billing and collections function to increase the likelihood of collecting every dollar the physician is entitled to receive.

Softbound with CD-ROM, 8-1/2"x11", 208 pages
Order #: OP318607CCW
ISBN: I-57947-867-0
Price: $75.95   AMA member price: $56.95

A Guide to Patient Safety in the Medical Practice

Discover a greater understanding of the risks, consequences of errors and adverse events in the medical practice. This book is designed to stimulate the evolution of a patient safety culture in today's physician practice. Readers are provided with an in-depth review of the practical patient safety process and available tools for providers and business cases for a safer physician practice is also discussed.

Softbound, 7"x10" 300 pages
Order #: OP401006CCW
ISBN: I-57947-674-0
Price: $59.95   AMA member price: $44.95

Other valuable practice management titles offered by the American Medical Association:

- Starting a Medical Practice
- Assessing the Value of the Medical Practice
- Managing the Medical Practice
- Buying, Selling and Owning a Medical Practice
- Financial Management of the Medical Practice
- Personnel Management in the Medical Practice

For more information on our practice success series or to review additional products and services visit *www.amabookstore.com* or call (800) 621-8335.

We have you covered!

HCPCS 2007 Level II

Stay up-to-date on the new HCPCS 2007 code changes that will impact code accuracy and claims submission!

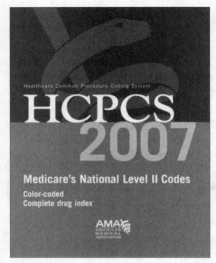

Your guide to Medicare's National Level II codes! Organized for efficiency and accuracy, with enhanced icons, detailed illustrations, quick-flip color tabs and dictionary-style headings. Additional features include:

- All HCPCS 2007 codes, modifiers and deleted codes—Includes the most up-to-date information found in the HCPCS, MPFS and OPPS files
- DMEPOS icon alerts—Feel confident and save time by knowing exactly what supplies should be submitted
- APC status indicators—Aids in learning which codes are payable under OPPS
- Age and sex edit icons
- AHA's *Coding Clinic for HCPCS*
- ASC designation symbols
- *National Coverage Manual* references and excerpts
- Expanded table of drugs

Available December 2006.
Softbound, 8-1/2" x 11", 380 pages
Order#: OP095107
ISBN: 1-57947-808-5
Price: $94.95
AMA member price: $74.95

HCPCS 2007 Level II ASCII Data Files

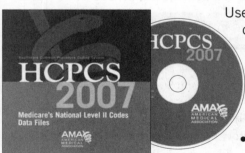

Use this CD-ROM data file to import 2007 HCPCS Level II codes and descriptions into your billing and claims reporting software.

- Contains all official 2007 HCPCS Level II codes
- Code status indicator alerts when a code was added or changed
- Indicates the MCM and CIM policy references, Medicare statues and Medicare coverage
- Two code description lengths: 35-character and full unabbreviated description

- Contains separate file with all HCPCS Level II modifiers
- One copy of the *HCPCS 2007* is included with the purchase of the data file
- Shipping included

Order #: OP096207
ISBN: 1-57947-809-3
Single User
Price: $199.95
AMA member price: $189.95

Order #: OP068807
ISBN: 1-57947-810-7
2-10 User License
Price: $275.00
AMA member price: $240.00

To order, call (800) 621-8335 or visit *www.amabookstore.com*.

AMA
AMERICAN
MEDICAL
ASSOCIATION

Monica Wehby, MD
Pediatric neurosurgeon
AMA member since 1986

DR. WEHBY HAS MADE A CAREER OF SAVING LIVES. NOW THE AMA IS FIGHTING TO SAVE HER CAREER.

Dr. Monica Wehby is being forced away from her patients. Without a liability cap, Oregon doctors are facing out-of-control insurance premiums. These costs have driven 20% of Oregon's neurosurgeons out of state, while many who stay can no longer perform brain surgery or treat children.

Dr. Wehby wants to stay...she wants to fight.

This is just one of the many reasons why Dr. Wehby is a member of the AMA. She knows that we won't rest while patients' lives are at risk. Dr. Wehby also knows that the AMA's strength lies in numbers. And that by joining together with her physician colleagues, she will not only be helping to save the lives of her patients, but the lives of millions of our nation's children, who are in need of a good doctor just like her. And just like you.

AMA
AMERICAN
MEDICAL
ASSOCIATION

Join Dr. Wehby and the AMA in our fight to help all patients.

Be a member of the AMA.
Contact your state or local medical society.

Together we are stronger.

www.ama-assn.org